Strategies for Collaborating With Children

Creating Partnerships in Occupational Therapy and Research

Strategies for Collaborating With Children

Creating Partnerships in Occupational Therapy and Research

Clare Curtin, PhD, OTR

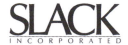
SLACK
INCORPORATED

www.Healio.com/books

ISBN: 978-1-63091-104-1

Copyright © 2017 by SLACK Incorporated

Published by: SLACK Incorporated
                  6900 Grove Road
                  Thorofare, NJ 08086 USA
                  Telephone: 856-848-1000
                  Fax: 856-848-6091
                  www.Healio.com/books

Contact SLACK Incorporated for more information about other books in this field or about the availability of our books from distributors outside the United States.

Library of Congress Cataloging-in-Publication Data

Names: Curtin, Clare, author.
Title: Strategies for collaborating with children : creating partnerships in
  occupational therapy and research / Clare Curtin.
Description: Thorofare, NJ : SLACK Incorporated, [2017] | Includes
  bibliographical references and index.
Identifiers: LCCN 2016024069 (print) | LCCN 2016024994 (ebook) | ISBN
  9781630911041 (softcover : alk. paper) | ISBN 9781630911058 (epub) | ISBN
  9781630911065 (web-ready)
Subjects: | MESH: Occupational Therapy | Child | Patient
  Compliance--psychology | Psychology, Child | Professional-Patient Relations
Classification: LCC RM735.3 (print) | LCC RM735.3 (ebook) | NLM WS 368 | DDC
  615.8/515--dc23
LC record available at https://lccn.loc.gov/2016024069

Printed in the United States of America.

Last digit is print number: 10 9 8 7 6 5 4 3 2 1

Dedication

This book is dedicated to the memories of…

John Nicholls, PhD, was my mentor and chair of my dissertation committee. He always treated me with respect even as he presented different viewpoints. Every time I left his office, I was eager to write. As we talked about the volume of research data I had gathered, he guided me in staying focused on the research question. John said I could describe all my findings in more detail in my book. He frequently said, "Save that for your book." The birth of this book started in my discussions with John.

So much of what I know about children and ways to approach them, I learned from my mother, Ann Curtin. I had a very happy and fun childhood. My mother had a great sense of humor and was a master at motivating us by using enticement. I remember her telling us we could roast marshmallows over a fire of burning leaves. All she did was buy a bag of marshmallows, and my brothers and I happily raked a large yard. She made it fun and not a chore.

Bill Curtin, my father, was outgoing and never at a loss for words. He was a top salesman in his company and had a wonderful way with people. He would skillfully put them at ease and engage them in conversation. Soon they would be captivated by his stories and laughing. I learned my people skills and how to be a storyteller from my father.

Nora Ann Dixon was a dear friend and an exceptional occupational therapist. She provided me with unwavering moral support and encouragement. Her editing suggestions made this a better book.

Contents

Acknowledgments

This book would not have been possible without the help of so many. I am grateful to…

My brothers, Tom and Charlie Curtin, and my cousin, Molly Horn, for their neverending love, encouragement, and belief in me.

My small writer's critique group: Angela Elliott, Ardelle Gifford, and Beth Kitely. For over 10 years we have met every 2 weeks to critique each other's writings. I have grown immensely from your friendship and edits.

All my friends, who have provided invaluable support and been there for me in countless ways: Donna and Joe Ashworth, Marion Bennett, Kim Bryze, Patrick Cabrera, Sandi Canuel, Theresa and David Conley, John Dixon, Amber Edwards, Rebecca Hawkins, Diana Healy, Devin Kelley, Kim and Rich Kelley, Nancy Kitely, Susie Lovercheck, Paula Malleck, Maria Morley-Bettler, Mary Ellen Myers, Lois Nicholson, Kathleen Paduano, Eileen Pappalardo, Kay Roberts, Laurie Rockwell-Dylla, James Theall, and Crystal Van Ocker.

Jeanette Langevin, for your friendship, assistance, expert advice, and helpful edits of the manuscript. Thank you for giving me permission to describe your Collaborative Consultation Model and for sharing your wonderful approaches with children, caregivers, and staff.

Livia Magalhaes, for your friendship and encouragement throughout this project. You have always supported my vision for this book and provided thoughtful guidance.

All the members of the Longmont Writer's Club. For the past 18 years, you have critiqued my stories and made me a better writer. I am proud to be a member of one of the oldest groups in Colorado.

To all the children (many of whom are now teenagers) for giving me written permission to use your photographs and drawings, and for providing your expertise in the children's panel. A special thanks to Courtney, Jennifer, and Christopher Ashworth; Jeremy, Spencer, and Emily Edwards; John Mitchell Healy; Sa'nyi Irving; and Jon and Julia Langevin.

Vivian and Dave Fauset, for your kindness and generosity in allowing me to use your "Hi! On a Windy Hill" mountain house for many writing retreats.

Mary Ann Foster and Mary Rose, for your guidance in helping me navigate the publishing world.

Courtney Ashworth, for your incredible artistic talent in creating the metaphorical drawings.

Steven Kaplan, for providing permission to reproduce material from the copyrighted book, *I Raise My Eyes to Say Yes*. Ruth Sienkiewicz-Mercer, whose life is briefly described in Chapter 1, was born a year before me but, sadly, died in 1998. Her co-author, Steven Kaplan, has reprinted their book as a memoir. I am glad this touching and powerful story is still available at iraisemyeyestosayyes.com.

I thank the excellent staff at SLACK Incorporated, particularly Brien Cummings, April Billick, Sarah Becker-Marrero, and Trevor Hirsh, for all their contributions in transforming my manuscript into a book. I appreciate their confidence in my work as well as their accessibility, respectful assistance, and collaborative approach.

In the spirit of the disability activists' slogan, "Nothing about us without us," I want to thank two friends with disabilities who reviewed the related sections.

All the children, caregivers, educational and hospital staff, therapists, and certified occupational therapy assistants with whom I have worked with over my 36 years as a therapist.

Words cannot express how appreciative I am.

About the Author

Dr. Clare Curtin has been an occupational therapist for 36 years. Her degree specialties include social work, occupational therapy, rehabilitation counseling, and educational psychology. Over the years, she has helped children in hospitals, psychiatric units, day treatment programs, and preschools and elementary schools. She has also worked in an outpatient pediatric oncology clinic.

In the 1990s, she designed and completed the first in-depth study of the occupational therapy collaboration process to highlight children's perspectives. Her research incorporated child-friendly, original, and playful participatory methods. Dr. Curtin has lectured extensively at the local, state, national, and international levels, emphasizing client-centered and strengths-based therapy. She has had intensive training in mediation, allowing her to provide expertise on resolving conflict. Throughout her career, she has advocated for children to have a voice in therapy and research. In her free time, she enjoys writing, photography, gardening, and traveling.

Introduction

This book is the culmination of my 36 years of practicing, exploring, and researching the process of collaboration. It has been my life's work to examine this process and discover how to give children a voice in therapy and research.

I often reflected:

What did I do that made a difference in helping children connect with me, open up, and become involved in therapy?

How can I discover what children want, especially if they are unable to speak?

What are the best ways to give a clear message to children that they are to be partners in therapy and research and that their perspectives are equally valued?

I wrestled with these questions and tried various methods to assist children in expressing their views about their lives, their dreams for the future, and what they wanted to address in therapy. The answers I found led to the creation of this book.

Experiences and Expertise

In my career, I have worked with a wide variety of children—some of whom were very challenging. I have been with children who were dying or suffering through painful treatments for cancer. There have been children who acted aggressively, such as the 5-year-old boy who, whenever he became angry, wrapped himself around my leg and tried to bite my knee. I always wore boots on the days I saw him! I have worked with children with limited body awareness, for whom a new task was often a major undertaking ending in failure. In the day treatment programs, I encountered children whose frequent refrain was, "I'm not doing this, and you can't make me." I have worked with children with autism who have a different way of seeing life, as well as children who only communicate with their eyes and by making different sounds. These are only a few examples of the many children whom I have had the pleasure of assisting.

My first job was in a private psychiatric hospital. The adolescents and adults were usually admitted for 3 weeks with diagnoses such as depression, bipolar disorder, or schizophrenia. As the department head, I experimented by creating various checklists to educate the adolescents and adults on what could be addressed in therapy and obtain their priorities for goals. Although challenging, I saw how therapy became meaningful and successful when I involved them in planning their treatment. During this time I worked on my Masters in rehabilitation counseling and studied client-centered therapy. This theory became a major influence in my practice, and the basis for many of the strategies and approaches in this book. In 1981, I also went on an occupational therapy study tour of China to learn about their culture, including their medical system and provision of therapy.

In my next job, I worked on a children's locked psychiatric unit. Many of them were hospitalized due to suicide attempts, psychotic episodes, defiance of authority figures, or violent actions. They usually stayed 3 months for assessment and treatment. On this unit, I observed and learned as much as I could from the close-knit and experienced staff. Because I believed in the value of collaboration and experienced success in collaborating with the adolescents and adults, I wanted to do the same with children. However, I found that it was more complicated. First of all, I had to learn *kid language*. For instance, to discuss the concept of concentration, I discovered they understood if I said, "Keep your mind on what you are doing." Again, I created different assessments to cue the children regarding what areas could be addressed in occupational therapy and have them decide what was important to them.

After that job, I spent the next 6 months travelling around the world. In Mumbai, India, I lectured in the occupational therapy department at the university and visited occupational therapy clinics. I observed sheltered workshops and a pediatric clinic where one therapist roamed a large room giving ideas to 20 mothers as they worked with their babies. My travels gave me a taste of different cultures and made me more cognizant of Western ways that affected my world view.

When I returned to the United States, my next job was in a children's hospital. There I worked on a unit with children who had a medical diagnosis but needed a psychosocial approach. This included babies who failed to thrive due to social reasons, children with diabetes who had difficulty taking their insulin, children with chronic pain, and adolescents with eating disorders. In addition to covering my unit, I performed developmental evaluations and sensory integration intervention on an outpatient basis and treated some children in the neonatal and pediatric intensive care units. For 1 year, I also worked 1 day a week as a consultant to the Sight Center Program for preschoolers who had low vision or were blind. During this period in the 1980s, I advocated for children by speaking at numerous national and state occupational therapy conferences on the topic of collaboration with children.

In 1988, I started a PhD program in special education. As part of the program, I provided treatment and conducted research in an early intervention program serving the needs of inner-city families. The next year I switched my major to educational psychology and became a university professor in the occupational therapy department. I taught classes in normal development, pediatric assessments, childhood occupations, and sociocultural aspects of therapy. I also started working part-time at the hospital's pediatric unit and created a program in an outpatient pediatric oncology clinic. In my last year at the university, I assisted in the creation of an outpatient clinic for children who were depressed or anxious.

In my dissertation, I examined how occupational therapists collaborated with children in treatment planning. I conducted a qualitative study following four cases by interviewing the children and therapists and videotaping the therapy. The results of my research provide the theoretical framework for the therapy chapters in this book.

For 17 years, I was employed by a large school district and worked with children in preschool classrooms through high school. I have been in a number of specialized programs. My school assignments included day treatment programs for children and adolescents with emotional difficulties. I also consulted for programs for children who were mainly nonverbal and had behavioral challenges. In these programs, I observed children who pulled hair, bit, or struck other people when they were in sensory overload. The importance of preventative approaches was critical. I also worked on an assessment team that evaluated children in private schools and residential treatment centers.

In 1997, I completed mediation training and learned how to manage conflict in a constructive manner. In 2000, I also pursued training in play therapy. During that internship, I was with a 3-year-old child who had undergone multiple heart surgeries. She put me in toy handcuffs and told me I was bad and I was going to jail. Then she opened the door for the police to take me. She reenacted this scenario until the end of her therapy, when she opened the door and told the police to go away. What became evident of course was that the jail represented the hospital and all she could determine was that she had been there because she was bad. Again, I was shown how important it is to talk with children and give them a voice. In 2001, my article, "Eliciting Children's Voices in Qualitative Research" was published in the *American Journal of Occupational Therapy*.

In addition, I have lectured three times about the collaboration process in conferences at the Federal University of Minas Gerais in Belo Horizonte, Brazil. There I had the pleasure to meet with occupational therapists and learn about their practices as well as their culture. I also have volunteered for 15 years helping a family with triplets, who were so tiny when they were born they could each put an arm through their dad's wedding ring. Thus, I have had the opportunity to learn an incredible amount about occupational therapy with children. Many people—children, caregivers, teachers, and clinicians—have taught me. In this book I share the lessons I have learned.

Purpose and Structure of the Book

Over the years as a professor and fieldwork supervisor, I often observed occupational therapy students becoming frustrated when their usual way of interacting did not work. For example, when they were stuck in power struggles with children, many had limited ideas of alternative approaches. I believed that my strategies and approaches were common knowledge, but the occupational therapy students showed me they were not generally known. They encouraged me to write about these practices. The purpose of this textbook, therefore, is to provide a detailed description of how to collaborate with children in occupational therapy and research. There is an emphasis on eliciting and strengthening children's voices while guiding them to make therapy meaningful, enjoyable, and successful.

In the first chapter, I describe the history of collaboration in occupational therapy. In the second chapter, I present a research-based conceptual model of collaboration with children, which is then used to organize the chapters regarding therapy. The theoretical underpinnings of this model emphasizing client-centered and strengths-based tenets are included. The third chapter is about how views of children's development, competencies, and rights have changed and ways to advocate for them using an ecological approach.

In Chapters 4 through 17, there are practical strategies covering the complexities of collaborating with those between 3 and 12 years old. The strategies are exemplified by easy-to-read short stories and are useful in any area of pediatric practice. Included are ways to do the following:

- Establish a collaborative frame
- Interview and promote stress-free testing
- Identify goals together
- Develop children's self-advocacy
- Set respectful limits
- Avoid power struggles
- Create challenging and fun experiences
- Improve the flow of therapy
- Create therapeutic endings

Also included are children's perspectives on what they think therapists should know, as well as what children said they themselves might be thinking at each stage of therapy.

The last chapter covers methods for doing research *with* children instead of *on* them. I present a variety of research methods that have been used in studies to enable preschool and school-age children to participate. Examples for how to involve children in various aspects of a research project are described. In addition, I outline creative ways for including children with disabilities as partners in the process.

At the end of each chapter, there are a list of key points to remember and review questions. The answers are provided in the back of the book.

The Approach

I chose storytelling as the main approach because stories are engaging. They capture your attention and pique your interest. Moreover they are easier to remember than a presentation of facts. Stories help you translate philosophical notions into everyday practice. An additional benefit is that they contain real dialogue. For instance, you know it is important to explain what occupational therapy is to all children, yet in practice you may wonder what words to use, especially with children who are very young or nonverbal.

The collaboration process is complex because what you say or do is different in each case. Therefore, a variety of strategies are provided to help you increase your repertoire. It is up to you to decide what strategies are best for a particular situation. Not every strategy works for every child.

Another important aspect is the involvement of children in writing this book. They were asked open-ended questions about what they thought you, as a therapist, should know. I also had two panels of children work with me to identify what they might be thinking during therapy, from the beginning to the end.

The Way Strategies Can Be Used

Experienced therapists develop a repertoire of approaches to use when their first strategy does not work. They learn that the right choice of words can convey respect, avoid power struggles, and promote thoughts about future possibilities. For instance, they learn to avoid saying, "It's time to go, okay?" when staying is not an option. Often the approach entails using subtle words or actions that would not be recognized by the casual observer. A professional dancer makes dancing look easy. Similarly, an experienced therapist makes therapy look easy.

There also are common scenarios that pediatric therapists always encounter. They need to know how to get and maintain children's attention, decide who will go first in a group, and help children start activities and face challenges. Also needed are strategies for helping children deal with mistakes or losing, and for stopping. Another aspect of working with children is being able to determine the *just-right challenge* with the *just-right amount of support*.

In this text, I make the "hidden practice" of collaboration explicit by identifying words and actions you can use. When you know a variety of strategies, you can prevent problems or quickly shift to a more productive one than what you are using in the moment.

This book is designed to be practical. It is useful if you are a student or a new therapist or if you have just switched to pediatric practice. As you begin to interact with children, you can refer to it for strategies such as how to help children deal with mistakes. Experienced therapists may use this text to gain new ideas on the challenging aspects of therapy such as how to involve children in setting goals or how to handle tough situations with children. For instance, I provide ideas on what you may do when children purse their lips, scrunch their faces, fold their arms, and refuse to budge. You may also refer to this resource for approaches to suggest to caregivers and teachers. As a fieldwork supervisor, you will find the detailed strategies helpful in providing constructive feedback to students.

Caveat

I believe that collaboration with families, educational staff, and communities is just as important as collaborating with children. However, because the process is different and less explored, this book zooms in and focuses on the intricacies of interacting with children.

In the book, I am using the term *caregiver* to refer to major adults in the children's lives. Because there are all kinds of families (e.g., grandparents raising grandchildren), I have chosen this generic term because it is more inclusive of such diversity. To maintain confidentiality, the children's names have been changed but their character remains intact.

Because I was raised and have practiced in the United States, my strategies and stories reflect a Western culture with its emphasis on values such as independence, self-determination, and self-advocacy. I recognize and respect that other cultures may have different values such as interdependence and family harmony. I do not advocate imposing the Western culture on others but instead want to emphasize the importance of collaborating to elicit the voices, values, and priorities of all children and their caregivers.

The Joy of Working With Children

One day in a preschool classroom, the teacher announced that they would get to use glitter in an activity. A 3-year-old boy jumped up with pure joy and spun around. I looked at him and thought, *I need to be more like you and enjoy the simple things in life.*

Children are full of energy, playfulness, and honesty. They provide a different perspective from adults, one that can be so jubilant. I have found that collaborating with them is an adventure. I hope this book will help you enjoy working with children as much as I do.

Clare Curtin, PhD, OTR

Section I

History, Theories, and Context of Collaboration With Children

WHY IS IT IMPORTANT TO HAVE STRATEGIES FOR COLLABORATING WITH CHILDREN?

The three chapters in Section I provide the answers to this question.

In Chapter 1, I trace the history of collaboration in occupational therapy. From the beginning of the profession, collaboration has been a core value and deemed an essential element of therapy. Students have been taught that occupational therapists *work with* not *on* clients. When the profession aligned with medicine, there was a shift to emphasizing an expert role. Eventually, leaders in the field argued that practice was not matching the core values and called for therapists to become more client centered and occupation based. In the same time period, activists in the disability rights movement demanded that they have a voice in therapy and research. Thus, when therapists work with children, they need to know HOW to be client centered with caregivers, teachers, and children.

In Chapter 2, I present theories that therapists may use to conceptualize the collaboration process, along with corresponding approaches. Theories are vital. They provide descriptions and plausible explanations of phenomena. Occupational therapy theories provide a framework that shapes therapists' understanding and provides the reasoning for choosing one action over another. Theories provide the reasons for WHY it is important to have collaboration strategies and determining which ones are best to apply in the moment.

First is a description of my research-based occupational therapy conceptual model of the collaboration process. It is based on an in-depth qualitative study, which entailed videotaping therapy sessions and interviewing children and therapists. Second, I outline what occupational therapy theorists and researchers describe as client-centered theory. Third, I propose incorporating a strengths-based model as part of the collaboration process.

In Chapter 3, I argue that perspectives regarding the need to collaborate with children are influenced by historical, cultural, and professional views of childhood, development, and competencies. These influences are not always recognized and yet play a pivotal role in determining whether and to what degree therapists consider involving children.

A second aim of this chapter is to highlight a worldwide children's rights movement. Internationally, there is the recognition that children's voices matter. Responding to the ratification of the United Nations Convention on the Rights of the Child, countries are exploring culturally acceptable ways to allow children to have a say in their lives, community, and government. There is a new focus on conducting research *with* children and being open to learning from their knowledge. These shifting attitudes and practices contribute to the justification for WHY collaborate with children.

A third purpose is to encourage therapists to maintain a broad ecological approach. Pediatric practice encompasses more than one-to-one interaction with a child. It is also crucial for therapists to engage in collaborative consultation with caregivers, teachers, and other meaningful adults. Another important role is being an advocate and changing systems to enhance families' and children's well-being.

In summary, these first three chapters provide the foundation and reasoning for the strategies presented later in the book.

1

Historical Review of Collaboration in Occupational Therapy

Chapter Overview

The purpose of this chapter is to trace how the history of occupational therapy has affected therapists' collaboration with clients. Over the years, the profession aligned with medicine, which changed their roles and the focus of therapy. The profession reached a crisis, prompting leaders to call for a return to the core values by becoming client centered and occupation based. People in the disability rights movement also challenged therapists to shift to focusing on their competencies and quality of life, and fixing society's barriers.

Introduction

He's going to die.

Brian, a skinny 9-year-old boy with solemn brown eyes and yellowish skin, was slowly dying of liver failure. In 1977, there was little that could be done for him. At that time I was an occupational therapy student at a children's hospital and assigned to help him stay independent in his daily activities. In the first two sessions, Brian went along with all my ideas as his mother watched on the sideline.

On the third day, Brian came from his hospital room alone into the occupational therapy clinic. He inched close to me and whispered, "Could you rub my feet?" I was surprised at his request but nodded and led him to a quiet corner of the clinic. Slowly I rubbed and kneaded his bony feet with deep pressure and abandoned the plan I had.

"I miss my mom today," Brian confided. I met his gaze as I continued massaging his feet. "My mom rubs my feet whenever I'm upset." After a minute, he continued, "I'm afraid of dying without her."

At that moment I realized Brian was telling me how I could help him the most. It was more important to listen and comfort him than to do what I had planned for therapy. He began my journey of learning how attuned children are to what they need and how important it is to listen to them. This book is about collaborating with all kinds of children, whatever their needs, including children like Brian.

What Is Collaboration?

A basic tenet of occupational therapy is that collaboration with clients is essential. As an occupational therapist, you use occupations to help people create and maintain a meaningful quality of life. One premise of our profession is that a healthy life entails the incorporation of valued occupations, such as play. The questions, "What is a meaningful life?" and "What are valued occupations?" are to be answered by the clients. Ethically, you have to embark on a discovery process to learn their visions of a good life. This exploration is not a simple process because every person and situation is unique. The process is ongoing and is not limited to just the first session. Therefore, I propose that *collaborative treatment planning is the process of working*

Curtin, C.
Strategies for Collaborating With Children: Creating Partnerships in Occupational Therapy and Research (pp. 3-12).
© 2017 SLACK Incorporated.

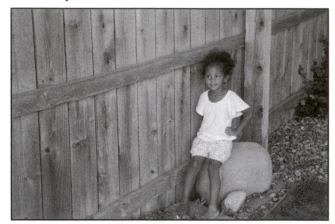

Figure 1-1. Children are experts about their lives.

together as partners to clarify a vision of a good life with meaningful occupations, and to identify and implement ways to create that life.

Collaboration also is required for determining the nature of therapy. You and the clients have different expertise that, when combined, create change. They know their lives and can assist you in clarifying what occupations are relevant and therapeutic for growth (Figure 1-1). You have knowledge regarding the power of occupations for changing lives. You also can be a catalyst in helping them reflect on their lives, identify their values, and explore future possibilities. The interweaving of the clients' and your knowledge establishes what is done for therapy. Collaboration is vital for this blending to occur.

HISTORICAL INFLUENCES ON THE ROLE OF OCCUPATIONAL THERAPISTS AND THEIR COLLABORATION WITH CHILDREN

When learning about a tradition, such as collaboration, it is essential to consider the history and context of that tradition. This is necessary because over the years, the practice of occupational therapy has been shaped by other professions, such as medicine and psychology. An examination of our history also provides an opportunity to highlight the underlying assumptions and taken-for-granted beliefs associated with the time period. The purpose of this historical review, therefore, is to show the transformation of the tradition of collaboration.

Core Values

Collaboration has been viewed as a necessity since the beginning of occupational therapy. Early leaders recognized that clients need to be active participants to identify and establish the meaningfulness of an occupation. Their perspectives were valued and considered critical for therapy. There also has been a long history of giving them choices and respecting their decisions. Early on, therapists were encouraged to be guides. "A therapist who is also a good guide … will stimulate and vitalize human energies so that the patient will achieve a level he [sic] had not suspected he [sic] could reach" (Carrington, 1946, p. 141).

Impact of the Positivist Paradigm

As the profession developed, there was an alignment with medicine and a shift in practice. To ensure job stability and professional credibility therapists embraced medicine's ideology, called the *medical model*. The major tenets of the medical model reflected the *positivist paradigm*. A *paradigm*, as defined by Fraser and Robinson (2005), "is a set of beliefs about the way in which a particular problem exist and a set of agreements on how such problems can be investigated" (p. 59). A paradigm contains views about reality and how to produce knowledge (Houghton, Hunter, & Meskell, 2012). In a positivist paradigm, knowledge was viewed as being constructed through scientific means. The discovery of facts meant the researchers were able to make definitive or positive statements, which resulted in the paradigm being called *positivism* (Fraser & Robinson, 2005).

Using the scientific methods of the natural sciences, medicine addressed the "problem" of how to cure illness and disease. Physicians investigated this "problem" through observations and experiments. They began a quest for descriptive and explanatory facts to determine causality. In medical studies, Sweeney and Kernick (2002) argued that physicians believed it was important to (a) examine the components of the body to understand bodily systems, (b) use linear thinking to link causes and effects, and (c) produce value-free and objective information. Another belief was that good science entailed studies that showed statistical significance and were replicated.

The Medical Model

The dependence on science led physicians to focus on the human body. A person's sick body came to be viewed like a machine with parts that needed to be fixed (Mattingly & Fleming, 1994). To cure or fix the body, physicians had to discover what was wrong. This required a search for deficits or dysfunctions within the individual. Specialties, such as cardiology and psychiatry, were developed. The practice of treating an illness or disease by focusing on a person's body down to the molecular level came to be known as *reductionism* (Rogers, 1982).

The clients' role during medical encounters was to provide details about their symptoms (e.g., When did the pain start? What type of pain is it?), passively accept the physician's diagnosis, and be compliant in the recommended treatment regime. The physicians were required to identify a constellation of symptoms, use their expert knowledge to diagnose the problem, and apply objective research results for treatment. They came to rely on factual tests such as electrocardiography and laboratory blood analysis.

More resources were devoted to addressing acute care (short-term) medical problems in which medications and surgery were the most effective. With long-term ailments, medical treatment addressed the body damage caused by chronic illnesses or disabilities. One type of approach for a child with cerebral palsy, for example, was surgery to release tight arm and leg muscles. Because of the many successful medical advances, application of the medical model became common practice.

Influence of the Medical Model on Views of People With Disabilities

Over the years, the medical model ideology also was applied to society's definition of disability. Prior to the shift, the cause of disabilities often was attributed to supernatural, spiritual, or moral causes leading to blaming and stigmatizing the individual (Baglieri & Shapiro, 2012). Use of the medical model was beneficial in demystifying disability and in changing approaches from punitive and persecuted to medical intervention and rehabilitation (Baglieri & Shapiro, 2012; Goodley, 2014).

Two other movements shaped physicians' and the rest of society's perspectives on disability. The Industrial Revolution and the rise of capitalism created a belief that one's value was determined by one's ability to work (Mallett & Runswick-Cole, 2014). This led to questioning the value to society of those who could not work. Coupled with the survival of the fittest ideas from Social Darwinism, the eugenics movement emphasized creating a society with the fittest citizens (Oliver & Barnes, 2012). This movement led to the inhumane treatment of society's "least-fit" citizens. Some of these treatments were involuntary sterilization to prevent the birth of more people with disabilities, removal from sight and placement in institutions, and medical experimentation without consent (Sabatello, 2014).

Disability came to be defined as an individual medical condition. This meant physicians, with their medical expertise, were believed to be the most qualified to determine what was a disability, the level of severity, the best course of treatment, and placement. They became the experts and often the main decision-makers.

Because disability was considered a health problem, the emphasis on preventing and curing illness was similarly applied to preventing and curing disability. Like disease, disability was considered an abnormality, a pathology, and a defect that needed to be prevented or treated (McDonald & Raymaker, 2013). Physicians were to maintain a professionally detached relationship and separate objective information from descriptions of subjective experiences (Mattingly & Fleming, 1994). If a cure was not possible, therapy was recommended. The scientific approach, which was so successful in saving lives, was highly valued.

The physician's diagnosis became an overarching frame that defined the disability, placed the person into a permanent patient role, and created a medical identity (Baglieri & Shapiro, 2012). The diagnosis became a label that medical professionals incorporated in all their descriptions. In addition, the diagnosis was used to dictate which therapies were provided.

For children with disabilities, the diagnosis was a major factor in determining where they lived and were educated. If, for instance, children were diagnosed as being "mentally retarded," up until the 1970s physicians often recommended placement in an institution. Many parents followed this advice trusting that physicians knew best. If physicians determined that children had potential, they may have recommended placement in rehabilitation centers, specialized schools, or classrooms.

Sadly, scores of children residing in institutions received no education and experienced dehumanizing and abusive treatment. The book, *What We Have Done: An Oral History of the Disability Rights Movement*, by Fred Pelka (2012), includes numerous stories exposing the appalling conditions children were forced to live in. In Michael Kennedy's (2014) book, *My Life in Institutions and My Way Out*, he told a similar story of atrocious treatment by the staff in the 1960s. He described, for example, a time when he was punished by having rope placed around his ankles and being hung upside down in a doorframe.

Children with disabilities in the United States were not guaranteed an education until 1975. For those who attended school, they tended to be grouped by their diagnosis (instead of their educational needs) and placed in specialized schools or classrooms (Baglieri & Shapiro, 2012). Schools were not required to make accommodations. Corbett O'Toole (Pelka, 2012) described her experiences as a child with polio who used crutches. She said she went to her local public school for kindergarten. The next year, however, the principal told her mother that she could not return because there were stairs to the first-grade classroom and it was "inappropriate" for her to be in a public school (p. 36).

Incorporation of the Medical Model in Occupational Therapy

As occupational therapists began to consider themselves as medical professionals, they incorporated many aspects of the medical model into their practice. Therapy became focused on the individual and, like a camera lens, they zoomed in on the client's body parts. Many therapists started to insist on the importance of addressing underlying components, such as muscle strength, joint range of motion, and emphasizing skill development for optimal functioning. They also attempted to show objective changes by using tests to measure development and other factors.

Similar to the physician's linear process—identify symptoms, diagnose disease, and treat—occupational therapists were taught to think of treatment planning as being a usually straightforward process: identify the problem (mainly a deficit or dysfunction within the person), determine goals to alleviate or fix the problem, and devise activities to achieve the goals. They also started using the medical diagnosis as a way of organizing what they did for treatment (Mattingly & Fleming, 1994). If, for example, they heard a child had a certain type of cerebral palsy, they would conjure up a host of principles and goals that were associated with that particular diagnosis. Another change was that therapists began to view the nature of practice as being the use of activities to address medical or psychiatric problems. For instance, some therapists used activities to elicit unconscious emotions that could then be dealt with in psychotherapy (Llorens & Young, 1960).

The therapist's role drifted from being a guide to being an expert, especially regarding participation in activities of daily living. The importance of independence was a guiding value, regardless of the client's culture. Once a deficit or dysfunction was labeled, therapists were to use their expert knowledge to help clients. Unlike the passive role in medical care, the clients were supposed to have an active involvement in occupational therapy. Often, however, therapists identified the problems and goals, and the clients were only given choices regarding the activities. For example, in one 1959 survey of 30 therapists, Choren (1959) found that only two of them involved clients in the development of goals.

In that time period, there were others who questioned the clients' level of involvement even in choosing the activities. Gordon and Wellerson (1954) contended that clients in acute care rehabilitation settings often only completed the recommended activity to oblige the therapist. They argued that many male clients did not see the value of arts and crafts and that a shortcoming of the profession was the "use of modalities unrelated to the patient's sense of values" (p. 239). Bateson (1956) made a similar argument that "mere good intentions towards the patient are not enough. He [sic] must also care about the modality…" (p. 188). Boynton (1954) also maintained that clients may only do an activity because they felt compelled. He emphasized the need to understand the clients' point of view, their motivation, and their own goals.

Whitehead (1956) advocated for a similar collaborative approach with children. She argued that:

> …we have a tendency to "do to" a child rather than be cognizant that true development comes only from within the child…. The child must have continuous active participation in the planning of his [sic] goals and the routes toward them… (p. 185).

Many elements of the medical model became part of occupational therapy's culture and an integral part of practice. But adoption of medicine's ideology eventually led to a crisis in occupational therapy.

The Story of Ruth

The story of Ruth Sienkiewicz-Mercer (Sienkiewicz-Mercer & Kaplan, 1996) exemplifies how the use of a scientific medical model failed a child with disabilities. Ruth was born in 1950 with a sound mind, but, as a result of encephalitis at 6 months, she only had the use of her eyes, ears, nose, and a few sounds from her vocal chords. She communicated by raising her eyes to say yes, curling her lips to indicate no, and making a small number of sounds to emphasize the intensity of her emotions. She was unable to use her hands, arms, or legs.

As an adult, Ruth told her life story through the use of her eyes and word boards. Steven Kaplan, a teacher with the Fundamental Right to Free Education program, assisted her by pointing to different rows of words until she raised her eyes for yes. Next, he would proceed across the row until Ruth focused on a word. He always checked if he was right and then combined the words into a sentence. At every stage, Ruth verified his accuracy.

In Ruth's younger days she lived with her loving family, who enjoyed her feisty personality and understood her nonverbal ways of speaking. The family sought help and, as a result, Ruth spent time in different rehabilitation centers. When she was a young child, physicians diagnosed cerebral palsy and she received intensive therapy. However, when over time she did not make observable and measurable changes such as starting to walk or feed herself, the therapies were discontinued.

From Ruth's perspective, she enjoyed being in school programs and was growing immensely both socially and educationally. This came to an end at age 10 after a newly graduated psychologist gave her an "objective" and standardized test of intelligence without adapting to her communication system. He incorrectly labeled her as an "imbecile" at a mental age of 4 months. She was then sent home and eventually the family followed medical advice to place her in an institution for the "mentally retarded" at the Belchertown (Massachusetts) State School. Ruth found herself living in subhuman conditions. She was placed in diapers even though she only needed assistance to transfer to the toilet and was force-fed while lying flat on her back. Because no one questioned the label assigned to her, it took years for the staff to realize that her mind was normal and she could communicate.

Her first short-lived experience with an occupational therapist was a dismal failure. The therapist, using a medical model, tried to get her to feed herself using an oversized spoon. The focus of therapy was on feeding skills instead of improving Ruth's life conditions including her total lack of meaningful occupations. After 4 months of many unsuccessful attempts, therapy stopped. Many years later, her second time with an occupational therapist was more valuable. The therapist designed her first customized wheelchair, which Ruth reported helped change her life.

With the emergence of the independent living movement, Ruth began to receive intensive speech therapy and expanded her communication by using word boards. With support, she moved out of the state institution and into an apartment, hired personal care assistants, and later married.

For a major part of Ruth's life, the professionals focused on just her body and lack of abilities, resulting in her being placed in deplorable living situations. Positive changes only occurred when, finally, the professionals first, recognized and enhanced Ruth's "voice"; second, appreciated her spirit; and third, focused on helping her leave the institution and create a fulfilling life.

Crisis in Occupational Therapy

Possibly, in response to cases like Ruth's, in the 1970s, Shannon (1977) wrote about the "derailment of occupational therapy" (p. 229). He emphasized that the profession had lost its original values and beliefs. In his view, occupational therapy practice had become too reductionistic when it aligned with medicine, had not adequately addressed the needs of the chronically ill, and had devalued arts and crafts. He contended that therapists viewed a client "... not as a creative being, capable of making choices and directing his [sic] own future, but as a mechanistic creature susceptible to manipulation and control via the application of techniques" (p. 233).

During this contentious time, therapists began to question their identity and theoretical frameworks (Figure 1-2). In the 1960s and 1970s, Mary Reilly and a group of her students began to recapture many of the basic beliefs about occupation and called their theoretical approach *occupational behavior* (Takata, 1980).

Other therapists also challenged the trend of declining client involvement. They advocated the view of clients as consumers with rights to participate in all aspects of treatment including treatment planning, program development, and evaluation (Bloomer, 1978; Johnson, 1977; Nixon, 1971). Matsutsuyu (1971) suggested that use of the occupational behavior frame of reference could assist the therapist in making the client "...an active partner in the identification of his [sic] problem, in acknowledging his[sic] strengths, and setting achievable goals, and implementing a course of action" (p. 293). Although many therapists advocated for the client to have full participation in treatment planning, there continued to be a range of approaches. Some therapists continued to set goals for the client after conducting an evaluation, whereas others engaged the

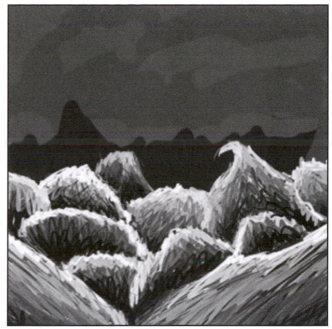

Figure 1-2. A clash emerged between the values and practice of occupational therapy.

client as an active partner in goal setting (Dunleavey, 1974; Heine, 1975; Kuenstler, 1976; McKenzie, 1970).

Disability Rights Movements

Discontent with the lack of a voice, the disability rights movement gained momentum in the 1970s. Seeing the effectiveness of the civil rights movement, people with disabilities in the United States began organizing and rebelling against the status quo (McDonald & Raymaker, 2013). They started a campaign that included speeches, marches, and civil disobedience. "Nothing about us without us," (Charlton, 1998) became the slogan for their movement. This slogan encapsulated their demand to have their voices included and heard in all areas affecting their lives, including their living situations, medical intervention, rehabilitation, disability theory, and research.

As the disability rights movement progressed, they began demanding more rights, especially the right to decide about their own lives. They rallied for equal citizenship. Parent groups, such as The United Cerebral Palsy Association and National Association for Retarded Children, supported them (Pelka, 2012). In 1975 The Education for all Handicapped Children's Act was passed, which ensured all children's right to an education in the United States.

Their efforts also led to the passage of the 1990 Americans with Disabilities Act (ADA). Months before in March, one of the organizations, The American Disabled for Public Transportation, which referred to their original cause, planned 3 days of demonstrations (Pelka, 2012). They marched to the Capitol. A large group left their wheelchairs at the bottom of the steep and inaccessible steps and crawled up. Other marchers chanted, "Access is our civil right" (Shapiro, 1994, p. 133). The next day a photo of 8-year-old Jennifer Keelan crawling up the steps was in newspapers across the country and was the "one photographic image from the ADA fight to register in the public's memory" (Shapiro, 1994, p. 133).

Similarly in the United Kingdom, people with disabilities demanded a change. In the 1970s the group, Union of the Physically Impaired Against Segregation, published a document containing a call to separate a "person with impairment" from society's creation of "disability" (Mallett & Runswick-Cole, 2014). This distinction eventually led to what became the *social model of disability* (Oliver & Barnes, 2012). In this model, activists and theorists argued that just because an individual had an impairment, it did not mean she or he was disabled. Rather, it was society's social, cultural, and physical barriers that created the disability. For example, many people who used wheelchairs could live and work independently if they had accessible living, transportation, and work accommodations. A political movement to remove society's barriers and oppression ensued. During this period, related changes also occurred elsewhere such as in Australia and the Scandinavian countries.

These movements centered on holding society accountable and insisting on change. Disability rights activists began writing about injustices and presented their perspectives on what it meant to be disabled. The field of disability studies emerged in academia. This resulted in a variety of new theories; all of them critiquing the limitations of the medical model.

Continuing with the cause, disability rights activists (Shapiro, 1994) and theorists (Goodley, 2014; Oliver & Barnes, 2012; Shakespeare, 2014a; Watson, Roulstone, & Thomas, 2014) presented common themes in their writings. The theorists included people with and without disabilities. These themes were also evident in the life stories of those with disabilities (Kennedy, 2014; Sienkiewicz-Mercer & Kaplan, 1996). First, they redefined disability. They argued that disability is a sociological, political, and cultural concept rather than an individual medical condition (Goodley, 2014). Disability, they said, also is a characteristic shared by all as they age over the life span, which needs to be viewed as a continuum versus all or nothing (Fleischer & Zames, 2011).

Second, activists and theorists commented on society's idealized notion of what is normal and able-bodied. They proposed that constantly judging people with disabilities with the "ideal" person as the norm created a normal-abnormal binary; either they were normal or not (Ferguson & Nusbaum, 2012). Society defined the norm without consideration of how people with disabilities felt about themselves or their lives. And, they maintained, the standards of normalcy were unattainable for those whose bodies or minds would never be considered normal.

In addition, they challenged the notion that they had to be able bodied to be full citizens and emphasized that this way of thinking created prejudice (Goodley, 2014).

Third, there was an insistence that efforts be shifted from fixing the person to fixing society. The activists said it was time to eliminate physical barriers (e.g., a lack of access to buildings and transportation); paternalistic and negative attitudes that created a culture of pity; denial of an education; and policies making them wards of the state versus full citizens with rights. They wanted an ending to segregation, exclusion, and discrimination.

Fourth, they highly criticized the approaches used by physicians and rehabilitation specialists. Oliver and Barnes (2012), sociologists with impairments, were especially vocal about this issue. Medical staff thought they were the experts. Although well-intentioned, they acted like they knew what was best for each individual. There was an unequal relationship in which the physicians and therapists had the power to decide who gets therapy and for how long. The people with disabilities objected to the focus on their deficits and the use of the diagnosis to determine services for all aspects of their everyday lives. Medicine, activists argued, needed to put more effort into improving their quality of life.

Rehabilitation specialists, including occupational therapists, were misaligned in focusing on their deficits and only trying to fix them without altering the environment and society. They asserted that people with disabilities were expected to do all the changing. They were supposed to learn to adapt, cope, and assimilate (Oliver & Barnes, 2012). Often the goal was to make them look normal versus creating a society that accepted differences.

Then even if therapists' goals did not match theirs, they were expected to cooperate. Occupational therapists' emphasis on full participation in activities of daily living, such as feeding and dressing, did not equate to their desired goal of independent living (Brown & Bowen, 1998). Therapists were too focused on discrete skills rather than total community involvement and integration. In addition, the value occupational therapists placed on independence and self-sufficiency did not take into account the value of interdependence.

Fifth, disability rights activists challenged the prevailing view of them as being damaged or undesirable individuals. They rejected the use of a medical label to define who they were as people and in the United States started using the phrase, "a person with...." They wanted to stop the culture of pity, the view of their lives as being "personal tragedies," and their being treated as passive victims (Barnes, 2014). They said to change the focus to their capacities versus their deficits and recognize their valuable contribution to society even if they could not work. They maintained that, contrary to others' views, they could view their disabled bodies and lives in a positive light and lead a good life (Shakespeare, 2014b).

Sixth, there was a demand to shift from only doing biomedical research with its focus on the elimination of disability to also having research that promoted their quality of life and health equity (McDonald & Raymaker, 2013). Rather than having rehabilitation sciences own the research about disability, they demanded inclusion (Ferguson & Nusbaum, 2012). "Nothing about us without us" meant that people with disabilities needed to provide consent, have a voice in research, and be included in the process, including deciding what was studied. Years later, there finally was a call for children with disabilities as well as adults to have a voice and be included in research.

Occupational Therapists' Continued Use of the Medical Model With Children

During the 1970s, therapists expanded their pediatric practice to new areas such as school systems and community health programs. They evaluated and provided treatment mostly to improve children's development of neurological functioning, perceptual-motor development, sensory processing, and participation in activities of daily living.

Neurodevelopmental treatment (NDT) and sensory integration (SI) were two pediatric treatment approaches described in the literature. In both approaches, the therapist instead of the child was primarily responsible for identifying the children's needs and defining therapy goals. In an NDT approach, since the concern was about children's quality of movement, the therapist was seen as needing to assume a directive role to provide children with more normal motor experiences. Therapists using an SI approach believed that children needed to have an active role in the choice of activities throughout the session.

Other therapists during this time conducted general developmental assessments and provided treatment for developmental delays. The therapists were seen as teachers, motivators, and role models who promoted the involvement of children in deciding on the activities (Banus, Hayes, Kent, Komick, & Sukiennicki, 1971). Although Coley (1972) recommended that therapists consider the children's point of view and develop a partnership in treatment, this was not highly valued by all therapists. For example, Gilfoyle and Hays (1979) conducted a national survey in which 294 therapists employed in school systems responded and rated the value of different evaluation tasks. Of 33 evaluation tasks, "interview for future plans and goals of a child" was 27th and given a weighted value of 2.6 whereas "observe developmental tasks" was given the highest value of 3.8 (p. 569). Even though therapists were challenging the approach to collaboration with adults, this did not occur with children.

A Call to Be Occupation Based, Client Centered, and Focused More on the Environment

In the 1980s, therapists wrote about the need to make changes and increase the consistency between the profession's core values and practice. In 1982, Rogers described the difference between two professions. Medicine focused on treating diseases whereas occupational therapy focused on treating dysfunctions in occupations. In 1984, West implored therapists to (a) return to the use of the term *occupation* versus the narrower term *activity*, (b) refer to the areas of concern as *occupational dysfunction* versus *disability*, and (c) consider the relationship between the mind-body-environment.

In the literature, therapists also talked more about negotiating with clients, making them active partners, and developing a model of mutual cooperation (Gilfoyle, 1987; Grady, 1990; Lloyd, 1986; Yerxa, 1980). Canadian therapists advocated for being client centered, developed a conceptual model, and created guidelines for this type of practice (Law, Baptiste, & Mills, 1995; Pollock, 1993). Frieden and Cole (1985) contended that therapists needed to change to a more supportive role. In addition, they said that instead of focusing on the use of activities to develop clients' abilities, therapists needed to shift to assisting clients in problem-solving the difficulties encountered while interacting with the environment.

The importance of collaboration was being emphasized. However, within therapists' descriptions of their practice, the level of collaboration, such as who determined the purpose of therapy, varied.

A Beginning Shift to Increase Children's and Families' Involvement in Determining the Purpose of Therapy

In the 1980s and 1990s, there was a move to become more family centered when working with children. When therapists centered their attention on just children, authors (Dunst, Trivette, & Deal, 1988, 1994) argued, they missed discovering and incorporating families' strengths, needs, and goals. Families needed to have a voice.

Another change was a description of the children's roles in pediatric practice models. Neurodevelopmental treatment and sensory integration continued to be common pediatric practice models described in the literature. The view of children's role in treatment planning changed little from the 1970s with therapists using an NDT approach. However, for therapists using an SI practice model, it was now recommended that children have an active role in planning treatment including the identification of problems and setting goals (Bundy, 1991). Therapists using models based on occupational behavior began to work with children to jointly identify their needs, goals, and methods for treatment (Curtin, 1992). Thus, the practice models used by the therapists seem to influence whether children were considered to be active participants in all aspects of treatment planning.

Occupational Therapists' Dilemma Between Using Biomedical and Phenomenological Frameworks

In the late 1980s, the American Occupational Therapy Foundation and Association funded a study of occupational therapists' clinical reasoning (Gillette & Mattingly, 1987). An anthropologist (Mattingly) and three occupational therapists (Fleming, Cohn, and Gillette), along with the involvement of different universities' faculty and students, conducted a 2-year ethnography that included participant observations, in-depth interviews, and videotaped treatment sessions (Mattingly & Gillette, 1991). After collecting the data, they incorporated components of an action-research design by including the therapists being studied in the analysis process.

In this groundbreaking study (Fleming, 1991; Mattingly, 1991; Mattingly & Fleming, 1994), the researchers found that therapists used four different types of reasoning: procedural, interactive, conditional, and narrative. One type, *procedural reasoning*, was used when determining how to address the client's disability or disease, and was similar to the problem-solving reasoning used by physicians. Therapists used this type when they described their sequence of identifying problems, setting goals, and planning treatment.

However, the other three types differed. They found there was a hidden humanistic practice reflecting the roots of the profession. In rehabilitation, therapists could not focus only on clients' bodies; they needed the clients' active participation to make therapy meaningful. To do this, they used *interactive reasoning* to understand, engage, and work with a particular individual. *Conditional reasoning* was used to consider (a) all aspects of a condition, such as how a disability affects an individuals' life; (b) what about the condition could change; and (c) how to engage the client in envisioning possible outcomes. They also used *narrative reasoning* by making connections and thinking in the form of a story, and with their clients tying together different events and perspectives to create new life stories.

Another finding in their research was that therapists assumed a *biomedical frame* yet also maintained a *phenomenological frame*. A biomedical view centered on the clients' bodies, medical conditions, and performance skills. A phenomenological view was evident when the therapists saw each client as an individual, considered each client's perspectives and experiences, and explored each client's values and goals.

At times, the therapists easily moved back and forth between the two frames. For instance, therapists often initiated conversation about the client's life and dreams (a phenomenological frame) while working on performance skills (biomedical frame). Other times, however, they found therapists experienced dilemmas. For instance, some therapists were in a quandary during the times they needed to advocate for the clients' own wishes when it was not in the normal course of medical treatment that they outwardly supported.

In this ethnographic study, therapists naturally wanted to be accepted in the medical setting and be reimbursed for their services. Consequently, they tended to document using biomedical terms and mainly described changes with the client's body or performance skills. What became evident was that by trying to align with medicine, a major part of occupational therapy's practice was hidden and undocumented.

In her article on clinical reasoning, Mattingly (1991) proposed that "perhaps occupational therapy as a profession needs to take its phenomenological tasks more seriously" (p. 986). She challenged the profession to change its language, teach courses on the phenomenological frame, and develop constructs that more accurately reflect therapists' practices. These changes were essential for articulating the value of occupational therapy.

SUMMARY

This historical review has highlighted the twists and turns of occupational therapy practice. Early leaders placed a high value on eliciting clients' perspectives, involving them in decision making, and ensuring they became active participants in therapy. The therapist's role was to be a guide. A core belief was occupational therapists work *with* clients not *on* them.

Then there was a significant change in practice. Therapists adopted the ideology of the medical model and defined themselves as medical professionals. Although the use of this model was effective for physicians, there were disadvantages for therapists in the long run. Many therapists shifted to an expert role, focusing more on clients' bodies and deficits, and defining goals with minimal or no clients' involvement. In addition, as disability rights activists argued, therapists spent all their time trying to change them and not trying to change society's barriers and oppression. Another consequence, seen in the study of clinical reasoning, was that therapists' humanistic practice was hidden and not documented.

Eventually, especially in the 1980s, leaders decried the direction in which the profession was going. Current practice, they said, was drifting away from the original core values and beliefs. They insisted that therapists define the profession by their knowledge of occupations, and return to being client centered and developing collaborative partnerships. They also challenged therapists to address society's injustices.

KEY POINTS TO REMEMBER

- Collaboration has always been a tenet of occupational therapy and considered essential.

- Occupational therapy's alignment with the medical model influenced the therapist's role, collaboration, and approaches with children.

- The profession reached a crisis when therapists' practices were not aligned with the profession's values.

- People with disabilities led the disability rights movement, criticized physicians and rehabilitation therapists for maintaining the medical model of disability, and demanded major changes.

- There was a call for occupational therapists to return to their core values by becoming more client centered and occupation based.

REVIEW QUESTIONS

1. A core belief of occupational therapy is that clients must be active participants in therapy. True or false.

2. Collaboration will look the same between all clients and therapists. True or false.

3. How did the profession of occupational therapy change when it aligned with medicine?

4. Name the four reasons Shannon (1977) gave for the "derailment of occupational therapy."

5. The medical model of disability considers a disability as an individual health problem. True or false.

6. What was the slogan for the disability rights movement in the United States?

7. Name at least five rights the disability activists demanded.

8. Many current disability theorists and activists view disability as being created by society's oppression and barriers. True or false.

9. In the 1990s study of clinical reasoning, what part of occupational therapy practice did Mattingly and Fleming find was hidden?

10. Name six changes leaders in occupational therapy called for in the 1980s to 1990s.

REFERENCES

Baglieri, S., & Shapiro, A. (2012). *Disability studies and the inclusive classroom: Critical practices for creating least restrictive attitudes.* New York, NY: Routledge.

Banus, B. S., Hayes, M., Kent, C. A., Komick, M. P., & Sukiennicki, D. A. (1971). *The developmental therapist: A prototype of the pediatric therapist.* Thorofare, NJ: Charles B. Slack.

Barnes, C. (2014). Understanding the social model of disability: Past, present and future. In N. Watson, A. Roulstone, & C. Thomas (Eds.), *Routledge handbook of disability studies* (pp. 12-29). New York, NY: Routledge.

Bateson, G. (1956). Communication in occupational therapy. *The American Journal of Occupational Therapy, 10*(4), 188.

Bloomer, J. S. (1978). The consumer of therapy in mental health. *The American Journal of Occupational Therapy, 32*(10), 621-627.

Boynton, B. L. (1954). Refining our resources. *The American Journal of Occupational Therapy, 8*(2), 45-47, 65.

Brown, C., & Bowen, R. E. (1998). Including the consumer and environment in occupational therapy treatment planning. *The Occupational Therapy Journal of Research, 18*(1), 44-62.

Bundy, A. (1991). The process of planning and implementing intervention. In A. Fisher, E. A. Murray, & A. Bundy (Eds.), *Sensory integration and practice* (pp. 302-320). Philadelphia, PA: F. A. Davis.

Carrington, E. M. (1946). Psychological foundations of occupational therapy. *Occupational Therapy and Rehabilitation, 25*(4), 141-144.

Charlton, J. I. (1998). *Nothing about us without us: Disability oppression and empowerment.* Berkeley, CA: University of California.

Choren, B. G. (1959). The initial interview as a treatment procedure in occupational therapy. *The American Journal of Occupational Therapy, 13*(2), 88-92, 106.

Coley, I. L. (1972). The child with juvenile rheumatoid arthritis. *The American Journal of Occupational Therapy, 26*(7), 325-329.

Curtin, C. (1992, March). *Collaborative treatment planning with children.* Paper presented at the annual national conference of the American Occupational Therapy Association, Houston, TX.

Dunleavey, E. (1974). Occupational therapist in home health. *The American Journal of Occupational Therapy, 28*(8), 484-487.

Dunst, C. J., Trivette, C. M., & Deal, A. G. (1988). *Enabling and empowering families: Principles and guidelines for practice.* Cambridge, MA: Brookline Books.

Dunst, C. J., Trivette, C. M., & Deal, A. G. (1994). *Supporting and strengthening families: Volume 1: Methods, strategies and practices.* Cambridge, MA: Brookline Books.

Ferguson, P. M., & Nusbaum, E. (2012). Disability studies: What is it and what difference does it make? *Research and Practice for Persons With Severe Disabilities, 37*(2), 70-80.

Fleischer, D. Z., & Zames, F. (2011). *The disability rights movement: From charity to confrontation.* Philadelphia, PA: Temple University.

Fleming, M. H. (1991). The therapist with the three-track mind. *The American Journal of Occupational Therapy, 45*(11), 1007-1014.

Fraser, S., & Robinson, C. (2005). Paradigms and philosophy. In S. Fraser, V. Lewis, S. Ding, M. Kellett, & C. Robinson (Eds.), *Doing research with children and young people* (pp. 59-77). Thousand Oaks, CA: Sage.

Frieden, L., & Cole, J. A. (1985). Independence: The ultimate goal of rehabilitation for spinal cord-injured persons. *The American Journal of Occupational Therapy, 39*(11), 734-739.

Gilfoyle, E. M. (1987). Creative partnerships: The profession's plan (presidential address). *The American Journal of Occupational Therapy, 41*(12), 779-781.

Gilfoyle, E. M., & Hays, C. (1979). Occupational therapy roles and functions in the education of the school-based handicapped student. *The American Journal of Occupational Therapy, 33*(9), 565-576.

Gillette, N. P., & Mattingly, C. (1987). Clinical reasoning in occupational therapy. *The American Journal of Occupational Therapy, 41*(6), 399-400.

Goodley, D. (2014). *Dis/ability studies: Theorising disablism and ableism.* New York, NY: Routledge.

Gordon, E. E., & Wellerson, T. L. (1954). Does occupational therapy meet the demands of total rehabilitation? *The American Journal of Occupational Therapy, 8*(6), 238-240, 275-276.

Grady, A. P. (1990). Collaborative relationships: Opportunities for occupational therapy in the 1990's and beyond. *The American Journal of Occupational Therapy, 44*(2), 105-108.

Heine, D. B. (1975). Daily living group: Focus on transition from hospital to community. *The American Journal of Occupational Therapy, 29*(10), 628-630.

Houghton, C., Hunter, A., & Meskell, P. (2012). Linking aims, paradigm and method in nursing research. *Nurse Researcher, 20*(2), 34-39.

Johnson, J. A. (1977). Humanitarianism and accountability: A challenge for occupational therapy in its 60th anniversary. *The American Journal of Occupational Therapy, 31*(10), 631-637.

Kennedy, M. J. (2014). *My life in institutions and my way out.* Victoria, BC, Canada: Friensen.

Kuenstler, G. (1976). A planning group for psychiatric outpatients. *The American Journal of Occupational Therapy, 30*, 634-639.

Law, M., Baptiste, S., & Mills, J. (1995). Client-centred practice: What does it mean and does it make a difference? *Canadian Journal of Occupational Therapy, 62*(5), 250-257.

Llorens, L. A., & Young, G. G. (1960). Case history: Finger painting for the hostile child. *The American Journal of Occupational Therapy, 14*(7), 306-307.

Lloyd, C. (1986). The process of goal setting using goal attainment scaling in a therapeutic community. *Occupational Therapy in Mental Health, 6*(3), 19-30.

Mallett, R., & Runswick-Cole, K. (2014). *Approaching disability: Critical issues and perspectives.* New York, NY: Routledge.

Matsutsuyu, J. (1971). Occupational behavior: A perspective on work and play. *The American Journal of Occupational Therapy, 25*(6), 291-294.

Mattingly, C. (1991). What is clinical reasoning? *The American Journal of Occupational Therapy, 45*(11), 979-986.

Mattingly, C., & Fleming, M. H. (1994). *Clinical reasoning: Forms of inquiry in a therapeutic practice.* Philadelphia, PA: F. A. Davis.

Mattingly, C., & Gillette, N. (1991). Anthropology, occupational therapy, and action research. *The American Journal of Occupational Therapy, 45*(11), 972-978.

McDonald, K. E., & Raymaker, D. M. (2013). Paradigms shifts in disability and health: Toward more ethical public health research. *American Journal of Public Health, 103*(12). 2165-2173. doi:10.2105/AJPH2013.301286

McKenzie, M. W. (1970). The role of occupational therapy in rehabilitating spinal cord injury patients. *The American Journal of Occupational Therapy, 24*(4), 257-263.

Nixon, R. A. (1971). The crisis and challenge of human services in the new decade. *The American Journal of Occupational Therapy, 25*(4), 187-192.

Oliver, M., & Barnes, C. (2012). *The new politics of disablement.* New York, NY: Palgrave Macmillan.

Pelka, F. (2012). *What we have done: An oral history of the disability rights movement.* Boston, MA: University of Massachusetts.

Pollock, N. (1993). Client-centered assessment. *The American Journal of Occupational Therapy, 47*(4), 298-301.

Rogers, J. C. (1982). Order and disorder in occupational therapy and medicine. *The American Journal of Occupational Therapy, 36*(1), 29-35.

Sabatello, M. (2014). A short history of the international disability rights movement. In M. Sabatello & M. Schulze (Eds.), *Human rights and disability advocacy* (pp. 13-24). Philadelphia, PA: University of Pennsylvania.

Shakespeare, T. (2014a). *Disability rights and wrongs revisited.* New York, NY: Routledge.

Shakespeare, T. (2014b). Nasty, brutish and short? On the predicament of disability and embodiment. In J. E. Bickenbach, F. Felder, & B. Schmitz (Eds.), *Disability and the good human life* (pp. 93-112). New York, NY: Cambridge University.

Shannon, P. D. (1977). The derailment of occupational therapy. *The American Journal of Occupational Therapy, 31*(4), 229-234.

Shapiro, J. P. (1994). No pity: People with disabilities forging a new civil rights movement. New York, NY: Times Books.

Sienkiewicz-Mercer, R., & Kaplan, S. (1996). *I raise my eyes to say yes: A memoir.* West Hartford, CT: Whole Health Books.

Sweeney, K., & Kernick, D. (2002). Clinical evaluation: Constructing a new model for post-normal medicine. *Journal of Evaluation in Clinical Practice, 8*(2), 131-138. doi:10.1046/j.1365-2753.2002.00312x

Takata, N. (1980). Introduction to a series: Occupational behavior for pediatric practice. *The American Journal of Occupational Therapy, 34*(1), 11-12.

Watson, N., Roulstone, A., & Thomas, C. (2014). *Routledge handbook of disability studies.* New York, NY: Routledge.

West, W. L. (1984). A reaffirmed philosophy and practice of occupational therapy for the 1980s. *The American Journal of Occupational Therapy, 38*(1), 15-23.

Whitehead, M. (1956). The patient as an individual. *The American Journal of Occupational Therapy, 10*(4), 184-185.

Yerxa, E. J. (1980). Occupational therapy's role in creating a future climate of caring. *The American Journal of Occupational Therapy, 34*(8), 529-534.

Theoretical Underpinnings of a Model of Collaboration

CHAPTER OVERVIEW

Practice is influenced by one's frame of reference that is developed through experiences, theories, and research. In this chapter, I present the theoretical underpinnings that shape collaboration in occupational therapy. A synopsis is given of my research on collaborative treatment planning with children that led to the development of a conceptual model called the *collaborative frame*. I include the children's interviews and the research methods used to elicit their voices. Next, I describe client-centered therapy and a strengths-based model that also contribute to the theoretical foundation of this book.

A STUDY OF COLLABORATION

In the early 1990s, as those in the profession began to reclaim the early leaders' core beliefs, I began my research on the collaboration process with children. I found that although it was common for therapists to collaborate with adults in the children's lives, it was much less common to collaborate with the children. I knew it was more challenging to include them. At that time, I was a university professor in an occupational therapy department and trying to teach students how to involve children. I found that the main description of treatment planning (identify problems, set goals to alleviate the problems, and determine activities

to achieve the goals) was limited. It did not explain how the client was involved in this process. At the same time, I worked 1 day a week in the pediatric oncology clinic and experienced the richness and power of occupational therapy that was not captured in that description. A search of the occupational therapy literature showed there was a lack of description and research on what the collaboration process with children entailed.

For this reason, I chose to focus on the intricacies of the therapist-child interactions to study the process in depth. I wanted to include the children's perspectives and learn from them. At that time, there were few studies in which children were research participants instead of subjects. The research question guiding my study (Curtin, 1995) was *How do occupational therapists collaborate with children in planning treatment?*

The study took place in an inner-city Midwestern general hospital. This hospital contained a pediatric unit and an outpatient sensory integration clinic. Three experienced occupational therapists were participants in four cases with children ranging from 8 to 12 years old. In one case, I was the therapist and a research assistant conducted the interviews. Two children were hospitalized and two came to a sensory integration clinic. The occupational therapy sessions were observed and videotaped. Interviews were conducted with the children and therapists immediately after each therapy session when possible. In addition to therapists and parents, the children also signed consent forms.

Curtin, C.
Strategies for Collaborating With Children: Creating Partnerships in Occupational Therapy and Research (pp. 13-35).
© 2017 SLACK Incorporated.

THE CHILDREN'S PERSPECTIVES AND RESEARCH METHODS USED

I have selected this section of the data to (a) provide a short summary of the four therapy stories, (b) share the children's perspectives, and (c) illustrate the use of participatory research methods used with these children.

In this study, the children's perspectives were obtained in the same room where therapy occurred. A variety of methods (e.g., role-play, drawing) were used, which shows how their voices could be elicited in different ways. The children were encouraged to describe what happened in therapy, and their thoughts and feelings regarding therapy and their therapist. They also were asked if they had suggestions for how therapists could be better at talking and working with children. Pseudonyms were used for the children and therapists.

Tony's Perspectives on Therapy While Being Hospitalized for Chemotherapy for a Brain Tumor

Ten-year-old Tony had recently had surgery, but the doctors were only able to remove part of his brain tumor. They reported that his type of cancer was usually terminal. After surgery, Tony had to learn how to adjust to double vision, hand tremors, and fatigue. Since the surgery, he had attended the pediatric oncology clinic where I was a therapist. Tony participated in the following interviews when he was hospitalized for 3 days of chemotherapy.

Lauren, a research assistant, videotaped the occupational therapy sessions and conducted the interviews. In this case, I was the therapist working with Tony. Prior to the first meeting, I had written the following script as one possible option Lauren could use in the interviews:

> You can make a movie and tell your story about what occupational therapy was like for you. In your movie, tell what happened when you were with [name of therapist]. What did you two do? How did you decide what to do for treatment? Also say what you were thinking and feeling during your time with [name of therapist].
>
> It may help if you pretend you are making this movie and telling your story to other kids, such as a friend, and you want them to know what it was like—though really only other therapists will see the movie.
>
> Also tell about any ideas that you may have on how therapists can talk better with kids or give ideas of what therapists could do with kids that would help them.

> You are the producer, and I'm your camerawoman. You are in charge of making your movie. Let me know what you want me to do. However, if you need my help, that is okay. I can help you. Just let me know. After each time you are with [name of therapist], we will meet and add to your movie. Have fun with it!

When Lauren met with Tony, she asked how he wanted to tell his story and said she also had an idea. He wanted to hear the idea, and she read him the script. He gave his description of therapy by looking into the camera and pretending to talk to his friend.

Tony began, "Well, Mack, this lady named Clare, she's from the OT department in the hospital I was in, you know? I told you about that. She asked me questions about how did it feel going back to school and playing with my friends again. She talked to me about what we do down in OT, all the crafts we'll be making and then, you know, stuff like that."

Lauren asked, "Did you like talking to her?"

"Yeah, she's real fun to talk to, and her friend, Lauren—she's fun to talk to too."

"So why do you think she was asking all those questions?"

"Well, uh, just to figure out what we could do. She was asking me what I was thinking about all the things that we did down in the OT room."

"So are you looking forward to it?"

"Yeah."

"What else do you think Mack would ask you?"

"Did I have fun and stuff like that."

"So did you have fun?"

"Yeah, we had fun. She was asking me the questions and I was telling her the answers. It was like fun doing that."

Lauren asked how he felt doing the tape as her final question.

"I had some good time. I get to talk about what just happened to me and Clare." He smiled at the camera and said, "We're in Hollywood."

Lauren again met with Tony after the second session and explored how he wanted to do the videotape. He began to reenact the session. Mimicking my voice, he said, "So Tony, how did it feel doing this, making this mobile?"

"It felt all right, Clare," he said in his voice. "I enjoyed doing it. It's just that the hard part was making the circle," referring to cutting out the cardboard pattern for the mobile. Then he waved at Lauren to help him.

She responded, "You want me to be Clare?" He nodded. Pretending to be me, she said, "You did a good job, Tony."

"Yeah, I guess so. I never knew that I could do things like this. I didn't."

Then Lauren switched to asking her own questions. "So what made you choose to do a mobile over the other things you got to choose from?"

"Because I can hang this over my niece's bed and she can play with it. So I'm making this for her."

Lauren continued, "What else do you think about the time you spent with Clare today?"

"It felt good spending time with her and you, and it makes me feel happy. I have somebody to play with. Today I was just in my room bored. I had nobody to play with."

"So you were waiting for this time to come?"

"Yeah, I kept asking everyone, 'What time is it? What time is it?' Now the time is here."

On the third day, Lauren asked him how he wanted to do the last tape. She asked if he wanted to talk or act. He decided to act. Lauren told him, "This is your chance at Hollywood again." Tony suggested that he pretend to talk to his friend named Roger. He told Roger that he added more yarn to the mobile and that we talked. Tony told Lauren that Roger left the room and directed Lauren to ask him some questions.

"So how was it working on the mobile today compared with yesterday?" Lauren asked.

"It was fun."

"Yeah? And easier? Harder?" Lauren asked

"Same. About the same."

"Say a therapist is just starting out, a new therapist, and she will be working with kids. What should she know? What have you found that you liked about working with Clare?"

"She's nice. She doesn't get mad if you don't do things right."

"So talking calm and not saying, 'Oh, you did this wrong or you did that wrong.'"

"Staying calm. Not, 'Put that there, boy,'" he said in a harsh tone.

"What else should an occupational therapist know when working with kids? What kind of projects should the occupational therapist think about doing?"

"Something she thinks they would like to do. That the kids would like to do," Tony replied. "Not something real hard or something she wants them to do and they don't want to do it because it's hard. Something easy or, you know, in between hard and easy."

"Do you think the kids should decide?"

"Yes."

"Anything else you want to tell Clare?"

"I enjoyed working with her. It was fun with you and her. I hope we can do it again sometime."

Before he was discharged, I gave Tony a videotape of our sessions. Later that week when he was readmitted to the hospital, I saw him and asked what he thought about the tape.

"I thought it was good."

"What did you like about it?" I asked.

"Me being on a videotape." He said he liked the way he was talking and sitting. "It was like I'm a real professional."

Then I told him I would be doing research with more children and asked if I should do anything differently. He said no. He liked the way it was. I also explained that I would need to use another name when I wrote about our time together. He thought that was "dumb" but told me to use the name Tony.

Julie's Perspective on Therapy in a Sensory Integration Clinic

When 11-year-old Julie entered the sensory integration clinic, the room had been transformed into a Hawaiian beach. Pictures of the sun, beach umbrellas, and tropical fish decorated the walls. Paper waves covered the side of the scooter board ramp. On one side of the room, next to a selection of balls, sat a large beach ball with a rope attached. On the other side was a sand pile with seashells, shovels, and sand toys in a plastic pool. The platform swing became a surfboard. Beach Boys music played in the background.

Over the phone, Julie's mother had previously told the therapist about Julie's learning disabilities and her diagnoses of attention deficit disorder with hyperactivity and cerebellar dysfunction. She said Julie had been hospitalized the year before when she tried to choke herself at school. Her child psychiatrist and mother emphasized her emotional and motor problems, including her lack of friends, frequent falling, and difficulty brushing her teeth, doing buttons, and riding a bike. The two current concerns, her mother reported, were Julie's difficulty expressing herself and getting ready in the morning.

Although Amy, her occupational therapist, heard all this, when she first met Julie, she saw her spirit. Her first thoughts were that she was a "very assertive, fairly happy girl who wasn't shy." She thought Julie did not need to hear another diagnosis emphasizing what was wrong with her. She said she wanted Julie to "feel good about what she can do." Amy addressed the concerns by actively engaging Julie in sensory integration therapy and building on her competencies. Julie, she said, was "like a hidden flower that hasn't opened yet. She has a lot of potential."

In this and the next two cases, I videotaped the sessions and conducted the interviews.

After her therapy session, Julie, her mother, and I met. She started the conversation saying, "I went to Hawaii."

"Did you have fun?"

"Yeah."

I explained that we could do the video any way she chose. She said she wanted to be on the surfboard. I expected Julie to be a verbal 11 year old, so I started by asking questions. I thought we could just talk and she would tell me what therapy had been like for her. I was not prepared when she responded to my questions with quietness and staring off into space. She gave a few short answers and encapsulated her responses in a few phrases.

"What did you do today?" I asked her.

"I played on the surfboard."

"What did you think about that?"

"Okay."

"How did it feel to do the trapeze?"

"Fine."

"Was it fun or was it scary?"

"Fun."

I told her that it looked hard to me, especially to hold on, and she added, "Not hard."

"Can you tell me more regarding what you thought about today?"

She paused. "Hmm, it's pretty hard to say."

I tried to explore why she thought she was doing all these activities, and she responded, "I don't know." Her mother asked if it was making her stronger, and she said, "Sort of."

"You worked hard," Julie's mother remarked.

I inquired if there was anything she wanted to tell us.

"No," Julie said.

Her mother suggested she tell about one game she liked.

Julie responded, "I liked them all."

I asked what she thought she would do next time, and she replied, "Same thing."

At this point, I felt our talking had turned into more of an interrogation, and I decided to stop.

Reflecting on our time together, I realized that Julie tended to use a few words to express everything she wanted to say. I was so anxious that I did not think to try different methods of getting her perspective, such as using drawing or puppets. When reflecting on the experience, I realized I had approached her like an adult and had not made any adaptations.

After this session, Julie did not return due to the cost of therapy.

Lisa's Perspectives on Therapy While Hospitalized for Kidney Failure

Due to kidney failure, 12-year-old Lisa was admitted to an intensive care unit on the pediatric floor of a general hospital. Noel, her occupational therapist, described how when they first met Lisa was "quiet, polite, friendly, and sweet." While talking with her, Noel discovered that Lisa did not know why she was hospitalized and getting tests.

Lisa had said, "They don't tell me nothin'."

Noel told her it was okay to speak up and ask, and she emphasized that Lisa had a right to know. Noel gave Lisa a notebook for her questions, and Lisa asked her to do the writing. Later, Lisa talked to the nurses, and her questions were answered.

During her hospitalization, there were multiple times medical staff came in her room and talked to each other but not to Lisa. Noel repeatedly brought Lisa into the conversation or explained what the staff was saying. As Lisa made presents for herself in occupational therapy (painting a wooden box and later stitching the edges of a leather bracelet), Noel inquired about how she was doing and if she needed anything. In her soft-spoken voice, Lisa responded in short phrases, her different tones of voice conveying her feelings.

A week later, her medical status became critical. She was placed on a ventilator for 5 days. She slowly recovered over the next few weeks, and Noel continued to see her during this time. She was able to go home while she waited for a kidney transplant.

When I met with Lisa after her therapy session, I came prepared with ideas and drawing supplies to make the interview more fun. After talking about the options, she chose to draw. When she finished her picture, I asked, "How was it for you today when you were working with Noel?"

"It was pretty good."

"What was good about it?"

"The stitching and the talking."

"What did you like about the stitching?"

"It gives me something to do when I'm bored."

"So it helps you get through your time here. What did you like about the talking?"

"It was good because when you stitching and when you talking, time goes faster."

"Noel told me about your first day together. What did you think about her?"

"I thought she was gonna be boring."

"How come?"

She shrugged her shoulders and said, "She's fun."

Next, I asked why she was doing these things, like painting her box and writing down questions.

"To help me find out what's wrong with me so you all can try to help me."

"What do you like about Noel?"

"She's fun. She's got a lot of neat things to do, and we talk. And that's it."

"Those are good things, especially since it is hard to be in the hospital away from your home and family."

"It's boring," she replied.

I brought up the time when the doctor was only talking to her dad and asked if she understood what was said. She shook her head.

"Were you listening and trying to?"

She nodded.

Then I asked what was important for us to know when we work with children.

"How to talk to them."

"Just make sure you can talk to them—that you do talk?"

"That they understand what you are saying," Lisa emphasized.

Three weeks later, after she came off of the ventilator and was strong enough, I met with Lisa again after therapy. She decided to draw another picture. "What to draw?" she asked me.

"Why don't you draw a picture of you being in OT?"

She drew a picture of Noel with a red and black sleeveless evening gown saying, "Come in." When she was through drawing, I asked Lisa how it had been the past few weeks with Noel.

"Fun."

"What did you like about it?"

"A lot of stuff—like activities."

"What did you like about today?"

She pointed to the bracelet she had just completed and, referring to her upcoming discharge, added, "The good news."

Tom's Perspectives on Therapy in a Sensory Integration Clinic

Prior to 8-year-old Tom coming to a sensory integration clinic, his mother conveyed her concerns. Gym class was difficult, and he could not keep up with his friends. She reported he was still using a Big Wheel, which had three wheels and was low to the ground. He could not ride a bike. Brushing his teeth seemed painful to him, and he was sensitive to seams in his socks and tags in his clothes. She added, "I just want him to be happy."

In the first session, Amy told Tom that children come to occupational therapy to do "fun activities that will help them get stronger and help them learn to do things that right now are hard for them, so they can keep up with friends in school and on the playground." As he tried different activities on a scooter board and swings, Amy tried to learn his cues for what he liked and disliked. Tom tended to be quiet and often responded to questions with silence or vague answers. At the end of the session, she told his mother, "I saw a lot of self-determination that he was really trying hard."

Over the next eight sessions, Amy encouraged Tom to make decisions and express himself. He gradually began initiating the activities and challenging himself. He also became more spontaneous and animated. Amy gently talked with his mother about being "competence based," suggesting she shift her focus from what he could not do to what he could. Amy highlighted what he was doing well.

The first time Tom and I talked, I described some options. He decided to draw a picture of when he was on a scooter board going down a ramp and knocking over cardboard blocks. When he was done, I asked him to tell me about it.

"I was going down the ramp and then I had to go back up by the rope—climbing on it."

"What did you like about it?"

"Going down and crashing."

"The crash and bang. Do you like going fast?"

"Yeah."

I asked him what he thought about his therapist.

"She's nice."

"Do you like working with her?"

"Yes."

"How come?"

"Because she does fun things."

I switched to talking about his experience on the scooter board. "I was really impressed. You had so many good ideas about how to make it harder and harder. Was that fun too?"

"Yeah."

"Trying to think of new things to make it even more challenging."

"Like that part where I pushed the ball into the blocks," he said, referring to his elaborate plan.

"That was a good idea."

"That was very good," his mother added.

"Should kids have a say in what they do?" I asked.

"Yeah. Then they can do lots of fun things—what they want to do."

"Is there anything else you think I should know that might be important?" I paused. "Any ideas for what therapists should do with kids?"

"No more," Tom replied. He started talking about his younger brother, and his mother asked if he thought his brother would benefit if he was in therapy.

"Yeah. He would like having fun."

In the following weeks, he drew more pictures, made puppets, conducted a puppet show, and did paint-with-water pictures. However, in the sixth session, he was barely saying anything. I had the feeling he was rushing to be done so he could leave. We had slipped into the routine where he did something and then I asked questions while his mother and brother watched. So I thought about how to change our time together to make it more fun. I tried to think of an idea that would take the pressure off his needing to talk.

The next time we met, I brought a gift-wrapped box that looked like a present.

"Oh my goodness," his mother said.

"Ah–a," Tom said as he laughed in delight while unwrapping the box.

I said, "Everybody's going to play. There are two games in here. Let me know which one you want to do. One's a guessing game. You pick a card and all of us will draw what we think is the answer to the question. If you have a different idea or if you want to change the game, let me know."

Then I described the matching game, where everyone would draw the different things Tom did in the session. I

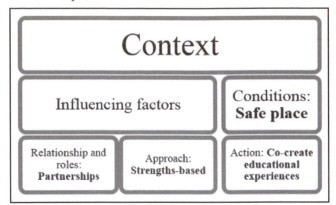

Figure 2-1. A broader picture of collaboration.

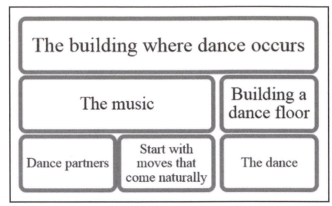

Figure 2-2. Collaboration as a dance.

said Tom could match the drawings to pictures of different facial expressions. Everyone chuckled as they looked at the faces.

Tom picked the guessing game and chose a card. It said "What did Tom like the best?" His mother and brother drew the car he drove through an obstacle course. I drew the map he had made. Tom drew the scooter board ramp.

"Yeah, that was a good one," I said. "You surprised us." He looked pleased to be the one to give the right answer, which also conveyed his perspective on therapy. I told him he could make up a card if he wanted. Another card said "Draw one thing Tom did that made Amy smile."

"Oh, I know, don't look," Tom said. When he finished drawing, he said, "This time, Mom goes first."

"Okay, when Tom was making the maps," she said.

"Yeah," Tom replied. When we were done with the 20 cards, I asked him what we should do next time. I also asked if he want me to think of new ideas. He said he wanted to make a puppet.

On the last day, we had a party with root beer and large cookies. Tom and his brother covered their cookies with frosting and sprinkles. To end our time together, we made puppets of football players, which he had previously mentioned wanting to do.

SUMMARY OF THE CHILDREN'S PERSPECTIVES

The children identified what they liked about their therapists and occupational therapy. Their descriptions clarified what they valued. It was important to them that the therapists were nice, understanding, and fun. They wanted therapists to stay calm and not get mad if they were not doing something the right way.

They thought therapists should talk with children, make sure they understand what is being said, and include them in making decisions. Therapy should involve doing

activities that were fun, based on what the children liked, and in between being hard and easy.

ANALYSIS OF THE RESEARCH DATA

After collecting all data, I transcribed and coded the videotaped sessions and interviews. Next, I conducted thematic and narrative analyses. I identified the themes by following Glasser and Strauss' (1967) constant comparative method. To address issues of credibility and trustworthiness, I followed guidelines suggested by Krefting (1991) and Lincoln and Guba (1985). For instance, I used triangulation of the data collection methods (observation and interviews), the data sources (children and therapists), and the analysis (by using a panel of therapists). The therapists in the study reviewed my writings (for member checking), and I made their suggested changes. I maintained a reflexive journal to increase my awareness of my influence on the data and wrote a detailed description of the research so others could make comparisons.

THEMES THAT EMERGED IN THE STUDY AND IMPLICATIONS FOR PRACTICE

In this section, in addition to describing the emergent themes, I have included what they mean for occupational therapy practice. I have chosen to do this because a conceptual model incorporating these themes is used to organize the therapy strategies chapters in this book. The broader picture of the dimensions of collaboration identified in the study is represented in Figure 2-1. Similarly, a way to view collaboration as a dance is captured in Figure 2-2.

The first theme was that the metaphor of dance could be used to conceptualize the interaction required for collaboration. The second theme was that therapists developed a frame to create the mentality that collaboration was desired. A frame is a message that conveys to children how to organize their perceptions (Bateson, 1987). Like a picture frame, Bateson argued that a psychological frame assists children in determining what aspects they will attend.

I found there were three interwoven processes within the frame: (1) creating a "safe place" for collaboration; (2) becoming partners, in which the therapists act as guides and elicit and strengthen the children's voices; and (3) co-creating educational experiences that are challenging and fun.

To create the partnerships, the therapists established a sense of:

- Togetherness, in which therapy was a joint effort.

- Mutual trust and respect, showing that what each said was viewed as important.

- Openness to each other's ideas.

- Connectedness and feeling comfortable with each other.

- Attentiveness by giving children their full attention and being in the moment together.

- Enjoyment of each other's personality and uniqueness.

- Hope that together they could create change.

The third theme was the therapists' descriptions of successful collaboration.

First Theme: Dance as a Generative Metaphor

Therapists in my study used the metaphor of dance to refer to the interactive nature of collaboration, in which the therapists and children were responsive to the moves of the other. When one therapist, for example, had difficulty understanding the child's nonverbal language, she said, "I'm having a hard time reading him, so it's not an automatic dance." After a more successful session she said, "He starts to do something, and I would just pick up on it, or I started to do something, he picked up on it or he would spontaneously change." She added that successful collaboration was like "dancing in step."

Implications for Practice: Be Open to the Dance

Schon (1979) argued that a metaphor can be viewed as a conceptual framework or perspective. He maintained that metaphors can be used to generate "new perspectives, explanations, and inventions" (p. 259). When this occurs, the generative metaphor assists with exploring new perspectives and broadening a person's conceptual understanding of a phenomenon or process.

The dance metaphor illuminates the process of collaboration because there are a number of similar characteristics. Dance and collaboration are experiences that unfold over time. Collaboration, like dancing, looks different with each group of participants.

When dancing with a new partner, each consciously thinks about where he or she is stepping in relation to the other person. However, as they learn each other's cues and ways of moving, dancing becomes more automatic and relaxed. Dancing together usually involves matching the moves of the other, such as doing similar dance steps. Many classical dances, such as the tango, require the partners to move as if they were one.

Similarly, when beginning to collaborate, the participants consciously observe each other to watch for signs on how to act. When each other's cues and styles of interaction are learned, collaboration can proceed more automatically and with increased ease.

Therefore, like building a dance floor, the therapist creates a foundation that allows the child to feel safe and in control. This promotes a partnership in which the therapeutic relationship can thrive. Next, there is a process to becoming dance partners, in which the therapist initially leads but teaches the child the dance steps and ultimately how to lead. Becoming dance partners involves learning each other's moves and body cues and being able to make the subtle adjustments needed to move together automatically. They also build on each other's strengths by starting with dance moves that come naturally to them. As partners practice dancing (and collaborating) together, they gradually begin to dance in step.

Second Theme: A Collaborative Frame

The therapists in my study created an image of therapy as a different world, and they gave messages to the children about what kind of place they hoped it would be. They did this by establishing a frame of collaboration. The therapists wanted the children to develop and maintain the perspective that (a) therapy would be a safe place, (b) the therapeutic relationship would be a partnership in which the children would have an important voice, and (c) together they would create educational experiences.

The Message: Occupational Therapy Is a Safe Place

The therapists referred to therapy as being as safe place, emphasizing emotional security and support. They were concerned that the children feel comfortable. One described how she avoided certain questions when talking with a child in the hospital. The child's father had not been able to visit for a few days. The therapist said she purposely did not ask any questions about her family. "I want this place to be really safe for her, so I did not want to bring up a lot of issues that I suspect are painful for her." Another told a child undergoing chemotherapy that "OT is a really good place to talk about how you are feeling—what you are going through with the hospital and what you are going through with all the changes with you too."

The therapists conveyed the notion of a safe place through various actions. They assumed a supportive and nonjudgmental approach. If the children made a mistake, the consequences were minimized. A protective stance was also taken by the therapists to ensure the children's physical safety. The therapists were sensitive to how the environment might be affecting the children and often reframed or adapted the environment to help the children feel more comfortable.

Implications for Practice: Establish That Therapy Is a Safe Place

For collaboration to occur, children must feel safe. They need to know that therapists will keep them physically, emotionally, and socially safe. To do this, therapists continually scan and change the environment to prevent physical harm. They work to create an atmosphere where children feel emotionally safe to talk, make decisions, and challenge themselves. The children's competencies are emphasized, and mistakes are minimized. By being empathetic and addressing any anxieties or worries, therapists can develop children's sense of security. The children can then be themselves and feel comfortable to take risks. Therapy also needs to be, as one child described it, a "no-bully zone."

By referring to therapy as a *place*, therapists convey that therapy is different from other places in the children's lives. It is to be a place where they belong, have a say, and have ownership. It is a place to gain the experience needed to develop a sense of mastery and lead to new visions of possibilities.

The Message: We Are Partners, and You Will Have a Voice

The therapists in the research conveyed their desire to have a partnership. They often used words like *we* and *together* in their discussions with the children, indicating that therapy would be a joint process. One therapist said to the child, "While you're here in OT, let's talk about what we plan to do." When interviewed later, the child indicated that he had received this message. He said the therapist was asking him what he was thinking "to figure out what we could do." Another way that partnership was suggested was by all the therapists telling the children they could say no and respecting it when the children did so. They also promoted joint decision making.

In this partnership, they described their role as a guide. One said how she wanted the children "to have an idea of what they want to do and how they want to play and then I can feed into it, guided and change it if I need to or modify it, but keep the essence of what they want."

The therapists guided by continually directing the therapy process, supporting the children, seeking an understanding, and communicating in a way the children would understand.

To enable the children to be partners, the therapists elicited and strengthened the voices of the children. The therapists learned each child's style of communication, which often included certain facial expressions, tones of voice, short phrases, and the use of silence. Children were engaged in conversations, involved in defining the purpose of therapy, and encouraged to lead conversations and therapy.

The therapists often told children that they wanted to hear their thoughts and feelings. There was an interactive back and forth between the children talking about their lives and the therapists explaining how therapy could relate. They elicited the children's concerns and desires, and together they defined therapy goals. Furthermore, they encouraged children to initiate and lead the conversations. One said that she did not bring up the topic of missing family with a hospitalized child. "I was very willing to address that, but I wanted it to come from her. I did not want to be leading." They also wanted children to lead and take charge of the therapy sessions. One therapist in a sensory integration clinic said, "I would rather have him be much more the initiator."

Implications for Practice: Become Partners

The rules for how to interact with each other are defined in the beginning moments of new relationships. In therapy, therapists convey that their role is to guide the process and set the limits needed to keep children safe. Their actions show that a partnership is desired in which children will have a voice. There will be shared decision making, negotiation, and the right to dissent. The expectation for the relationship is that each will be treated with respect.

The Message: We Will Create Educational Experiences That Are Challenging and Fun

In the study, the therapists wanted the children to keep learning even when they were in difficult situations. They were concerned about the children's present experience and maintaining the children's motivation to learn. One said about a child in a sensory integration clinic, "I was concerned with what extent all that frustration would impact on her motivation to keep trying and to keep challenging herself…. I'm concerned that there's motivation to keep learning." They emphasized the criteria of challenge and fun for the experience in therapy. They hoped the children would learn from their experiences in therapy and apply their knowledge in the future.

Implications for Practice: Co-Create Educational Experiences

Co-creating educational experiences is collaboration in action. The following are criteria for an educational experience: (a) starts with children's desires, (b) addresses their present experiences, (c) connects to their other life experiences, (d) explores future possibilities, and (e) is challenging and fun. For the therapy experience to be meaningful to children, they need to be included in defining the purpose of therapy and deciding on the activities. There also needs to be a connection to their immediate and future desired experiences.

In addition, the treatment planning process involves working together to create experiences that are an interplay between challenge and fun. Some sessions emphasize one more than the other. At times, even in one activity, there is a weaving back and forth between the amount of challenge and fun. Both are equally important. Challenge without any experience of fun has the potential to be stressful or overwhelming. Fun without challenge may not promote growth and change. The ultimate goal is that after therapy children will increase their ability to direct their own educational experiences.

An Additional Message: Your Strengths Will Be Acknowledged and Emphasized

Based on the themes that emerge from this research and the application of related theories, I developed a model of collaboration with children in occupational therapy. When I returned to working with children full time, I applied this model. I continually reflected on and analyzed my practice by identifying collaborative strategies and corresponding stories, described in the following chapters. In 2005, I added the strengths-based approach to the model and presented this information at our Colorado Occupational Therapy State Conference. I incorporated this approach into my practice.

When I reexamined the data from my study, I discovered this message was also given by the therapists. The children's competencies were frequently discussed and highlighted throughout the therapy sessions. Their main focus was on what children could do, as well as their potential. And one therapist even referred to her approach as being "competence based."

Implications for Practice: Use a Strengths-Based Approach

Therapists start by learning the children's and caregivers' current strengths, strategies, concerns, and dreams. After identifying the purpose of therapy, together they build on competencies and aim toward what is wanted. This is different from a problem-solving process, with the mentality of fixing deficits. Instead, the emphasis shifts to discovering and highlighting strengths. The focus is on achieving what is desired for the future instead of fixing what was considered a problem in the past. This exploration of new possibilities versus remediation of problems widens the range of future solutions and changes.

Third Theme: Indications of Successful Collaboration

The therapists in the study identified the signs of effective collaboration. They said there was a sense of "flow" between them and the children, as well as within sessions and between sessions. They reported "being on the right track" to reflect progress. The other signs were seeing children being self-directed, engaging in the process, challenging themselves, displaying positive nonverbal cues, and expressing themselves.

Implications for Practice: Indications of Successful Collaboration

Throughout the sessions, therapists look for signs of successful collaboration. One indication of a working partnership is having a sense of connectedness, togetherness, and comfort. Another indication is seeing progress leading to a feeling of being on the right track. A third indication is that children's actions are signs that they are directing their own educational experiences and showing enjoyment. For example, the children are absorbed, self-directed, and challenging themselves at levels that match their skills. The last indication is a sense of ease in working together, often expressed with the word *flow*. There is a flow between individuals, representing a sense of working together. Additionally, there is a flow between and within sessions, creating a sense of momentum and connection between events.

A CONCEPTUAL MODEL: THE COLLABORATIVE FRAME

The concepts reflected by the themes found in the research were linked together into a conceptual model to explain the process of collaboration. A diagram of this conceptual framework was developed, and the metaphor of a pictorial frame was incorporated to represent the collaborative frame (Figure 2-3) used by the therapists.

The model encapsulates the research findings into a framework that is easy to understand and apply in occupational therapy practice. It provides a more detailed and different way to conceptualize the collaboration process, which in the past has been described in more general terms. This collaboration model is to be used in the following two ways: (1) to define what messages are given to children to create a collaboration mindset and (2) to then guide therapists' actions. In later chapters of this book, I show what this model looks like in everyday practice.

First a caveat: This model was created based on research conducted in the United States and its Western culture. It is based on the premise that children and adults are experts

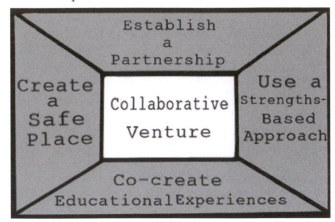

Figure 2-3. The collaborative frame.

on their own lives, and eliciting their perspectives is crucial for treatment planning. Applicability to other cultures and countries needs further investigation.

It is also important to acknowledge that interactions between people are shaped and affected by the context in which they live. This can include their social, cultural, economic, political, and physical environments. In addition, there are always multiple influencing factors that affect the relationship. The therapist's workplace, caseload, and years of experience are just a few examples. Further research, such as conducting institutional ethnographies, recommended by Townsend, Langille, and Ripley (2003), would be beneficial. Collaborative consultation with the adults in the children's lives is discussed in Chapter 3. Like using a magnifying glass, this model zooms in to capture the intricacies of interacting with children.

For all clients, treatment planning is continuous throughout the sessions. The level and amount of collaboration is negotiated between therapists and clients. Collaboration can be viewed as a continuum that looks different in various situations. Collaborative treatment planning, however, requires that at least (a) therapy is based on what the clients and therapists think is best and (b) the clients understand the purpose and process of therapy.

In summary, the establishment of a collaborative frame is used to give children the message that collaboration is desired and to direct therapists' actions. There are four dimensions: (1) create a safe place, (2) become partners, (3) use a strengths-based approach, and (4) co-create educational experiences that are challenging and fun. In other words, collaborative treatment planning encompasses the following:

- Creating an emotional climate so that occupational therapy is a *safe and comfortable place.*
- *Defining the roles and developing a partnership* with the occupational therapist as a guide, and the children and caregivers having a voice.

- Using a *strengths-based approach* that starts with a focus on competencies.
- *Co-creating educational experiences*, in which the children learn from their experiences in therapy.

CLIENT-CENTERED OCCUPATIONAL THERAPY

One of the main theories underlying the collaborative frame is client-centered occupational therapy. This theory best describes the type of interaction, and clients and therapists' roles that are inherent in the collaboration process. Therapists applying this theory ensure that clients are active participants, which is a tenet of the profession.

Client-Centered Therapy

Carl Rogers (1939, 1951), a clinical psychologist and pioneer in the humanistic psychology movement, was the first to describe *client-centered therapy.* He advocated for a new paradigm that emphasized people's competencies instead of focusing on their faults or problems. He conveyed his belief in people's resiliency. Rogers (1980) also challenged those in the American Psychological Association to develop a "future-oriented preventative approach" versus a "past-oriented remedial" one (p. 240).

Rogers argued that client-centered therapy (also referred to as *person-centered therapy*) was based on a number of core beliefs. The first one was that everyone had a tendency toward self-actualization. They were drawn to self-exploration, discovery, and healing, which led to personal growth. A second belief was that everyone had within him- or herself the inner resources and competencies to address his or her difficulties. A third belief was that given a supportive psychological environment, those who needed help "were capable of releasing undreamed of potentialities" (Rogers, 1980, p. 201).

For therapy to be effective, Rogers maintained that the therapeutic relationship was a key component. The therapist needed to convey the following three attitudes (Rogers, 1980): genuineness, unconditional positive regard for the client, and empathetic understanding of the client's perspectives and experiences. To create an atmosphere of trust, the therapist needed to be sincere, accepting, and understanding. Therapy started with the client's concerns. In a responsive and nondirective manner, the therapist assisted the client in tapping into inner resources. The focus was to promote individual growth instead of fixing problems. Importantly, there was to be shared power within the relationship.

What Is Client-Centered Occupational Therapy?

In the 1980s, Canadian occupational therapists proposed applying a client-centered approach to their practice. Their national association developed guidelines about what this type of practice would entail. In the following years, various theorists and researchers have further defined this approach.

In 1995, Law, Bapiste, and Mills were the first to identify the essential components of client-centered occupational therapy. Therapists, they said, needed to respect clients' autonomy, identify clients' strengths, and develop a partnership. Clients needed to make decisions regarding their occupational needs. Finally, services needed to be accessible and fit within the context of the clients' lives (p. 253). They maintained that the values of Rogers' client-centered therapy were congruent with occupational therapy's theoretical framework. Although based on Rogers' theory, client-centered occupational therapy was conceptualized and broadened to include the role of the environment and social policy (Law, 1998).

Clients' Perspectives on What Client-Centered Therapy Entails

Whalley Hammell (2006) argued that in order for occupational therapy to be truly client centered, it was necessary to discover what clients say this approach encompasses. To gain this information, a number of researchers elicited clients' perspectives through the use of *qualitative interviews* (Blank, 2004; Corring & Cook, 1999; Doig, Flemming, Cornwell, & Kulpers, 2009; Maitra & Erway, 2006; Palmadottir, 2006; Rebeiro, 2000; Sumsion, 2005), *focus groups* (Cott, 2004; Gan, Campbell, Snider, Cohen, & Hubbard, 2008), and a *telephone survey* (McKinnon, 2000). In 2007, Whalley Hammell conducted a meta-synthesis of studies done with people with spinal cord injuries about their experiences in rehabilitation (2007a). This resulted in summarizing the views of a 123 people. Similarly, in 2014, Thorarinsdottir and Kristjansson conducted a conceptual synthesis on person-centered care by reviewing qualitative studies of patients' perspectives on their experiences in the health care system.

Within these different studies, consistent themes emerged regarding what clients said they found beneficial and what they liked, disliked, and desired. The first and most prominent theme was the value placed on staff qualities and actions. Frequently mentioned were personal characteristics. They appreciated therapists who were warm, friendly, welcoming, approachable, and calm. They wanted therapists to be kind, caring, and concerned about them. It was important, they thought, for therapists to listen and be attentive, nonjudgmental, sensitive, and empathetic. The other qualities mentioned were for therapists to be supportive, encouraging, helpful, honest, and available.

The clients in these studies also described their desired type of mentality and actions. They wanted therapists to do the following:

- View each one of them as an individual—a unique and equal person.

- Value and respect their perspectives.

- Recognize their knowledge, including knowledge obtained from experience. One client said, "The only person who is an expert on me is me" (Rebeiro, 2000, p. 12).

- Recognize their strengths, acknowledge their resourcefulness, and believe in their potential.

- Challenge stereotypes. Stop the preoccupation with their limitations and focus on what they can do in the present and the future.

- Be knowledgeable, engender hope, and address their concerns and wishes.

- Be visionary by envisioning new possibilities for their future life.

- Be an advisor or guide who treats them with respect and dignity.

- Provide information, explain, and take time to talk with them.

- Use language they understand, explain, and be willing to answer any questions.

- Involve them in defining their needs, goals, and priorities. Individualize therapy and allow shared decision-making when desired.

- Prepare them for the real world, address more than their physical functioning, connect their past with their future life, and follow up with them after discharge (Whalley Hammell, 2007a).

- Provide choices, give ideas and suggestions, and go at their pace.

- Go out of the way to solve other problems outside of therapy.

Client-centered therapists, according to the children's perspectives in my study (Curtin, 1995), would add the following:

- Be nice, be fun, and be understanding.

A second major theme in these studies (Corring & Cook, 1999; Rebeiro, 2000; Thorarinsdottir & Kristjansson, 2014) was the need for therapists to create an inviting, supportive, and accepting atmosphere. These results correspond with my study's finding that part of the collaboration process is establishing that therapy is a safe place.

A third major theme was the importance of involving families and peers in rehabilitation (Cott, 2004; Whalley

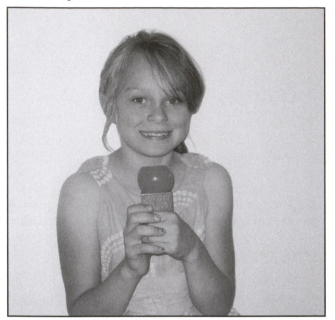

Figure 2-4. Children are clients too and should have a voice in therapy.

Hammell, 2007a). Families, they said, provided critical emotional, physical, and practical support. Peers, especially those with similar conditions, were good mentors and motivators.

The fourth theme was the desire to have a health care system that was individualized and flexible and addressed their needs (Corring & Cook, 1999; Cott, 2004; Maitra & Erway, 2006; Whalley Hammell, 2007a). They also wanted reasonable availability and proximity of services and easy access (McKinnon, 2000).

Therapists' Perspectives on What Client-Centered Therapy Entails

When occupational therapists were interviewed in qualitative studies (Aquilar, Stupons, Scutter, & King, 2013; Morrison & Smith, 2013; Sumsion, 1999; Sumsion & Law, 2006; Sumsion & Lencucha, 2006, 2009), they defined client-centered therapy in a similar manner as the clients. The therapists emphasized the need for respect, collaboration, and negotiation. They said a partnership was essential and highlighted the importance of involving families. An important part of client-centered practice, they said, was the recognition of clients' strengths, resources, and supports. The clients' environments needed to be identified, acknowledged, and changed if necessary.

As therapists began implementing this approach, they expanded the definition of client-centered therapy. First, they (Pollock & McColl, 1998; Whalley Hammell, 2013) clarified that a client can be a person, group, family, organization, or even a community. Children (Missiuna & Pollock, 2000) (Figure 2-4), youth (Gan et al., 2008), and people with cognitive impairments (Hobson, 1996; Moats,

2007) are also clients. Hobson (1996) argued that "it is both possible and desirable to practice client-centered occupational therapy with clients with cognitive impairments, including those who have been legally declared incompetent" (p. 136).

Mortensen and Dyck (2006) argued that collaboration should be considered as a continuum versus an all-or-nothing process. Hobson (1996) stressed that because occupational therapists have expertise in grading activities, they could use the same skills to adapt the collaboration process. With these changes, clients could be involved in decision-making to the best of their abilities. Similarly, Missiuna and Pollock (2000) maintained that with adaptations, such as using picture cues, young children could provide their views and participate in goal setting. They emphasized the importance of including children because their goals and priorities often differed from those of their parents.

Second, they (Mortenson & Dyck, 2006; Restall, Ripat, & Stern, 2003; Townsend, 2003; Townsend et al., 2003; Whalley Hammell, 2007b) contended that client-centered therapy entailed addressing and changing environments, institutions, and systems. The importance of this became especially evident in the institutional ethnography conducted by Townsend, Langille, and Ripley (2003). In their study, they found clients' choices were severely limited by the structure, policies, and management of the institution. Therapists, Townsend (2003) asserted, may not be aware of these invisible and taken-for-granted constraints and by upholding their employers' policies perpetuate the power imbalance. This meant that to truly collaborate with clients, therapists had to advocate for increasing clients' power by promoting constructive change within their social institutions. Disability rights activists made the same argument that to meet their needs and desired goals, therapists were required to change environmental and societal barriers and oppression (Oliver & Barnes, 2012; Whalley Hammell, 2006).

Third, in this type of therapy, therapists must share power with clients (Mortenson & Dyck, 2006; Sumsion, 1999; Sumsion & Law, 2006; Townsend, 2003; Whalley Hammell, 2013). The therapists' assumption of an expert role, with an I-know-what-is-best-for-you mentality, placed them in a position of dominance. There needed to be recognition of the power differential that existed between professionals and clients. To be client centered, therapists had to recognize the extent of their control, change their role, and realign the imbalance of power in their interactions.

Fourth, another addition to the definition was for therapists to be culturally sensitive to clients' beliefs, needs, and goals (Kjellberg, Kahlin, Haglund, & Taylor, 2012; Stedman & Thomas, 2011; Whalley Hammell, 2011, 2013). Overall, the major conceptions underlying this theory, the therapists proposed, were based on Western notions and values, focused on individuals, and emphasized independence. Instead, Stedman and Thomas (2011) argued that client-centered occupational therapy required therapists to use "culturally safe practices" that involve "recognizing, respecting and nurturing a client's cultural identity to address client needs, expectations and rights safely" (p. 44). Whalley Hammell (2013, 2015) added that this approach required therapists to recognize underlying assumptions and biases, be open to learning from different cultures, support the clients' wishes to make decisions in consult with others, and respect the clients' cultural values of interdependence, belonging, and reciprocity.

Fifth, they (Hammell, Miller, Forwell, Forman, & Jacobsen, 2012; McKinnon, 2000; Whalley Hammel, 2001, 2002, 2006, 2007c) asserted that to be client centered, it was imperative to involve clients in the research process. Hammell et al. (2012) emphasized this point, saying, "By enabling clients to share in establishing research agendas, and by engaging in collaborative research, occupational therapists are more likely to develop evidence-based theories and interventions that are informed by, and relevant to, clients' lives, values, and priorities" (p. 302).

Through collaboration, combining researchers' and clients' expertise would expand the parameters of occupational therapy's knowledge base. The development of a partnership would lead to the sharing of power and respecting the disability rights activists' demand of "nothing about us without us." This meant that clients needed to be involved in the development of theory, assessments, and outcome measures. They also needed to participate in progress monitoring, program evaluations, and research needed to support evidence-based practice.

To summarize, therapists would add the following to the clients' definition of client-centered occupational therapy:

- Recognize that a client can be an individual (including a child, youth, or a person with a cognitive impairment), group, family, institution, or even a community.

- Address and change environments, institutions, and systems to increase clients' voices and meet their needs.

- Share power with clients and increase their power within institutions and systems.

- Be culturally sensitive and respectful.

- Involve clients in research and program evaluations, including the development of theory, assessments, and outcome measures.

STRENGTHS-BASED THERAPY

A *strengths-based model* (Jones-Smith, 2014; Rapp & Goscha, 2012) provides the second cluster of theoretical constructs underlying the collaborative frame. This perspective developed as the result of various disciplines' concerns with preventing health problems, enhancing wellness, and promoting well-being (Gottlieb, 2013).

A Competency Movement

In the 1970s, researchers studying resilient children found themselves shifting from examining deficits to identifying children's strengths. In a similar vein, Seligman and Csikszentmihalyi (2000) advocated for the rise of *positive psychology* to gain an understanding of and to amplify clients' virtues and strengths. Starting in the 1980s and expanding in the early 1990s, social workers embraced and integrated strengths-based principles into their practice (Rapp & Goscha, 2012).

In other professions, advocates in counseling psychology (Smith, 2006), educational psychology (Nickerson & Fishman, 2013), early childhood special education (Lickey & Powers, 2011), and nursing (Gottlieb, 2013) have promoted a strengths-based approach. In medicine, a movement for whole-person care reflects a similar perspective (Gottlieb, 2013). Emerging in the field of mental health is a person-centered and strengths-based *collaborative recovery model* (Oades, Crowe, & Nguyen, 2009). An asset-based community development approach for health promotion is now being developed within public health (Durie & Wyatt, 2013). In addition, *appreciative inquiry* is being used as an approach to promote organizational change (Davies & Lewis, 2013).

A strengths-based perspective gained momentum as the result of research on resilient children (Saleebey, 2002). What became evident in this body of research (Masten, 2014; Masten & Obradović, 2006) was that all children who experienced hardship, such as abuse, were not doomed to a life of failure. On the contrary, many children persevered and thrived without receiving intervention. They became productive, well-functioning adults. These findings led researchers to ask questions: What helped these children survive and thrive? How did they develop resiliencies while facing adversity? Could those factors that seemed to protect children be fostered as part of intervention? Researchers started to study children's competencies instead of deficits.

Resiliency

According to Masten and Obradović (2006), behavioral scientists in the 1970s began identifying and describing the assets found within resilient children and related protective factors. In the following years, researchers expanded their focus to studying resiliency processes, policies, prevention, and intervention. They recognized the necessity of improving children's environments and communities to support their adjustment and adaptation. In addition, Masten and Obradović (2006) maintained that with the development of prevention science, the promotion of competencies became an important strategy in addressing emotional and behavioral problems.

In their book *The Resilient Self*, Wolin and Wolin (1993) described their findings from their interviews of "survivors of troubled families." They presented what they referred to as the *damage* and *challenge models*. When therapists and survivors applied the damage model, they assumed that the harm done to children created pathology. Then considered damaged, children were automatically expected to have difficulties functioning as adults. These children were viewed as being vulnerable, passive, and helpless victims.

Wolin and Wolin (1993) proposed that a different mindset was to view adversity as a challenge. There was the acknowledgment that hardship had harmful effects and had created wounds. At the same time, however, there was the recognition that hardship could be an opportunity for growth. The resilient survivors, for instance, had an active role in deciding how to deal with difficult situations and, as a result, developed new strengths. A friend of mine exemplifies this point. She told me that when she was 7 years old, she dealt with her alcoholic and verbally abusive father by telling herself he was crazy and staying away from him when he was drinking. That helped her survive, and she is now a strong person.

Wolin and Wolin (1993; Wolin, 2003) identified seven possible strengths they found to be associated with resilience. With the first one, *insight*, children had increased awareness of the strangeness of their family and questioned the normality of their situation. Second, by establishing *independence*, they defined boundaries between themselves and their situation. With a third strength, seeking *relationships*, children obtained help from benevolent and trustworthy adults. Fourth, through *initiative*, they found ways to take charge of the situation. Fifth and sixth, applying *creativity and humor*, they used their imagination to deal with the hardship. Finally, acknowledging *morality*, they recognized what was right and wrong and held onto a vision of a better life.

Hence, those maintaining a challenge model perspective believed that people had the capacity to help themselves. Children could create buffers from their difficulties by developing new competencies. For those who needed intervention, a vital part of therapy would be a focus on their assets and a belief in their potential.

Positive Psychology

Building on the work of humanistic psychologists such as Maslow, in 1998 Seligman called for a change in psychology (Shogren, 2013). As president of the American Psychological Association, he stressed the need for a positive psychology. Seligman stated that "psychology is not just the study of disease, weakness and damage; it also is the study of strength and virtue" (Seligman, 2002, p. 4). He said it was time for a "new science of strength and resilience" and argued that "by identifying, amplifying and concentrating on these strengths in people at risk, we will do effective prevention" (p. 5). In 2000, Seligman and Csikszentmihalyi further described the constructs of

positive psychology in their seminal article in *American Psychologist*. They proposed that there were three underlying pillars: (1) subjective experiences and well-being, (2) positive traits, and (3) civic virtues and positive, supportive institutions. Since then, positive psychology has become an established part of their profession, including publishing their own *Journal of Positive Psychology*, numerous texts, and supporting research studies (Shogren, 2013).

Solution-Focused Brief Therapy

Solutions-focused therapy evolved from the 1980s work done at the Brief Family Therapy Center in Milwaukee (DeShazer, 1994). De Shazer and Berg were dissatisfied with the problem-based mentality used in their profession of psychotherapy (Bond, Woods, Humphrey, Symes, & Green, 2013). They (Berg, 1994; DeShazer, 1985) proposed and described a brief, solution-focused approach. Believing in people's capacities for finding solutions, they argued that therapists needed to assist clients in identifying future possibilities. Instead of trying to fix past problems, they emphasized shifting attention and efforts to defining the clients' desired future.

They encouraged therapists to use reflective techniques to assist clients to envision changes. For example, therapists could ask the client to think of exceptions—times when they were doing well and what their life would look like if a miracle occurred. Therapists could encourage clients to increase use of their own successful solutions and strategies. By focusing on the future and not past problems, they broadened the range of possible solutions. Then, together in a partnership, clients and therapists could move to exploring solutions. De Shazer (1985) and Berg (1994) maintained that with this practical and concentrated focus, therapy could often be done on a short-term basis.

The Dissatisfaction With Deficit-, Damaged-, and Dysfunction-Based Thinking and Practices

Deficit-based thinking is the norm in our Western society (Gottlieb, 2013). This perspective has become a natural, taken-for-granted way to view individuals, families, and communities. When change is needed or desired, practitioners tend to focus on what is wrong and how to fix it. As a result, they look for clients' inabilities, inadequacies, and/or dysfunction. Applying this type of thinking, it is assumed that when experts define the problem and identify underlying causes, they will know how to intervene. A second assumption is that the most efficient method to create change is to get to the heart of the problem. The next assumption is that, of course, resolving problems will make clients' lives better.

This linear and rational way of thinking appeared logical and became a prevalent mindset, especially in health care, educational, and reimbursement systems. Gradually, however, advocates in various disciplines identified and examined the shortcomings associated with deficit-based thinking and practice. They maintained that the tendency to dwell on problems affected assessment, intervention, community development, and research.

Advocates (Gottlieb, 2013; Jones-Smith, 2014; Rapp & Goscha, 2012; Saleebey, 2013) voiced a major concern with those who maintained a mentality that emphasized weakness, failures, and pathology. They objected to the narrow and negative lens used for exploring problems and defining goals. There were objections to the centrality of problems and the use of a reductionistic approach. Saleebey (2013) argued that this type of thinking implied that the client was flawed or weak, with questionable abilities to cope. Another implication was that an expert was needed to identify the problem and possible solutions. Although practitioners using this framework could collaborate with clients in defining the purpose of therapy and goals, it was not required.

A second major concern was the assessment process. Practitioners tended to interview clients about their past problems and possible causes. Problem-saturated discussions dominated the discourse. If asked at all, there were often minimal inquiries about the clients' strengths, resources, and supports. This led practitioners to miss or underestimate clients' competencies. The spotlight was on the individual, without always considering influencing contextual factors. Practitioners also used tests to try to discover what was wrong.

Then practitioners were the main ones to name the problem, usually in professional language (Rapp & Goscha, 2012). Explanations for the problems tended to center on the client, which often led to blaming the individual. Practitioners' diagnoses also centered more on the individual and did not always include outside contributing factors (Jones-Smith, 2014). These explanations led to the belief that it was the individual who needed to change. With the focus on them, some clients came to see themselves as a "cluster of deficits" (Bozic, 2013, p. 19).

In practitioners' documentation and meetings, they emphasized what the client could not do, resulting in the use of language that centered on failure. Additionally, problems were often stated without describing the context. Weishaar (2010) cautioned against past practices that attributed difficulties to children's personalities (such as saying a child was aggressive) instead of detailing the circumstances where and when the behavior occurred. The role of outside factors (such as a chaotic and noisy classroom) were not always considered or described.

A fourth major concern was the look-for-shortcomings approach for community development. Durie and Wyatt (2013) argued that instead of seeing assets, deficit-based approaches viewed communities as lacking the competence to address their own health problems. This approach implied outside experts were needed to define the community's problems and solutions.

A fifth concern was researchers' focus on dysfunction, damaging factors, and negative outcomes. According to Gottlieb (2013), researchers have often used a deficit-based perspective when studying different phenomena. This concern especially became known when researchers discovered the importance of studying protective factors of resilient children. Additionally, McMahon, Kenyon, and Carter (2013) maintained that researchers' primary focus on the individual as the most powerful force for change limited the study of organizations, communities, and related contextual factors.

Restoring the Balance: Strengths-Based Thinking and Practice

A strengths-based model (Jones-Smith, 2014: Rapp & Goscha, 2012) or perspective (Saleebey, 2013) is a different philosophy from deficit-based thinking. There are differences in the perceptions of clients' knowledge and potential and how to facilitate change. These practitioners use different language and emphasize clients' competencies throughout assessment and intervention. As with client-centered therapy, clients can be children, adults, families, and/or communities.

Practitioners using this holistic model recognize the uniqueness and complexity of each client, including his or her capabilities and vulnerabilities (Blundo, 2013). Their predominant focus is on strengths, which places the client, instead of the problem, in the center of practice (Krishardt, 2013). They accentuate the clients' assets and honor their wisdom, resourcefulness, and potential. To promote change, practitioners assist clients in (a) identifying their vision of a good life, (b) creating hope, and (c) expanding their internal and external resources to achieve that vision.

What Are Strengths?

According to Brownlee et al. (2013), strengths are the characteristics and competencies needed for clients' well-being and development. Gottlieb (2013) maintained that strengths include "assets, attitudes, capacities, competencies, resources, skills, talents and traits" (p. 105). She added that there is a wide range of strengths and they can be subjective, social, psychological, and biological.

Strengths may include the resources offered by families and communities. These resources are often protective factors, such as having a social network and support. Additionally, each client has strengths derived from his or her heritage and experiences within his or her culture. Clients holding a minority status may develop strengths from dealing with adversity. Practitioners applying this model listen for the values of the clients' cultures and recognize that what are considered strengths varies in each culture. For instance, a strength in Eastern culture would be actions that promote harmony and benefit families and the communities. Jones-Smith (2014) argued that a strengths-based model has universal appeal because practitioners "search for the best rather than the worst" in clients (p. 99).

Changing the Emphasis From Problems to Strengths

It is important to note that the clients' pasts, problems, suffering, and adversity are not ignored in a strengths-based model. Deficits, difficulties, and current challenges are not downplayed. They are acknowledged and addressed. Rather, what is different from a problem-solving model is that this model incorporates a more balanced view of the client. Practitioners recognize that clients have strengths and resources as well as problems. Their strengths coexist with deficits (Gottlieb, 2013).

Another difference is that the emphasis shifts to clients' assets. Strengths are in the forefront, and problems are in the background (Davidson, 2014). Practitioners direct their attention to and build upon clients' competencies. They assist clients in identifying their strengths, which can be used to both address the problem and, more importantly, create movement toward the clients' desired lives.

Rapp and Goscha (2012) maintain that solving problems just returns clients to their previous state of equilibrium, whereas expanding their strengths and resources leads to greater growth (p. 54). Consequently, those using this model spend more energy on exploring ways to create change instead of trying to determine the causes of the problem. The main focus is on defining the vision instead of the problem (Davidson, 2014). Practitioners ask clients what they want their lives to be and, in doing so, shift the spotlight from past difficulties to future possibilities.

Additionally, practitioners move from exploring what is wrong to what is right with the clients. They delve into the clients' repertoires of successful strategies and skills. As a result, the strengths-based model, according to Rapp and Goscha (2012) "is more concerned with achievement than solving problems; with thriving more than just surviving; with dreaming and hoping rather than just coping; and with triumph instead of just trauma" (pp. 38-39).

Fundamental Beliefs

One core belief of the strengths-based model is that clients have the innate capacity to learn, develop, and be resilient. They have a natural self-righting tendency in which they draw upon their inner strengths to adapt and heal themselves (Jones-Smith, 2014). They also have dormant capabilities that have yet to be tapped and should not be underestimated (Rapp & Goscha, 2012).

A second basic belief is that clients are competent and know what helps and hinders them in their lives. They have

the right to define their vision of a good life for themselves and make decisions. They are the "rightful architects of their own destinies" (Davidson, 2014, p. 13). When seeking assistance, clients are the ones to determine the type of help they want. Although practitioners provide guidance, clients are responsible for discovering which strategies and solutions work for them.

A third fundamental belief is that individuals are interconnected with their families, friends, and communities. Their cultural values influence their perceptions and actions. Situational circumstances and the environment are additional factors. Hence, those applying this model look for the assets and resources in all of these areas.

A fourth major belief is that clients are motivated to change when they have awareness of their strengths, determine their goals, and have positive expectations. Practitioners start the change process by exploring clients' interests, competencies, aspirations, and resources. This type of discussion promotes a strengths versus a deficit mindset (Jones-Smith, 2014). As clients shift from talking about their problems to talking about their effective strategies, they learn more about the success of their own efforts. They develop a sense of confidence once they recognize that because they were able to adapt in the past, they can also do so in the future. This discussion enables them to envision positive changes, generate hope, and create the optimism needed to take action.

Creating a Partnership

To apply a strengths-based model, practitioners have to develop a collaborative partnership with clients (Krishardt, 2013). To create this type of relationship, they start by acknowledging clients' expertise, wisdom, and knowledge and respecting clients' vision of a good life. Their role is to facilitate change by assisting and supporting the client. They create the safe conditions that encourage the exploration and discovery of internal and external resources.

As partners, practitioners also share their knowledge, expertise, and wisdom. They first elicit the clients' perspectives and goals. If they have concerns, they need to discuss these with the clients. Practitioners have the right to set limits on what they can do. They must abide by the ethics and guidelines of their profession.

Applying a Strengths-Based Model While Working Within Deficit-Based Systems

Health care, educational, and reimbursement systems currently are based on the identification and remediation of deficits. The more problems an individual has, the greater the need and justification for services. The majority of practitioners work within these systems.

The challenge then becomes how to apply a strengths-based model while working in these deficit-based systems. Saleebey (2013) argued that it is possible. He maintained that practitioners can choose how to view clients and can make a commitment to identifying and incorporating their strengths and resources in assessment, documentation, and intervention.

Assessment and Intervention

Strengths-based assessment is broader than problem-based assessment. In addition to hearing clients' concerns, the process entails gathering detailed information regarding clients' interests, dreams, and competencies (Oliver, 2014). Hence, the main focus in interviews is on past and current strengths, skills, and solutions and the potential for developing new ones. When problems are mentioned, practitioners elicit details regarding the surrounding context and circumstances. Additionally, practitioners include assessments that directly identify and measure abilities, strengths, and environmental resources.

The language used in the discussions and reports is positive. By using words that affirmed clients' dignity, resourcefulness, and potential, practitioners create a language of hope (Gottlieb, 2013). The clients' own words, abilities, and recently mastered skills are included in the documentation. The reporting of concerns and problems is always described within a certain context and circumstances.

Practitioners and clients then collaborate to determine the purpose and goal of intervention. Together, they define goals and steps after clarifying the clients' vision of a good life and drawing upon internal and external resources. Common areas of concern in this model are the improvement of life satisfaction, quality of life, participation, and achievement (Rapp & Goscha, 2012).

Intervention starts by expanding the successful skills, strategies, and solutions already in the clients' repertoires. Practitioners can encourage them to increase their usage or apply them to other areas of their lives. Another aspect of intervention is assisting clients in accessing and increasing their use of external resources.

For some clients, intervention may focus on changing their beliefs about their abilities. Practitioners can help clients reframe weaknesses into strengths or minimize their deficits to "allow a strength to shine forth" (Gottlieb, 2013, p. 366). Often, intervention includes developing new skills and strategies.

Community Development

The same strengths-based principles and beliefs apply when the community is the client (Durie & Wyatt, 2013). The primary emphasis is on discovering and expanding community members' competencies and resources. They, rather than outside experts, define what is needed and wanted to improve their community. Practitioners work as partners with the members to facilitate change. A guiding belief is that it is more beneficial to enhance a community's assets than to try to eliminate dysfunction.

Changing the Focus of Research

Researchers who apply a strengths-based model center their interests in prevention and wellness. They broaden their investigations to include studies of competencies, adaptation, and positive factors, not just deficits and pathology (McMahon et al., 2013). They study what *promotes*—versus what *hinders*—development and growth. Their research is expanded to include an examination of organizations, communities, and environments, as well as individual factors. Finally, as promoted by Cerecer, Cahill, and Bradley (2013), researchers present their findings in a way that raises awareness and promotes action rather than supporting deficit-based thinking (p. 221).

STRENGTHS-BASED OCCUPATIONAL THERAPY

The tenets of a strengths-based model match occupational therapy's humanistic values and practices. Those using this framework view people in a positive light, as well as identify and build upon client's strengths and resources. Similarly, occupational therapists have recognized that effective therapy requires a belief in clients' potential and capitalizing their strengths. This view has been articulated by the founders and subsequent leaders in the profession.

In the early 1900s, the founders of occupational therapy stressed the need for holistic and humanistic practice (Bing, 1981; Schwartz, 2009). They recognized the importance of occupations on clients' quality of life and well-being and the necessity of addressing environmental factors (Reitz, 1992; Schwartz, 2009). They saw people's assets and potential (Yerxa, 1998). Their philosophical stance included the promotion of health, wellness, and preventive practices (Reitz, 1992).

In the following years, as occupational therapy aligned with medicine, leaders cautioned them about the importance of maintaining their core values. In the Eleanor Clarke Slagle lectures, presidential addresses, and other articles, these leaders described themes that correspond with the values and beliefs underpinning the strengths-based model. They contended that occupational therapy entails (a) an emphasis on clients' strengths and potential, (b) the promotion of health and wellness, (c) the enhancement of self determination and well-being to create a good life, (d) the importance of a partnership in the collaborative quest to identify and create desired changes, (e) a belief in the mind-body-environment connection, and (f) the inclusion of different ways of knowing, such as the additional use of qualitative research to learn about clients' experiences.

Occupational Therapists' Emphasis on Clients' Strengths and Potential

Strengths-based model: The primary emphasis is on client's strengths and adaptability.

Occupational therapy: According to Yerxa (1992), historically occupational therapists have maintained an optimistic perspective of human nature and focused on clients' abilities, competencies, and assets. She later stated that "occupational therapists discover a person's resources and emphasize what that person can or might be able to do instead of the person's incapacities; what's right instead of what's wrong" (Yerxa, 1998, p. 413). Abreu (2011) and Dunn (2001) similarly asserted that therapy involved keeping a positive perspective, promoting hope, and accentuating clients' assets.

Other leaders articulated essential elements needed to explore and enhance clients' strengths and potential. Therapists needed to "step into the lives of others to find possibilities" and then help them discover or regain their strengths (Peloquin, 2005, p. 476). Likewise, Baum (1980) argued that by reaching out with empathy and caring, therapists assisted clients in finding their strengths.

Therapists, as described by Yerxa (1998), were "'search engines' for potential" (p. 412). They recognized potential in people, including those with disabilities, and envisioned future possibilities. They conveyed their vision by providing "glimpses of what is possible, what can be done, and what it will take to get there" (Burke, 2010, p. 858). And, as Rogers (1983) maintained, by ascertaining clients' intentions and potential, therapists helped them "discover the health within themselves" (p. 616).

The leaders decried overreliance on deficit-based thinking. Fine (1991) stated that "the snapshot approaches to capacity failed to reflect the unique adaptive style and potential of each person" (p. 500). Yerxa raised many concerns. The rehabilitation system was not fostering the "strength and resiliency of the human spirit" (2000, p. 194). The "fix and cure approach" treated the person as a "deficient object" (2009, p. 492). Therapists were admonished to not become preoccupied with pathology and attaining normality because many clients would never be "normal" in society's eyes (1991). To avoid having a skewed and negative perception of clients, Fisher (1998) and Rogers (1983) maintained that clients' strengths needed to be included in assessments and treatment plans. Rogers (1983) added that "knowing a person's problems or deficits tells us little about his or her strengths" (p. 604).

The Role of Occupational Therapy in Promoting Health and Wellness

Strengths-based model: There is an emphasis on preventing health problems and fostering wellness.

Occupational therapy: Gilfoyle (1984) maintained that occupational therapy's values are based on a wellness paradigm and advocated for shifting from a medical model to a "model of healthfulness where patients influence their own state of health" (p. 356). West (1968) stated a similar stance by encouraging therapists to broaden their role. She proposed that they shift from being a profession that identified with medicine to one that emphasized meeting the health needs of people and included a focus on prevention.

More recently, with the changing health care systems in the United States, Hildenbrand and Lamb (2013) maintained that this is a prime time for occupational therapists to commit to and expand their practice in the areas of health promotion, wellness, and prevention. They called for a "greater focus on the strengths of and possibilities for an individual or community instead of the concentrated attention to deficits and limitations that in some ways restricts the public's image and understanding of occupational therapy" (p. 267).

Enhance Self-Determination and Well-Being to Create a Good Life

Strengths-based model: Foster client's self-determination to help them create a better life.

Occupational therapy: Since the beginning of the profession, the client's right to self-determination has been a core value (Grady, 1992). Occupational therapists have made an ethical commitment to improving the well-being and quality of life for all clients (Yerxa, 1991). They believed that even if clients had disabilities, they could lead meaningful and healthy lives (Yerxa, 1998). Rogers (1983) argued that it was also important that the treatment plan and therapy be congruent with the client's "concept of the 'good life'" (p. 602).

Occupational therapists' unique role has been to apply their knowledge and use of occupations to promote health, well-being, and quality of life (Royeen, 2003). Christiansen (1999) asserted that although health was important for participation in occupations, the ultimate goal of therapy was to help clients achieve well-being. To promote this outcome, Stoffel (2014) challenged therapists to make occupational therapy a "health profession" that helps clients identify "what makes life worth living" and assists them in "living life to the fullest" (p. 629).

Dige (2009) contended that the concept of well-being, more than the concept of wellness, provided a "broader understanding of a good human life" (p. 91). Well-being, as described by Whalley Hammell and Iwama (2012) in a synthesis of different theorists, was being content or in harmony with one's physical, emotional, mental, and spiritual health; economic and personal security; self-worth; sense of belonging; opportunities for self-determination; sense of hope; and opportunities to engage in purposeful and meaningful activities (p. 387).

Aldrich (2011), in her review of various definitions of well-being in the occupational therapy literature, found generalizations about this concept. She asserted that well-being involved objective and subjective aspects; had psychological and physical health factors; was influenced by environmental conditions and opportunities, especially being able to participate in a variety of meaningful activities; focused on quality and satisfaction; and was evident by the indicators of control, coherence, and success (p. 95). When evaluating well-being, Doble and Caron Santha (2008) argued that therapists needed to consider if the clients' occupational needs of agency, affirmation, accomplishments, coherence, pleasure, companionship, and renewal were being met.

By promoting self-determination and wellness, therapists assisted clients in creating or regaining their desired lives. A central belief of occupational therapists, Dige (2009) contended, was that a "good life must be imbued with activity and participation" (p. 91). Radomski (1995) argued that, "If the ultimate treatment aim of occupational therapy is good quality of life, our evaluation procedures must *illuminate* the patient's definition of a good life so we will know when our work is complete" (pp. 488-489).

The Importance of a Partnership in the Collaborative Quest to Identify and Create Desired Changes

Strengths-based model: Clients are competent and have the right to make decisions about their lives.

Occupational therapy: As described in Chapter 1, leaders insisted that occupational therapy required a partnership and collaboration. A collaborative partnership was crucial for effective treatment (Fisher, 1998). Therapists could be facilitators, advisors, guides, coaches, or, at times, advocates (Rogers, 1983; Stoffel, 2014; Yerxa, 1980). They had an ethical responsibility to discover and respect clients' goals and to present their perspectives (Yerxa, 1991). The client, according to Rogers (1983), needed to be actively involved in deciding therapy goals and methods and was the "agent of change" (p. 608).

A Belief in the Mind-Body-Environment Connection

Strengths-based model: Individuals are interconnected with their families, communities, and environments.

Occupational therapy: Occupational therapists, according to Gilfoyle (1984), needed to recognize the interplay of clients' minds, bodies, and environments. They needed to consider the environmental influences on performance of occupations and modify these influences when they were hindrances (Yerxa, 1998). In addition, Hasselkus (2006) urged therapists to promote social transformation by reorienting from a focus on individuals to a focus on "the social forces that affect whole communities and populations" (p. 635).

The Inclusion of Different Ways of Knowing

Strengths-based model: Research focuses on assets, adaptation, and positive factors within individuals, communities, and environments.

Occupational therapy: Coster (2008) maintained that occupational therapists were concerned with clients' observable performances and their experiences, which included "the phenomena we call meaning, feeling, being, and quality of life" (p. 744). She advised therapists to develop instruments that captured and measured the complexity of therapy and could be used for outcome studies.

Yerxa (1991) made a similar argument that to be true to clients ethically, therapists needed to "seek or invent new ways of knowing" (p. 200), such as the use of qualitative research. She emphasized that occupational therapy's knowledge base, which included the humanities, social sciences, and evolutionary biology, differed from medicine's science foundation. Yerxa (1992) encouraged therapists to expand their knowledge base by building on the tradition of optimistic and positive views of people. Schwartz (2009) recommended they create a bridge between and incorporate both the humanistic and scientific paradigms. She stated, "The challenge the profession faces is to be scientific in its interventions, documentation, and measurement of outcomes and still hold true to its original humanistic values" (p. 688).

COMBINING CLIENT-CENTERED AND STRENGTHS-BASED THERAPY

The strengths-based model matches and enhances the profession's humanistic values and beliefs. It is complementary and compatible with client-centered occupational therapy. Client-centered theory emphasizes the importance of obtaining and respecting clients' voices in therapy and research. A strengths-based model provides more details about a mindset therapists may use when listening to clients and as they collaborate in determining the focus of therapy. For example, instead of listening for clients' past problems and thinking of ways to fix them, therapists would listen for what is desired in the future and help clients achieve their visions of a good life.

SUMMARY

In this chapter, I presented a collaborative frame, which is a new way of thinking about collaborative treatment planning. I outlined the theoretical underpinnings by describing what is considered client-centered and strengths-based occupational therapy. The values, beliefs, and assumptions contained in these approaches are the foundation for the strategies presented in the following chapters.

KEY POINTS TO REMEMBER

- A conceptual model was developed based on a qualitative study of the collaboration process with children in occupational therapy.

- The model, called a collaborative frame, has four dimensions: create a safe place, establish a partnership, use a strengths-based approach, and co-create educational experiences.

- By being client-centered in therapy, occupational therapists stay true to their core values.

- Clients can be an individual (including children, youth, and people with cognitive impairments), families, organizations, or communities.

- Collaboration can be viewed as a continuum versus an all-or-nothing process.

- Occupational therapists have the expertise needed to develop adaptations to make collaboration possible.

- A strengths-based perspective has a different focus than a problem-solving/deficit-based approach.

- A strengths-based model restores the balance by recognizing clients' competencies and resources as well as their difficulties.

- A strengths-based approach shifts thinking about past problems to future potential and possibilities.

- A strengths-based model is being used by a variety of disciplines and matches occupational therapy's beliefs and values.

REVIEW QUESTIONS

1. Name four personal qualities children in the study of collaboration believed therapists should have.

2. Name three actions children in the collaboration study said they want therapists to do.

3. Name three crucial elements of activities within therapy the children in the collaboration study identified.

4. If therapy is to be meaningful and effective, therapists must use a client-centered approach. True or false.

5. Children are too young to have a voice in therapy. True or false.

6. Clients with cognitive impairments are unable to collaborate with therapists. True or false.

7. It is possible to use a strengths-based approach while working in a deficit-based system. True or false.

8. Clients' problems are not addressed in a strengths-based approach. True or false.

9. A strengths-based approach to research centers on what is hindering children from developing normally. True or false.

10. A strengths-based approach is not compatible with the demands of current occupational therapy practice. True or false.

REFERENCES

Abreu, B. C. (2011). Accentuate the positive: Reflections on empathetic interpersonal interactions. *The American Journal of Occupational Therapy, 65*(6), 623-634.

Aguilar, A., Stupans, I., Scutter, S., & King, S. (2013). Towards a definition of professionalism in an Australian occupational therapy: Using the Delphi technique to obtain consensus on the essential values and behaviours. *Australian Occupational Therapy Journal, 60*, 206-216. doi:10.1111/1440-1630.12017

Aldrich, R. M. (2011). A review and critique of well-being in occupational therapy and occupational science. *Scandinavian Journal of Occupational Therapy, 18*, 93-100. doi:10.3109/11038121003615327

Bateson, G. (1987). *Steps to an ecology of mind* (Rev. ed.). Northvale, NJ: Jason Aronson.

Baum, C. M. (1980). Occupational therapists put care in the health system. *The American Journal of Occupational Therapy, 34*(8), 505-516.

Berg, I. K. (1994). *Family-based services: A solution-focused approach.* New York, NY: Norton.

Bing, R. K. (1981). Eleanor Clarke Slagle Lectureship—1981: Occupational therapy revisited: A paraphrastic journey. *The American Journal of Occupational Therapy, 35*(8), 499-518.

Blank, A. (2004). Clients' experience of partnership with occupational therapists in community mental health. *British Journal of Occupational Therapy, 67*(3), 118-124.

Blundo, R. (2013). Learning and practicing the strengths perspective: Stepping out of comfortable mind-sets. In D. Saleebey (Ed.), *The strengths perspective in social work practice* (pp. 25-52). Upper Saddle River, NJ: Pearson.

Bond, C., Woods, K., Humphrey, N., Symes, W., & Green, L. (2013). Practitioner review: The effectiveness of solution focused brief therapy with children and families: A systematic and critical evaluation of the literature from 1990-2010. *Journal of Child Psychology and Psychiatry, 54*(7), 707-723. doi:10.1111/jcpp.12058

Bozic, N. (2013). Developing a strength-based approach to educational psychology practice: A multiple case study. *Educational and Child Psychology, 30*(4), 18-29.

Brownlee, K., Rawana, J., Franks, J., Harper, J., Bajwa, J., O'Brien, E., & Clarkson, A. (2013). A systematic review of strengths and resilience outcome literature relevant to children and adolescents. *Child and Adolescent Social Work Journal, 30*, 435-459. doi:10.1007/s10560-013-0301-9

Burke, J. P. (2010). What's going on here? Deconstructing the interactive encounter (Eleanor Clarke Slagle Lecture). *The American Journal of Occupational Therapy, 64*(6), 855-868.

Cerecer, D. A. Q., Cahill, C., & Bradley, M. (2013). Toward critical youth policy praxis: Critical youth studies and participatory action research. *Theory Into Practice, 52*, 216-223. doi:10.1080/00405841.2013.804316

Christiansen, C. H. (1999). Defining lives: Occupation as identity: An essay on competence, coherence, and the creation of meaning, 1999 Eleanor Clarke Slagle lecture. *The American Journal of Occupational Therapy, 53*(6), 547-558.

Corring, D., & Cook, J. (1999). Client-centred care means that I am a valued human being. *Canadian Journal of Occupational Therapy, 66*(2), 71-82.

Coster, W. J. (2008). Embracing ambiguity: Facing the challenge of measurement. *The American Journal of Occupational Therapy, 62*(6), 743-752.

Cott, C. A. (2004). Client-centred rehabilitation: Client perspectives. *Disability and Rehabilitation, 26*(2), 1411-1422. doi:10.1080/09638280400000237

Curtin, C. (1995). *Collaborative treatment planning with children* [Unpublished doctoral dissertation]. Chicago, Illinois: University of Illinois at Chicago.

Davidson, T. (2014). Strength: A system of integration of solution-oriented and strength-based principles. *Journal of Mental Health Counseling, 36*(1), 1-17. doi:10.17744/mchc.36.1.p0034451n14k4818

Davies, O., & Lewis, A. (2013). Children as researchers: An appreciative inquiry with primary-aged children to improve "Talking and Listening" activities in their class. *Educational and Child Psychology, 30*(4), 59-74.

De Shazer, S. (1985). *Keys to solution in brief therapy.* New York, NY: Norton.

De Shazer, S. (1994). *Words were originally magic.* New York, NY: Norton.

Dige, M. (2009). Occupational therapy, professional development, and ethics. *Scandinavian Journal of Occupational Therapy, 16*, 88-98. doi:10.1080/11038120802409754

Doble, S. E., & Caron Santha, J. (2008). Occupational well-being: Rethinking occupational therapy outcomes. *Canadian Journal of Occupational Therapy, 75*(3), 184-190.

Doig, E., Flemming, J., Cornwell, P. L., & Kulpers, P. (2009). Qualitative exploration of a client-centered, goal-directed approach to community-based occupational therapy for adults with traumatic brain injury. *The American Journal of Occupational Therapy, 63*(5), 559-568.

Dunn, W. (2001). The sensations of everyday life: Empirical, theoretical, and pragmatic considerations. *The American Journal of Occupational Therapy, 55*(6), 608-620.

Durie, R., & Wyatt, K. (2013). Connecting communities and complexity: A case study in creating the conditions for transformational change. *Critical Public Health, 23*(2), 174-187. doi:10.1080/09581596.2013.781266

Fine, S. B. (1991). Resilience and human adaptability: Who rises above adversity? 1990 Eleanor Clarke Slagle Lecture. *The American Journal of Occupational Therapy, 45*(6), 493-503.

Fisher, A. G. (1998). Uniting practice and theory in an occupational framework. *The American Journal of Occupational Therapy, 52*(7), 509-521.

Gan, C., Campbell, K. A., Snider, A., Cohen, S., & Hubbard, J. (2008). Giving youth a voice (GYV): A measure of youths' perceptions of the client centeredness of rehabilitation services. *Canadian Journal of Occupational Therapy, 75*(2), 96-104.

Gilfoyle, E. M. (1984). Transformation of a profession. *The American Journal of Occupational Therapy, 38*(9), 575-584.

Glasser, B. G., & Strauss, A. L. (1967). *The discovery of grounded theory: Strategies for qualitative research.* Chicago, IL: Aldine.

Gottlieb, L. N. (2013). *Strengths-base nursing care: Health and healing for person and family.* New York, NY: Springer.

Grady, A. P. (1992). Occupation as vision. *The American Journal of Occupational Therapy, 46*(12), 1062-1065.

Hammell, K. R. W., Miller, W. C., Forwell, S. J., Forman, B. E., & Jacobsen, B. A. (2012). Sharing the agenda: Pondering the politics and practices of occupational therapy research. *Scandinavian Journal of Occupational Therapy, 19*, 297-304. doi:10.3109/11038128.2011.574152

Hasselkus, B. R. (2006). 2006 Eleanor Clarke Slagle lecture—The world of everyday occupation: Real people, real lives. *The American Journal of Occupational Therapy, 60*(6), 627-640.

Hildenbrand, W. C., & Lamb, A. J. (2013). Occupational therapy in prevention and wellness: Retaining relevance in a new health care world. *The American Journal of Occupational Therapy, 67*(3), 266-271.

Hobson, S. (1996). Being client-centred when the client is cognitively impaired. *Canadian Journal of Occupational Therapy, 63*(2), 133-137.

Jones-Smith, E. (2014). *Strengths-based therapy: Connecting theory, practice, and skills.* Thousand Oaks, CA: Sage.

Kjellberg, A., Kahlin, I., Haglund, L., & Taylor, R. (2012). The myth of participation and occupational therapy: Reconceptualizing a client-centered approach. *Scandinavian Journal of Occupational Therapy, 19*, 421-427. doi:10.3109/11038128.2011.627378

Krefting, L. (1991). Rigor in qualitative research: The assessment of trustworthiness. *The American Journal of Occupational Therapy, 45*(3), 214-222.

Krishardt, W. E. (2013). Integrating the core-competencies in strengths-based, person-centered practice: Clarifying purpose and reflecting principles. In D. Saleebey (Ed.), *The strengths perspective in social work practice* (pp. 53-78). Upper Saddle River, NJ: Pearson.

Law, M. (1998). *Client-centred occupational therapy.* Thorofare, NJ: SLACK Incorporated.

Law, M., Baptiste, S., & Mills, J. (1995). Client-centred practice: What does it mean and does it make a difference? *Canadian Journal of Occupational Therapy, 62*(5), 250-257.

Lickey, D. C., & Powers, D. J. (2011). *Starting with their strengths: Using the project approach in early childhood special education.* New York, NY: Teachers College.

Lincoln, Y. S., & Guba, E. G. (1985). *Naturalistic Inquiry.* London, UK: Sage.

Maitra, K. K., & Erway, F. (2006). Perceptions of client-centered practice in occupational therapists and their clients. *The American Journal of Occupational Therapy, 60*(3), 298-310.

Masten, A. S. (2014). Global perspectives on resilience in children and youth. *Child Development, 85*(1), 6-20. doi:10.1111/cdev.12205

Masten, A. S., & Obradović, J. (2006). Competence and resilience in development. *New York Academy of Sciences, 1094*, 13-27. doi:10.1196/annals.1376.003

McKinnon, A. L. (2000). Client values and satisfaction with occupational therapy. *Scandinavian Journal of Occupational Therapy, 7*, 99-106. doi:10.1080/110381200300006041

McMahon, T. R., Kenyon, D. B., & Carter, J. S. (2013). My culture, my family, my school, me: Identifying strengths and challenges in the lives and communities of American Indian youth. *Journal of Child and Family Studies, 22*, 694-706. doi:10.1007/s10826-012-9623-z

Missiuna, C., & Pollock, N. (2000). Perceived efficacy and goal setting in young children. *Canadian Journal of Occupational Therapy, 67*(2), 101-109.

Moats, G. (2007). Discharge decision-making, enabling occupations, and client-centred practice. *Canadian Journal of Occupational Therapy, 74*(2), 91-101.

Morrison, T. L., & Smith J. D. (2013). A working alliance development and occupational therapy: Across-case analysis. *Australian Occupational Therapy Journal, 60*, 326-333. doi:10.1111/1440-1630.12053

Mortenson, W. B., & Dyck, I. (2006). Power and client-centred practice: An insider exploration of occupational therapists' experiences. *Canadian Journal of Occupational Therapy, 73*(5), 261-271.

Nickerson, A. B., & Fishman, C. E. (2013). Promoting mental health and resilience through strength-based assessment in US schools. *Educational & Child Psychology, 30*(4), 7-17.

Oades, L. G., Crowe, T. P., & Nguyen, M. (2009). Leadership coaching transforming mental health systems from the inside out: The Collaborative Recovery Model as person-centred strengths based coaching psychology. *International Coaching Psychology Review, 4*(1), 25-36.

Oliver, C. (2014). The fundamental of strengths-based practice. *Relational Child and Youth Care Practice, 27*(3), 46-50.

Oliver, M., & Barnes, C. (2012). *The new politics of disablement.* New York, NY: Palgrave Macmillan.

Palmadottir, G. (2006). Client-therapist relationships: Experiences of occupational therapy clients in rehabilitation. *British Journal of Occupational Therapy, 69*(9), 394-401.

Peloquin, S. M. (2005). The 2005 Eleanor Clarke Slagle Lecture: Embracing our ethos, reclaiming our heart. *The American Journal of Occupational Therapy, 59*(6), 611-625.

Pollock, N., & McColl, M. A. (1998). Assessment in client-centred therapy. In M. Law (Ed.), *Client-centred occupational therapy* (pp. 89-105). Thorofare, NJ: SLACK Incorporated.

Radomski, M. V. (1995). There is more to life than putting on your pants. *The American Journal of Occupational Therapy, 49*(6), 487-490.

Rapp, C. A., & Goscha, R. J. (2012). *The strengths model: A recovery-oriented approach to mental health services.* New York, NY: Oxford Press.

Rebeiro, K. L. (2000). Client perspectives on occupational therapy practice: Are we truly client-centred? *Canadian Journal of Occupational Therapy, 67*(1), 7-14.

Reitz, S. M. (1992). A historical review of occupational therapy's role in preventive health and wellness. *The American Journal of Occupational Therapy, 46*(1), 50-55.

Restall, G., Ripat, J., & Stern, M. (2003). A framework of strategies for client-centred practice. *Canadian Journal of Occupational Therapy, 70*(2), 103-112.

Rogers, C. R. (1939). *The clinical treatment of the problem child.* Boston, MA: Houghton Mifflin.

Rogers, C. R. (1951). *Client-centered therapy.* Boston, MA: Houghton Mifflin.

Rogers, C. R. (1980). *A way of being.* Boston, MA: Houghton Mifflin.

Rogers, J. C. (1983). Eleanor Clarke Slagle Lectureship—1983; Clinical reasoning: The ethics, science, and art. *The American Journal of Occupational Therapy, 37*(9), 601-616.

Royeen, C. B. (2003). The 2003 Eleanor Clarke Slagle Lecture: Chaotic occupational therapy: Collective wisdom for a complex profession. *The American Journal of Occupational Therapy, 57*(6), 609-624.

Saleebey, D. (2002). *The strengths perspective in social work practice.* Boston, MA: Allyn & Bacon.

Saleebey, D. (2013). *The strengths perspective in social work practice.* Upper Saddle River, NJ: Pearson.

Schon, D. (1979). Generative metaphor: A perspective on problem-setting in social policy. In A. Ortony (Ed.), *Metaphor and thought* (pp. 254-283). Cambridge, UK: Cambridge University.

Schwartz, K. B. (2009). Reclaiming our heritage: Connecting the founding vision to the centennial vision. *The American Journal of Occupational Therapy, 63*(6), 681-690.

Seligman, M. E. P. (2002). Positive psychology, positive prevention and positive therapy. In C. R. Snyder & S. J. Lopez (Eds.), *Handbook of positive psychology* (pp. 3-12). New York, NY: Oxford Press.

Seligman, M. E. P., & Csikszentmihalyi, M. (2000). Positive psychology: An introduction. *American Psychologist, 55*(1), 5-14. doi:10.1037//0003-066x55.1.5

Shogren, K. A. (2013). Positive psychology and disability: A historical analysis. In M. L. Wehmeyer (Ed.), *The Oxford handbook of positive psychology and disability* (pp. 19-33). New York, NY: Oxford University.

Smith, E. J. (2006). The strengths-based counseling model: A paradigm shift in psychology. *The Counseling Psychologist, 34*(1), 134-144. doi:10.1177/001000005282364

Stedman, A., & Thomas, Y. (2011). Reflecting on our effectiveness: Occupational therapy interventions with indigenous clients. *Australian Occupational Therapy Journal, 58*, 43-49. doi:10.1111/j.1440-1630.2010.00916.x

Stoffel, V. C. (2014). Presidential address: Attitude, authenticity, and action: Building capacity. *The American Journal of Occupational Therapy, 68*(6), 628-635.

Sumsion, T. (1999). A study to determine a British occupational therapy definition of client-centred practice. *British Journal of Occupational Therapy, 62*(2), 52-58.

Sumsion, T. (2005). Facilitating client-centred practice: Insights from clients. *Canadian Journal of Occupational Therapy, 72*(1), 13-20.

Sumsion, T., & Law, M. (2006). A review on the conceptual elements informing client-centred practice. *Canadian Journal of Occupational Therapy, 73*(3), 153-162.

Sumsion, T., & Lencucha, R. (2006). Balancing challenges and facilitating factors when implementing client-centered collaboration in a mental health setting. *British Journal of Occupational Therapy, 70*(12), 513-520.

Sumsion, T., & Lencucha, R. (2009). Therapists' perceptions of how teamwork influences client-centred practice. *British Journal of Occupational Therapy, 72*(2), 48-54.

Thorarinsdottir, K., & Kristjansson, K. (2014). Patients' perspectives on person-centred participation in healthcare: A framework analysis. *Nursing Ethics, 21*(2), 129-147. doi:10.1177/0969733013490593

Townsend, E. (2003). Reflections on power and justice in enabling occupation. *Canadian Journal of Occupational Therapy, 70*(2), 74-87.

Townsend, E., Langille, L., & Ripley, D. (2003). Professional tensions and client-centered practice: Using institutional ethnography to generate understanding and transformation. *The American Journal of Occupational Therapy, 57*(1), 17-28.

Weishaar, P. M. (2010). What's new in …twelve ways to incorporate strengths-based planning into the IEP process. *The Clearing House, 83*, 207-210. doi:10.1080/00098650903505381

West, W. (1968). Professional responsibility in times of change. *The American Journal of Occupational Therapy, 22*, 9-15.

Whalley Hammell, K. (2001). Using qualitative research to inform the client-centred evidence-based practice of occupational therapy. *British Journal of Occupational Therapy, 64*(5), 228-234.

Whalley Hammell, K. (2002). Informing client-centred practice through qualitative inquiry: Evaluating the quality of qualitative research. *British Journal of Occupational Therapy, 65*(4), 175-184.

Whalley Hammell, K. (2006.) *Perspectives on disability and rehabilitation: Contesting assumptions; Challenging practice.* New York, NY: Churchill Livingstone.

Whalley Hammell, K. (2007a). Experience of rehabilitation following spinal cord injury: A meta-synthesis of qualitative findings. *Spinal Cord, 45*, 260-274. doi:10.1038/sj.sc.3102034

Whalley Hammell, K. (2007b). Client-centred practice: Ethical obligation or professional obfuscation? *British Journal of Occupational Therapy, 70*(6), 264-266.

Whalley Hammell, K. (2007c). Reflections on… A disability methodology for the client-centred practice of occupational therapy research. *Canadian Journal of Occupational Therapy, 74*(5), 365-369.

Whalley Hammell, K. (2011). Resisting theoretical imperialism in the disciplines of occupational science and occupational therapy. *British Journal of Occupational Therapy, 74*(1), 27-33.

Whalley Hammell, K. (2013). Client-centred occupational therapy in Canada: Refocusing on core values. *Canadian Journal of Occupational Therapy, 80*(3), 141-149.

Whalley Hammell, K. (2015). Respecting global wisdom: Enhancing the cultural relevance of occupational therapy's theoretical base. *British Journal of Occupational Therapy, 78*(11), 718-721.

Whalley Hammell, K. R., & Iwama, M. K. (2012). Well-being and occupational rights: An imperative for critical occupational therapy. *Scandinavian Journal of Occupational Therapy, 19*, 385-394. doi:10.3109/11038128.2011.611821

Wolin, S. (2003).What is a strength? *Reclaiming Children and Youth, 12*(1), 18-21.

Wolin, S., & Wolin, S. (1993). *The resilient self: How survivors of troubled families rise above adversity.* New York, NY: Villard Books.

Yerxa, E. J. (1980). Occupational therapy's role in creating a future climate of caring. *The American Journal of Occupational Therapy, 34*(8), 529-534.

Yerxa, E. J. (1991). Nationally speaking: Seeking a relevant, ethical, and realistic way of knowing for occupational therapy. *The American Journal of Occupational Therapy, 45*(3), 199-204.

Yerxa, E. J. (1992). Some implications of occupational therapy's history for its epistemology, values, and relation to medicine. *The American Journal of Occupational Therapy, 46*(1), 79-83.

Yerxa, E. J. (1998). Health and the human spirit. *The American Journal of Occupational Therapy, 52*(6), 412-418.

Yerxa, E. J. (2000). Confessions of an occupational therapist who became a detective. *British Journal of Occupational Therapy, 63*(5), 192-199.

Yerxa, E. J. (2009). Infinite distance between the I and the It. *The American Journal of Occupational Therapy, 63*(4), 490-497.

An Ecological Approach to Enhancing Children's Competencies and Participation

CHAPTER OVERVIEW

The belief that children should have a voice in therapy and research is based on different conceptualizations of childhood and development from a traditional view. Previously, a widely held perspective was that all children develop in predictable stages, based mainly on their age. Current theories include recognition that childhoods differ depending on experiences and culture and that children are active agents in their own development. This shift in theories, along with the new academic field of childhood studies and the 1989 United Nations Convention on the Rights of the Child, led to the acknowledgment of their rights and recognition of the importance of their knowledge. Therapists can be advocates by maintaining a collaborative mentality, bolstering their participation, supporting the meaningful adults in their lives, and promoting system changes.

A TRADITIONAL VIEW OF CHILDREN AND CHILDHOOD

At the same time that occupational therapy aligned with medicine, therapists were influenced by developmental psychology and sociology. Based on the theories and research of these two professions, our Western society developed a certain image of children and beliefs regarding how and at what age normal development occurs. These beliefs were incorporated into our Western culture and became commonplace and taken for granted.

Developmental psychology's theories became the most dominant influence on our attitudes toward children and affected parenting, education, intervention, and laws (Burman, 2008). The root of these theories, according to Freeman and Mathison (2009), was Darwin's perspective on evolution. Thereafter, those who studied children were shaped by the mindset that development follows a natural, biologically determined course. The focus of the research became centered on identifying milestones, explaining underlying developmental processes, and examining environmental factors (Woodhead, 2011). At the same time, sociology's theories became a dominant influence on views of socialization.

Influential Researchers and Theorists of Children's Development

In the early 1900s, Arnold Gesell founded a clinic with a glass observation room and used a movie camera to collect extensive information on children's behavior at different ages (Woodhead, 2011). From this research, he identified a schedule of developmental milestones, which specified what children should be able to do within each age group. These milestones were then used for assessing whether their development was normal or delayed.

Curtin, C.
Strategies for Collaborating With Children: Creating Partnerships in Occupational Therapy and Research (pp. 37-50).
© 2017 SLACK Incorporated.

Jean Piaget, whom James and James (2012) referred to as the "founding father of developmental psychology" (p. 40), was another prominent researcher. His research and theories were considered humanist in stark contrast to the prevailing Behaviorism movement of his time (Burman, 2008). Behaviorists, such as B. F. Skinner, focused on examining the effects of observable environmental reinforcements. Applying his visionary and creative approach, Piaget used semi-structured interviews and experimental tasks to examine children's thinking. He showed utmost respect for children by truly listening and taking what they said seriously (Woodhead, 2015). By using this approach, he was able to demonstrate that children's thinking was different from that of adults.

Based on his research, he developed an *ages and stages model* to describe the changes in children's ways of thinking (Wyness, 2012). He argued that children had an active role in their learning and adapting to their environment. His emphasis on adaptation, according to Burman (2008), was instrumental in bringing evolutionary theory into psychology (p. 244).

Piaget maintained that children's cognitive competencies increased at certain ages. He defined each stage of intellectual development that occurred in a linear and universal sequence. Western society came to rely on these ages and stages to define what constituted normal cognitive development. From then on, expectations regarding children's competencies were based upon their ages.

Main Features of a Traditional View of Childhood and Development

The first belief within a traditional view is that as children grow, there is a natural progression of biological changes. These physical and mental changes take place in the same sequence. Children, for example, learn to walk before being able to run. There are also developmental milestones that describe exactly what they can do for every year they grow older. Delays in achieving these normal milestones are usually an indication that intervention is needed.

A second belief within a traditional view is that because childhood is universal, there can be a general, unitary model of development (Smith, 2011). Hence, a major objective for researchers is to discover and examine the universal laws of development (Hogan, 2005). Any findings from the research can then be applied to all children.

A third belief is that childhood is a time of preparation for becoming a mature adult. Younger children have limited reasoning, are egocentric, and can be irrational. They become more competent as they get older. When they become adults, they are considered mature, rational, socially sophisticated, and capable of complex thinking.

A fourth belief is that children belong to a family and the adults in their lives know what is best for them. As minors, they are passive and dependent on others. When problems occur, the focus needs to be on addressing the individual issues of the child.

The last major belief is that researchers need to concentrate their efforts on studying what is normal development at different ages. They should ensure objectivity by applying the principles of good science, reflecting their positivist paradigm. To conduct value-free research, it is best to study children in a controlled laboratory setting. This allows researchers to limit and account for any influencing factors.

A Traditional View of Children's Socialization

Talcott Parsons' (1951) theoretical work in sociology provided the main concepts for the traditional view of the ways children are socialized (Wyness, 2012). He conceptualized socialization as being the process by which children become functioning adult members of society. In the traditional view, children are blank slates who are unsocialized and unaware of the norms and rules of society. It is the role of key social institutions, such as families and schools, to impart the knowledge needed for children to conform to society's norms. These institutions, especially parents, assist children in internalizing crucial values and acceptable actions. Therefore, it is a priority for researchers in sociology to study these important key institutions to increase understanding of the process.

DECONSTRUCTING THE TRADITIONAL VIEWS

The core beliefs described became ingrained in Western society's mentality about and the treatment of children. These traditional ways of thinking appeared to be common sense and were easily accepted as truths. In the 1970s to 1980s, however, theorists and researchers challenged multiple aspects and assumptions underlying the traditional view.

Influential Researchers and Theorists

Lev Vygotsky (1978), a Russian psychologist and contemporary of Piaget, articulated a different theory about how children develop and learn. His *sociocultural theory*, which has also been called a *cultural-historical theory*, was translated into English in the 1978 book, *Mind in Society*. He posited that in addition to biological maturation, culture played a major role in shaping children's development. The knowledge of past generations, he argued, was passed on through social interaction and activities done with others (Corsaro, 2015). There was a continuation of culture when children learned and used language. Higher mental functions matured when children internalized the cultural tools, such as language. Instead of viewing development as linear and evolutionary, he believed there were *qualitative transformations* leading to revolutionary changes (Mann, 1999). He maintained that children had an active role in their learning but stressed that it was a collective versus an individual process, as outlined by Piaget (Corsaro, 2015).

In 1979, Urie Bronfenbrenner published his book, *The Ecology of Human Development: Experiments in Nature and Design.* In his new theory of human development, he described nested layers of contexts (e.g., communities, schools, families) that played a role in children's development. He proposed that as children develop, they interact with and are influenced by their families and teachers, who are part of the community, which is situated within a certain society and culture. He argued that research needed to be conducted in children's natural settings instead of laboratories. In his book, he stated, "Much of developmental psychology, as it now exists, is the science of the strange behavior of children in strange situations with strange adults for the briefest possible periods of time" (1979, p. 19). Bronfenbrenner also advocated for policy changes to support families and was an advisor in the development of Head Start (Weisner, 2008).

In later years, he emphasized developmental processes, including changes in the biopsychological characteristics of children, and named his revised theoretical framework the *bioecological model* (Bronfenbrenner & Morris, 2006). He also described four interrelated components (Process-Person-Contexts-Time), which he maintained were the main mechanisms for producing development.

Margaret Donaldson (1978), in her book, *Children's Minds*, described studies that replicated Piaget's work but made child-friendly adaptations. In a study by Piaget, younger children had difficulty assuming the perspective of a doll looking at a model of mountains. Yet, as described by Donaldson, when one researcher asked children where a boy should hide from a policeman, they were able to identify the policeman's point of view and accurately hide the boy. The children understood the concept of hiding when they were bad. When adaptations were made in other studies (e.g., using "naughty teddies"), children continued to show a higher level of reasoning than was suggested by Piaget's work.

A key difference, Donaldson argued, was that when the questions and activities made sense to the children, the studies were a more accurate reflection of their competencies. In addition, Woodhead and Faulkner (2008) maintained that these studies by Donaldson and colleagues showed that instead of having immature reasoning, the children were "ingenious" in their attempts to make sense of what to them were "nonsensical situations and contexts" (p. 26).

Studies on resilient children, as described in Chapter 2, were being conducted during this time. The research highlighted resilient children's competencies and growth when dealing with adversity. This line of research contributed to the recognition that children were active, not passive, agents in their development.

A shift in sociological theories reflected a similar theme. Children were active, not passive, members of society. Of course, they learned the ways and norms of their community and society from others, but their interactions changed their families, communities, and society. Socialization was not a unidirectional process. Traditionally, sociologists had focused on the family with little interest in children or childhood (Mayall, 2013). In the 1980s, Jens Qvortrup, a Danish sociologist, challenged his colleagues to include children and childhoods in their theories and research. In his later writings, he argued for the need to view children as "human beings" instead of "human becomings," and to study the structure of childhood (Qvortrup, 1994, p. 18; 2011). Rather than viewing childhood as an individual child's transitional passage to adulthood, he contended that childhood, like social class, could and should be viewed as a structural form. A deeper and more thorough understanding of childhood was vital.

These new theories and research emphasized the need to account for the following:

- The role of culture, social interactions, and language.
- The interrelationships between children and all their contexts (such as families, schools, and communities) over time.
- The need to study children in their naturalized settings.
- The use of research methods that made sense to children when studying their development.
- The importance of studying children's competencies and their active role in their development.
- Children's active role in society.

Challenges and Changes to the Traditional Views, Practices, and Research

Building upon the alternative perspectives, theories, and research of the 1970s to 1980s, there continued to be challenges to the status quo. There were critiques of the assumptions about and descriptions of the developmental process. Others began to embrace another philosophy regarding the nature and construction of knowledge. They promoted the adoption of a *social construction paradigm* that differed from the widely accepted positivist paradigm. The professions of developmental psychology and sociology changed.

Criticisms of the Traditional Views

The first criticism was that biological maturation was not the only factor determining children's development. Children did undergo similar physical changes (e.g., getting taller, increased mobility); however, physical growth did not account for all aspects of their social, language, emotional, and cognitive development. Their culture, environments, social relationships, and experience were also major factors. In addition, theories that centered on the children implied that their environments were only in the background instead of being intertwined (Wyness, 2012).

The second criticism was that the traditional views were acultural and ahistorical (Mayall, 2013). The theories and descriptions did not explain the role of cultural, social, and physical contexts. They did not consider the individuality of children and the diversity of cultures. The theories were based mainly on research of White, middle-class children in the United States and Europe but generalized the findings to other countries and cultures. There needed to be acknowledged that these theories and studies were based upon a Western conceptualization of childhood within a certain historical and political period.

A third criticism was that a universal childhood and a unitary model of development did not exist. Burman (2008), a psychologist, argued that the so-called normal child was a "fiction or a myth" that was "distilled from the comparative scores of age-graded populations" and contended that it was an abstraction and that "no individual child lies at its base" (p. 22). The view that a certain type of childhood was universal limited the exploration and understanding of the diversity of childhoods (Goodyer, 2011). Another limitation was that the traditional description of normal development did not explain the trajectory of children with disabilities who grew but could not follow the same pathway. James and James (2012) asserted that there was not a single global model of development that covered every child in every country in every culture in every period.

A fourth criticism was that the traditional view promoted binary thinking. Children were either normal or abnormal. They were viewed as the opposite of adults: immature, irrational, and incompetent. The focus was on what they could not do as compared with adults. Wyness (2012) stressed that in this view childhood became a "deficit model of adulthood" (p. 82). And yet, Mayall (2000) pointed out that ironically not every adult is mature, rational, and competent!

A fifth criticism was about the narrow perspective of children. Children were not passive, blank slates and invisible members of their families. They had an active role in their development, families, and socialization. They had their own thoughts and feelings that often differed from their parents' thoughts and feelings. They needed to be valued for their individuality and knowledge.

The sixth criticism was that the focus of interventions and research needed to be broadened. Instead of only studying White, middle-class children in Western countries, researchers needed to include children of different races, countries, and cultures. Because the children's social, cultural, and physical environments played a vital role in their development, children needed to be studied in their natural settings instead of just laboratories. Rather than focusing only on children, interventions and research needed to have an ecological approach and examine the interrelationships between children and various contexts. Researchers also needed to learn more about children's perspectives, knowledge, experiences, and everyday activities.

A Different Paradigm: Social Construction

Another catalyst for change was the embracing of the social construction paradigm by many theorists and researchers. This paradigm, as defined by James and James (2012), is "a theoretical perspective that explores the ways in which 'reality' is negotiated in everyday life through people's interactions and through sets of discourses" (p. 116).

In contrast to the beliefs of the positivist paradigm that there are truths out there that can be observed and discovered, social constructionists believe the development of knowledge and what is viewed as reality occurs through social interactions within certain traditions (Gergen, 2015). For example, what is considered childhood varies across cultures and historical time periods. Each person's version of childhood develops through his or her interactions with others and is shaped by his or her own history, education, experiences, and culture (Jones, 2011). (See Gergen's [2015] readable and easy-to-follow book, *Invitation to Social Construction*, for an in-depth explanation of this paradigm.)

Changes in Developmental Psychology

With the inclusion of theorists such as Bronfenbrenner and Vygotsky, developmental psychologists broadened their focus. There was more emphasis on social relationships, and socioeconomic and cultural contexts (Tisdall & Punch, 2012). They shifted to doing more research in natural settings. Mayall (2013) suggested that both an increased number of women researchers and greater access to children in day care settings may have contributed to these changes.

Changes in Sociology: The New Sociology of Childhood

The *new sociology of childhood* emerged with the coming together of multiple theorists and researchers with a similar and radical (for that time) point of view regarding children. A cohort of mainly sociologists and anthropologists were the most vocal in challenging the traditional views. Following a series of workshops on ethnography with children, James and Prout (1990, 1997) edited the book *Constructing and Reconstructing Childhood*, which encapsulated different conceptualizations of children. They criticized the current view that was being perpetuated by developmental psychology.

Prout and James (1997) defined six key tenets of this new branch of sociology. First, childhood is socially constructed; its structures vary in different cultures. Second, childhood is intertwined with social factors such as gender and class; there is not one universal conceptualization that applies to all. Third, the cultures, social relationships, and lives of children are worth studying. Fourth, children are viewed as active in constructing and determining their lives and influencing their families and societies; they have agency and are not passive. Fifth, ethnography is a beneficial methodology because it provides an opportunity for children to have a voice and participate in research. Sixth, conceptualizations of childhood and types of research need to be reconstructed in society; a new sociology can contribute to these changes.

In addition to Alan Prout and Allison James, Smith and Greene (2014) identified many of the other sociologists and anthropologists contributing to the growth of this branch, including Leena Alanen, Pia Christensen, William Corsaro, Judith Ennew, Chris Jenks, Berry Mayall, Jens Qvortrup, and Barrie Thorne.

With this new sociology, children became more visible in theories and research and were no longer hidden in the margins of society. Mayall (2013) emphasized that it was important for sociologists to include a subsection on childhood because children are part of the social structure and play a role in maintaining and changing societies. Additionally, it was recognized that to gain a thorough understanding of childhood, they needed to learn from children themselves (Figure 3-1).

A New Academic Field: Childhood Studies

Although sociologists and anthropologists were pivotal in developing the sociology of childhood, scholars in other professions were developing similar viewpoints and ways of doing research with children. The other disciplines included social work, geography, history, and education. These professions joined together with sociology and anthropology, and their interest in children and childhood led to the creation of a new academic field called *childhood studies*. According to Smith and Greene (2014), additional influential contributors were Priscilla Alderson, Daniel Cook, Ivar Frønes, Robbie Gilligan, Roger Hart, Henry Hendrick, Mary Kellett, Irene Rizzini, Nigel Thomas, and Martin Woodhead.

As the field of childhood studies has evolved, it has continued to embrace the major tenets initially proposed by Prout and James (Tisdall & Punch, 2012). There are multidisciplinary perspectives and approaches focusing on childhood as a social category, children's agency, and the value of including children in research and as co-researchers. There is an emphasis on addressing and weaving

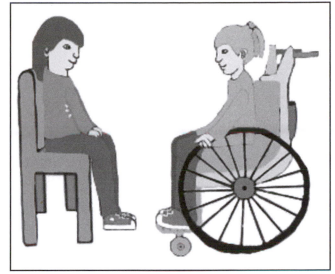

Figure 3-1. In the early 1990s, there was a shift to focusing on children's competencies and their knowledge.

together the commonalities of childhood (structure) with the plurality of individual childhoods and children's agency (James, 2010). In addition, there is an examination of the development, benefits, and challenges of children's agency, as well as limiting contexts and circumstances (Tisdall & Punch, 2012).

In the past decade, scholars in childhood studies have advocated for changes in their field. They are emphasizing the importance of supporting theorists and researchers globally (Smith & Greene, 2014). They assert that this is necessary to increase understanding of childhood in diverse cultures and countries. There is a call to create a conceptual bridge between (a) developmental psychology's emphasis on the developmental process and (b) childhood studies' emphasis on the sociological understanding of children and the child as an active agent in his or her life (James, 2010; Mayall, 2013; Woodhead, 2011, 2015).

Rather than emphasizing the adult/child dichotomy, there is now a shift to viewing the differences as a continuum and focusing more on relationships and understanding interdependency (James, 2010; Tisdall & Punch, 2012). Furthermore, alternative paradigms are being explored, such as critical realism as described by Alderson (2013) in her book, *Childhoods Real and Imagined: Volume 1: An Introduction to Critical Realism and Childhood Studies.*

Departments of childhood studies are located in universities worldwide, and a body of scholarly work is developing, often published in children-focused journals such as *Childhood*, *Children's Geographies*, and *Children and Society*. Research with children and including them as co-researchers has increased. In addition to ethnography, a multitude of creative research methods are being used to study their perspectives and experiences. There is growing recognition of the value and need for research with children with disabilities, including those who are nonverbal (Richards, Clark, & Boggis, 2015; Tisdall, 2012). Additionally, scholars (Kellett, 2014; Woodhead, 2014) are stressing the importance of incorporating knowledge generated by nongovernmental organizations and linking research to the promotion of children's rights and well-being.

CHILDREN'S RIGHTS

At the same time that developmental psychology and sociology were changing in the 1970s to 1980s, there was a movement to explicitly define children's rights. Perceptions of children and childhood began to shift as a result of (a) changes in theories of development, (b) the new field of childhood studies, and (c) the influence of the children's rights movement. The necessity and importance of their participation became a prominent theme.

Hence, after 10 years of negotiation, in 1989 all countries belonging to the United Nations, except Somalia and the United States, ratified the United Nations Convention on the Rights of the Child (UNCRC). This human rights treaty was the "world's first international legal instrument of children's rights" (Freeman, 2000, p. 227). Countries worldwide came to an agreement that children were citizens with social, civil, political, and cultural rights. This legally binding document held the signing countries accountable through a monitoring system to ensure the rights of their youngest citizens.

The UNCRC was monumental. It was the first time that:

- Children were identified as subjects with rights rather than just objects of concern who needed protection (Freeman, 2011; Hanson & Nieuwenhuys, 2013)

- Children were viewed as individuals with their own perspectives and needs rather than being considered "owned" by their parents (Alderson, 2008, p. 87)

- The rights of children with disabilities were specified internationally in human rights law (Lansdown, 2010).

United Nations Convention on the Rights of the Child

The UNCRC applies to all children, from birth to 18 years old. The 54 articles cover four main principles. First, countries (referred to as "States") need to protect children from all types of discrimination (Article 2). Second, actions undertaken by private and public bodies need to make children's best interests primary (Article 3). Third, children have a right to life, and States are obligated to ensure survival and development as much as possible (Article 6). Fourth, children have a right to express their views and be given serious consideration.

Overall, three main types of children's rights are described (Alderson, 2008):

1. Provision of essential needs (e.g., a name, nationality, economic welfare, education, health care, and a right to stay with their family, rest, and engage in play)

2. Protection (e.g., from abuse and neglect)

3. Participation (e.g., to express views, receive information, and participate within the community)

Parents' rights are emphasized in Article 5:

> "States Parties shall respect the responsibilities, rights and duties of parents or, where applicable, the members of the extended family or community as provided for by local custom, legal guardians or other persons legally responsible for the child, to provide in a manner consistent with the evolving capacities of the child, appropriate direction and guidance in the exercise by the child of the rights recognized in the present convention."

Article 12 emphasizes children's participation rights:

> "States Parties shall assure to the child who is capable of forming his or her own views the right to express those views freely in all matters affecting the child, the views of the child being given due weight in accordance with the age and maturity of the child."

With the adoption of the UNCRC, governments attended more to children's issues, debated what were children's rights in their culture, and created new policies and laws to enhance children's lives (Levesque, 2014). The convention promoted social justice by advancing the cause of children's rights movements, such as the increased development of working children's organizations in India, Latin American, Africa, and Asia (Saadi, 2012; Smith, 2015). The view that children have competencies to participate supported the tenets of childhood studies and led to the inclusion of children's rights studies within departments of childhood studies (Reynaert, Bouverne-De Bie, & Vandevelde, 2012).

United Nations Convention on the Rights of Persons With Disabilities

In 2001, members of the United Nations as well as adults and children with disabilities started developing a document that became the United Nations Convention of the Rights of Persons with Disabilities (UNCRPD). It was enacted in 2008 (the United States signed it but has yet to ratify it). The 1989 UNCRC had outlined the human rights of all children, including those with disabilities. The 2008 UNCRPD introduced detailed government obligations to make those rights reality (Lansdown, 2009).

Article 7 is entirely devoted to children with disabilities:

1. States parties shall take all necessary measures to ensure the full enjoyment by children with disabilities of all human rights and fundamental freedoms on an equal basis with other children.

2. In all actions concerning children with disabilities, the best interests of the child shall be a primary consideration.

3. States Parties shall ensure that children with disabilities have their right to express their views freely on all matters affecting them, their views being given due weight in accordance with their age and maturity on an equal basis with other children, and to be provided with disability and age-appropriate assistance to realize that right.

Article 21 especially pertains to children who are nonverbal. It is stated that governments are to take adequate measures to provide information in accessible formats and technologies and to accept and facilitate communication modes chosen by people with disabilities. This includes sign language, Braille, argumentative, and alternative communication modes.

First Concern: The Relationship Between Parental and Children's Rights

During the countries' debates about the role and implementation of the 1989 UNCRC, one main concern centered on the relationship between children's and parents' rights. Some worried that if children had rights, it would be detrimental to their families.

In response, Alderson and Montgomery (1996) identified four levels in which children could be involved in making decisions. They could (1) be informed, (2) express a view, (3) influence the decision, or (4) be the main one to make the decision. Alderson (2008) maintained that the children's participation rights in the UNCRC referred to the first three levels; parents still made the final decisions. She also argued that although children want their perspectives heard, they often want their parents to make the major decisions. Governments would only intervene if children's safety was in jeopardy.

Another response to this concern was that listening to children's views would help parents make better-informed decisions. Furthermore, the practice of listening to each other would teach respect, and the handling of conflicting views would teach negotiation skills (Gal & Duramy, 2015; Krappmann, 2010).

Second Concern: The Competence of Children to Participate

The second issue raised was whether children have the competencies needed to participate. A number of scholars (Freeman, 2007; Lansdown, 2010) addressed this issue, contending that all children can express their views. Although their verbal and nonverbal means of communication may differ from adults', their messages are still valid and important. Gal and Duramy (2015) added that a cycle is created when adults assume children are incompetent and do not give children the opportunity to develop their skills or prove that they are competent. Alderson (2008) advocated for adults to change the question of "Do they either understand or not?" to "Do they understand enough? And, if not, could they understand enough if they had more information or if they were asked in a different way?" (p. 24). Based on her research, she argued that children's competence is based more on their experiences, family life, and culture rather than their age.

What Are Considered Children's Rights?

Freeman (2007) argued that all children have rights and that most would agree, for instance, that they have the right to not be abused. Without rights, they are at the mercy of others. Rights preserve their humanity, dignity, and autonomy.

However, there continues to be a debate about what specific rights children have. There is a general consensus that children are entitled to basic human rights. The UNCRC was an attempt by the international community to further clarify the specifics. Others maintain that in addition to the UNCRC top-down approach, there needs to be a bottom-up approach, also referred to as *living rights* (Hanson & Nieuwenhuys, 2013; Liebel, 2012). This entails having children identify their own needs and corresponding rights unique to their situation and context. For example, child workers in Asia and Africa might emphasize their right to safe working conditions, whereas full-time students in the United States might emphasize their right to be free from bullying. Similarly, Mannion (2007) maintained that identifying and researching children's rights requires a relational and spatial approach. It is the child-adult relationship and the spaces they occupy that shape what are considered essential rights.

Occupational Justice and Rights

Occupational therapists can support children's rights and work toward social justice. They have an extensive knowledge of occupations that can be used for the betterment of children, families, communities, and society.

Because the core premises of the profession are based on a social justice framework (Nilsson & Townsend, 2010), occupational therapy philosophy can be a guide for advocacy. For instance, to promote social justice requires a belief in (a) the equal worth of all people, (b) people's ability to change, (c) the necessity of collaboration, and (d) the importance for all to have a voice and be able to represent themselves (Townsend, 1993). Therapists share these same beliefs.

This type of advocacy in occupational therapy practice has come to be called an *occupational justice approach.* Occupational justice, a concept that expands the focus of social justice, was developed by Townsend and Wilcock (2004; Wilcock, 2006) and further described in a *participatory occupational justice framework* by Townsend and Whiteford (2005) and Whiteford and Townsend (2011). Central to this approach are the perspectives that people are occupational beings and that "satisfying and meaningful participation in occupation" can determine well-being, health, and quality of life (Wilcock, 2006, p. 253). Those using this approach advocate for equal access to opportunities, choices, and conditions that support participation in health-promoting occupations (Townsend & Wilcock, 2004).

Occupational injustices occur when "participation in occupations is barred, confined, restricted, segregated, prohibited, undeveloped, disrupted, and alienated, marginalized, exploited, excluded or otherwise restricted" (Townsend & Wilcock, 2004, p. 77). Stadnyk, Townsend, and Wilcock (2010) described the following four types of injustices that can occur with groups of people:

1. *Occupational alienation* refers to the lack of resources or opportunities to participate in meaningful occupations, possibly affecting self-identity or leading to emptiness or isolation.

2. *Occupational deprivation* occurs when people are denied opportunities to participate in certain occupations, such as play, due to external forces.

3. *Occupational marginalization* refers to limited opportunities to make choices regarding occupations affecting autonomy.

4. *Occupational imbalance* is seen when people are underoccupied or overoccupied.

In a similar vein, Whalley Hammell (2008) advocated for therapists to focus on and address people's occupational rights, which she defined as "the right of all people to engage in meaningful occupations that contribute positively to their own well-being and the well-being of their communities" (p. 61). Whalley Hammell (2015) and Whalley Hammell and Iwama (2012) argued that the right to occupation is a human right, and the profession needs to work to ensure those rights for all.

As proposed by these leaders in the profession, occupational therapy practice is not limited to working with individual children. Therapists have valuable knowledge that when partnered with others can create change in broader areas.

AN ECOLOGICAL APPROACH: SUPPORTING CHILDREN AT DIFFERENT LEVELS

As a therapist, you can support children and families at different levels by (1) maintaining a respectful mindset, (2) bolstering their participation and efforts for change, (3) engaging in collaborative consultation with caregivers and educational staff, and (4) changing systems, communities, and policies to improve children's well-being.

An Ecological Approach

It is just as important to collaborate with caregivers, educational staff, and communities as it is to collaborate with children. As a therapist, you can enhance children's participation, consult with caregivers and educational staff, and advocate for changes on the children's behalf.

To apply an ecological approach means you stay cognizant of children's social and cultural contexts when working or doing research with them. For instance, if children are getting bullied at school, you could talk with them about their successful strategies and, if necessary, teach additional ways to address the situation. However, you would not stop there. You would consider the role of classroom and school environment, and work with staff to create a safer place.

A client-centered, strengths-based approach can be used when you are a consultant or advocate. As described in Chapter 2, you would establish partnerships with community members, educational staff, and caregivers. The process would always include identifying their strengths, building on their assets, and addressing their desired changes.

First Level: Advocate for Children at a Personal Level Through Your Thoughts, Words, and Actions

The first step in advocating for children starts with you. Your mindset guides your actions. How you view children and their competencies influences if you will even advocate and, if so, how you will consult for them. Ask yourself the following:

- Do you believe children should have a say regarding their lives, therapy, and research?

- Do you value their perspectives?

- Is your attention more on what they can do instead of what they cannot do?

- Do you talk about them in nonjudgmental terms?

- Do you always consider the social and cultural contexts?

These same questions apply for caregivers and educational staff.

An Example of Advocating at a Personal Level

In one of my schools, specialists were called in to aid the functioning of a 9-year-old boy in the classroom. They created a system to increase his compliance and completion of schoolwork. He was to be reinforced by rewards if he finished his work without outbursts.

Meanwhile, his teacher told me that she wondered if sensory issues were contributing factors. The next day, I was in the class and saw him looking upset as he struggled with the assignment. Before discussing my observations with his teacher, I wanted to find out his concerns. I valued his perspective. In talking with him, I discovered that he was not trying to be defiant; he was just overwhelmed with how difficult the work was. I shared his concerns with his teacher. She adapted the assignment, and he calmly finished it.

Second Level: Bolster Children's Participation and Efforts for Change

A second way you can support children is to increase their level of participation and assist their efforts for change. The key factor is that they have opportunities to choose whether and how much they would prefer to be involved. There is a range of opportunities that can be matched to their desired level.

In 1992, Hart created a seminal model of degrees of children's participation using the metaphor of a ladder. In the bottom three rungs indicating nonparticipation were (1) manipulation, (2) decoration, and (3) tokenism. The next five levels progressing to a higher level were (4) assigned but informed, (5) consulted and informed, (6) adult-initiated and shared decisions with children, (7) child-initiated and directed decisions, and (8) child-initiated and shared decisions with adults (p. 8). He advocated using it as a guide for reflecting on children's involvement in making decisions in projects with adults. Hart (1997) stipulated that one upper level was not better than another because involvement depended upon the children's interest and abilities.

In 2007, Lundy described a different model of enabling children's participation as outlined in the UNCR. She described the following four key factors: (1) giving children *space* to share their perspective, (2) facilitating the expression of their *voices*, (3) having an *audience* that listens, and (4) ensuring their perspectives have an *influence*. Lundy emphasized that it is not enough to just listen. Rather, children need to see that their input can make a difference in their or others' lives.

An Example of Bolstering Children's Participation

In one preschool classroom, the children and teacher knew me well because I was able to be there an entire morning once a week. The teacher and I talked about finding out what the children, including those with disabilities, thought about their current centers, which had a fairy tale theme. By discovering what interested them and helped them learn, I would be better able to suggest ideas to promote motor skills and sensory processing. I volunteered to collect this information. First, I took photos of all the centers: (1) Three Little Pigs in the blocks area, (2) Little Mermaid at the water table, (3) Ye Royal Library in the books section, (4) Elves and the Shoemaker at the arts and craft table, (5) Goldilocks and the Three Bears in dramatic play, and (6) the Castle in the science area.

I attached one photo to each page and wrote the children's comments underneath. I asked them, "What do you like about [name of the center]?" and, "What would you add or what else would you put in this center?" The children looked at the photos and watched me write their statements; this was done for each center. For the Little Mermaid center, the children said they liked playing with toys in the water. They recommended adding sharks, shells, more mermaids, and toys. Afterwards, their teacher made those additions.

To get more feedback, I brought in a camera and had the children take three pictures:

1. My favorite thing to play with at school is…
2. My favorite center is…
3. I want to take a picture of…" (free choice)

As they took the pictures, I wrote down their answers. I gave copies of their photos and answer sheets to the children to take home. The teacher and I looked at their answers. We were pleased that for the free choice picture, the majority of them took pictures of their friends playing, which included all the children with disabilities. To us that indicated that the children valued the friendships they had made in preschool and were accepting of diversity.

Third Level: Support the Meaningful Adults in Children's Lives

Another essential way to help children is to provide support to the meaningful adults in their lives, especially their caregivers and educational staff. Through a collaborative consultation process, you work together as partners to improve children's and adults' lives. Additionally, as a consultant, you may assist them in their efforts to advocate for their children or children's causes.

Collaborative Consultation

Traditionally, people think of consultation as a process of an expert giving ideas to a consultee on what to do. Yet there is much more to this process than just walking into a class or home and providing ideas and recommendations. It is not that simple. The consultant needs to learn and adapt to the consultee's social and cultural contexts. There is a relationship-building process, negotiations, and learning how to get in synchrony with each other. There is sharing of knowledge between the consultee and consultant.

Consultation also tends to be described as a problem-solving process that begins with the identification of

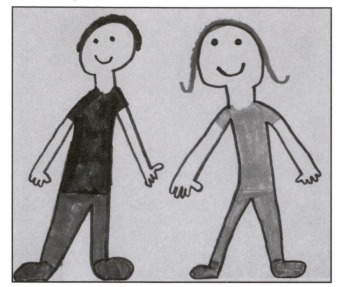

Figure 3-2. Collaborative consultation with caregivers and teachers is vital.

problems. On the surface, this approach appears sensible. But as highlighted in Chapter 2, there are limitations. When talking about problems, the focus is oriented toward deficits and past actions. This often results in blaming and may hinder thinking about solutions not related to the problem.

On the other hand, a strengths-based approach guides therapists to be future oriented, discover the consultees' desired changes, and build on their competencies and successful strategies. Collaboration, rather than problem solving, is the main focus (Figure 3-2). There is not one right method of consultation. To be client centered, therapists have to discover what type of consultation is desired. Some consultees may want you to give them quick and easy ideas of what to do. Others, however, may want a more interactive exploration of ideas and strategies for change.

In 2005, Deaver conducted a qualitative study examining the process of collaborative consultation between mental health practitioners and early childhood educators. She interviewed 24 teachers about their experiences with the consultants. Then, based on the identified themes and building on theories of adult learning and Bandura's (1995) theory of self-efficacy, she developed a conceptual model of the process.

As described in Deaver's model, the process begins with identifying the consultee's compelling needs. There is a discovery process of finding out what is important to the consultee, what is the desired outcome, and what she or he wants from the consultation. There is clarification whether a directive or nondirective approach is preferred. The practitioner recognizes the consultee's competencies and continually checks and responds to how the consultation process is affecting him or her.

Collaborative consultation, as posited by Deaver, then involves a certain style and technique of interaction. Together these can lead to changes in the situation and achievement of desired outcomes. An additional and just-as-important outcome is changes in the consultee's self-efficacy, which are the feelings and beliefs of being effective in one's environment.

The style of interaction refers to three unifying conditions needed to develop a relationship and create a foundation for teamwork: authentic caring, respectful communication, and nonjudgmental support.

To demonstrate authentic caring, practitioners are present, genuine in their caring, accessible, approachable, and willing to help and spend time with the consultee.

Respectful communication is shown by developing a reciprocal relationship, being understanding and empathetic, learning the consultee's likes and dislikes, and inviting discussion through words and actions.

The last condition, nonjudgmental support, is seen when practitioners listen, provide validation, step in without judgment, and provide physical support when needed.

The technique of interaction refers to how the practitioner creates a learning environment for the consultee to increase self-efficacy. The practitioner believes in the consultee's competence, builds on previous successes, and assists him or her in increasing a toolbox of effective approaches and strategies. In a nondirective approach, ideas are elicited (from children too when possible), explored, and negotiated. Expertise and resources are shared, which often leads to adapting or generating new ideas. If a directive approach is desired, the practitioner provides suggested ideas that are practical, realistic, simple, and easy to implement.

Another aspect of creating a learning environment is for the practitioner to provide the consultee with vicarious experiences where they learn by watching and/or promoting enactive experiences where they learn by trying. The practitioner provides performance feedback and, by using simple prompts and positive observations, encourages the consultee to reflect on his or her current actions. Successful consultation would lead to changes in self-efficacy, as seen by increased positive thinking, gains in self-confidence, and a greater range of practices.

An Example of Applying Deaver's Collaborative Consultation Model to a Program

After working 8 years for the school district, I was assigned to be the therapist at a specialized school for children and adolescents with severe behavioral challenges. On the first day, I saw teachers wearing thick arm guards to protect them from being scratched or bitten. As they talked with me, they emphasized the need to be cautious because many of the children had a history of eye-poking, hair-grabbing, biting, or hitting. I went to each classroom and then to the staff lounge. Although I was a seasoned therapist, I realized I was scared! I wondered how I was going to do this job. I kept taking deep breaths and telling myself I would be okay.

Later at a staff meeting, I met with the teachers, psychologist, vocational coach, and program director. First thing they told me was that they did not have an extra room to take students when it became too noisy. I discovered the previous occupational therapist had made that recommendation. They said they wanted to know more about sensory processing and ways to help the students stay calm. They wanted to avoid restraining the students.

When I returned to the school a week later (I was also responsible for seven other schools), I spent time in each classroom. In talking with the teachers, I acknowledged how stressful their job must be and that I was open to learning from them. I told them they were familiar with the students and to please let me know what I should or, especially, should not do with certain students. I did not want to get hurt.

As I watched the class and took notes, I looked for what was going well and what were the teachers' and students' strengths. In one class, however, I thought one of the teaching assistants was a little forceful in her words and actions with one boy. After school, I gave an in-service on sensory processing, describing all the senses and ways to prevent and deal with sensory overload. I wove in sensory-related observations of what I had seen them doing that had helped.

On my next visit, I brought some weighted lapbags and vests. On the playground I saw the children having fun but at the same time winding up and almost becoming agitated. I casually mentioned to their teacher that dimming the lights and playing soft music when they returned inside would help them become calmer. She followed my suggestions and had success. She then began using those strategies routinely.

Because I wanted to learn from all the staff, I decided to interview each one and compile all their ideas into a handout. I asked for their ideas on how to avoid power struggles and help the students to be successful. The staff members smiled and were animated as they shared strategies and stories about their successes. I listened closely, showing that I cared, was open to their ideas, and was not there to judge them.

When I talked with the staff member whom I was concerned about, I discovered she only had the one strategy she was using. I reframed my thinking and realized she did not know any other way. I made the handout and did another in-service to share everyone's expertise. It was a collective endeavor, and, most importantly, there were useful ideas that would work in their school. As I presented each strategy, I identified who had given the idea.

Our relationship changed after that. There was a mutual openness and respect. We had learned from each other. I became more comfortable and began enjoying the students' personalities. After a while, I thought it would help to have a more consistent use of a visual schedule. Instead of telling them what to do, I met with them at another staff meeting and explored their concerns about having this type of schedule.

They said it was too hard to keep track of all the picture symbols when they were attached to a notebook. A constant turnover of staff was another problem. We talked about the benefits of visual schedules and brainstormed what might work. The group came up with the idea of having picture symbols of each school activity put on a key ring attached to a clip. Every staff member would have one. The key rings were made, and they began using them.

What started as a scary experience ended up being very rewarding. I learned that as a consultant I was more effective as a facilitator rather than an expert. By building on the staff's strengths and collaborating with them, we became a real team.

Fourth Level: Creating System Changes to Help Children

The thought of changing systems, communities, and policies can be daunting. It may feel overwhelming and too difficult a challenge. Often it seems easier to focus on interactions with children. And yet by branching out you can impact multitudes of children. Even starting in small ways, such as being on a community board, speaking at your city council meetings, or supporting a children's issue on social media, can blossom.

An Example of Creating Change in a School District

When I first started working in the school district, I was told that occupational therapists only did "motor" and not "sensory" therapy. I thought it was a narrow role and a limited use of our expertise. However, being new, I focused on learning what was expected, how to work in each school, and everything I could about motor development and therapy. Gradually, I began teaching students and teachers sensory strategies, especially at the day treatment programs.

A few years later, a group of occupational therapists met to discuss how to address sensory issues in the schools. The administrators equated *sensory* with sensory integration clinics. Our group talked about how we had been addressing sensory issues behind the scenes. We decided that we needed to define our role and use our expertise more openly. I volunteered to collate all our information and literature and be the spokesperson for the group. They gave me their resources, and, with my notes from our discussions, I wrote up a description of how occupational therapists could address children's sensory needs affecting their school functioning. I created a notebook that included sensory strategies and case examples.

Then it came time to meet with the administrators. Their first response was, "Oh no, this is going to open the flood gates." They were worried there would be too many referrals. Then they said it was impossible to have sensory integration clinics in the schools. They thought we were going to ask for hooks in every school's ceilings so we could have therapy swings.

I responded, with the support of two other therapists, by clarifying that we were not trying to set up clinics. I explained how a school therapist could address sensory issues in a different way from therapists working in an outpatient or hospital-based clinic. I provided multiple examples of how we could and had helped children learn and be successful in school.

It took some discussion, but it was finally agreed that this could be part of our role. I was then asked to do a presentation to all special education staff (around 60 people) to describe our role, our expertise, and what we could offer. It is now widely accepted that occupational therapists offer this valuable service.

SUMMARY

This chapter covered the changing conceptions about children, development, and childhood. The traditional view of development seemed like common sense in that children's development changed as they grew older. Yet the addition of new theories and perspectives demonstrated the limitations of this way of thinking; biological development was only one factor. Other major factors, such as the role of family experiences, culture, and different environments, came to light.

Another major change was the recognition and value of children's active role in their development and socialization. This led to more explicit descriptions of their rights and an emphasis on doing research *with* children.

With their knowledge of occupations, therapists can play a vital role in promoting occupational justice and rights. Applying an ecological approach, they can support caregivers and educational staff and advocate for children at community and national levels.

KEY POINTS TO REMEMBER

- The main emphasis of a traditional view of children's development was on their age–related biological development.

- The main emphasis of a traditional view of socialization was on how key institutions, such as families and schools, taught society's norms to children, who were considered blank slates.

- Theorists such as Bronfenbrenner and Vygotsky challenged the traditional views.

- There was a shift to account for the role of culture, social relationships, and context in children's development.

- Another shift was the recognition that children play an active role in their development and socialization.

- Developmental psychology changed and a new sociology of childhood emerged.

- A new multidisciplinary academic field of childhood studies came into existence.

- The children's rights movement also gained momentum following the 1989 United Nations Convention of the Rights of the Child and the 2008 United Nations Convention for the Rights of Persons With Disabilities.

- The acknowledgment of children's competencies and the importance of their participation came to the forefront.

- Occupational therapists can make a valuable contribution by promoting occupational justice and rights with a broader ecological approach.

- Therapists can advocate for children by maintaining a collaborative mindset, promoting their participation, consulting with the meaningful adults in their lives, and working to change systems and policies to enhance children's lives.

REVIEW QUESTIONS

1. There is a universal model of children's development. True or false.

2. Children are blank slates who are primed for learning from adults. True or false.

3. The application of a positivist paradigm is the best way to conduct research. True or false.

4. The new sociology of childhood and childhood studies share the same core tenets. True or false.

5. The UNCRC was the first legal instrument to identify children as subjects with rights. True or false.

6. Children and adults with disabilities contributed to the development of the UNCRPD. True or false.

7. Giving children rights will negatively impact parental rights. True or false.

8. The main focus of pediatric occupational therapy needs to center on individual children. True or false.

9. Just as important as listening to children is making sure their voices influence decisions and actions. True or false.

10. Occupational therapists' jobs are too demanding to consider making system changes. True or false.

REFERENCES

Alderson, P. (2008). *Young children's rights: Exploring beliefs, principles and practice* (Rev. ed.). Philadelphia, PA: Jessica Kingsley.

Alderson, P. (2013). *Childhoods real and imagined: Volume 1: An introduction to critical realism and childhood studies.* New York, NY: Routledge.

Alderson, P., & Montgomery, M. (1996). *Health care choices: Making decisions with children.* London, UK: Institute for Public Policy Research.

Bandura, A. (1995). Exercise of personal and collective efficacy in changing societies. In A. Bandura (Ed.), *Self efficacy in changing societies* (p. 1-45). Cambridge, UK: Cambridge University.

Bronfenbrenner, U. (1979). *The ecology of human development: Experiments by nature and design.* Cambridge, MA: Harvard University.

Bronfenbrenner, U., & Morris, P. A. (2006). The bioecological model of human development. In W. Damon & R. M. Lerner (Eds.), *Handbook of child psychology* (pp. 793-828). Hoboken, NJ: John Wiley.

Burman, E. (2008). *Deconstructing developmental psychology.* New York, NY: Routledge.

Corsaro, W. A. (2015). *The sociology of of childhood.* Thousand Oaks, CA: Sage.

Deaver, J. (2005). *A model of collaborative consultation to raise teachers' self efficacy* [Unpublished doctoral dissertation]. Denver, CO: University of Colorado at Denver.

Donaldson, M. (1978). *Children's minds.* New York, NY: W. W. Norton & Company.

Freeman, M. (2000). The future of children's rights. *Children & Society, 14,* 277-293. doi:10.1111/j.1099-0860.2000.tb00183.x

Freeman, M. (2007). Why it remains important to take children's rights seriously. *International Journal of Children's Rights, 15,* 5-23. doi:10.1163/092755607X181711

Freeman, M. (2011). Children's rights as human rights. In J. Qvortrup, W. A. Corsaro, & M. Honig (Eds.), *The Palgrave handbook of childhood studies.* (pp. 377-393). New York, NY: Palgrave Macmillan.

Freeman, M., & Mathison, S. (2009). *Researching children's experience.* New York, NY: Guilford Press.

Gal, T., & Duramy, F. (2015). Enhancing capacities for child participation: Introduction. In T. Gal & F. Duramy (Eds.), *International perspectives and empirical findings on child participation: From social exclusion to child-inclusive policies* (pp. 1-16). New York, NY: Oxford University.

Gergen, K. J. (2015). *An invitation to social construction.* Thousand Oaks, CA: Sage.

Goodyer, A. (2011). *Child-centred foster care: A rights-based model for practice.* Philadelphia, PA: Jessica Kingsley.

Hanson, K., & Nieuwenhuys, O. (2013). Living rights, social justice, translations. In K. Hanson & O. Nieuwenhuys (Eds.), *Reconceptualizing children's rights in international development: Living rights, social justice, translations* (pp. 3-25). Cambridge, UK: Cambridge University.

Hart, R. (1992). *Children's participation: From tokenism to citizenship.* Florence, Italy: International UNICEF Child Development Centre.

Hart, R. (1997). *Children's participation: The theory and practice of involving young citizens in community development and environmental care.* London, UK: Earthscan.

Hogan, D. (2005). Researching "the child" in developmental psychology. In S. Greene & D. Hogan (Eds.), *Researching children's experience* (pp. 22-41). Thousand Oaks, CA: Sage.

James, A. (2010). Competition or integration? The next step in childhood studies? *Childhood, 17*(4), 485-499. doi:10.1177/0907568209350783

James, A., & James, A. (2012). *Key concepts in childhood studies.* Thousand Oaks, CA: Sage.

James, A., & Prout, A. (1990). *Constructing and reconstructing childhood: Contemporary issues in the study of childhood.* London, UK: Routledge Falmer.

James, A., & Prout, A. (1997). *Constructing and reconstructing childhood: Contemporary issues in the study of childhood* (Rev. ed.). London, UK: Routledge.

Jones, P. (2011). What are children's rights? Contemporary developments and debates. In P. Jones & G. Walker (Eds.), *Children's rights in practice* (pp. 3-16). Thousand Oaks, CA: Sage.

Kellett, M. (2014). Mary Kellett. In C. Smith & S. Greene (Eds.), *Key thinkers in childhood studies* (pp. 139-147). Chicago, IL: Policy Press.

Krappmann, L. (2010). The weight of the child's view (Article 12 of the Convention on the Rights of the Child). *International Journal of Children's Rights, 18,* 501-513. doi:10.1163/157181810X528021

Lansdown, G. (2009). *See me, hear me: A guide to using the UN Convention on the Rights of Persons with Disabilities to promote the rights of children.* London, UK: Save the Children.

Lansdown, G. (2010). The realisation of children's participation rights: Critical reflections. In B. Percy-Smith & N. Thomas (Eds.), *A handbook of children's and young peoples' participation: Perspectives from theory and practice* (pp. 11-23). New York, NY: Routledge.

Levesque, R. J. R. (2014). Childhood as a legal status. In G. B. Melton, A. Ben-Arieh, J. Cashmore, G. S. Goodman, & N. K. Worley (Eds.), *The sage handbook of child research* (pp. 38-53). Thousand Oaks, CA: Sage.

Liebel, M. (2012). *Children's rights from below: Cross-cultural perspectives.* New York, NY: Palgrave Macmillan.

Lundy, L. (2007). "Voice" is not enough: Conceptualizing article 12 of the United Nations Convention on the Rights of the Child. *British Educational Research Journal, 33*(6), 927-942. doi:10.1080/01411920701657033

Mann, H. (1999). Vygotsky's methodological contribution to sociocultural theory. *Remedial and Special Education, 20*(6), 341-350. doi:10.1177/07193259902000607

Mannion, G. (2007). Going spatial, going relational: Why "listening to children" and children's participation needs reframing. *Discourse: Studies in the Cultural Politics of Education, 28*(3), 405-420. doi:10.1080/01596300701458970

Mayall, B. (2000). The sociology of childhood: Children's autonomy and participation rights. In A. B. Smith, M. Gollop, K. Marshall, & K. Nairn (Eds.), *Advocating for children: International perspectives on children's rights* (pp. 126-140). Dunedin, NZ: University of Otago.

Mayall, B. (2013). *A history of the sociology of childhood.* London, UK: Institute of Education Press.

Nilsson, I., & Townsend, E. (2010). Occupational justice: Bridging theory and practice. *Scandinavian Journal of Occupational Therapy, 17,* 57-63. doi:10.3109/11038120903287182

Parsons, T. (1951). The social system. London, UK: Routledge & Kegan Paul.

Prout, A., & James, A. (1997). A new paradigm for the sociology of childhood? Provenance, promise and problems. In A. James & A. Prout (Eds.), *Constructing and reconstructing childhood: Contemporary issues in the study of childhood* (Rev. ed.) (pp. 7-33). London, UK: Falmer Press.

Qvortrup, J. (1994). Childhood matters: An introduction. In J. Qvortrup, M. Brady, G. Sgritta, & H. Wintersberger (Eds.), *Childhood matters: Social theory, practice and politics* (pp. 1-23). Brookfield, VT: Ashgate.

Qvortrup, J. (2011). Childhood as a structural form. In J. Qvortrup, W. A. Corsaro, & M. Honig (Eds.), *The Palgrave handbook of childhood studies* (pp. 21-33). New York, NY: Palgrave Macmillan.

Reynaert, D., Bouverne-De Bie, M., & Vandevelde, S. (2012). Between "believers" and "opponents": Critical discussion on children's rights. *International Journal of Children's Rights, 20,* 155-168. doi:10.1163/157181812X626417

Richards, S., Clark, J., & Boggis, A. (2015). *Ethical research with children: Untold narratives and taboos.* New York, NY: Palgrave Macmillan.

Saadi, I. (2012). Children's rights as "work in progress": The conceptual and practical contributions of working children's movements. In M. Liebel, K. Hanson, I. Saadi, & W. Vandenhole (Eds.), *Children's rights from below: Cross-cultural perspectives* (pp. 143-161). New York, NY: Palgrave Macmillan.

Smith, A. (2011). Respecting children's rights and agency: Theoretical insights into ethical research procedures. In D. Harcourt, B. Perry, & T. Waller (Eds.), *Researching young children's perspectives: Debating the ethics and dilemmas of educational research with children* (pp. 11-25). New York, NY: Routledge.

Smith, A. (2015). Rights, research and policy. In A. Smith (Ed.), *Enhancing children's rights: Connecting research, policy and practice.* New York, NY: Palgrave Macmillan.

Smith, C., & Greene, S. (2014). *Key thinkers in childhood studies.* Chicago, IL: Policy Press.

Stadnyk, R., Townsend, E. A., & Wilcock, A. (2010). Occupational justice. In C. H. Christiansen & E. A. Townsend (Eds.), *Introduction to occupation: The art and science of living* (pp. 329-358). Upper Saddle River, NJ: Prentice Hall.

Tisdall, E. K. M. (2012). The challenge and challenging of childhood studies? Learning from disability studies and research with disabled children. *Children & Society, 26*(3), 181-191. doi:10.1111/j.1099-0860.2012.00431.x

Tisdall, E. K. M., & Punch, S. (2012). Not so "new"? Looking critically at childhood studies. *Children Geographies, 10*(3), 249-264. doi:10.1080./14733285.2012.693376

Townsend, E. (1993). 1993 Muriel Driver lecture: Occupational therapy's social vision. *Canadian Journal of Occupational Therapy, 60*(4), 174-184.

Townsend, E., & Whiteford, G. (2005). A participatory occupational justice framework: Population-based processes of practices. In F. Kronenberg, S. Simó Algado, & N. Pollard (Eds.), *Occupational therapy without borders: Learning from the spirit of survivors* (pp. 110-126). New York, NY: Elsevier Churchill Livingstone.

Townsend, E., & Wilcock, A. A. (2004). Occupational justice and client-centered practice: A dialogue in progress. *Canadian Journal of Occupational Therapy, 71*(2), 75-87.

United Nations. (1989). *Convention on the Rights of the Child.* Geneva, Switzerland: Author.

United Nations. (2008). *Convention on the Rights of Persons with Disabilities.* Geneva, Switzerland: Author.

Vygotsky, L. S. (1978). *Mind in society.* Cambridge, MA: Harvard University.

Weisner, T. S. (2008). The Urie Bronfenbrenner top 19: Looking back at his bioecological perspective. *Mind, Culture, and Activity, 15,* 258-262. doi:10.1080/10749030802186785

Whalley Hammell, K. (2008). Reflections on…well-being and occupational rights. *Canadian Journal of Occupational Therapy, 75*(1), 61-64.

Whalley Hammell, K. (2015). Participation and occupation: The need for a human rights perspective. *Canadian Journal of Occupational Therapy, 82*(1), 4-8.

Whalley Hammell, K. R., & Iwama, M. K. (2012). Well-being and occupational rights: An imperative for critical occupational therapy. *Scandinavian Journal of Occupational Therapy, 19,* 385-394. doi:10.3109/11038128.2011.611821

Whiteford, G., & Townsend, E. (2011). Participatory occupational justice framework (POJF 2010): Enabling occupational participation and inclusion. In F. Kronenberg, N. Pollard, & D. Sakellariou (Eds.), *Occupational therapy without borders: Vol. 2: Towards an ecology of occupation-based practices.* New York, NY: Elsevier Churchill Livingstone.

Wilcock, A. A. (2006). *An occupational perspective of health.* Thorofare, NJ: SLACK Incorporated.

Woodhead, M. (2011). Child development and the development of childhood. In J. Qvortrup, W. A. Corsaro, & M. Honig (Eds.), *The Palgrave handbook of childhood studies* (pp. 46-61). New York, NY: Palgrave Macmillian.

Woodhead, M. (2014). Martin Woodhead. In C. Smith & S. Greene (Eds.), *Key thinkers in childhood studies* (pp. 229-238). Chicago, IL: Policy Press.

Woodhead, M. (2015). Childhood studies: Past, present and future. In M. J. Kehily (Ed.), *An introduction to childhood studies* (3rd ed., pp. 19-33). New York, NY: Open University.

Woodhead, M., & Faulker, D. (2008). Subjects, objects or participants: Dilemmas of psychological research with children. In P. Christensen & A. James (Eds.), *Research with children: Perspectives and practices* (pp. 10-19). New York, NY, Routledge.

Wyness, M. (2012). *Childhood and society: An introduction to the sociology of childhood* (Rev. ed.). New York, NY: Palgrave Macmillan.

Section II

Putting Collaboration Into Practice

The chapters in this second section describe strategies that therapists may use to collaborate with children in therapy and research. Similar to looking through a magnifying glass, the main focus of this book zooms in on the challenges and ways of creating partnerships with children. These interactions occur at the same time therapists are collaborating with caregivers and educational staff. Many, such as the interview strategies, but not all of the ideas may be incorporated during interactions with adults.

The purpose for identifying them is to make explicit what experienced therapists know. These thoughtful and often subtle strategies are usually unnoticed by casual observers. These ways of working with children as partners make therapy appear easy and fun. Yet, the collaboration process is complex. Thus, one aim of this section is to show WHAT client-centered and strengths-based collaboration entails.

A second purpose for this section is to increase therapists' repertoire of actions they can take to facilitate collaboration. Guided by occupational therapy theories, interactive clinical reasoning, and therapeutic use of themselves, therapists choose which combination of strategies to apply within a certain interaction. To do this they need to have a range of ideas in their "toolbox."

The third purpose is to advocate for and show how to apply them with children. At times, children's competencies are underestimated. When approaches used with adults are unsuccessful with children, some believe the cause is a lack of competence. However, if therapists adapt and use child-friendly approaches, children's competencies become evident. Described in this section is HOW to make approaches client centered, strengths based, and child friendly.

The fourth purpose is to show what collaboration looks like from the beginning to the ending of therapy. In addition to eliciting and strengthening children's voices, the therapists' role in the partnership is to be a guide. For instance, the chapters on setting respectful limits, avoiding power struggles, and making smooth transitions clarify how therapists may avoid being authoritarian and instead work as partners.

The last purpose of this section is to describe ways to collaborate, adapt, and involve children in research. Details and examples are provided for how to do studies *with them* versus *on them*. This is important because occupational therapists have the potential to use their expertise to gain knowledge from a variety of children, including those with disabilities.

This art of collaborating in therapy and research is essential for meaningful and effective practice. Occupational therapists often are strong advocates for all children, especially those who are nonverbal. By knowing how to collaborate, therapists can strengthen children's voices and assist them in changing their lives.

4

Introduce Yourself and Explain Therapy

CHAPTER OVERVIEW

When you first meet children to start therapy, you have to convey by your words and actions that collaboration is desired. In this chapter, there are strategies you may use when you introduce yourself, explain therapy, and start conversations. Also described are considerations for matching your approach to children's desired level of emotional involvement, and creating a common language that is understood by all.

CHILDREN'S DESCRIPTIONS OF WHAT THEY THINK YOU SHOULD KNOW

Dr. Clare: "When therapists first meet children, how can they make them feel comfortable?"

Noah (age 8): "Introduce yourself."

Raquel (age 10): "Try to be friendly."

Sam (age 10): "They can make me feel comfortable by saying nice things."

Debbie (age 11): "Ask the kids, 'What is your day like at school?'"

Joe (age 11): "Find out as much as you can about the children. Find out if they know Spanish or English."

Dr. Clare: "If you had fun the first time you are with a therapist, what would you think about coming back?"

Nicole (age 12): "I would want to come back because I would know that I was going to have fun instead of just listening to that person talk."

Elena (age 11): "I would feel really excited because it meant I was going to have fun and not be bored the whole time."

BEGINNINGS

The first time you meet children, they will try to determine what kind of person you are and if they want to be in therapy. They will wonder if you are going to be nice or mean. They will question the purpose and nature of therapy, and especially wonder whether they will like it. First impressions count. Use your words and actions to convey a "come join me" message and encourage them to symbolically make the first step into the world of occupational therapy, a place of new possibilities.

Introduce Yourself and Describe Therapy

In the beginning, warmly welcome children and start to discover their uniqueness and positive attributes. Show them that you are a nice and caring person, and that therapy will be challenging and fun. Pique their interest.

Curtin, C.
Strategies for Collaborating With Children: Creating Partnerships in Occupational Therapy and Research (pp. 53-76).
© 2017 SLACK Incorporated.

Greet the Child and Explain Therapy

> **Children might be thinking:**
> *Who are you? What is your name?*
> *Are you like anybody I know? Are you mean or nice?*
> *What are you doing here?*
> *Why am I here?*
> *Am I in trouble? Did I do something wrong? I feel nervous.*
> *What are we going to do? Am I going to have to work?*
> *Will this be hard? Boring? Fun? Will I like it?*

The first messages to give are that children are welcome and you want to be with them. When you acknowledge people, you reflect their worth and importance, whereas to ignore them implies they are not valued. Therefore, it is critical to greet them, as well as caregivers. This allows them to perceive you as being attentive to them and to others. Children, like adults, want to be heard and understood. Most of them like having the complete attention of an adult who truly listens, but they do not want to be pressured to talk if they do not feel like it. Those who are nonverbal also want to be recognized as a person and have their own way of communicating acknowledged as their voice, whether it is the use of sounds, gestures, or eye movements.

Another reason to acknowledge children is to minimize the power differential. They know and expect that adults will tell them what to do. They have learned that in certain situations they are to be quiet and not interrupt adults. Often they find that their voices are downplayed and discounted. They may not know that you, an adult, want and expect them to talk. Your words and actions need to show them that it is safe to converse with you and share their perspectives.

Children will try to make sense of who you are and will rely on their history with other adults to do so. They will wonder if you are like anyone else they know. For example, the first time you walk into a kindergarten room, they often ask if you are a teacher or someone's mom or dad. These roles are familiar, and they know how to act with parents and teachers.

They also may automatically assume that you are like the other adults in their life. One time, a friend took his 5-year-old son with him to buy a motorcycle. His son wandered over to a burly guy in a black leather jacket and, to the man's surprise, asked him, "Whose daddy are you?" The son assumed that all men were fathers like his dad. Similarly, children also develop expectations based on their experiences that influence their initial perception of you. The information gathered from these previous adult relationships color children's expectations before they even meet you.

Your style of interaction additionally influences their perceptions of you. I have found that they have their own classification system. When they first meet you, they look for signs of whether you fit in their category of being a nice or mean person. I interviewed children on what they thought nice or mean adults would say or do. Their answers clearly delineate the differences (Table 4-1). In the first session, expect that they will be continually evaluating you to determine that you are a nice person. They will rely on their perceptions to decide whether therapy is a good place to be and to weigh whether they want to stay.

As you begin to spend time with children, be open to learning who they are as individuals. Before meeting them, you may have an image of them that is based upon others' descriptions or written reports. Let children tell and show you who they are. View them in a positive light. Some, for instance, may be described by other staff as being difficult and noncompliant. Rather than assuming the same viewpoint, approach them with the intent of understanding their lives from their perspectives. Learn about their unique talents and abilities. Also consider what life circumstances and other environmental factors may contribute to their way of being.

Give a Warm Greeting and Introduce Yourself

The type of greeting you choose may range from just eye contact and waving hello from a distance to saying "Hi" and directly asking the children questions. You ordinarily start the interaction with a warm greeting that is tailored to their easiest method of learning. If, for example, they have limited vision and hearing, you may want to greet them by signing in their hands. If possible, use communication systems to create ways for those who are nonverbal to respond.

Then introduce yourself in a way that enhances their comfort level and tell them your name. Do this with all even if you question their comprehension. Whether you use your first or last name gives them a clue about how formal or casual you wish the relationship to be. Children are used to calling teachers by their last names. To call an adult by the first name in settings like schools is more unusual and signals that this may be a different kind of adult-child relationship. However, it is your personal and cultural choice on what name you wish to be called.

If they are from a different culture than your own, learn their rules to establish how children and adults are supposed to greet and interact with each other. Otherwise, if you impose a Western-style greeting, you could create a dilemma for the children, making them unsure of how to respond. Also consider what their life experiences may have taught them about adults. Some families who are refugees due to persecution have learned to rely only on themselves and to be distrustful of authority figures. Children may have been cautioned about talking to strangers. Let them know that you want to be respectful of their feelings and learn about their customs. Be sensitive and recognize that you may make mistakes in your approach. Ask them to please inform you if what you do or say is upsetting or

TABLE 4-1

CHILDREN'S QUOTES ON THE DIFFERENCES BETWEEN NICE AND MEAN ADULTS

NICE ADULT	MEAN ADULT
Says, "Hi" to you.	Ignores you.
Smiles.	Makes a bad or mean face—like this [scrunches face into a scowl].
Is funny, always happy.	Always mad, gets mad at you.
Does not yell at you.	Yells, yells for no reason.
Helps you, shows you what to do or how to do stuff, says helpful things.	Says, "I'm not helping you." Does not give help.
Does fun things, plays games, shares toys, surprises you.	Is boring.
Says nice stuff like, "Please" and "Thank you." "Nice job." "You did a great job." "You've been doing good."	Says bad words like, "Stupid" or cuss words. Says mean stuff like, "Shut up," "Stupid kid," or "I don't like that kid."
Tries to makes friends with everybody.	Is a grown-up bully.
Says, "Please would you sit down."	Says (in a harsh tone of voice), "Sit down."
Listens.	Is rude, interrupts, talks out of turn.
Can't be mean.	Hurts your feelings.
Says yes.	Says no all the time.
Gives rewards.	Gets you in trouble, gives detention for no reason, tells on you.
Gives you things (candy, snacks, prizes, awards).	Says, "You can't have…."
Lets you do what you want.	Does not let you do what you want.
Gives first graders first-grade work.	Gives first graders sixth-grade work.
If adults are super nice, they let kids be a teacher.	They never listen, just talk.

awkward for them. If you do not speak their native language, have them or other bilingual children teach you how to say hello.

It also is important to extend common courtesy to children. Discover what name they like to be called and what is the correct pronunciation, if you are uncertain. Some families refer to children by their nicknames. Other children may use their middle name, initials, or a variation of the name if they have the same name as a parent.

Fabulous Five: Greet Children and Introduce Yourself

- **Tell children your name and who you are.**

"We need to do an occupational therapy evaluation with Todd," the occupational therapy student said to the second-grade teacher.

His teacher pointed to a curly-haired child and beckoned him. "Todd."

He sat paralyzed for 10 seconds and swallowed several times. "Am I in trouble?"

"No," his teacher reassured him.

He shuffled his feet as he followed us down the hall.

I waited for the occupational therapy student to do introductions. She looked to me for help, so I stooped until my eyes met Todd's and said, "Hi. My name is Dr. Clare. I'm an occupational therapist. This is Sue. She is an occupational therapy student—like a student teacher. Your mom wanted us to check on how you are doing with coloring, cutting, and writing. Sometimes we can help you discover ways to make school easier." As I spoke, the tightness in his shoulders eased.

- **Acknowledge all children, even if you are unsure whether or not they understand.**

When I entered the classroom, I saw 9-year-old Kathy sitting with her head tilted to the right side and her eyes fixated on the wall. Her mouth hung open in an oval shape and drool covered her chin. I moved into her line of vision and said in a soft voice, "Hi, Kathy. My name is Dr. Clare and I'm going to spend some time with you to learn what you like. One thing your teacher said is that you enjoy looking at the computer. Together, we can try and see if there are easier ways for you to use the computer." Kathy's eyes blinked, although I was unclear if her reaction was a response.

- **Greet children using their easiest channel for learning.**

"Katrina is good at dancing," her teacher said, referring to Katrina's bobbing head movements. "So the sign for her name is the letter 'K' dancing on the arm. She has limited hearing and loves to talk with her eyes."

On Katrina's first day, I sat facing the petite 6 year old who was upright in a stander. First, I smiled and waved hello. Next, I signed her name by raising my index and middle finger and placing my thumb between them. Then I bounced my hand as if dancing on my extended arm. She responded with her happy clicking sound. "My name is Dr. Clare," I continued and signed my name by curling my fingers into a 'c' and tapping my wrist as the sign for doctor.

- **Greet children in their native language if possible.**

"¡Hola! ¿Cómo estas?" I said to 10-year-old Maria.

"Bien," she replied with a smile.

Pinching my index finger and thumb together to let her know I only spoke a little Spanish, I said, "Yo hablo un poquito español."

- **Use a communication device so children may greet you back.**

I pushed the button of the communication device and recorded, "Hi. My name is Trish." When 7-year-old Trish maneuvered her electric wheelchair into the room, I greeted her. Then I showed her the red button and said, "You can say hi too." She followed my cue and pressed. A smile spread across her face as the message played. "It's nice to meet you," I responded.

Explain Therapy

Another important part of introductions is to provide a general description of therapy. Many children do not know what occupational therapy entails. Until they are given information, they will create their own theory. They will wonder what it is like and may worry about being with you. Once you provide an explanation and clarify your role, you decrease the likelihood of misunderstanding and may prevent distress.

It is essential to explain therapy even when you are unsure if the children understand. It is always best to assume they comprehend everything, whether they are able to respond or not. It is common for children who are nonverbal to have experiences where adults talk with each other as if they were not there. People often expect that children who lack control of their bodies also lack awareness of what is being said.

Determine quickly how you may help children and tailor the discussion to each individual's circumstances. For example, how you define therapy is different for children with cancer than for those with fine motor difficulties. To create your description, you may use your knowledge about the impact of illness or disability on occupational functioning. Another method is to discuss therapy using information gleaned from caregivers' interviews or based on your observation of the children's interests, desires, or even frustrations.

Start by giving a simple explanation like you would with adults, making sure to use words children understand (Figure 4-1). In one to two sentences, describe the purpose for being together. For children who are nonverbal, you may want to explain therapy with the exact words you would use with a same-aged peer and then provide a simpler description to give the children every opportunity to comprehend. Your initial description of therapy also will be in broad terms such as "to help figure out ways to make school easier." As time progresses, you will work with children, caregivers, and educational staff to determine the specific purpose and meaning of their therapy. In this instance, you would explore what specific aspects of school the children and caregivers want to change.

A discussion about therapy in child-friendly terms lets them know that you respect them. Providing information regarding the nature of therapy also shows children that you intend to be honest and upfront with them. Your truthfulness about what will happen and why you are meeting facilitates the development of trust and confidence in you. Hence, the more you help children understand what therapy involves, the better the relationship will be.

Fabulous Five: Provide a Broad Description of Therapy

- **Provide a description of therapy based on your experience with children having a similar disability.**

"Hi, Deana! My name is Dr. Clare and I am an occupational therapist. I'm on your right side."

"Doc-tor Clare," the preschooler with limited vision responded. She raised her arm, searching for my face.

When she touched my cheek, I said, "We get to spend some time together and can work on helping you do things by yourself. We'll do some fun activities to help you get stronger and feel more comfortable getting dressed and touching all kinds of toys. I'm glad I get to be with you!"

- **Explain therapy based on your knowledge of an illness or condition.**

Eight-year-old Abby peeked through her long blonde bangs, checking the toys and games in the oncology clinic's therapy room. I smiled and said, "In occupational therapy we use activities to help you learn ways to help yourself. Kids usually enjoy it. I know you've been very sick and you may not be able to do everything like you did before. Together, we can find fun things for you to do now."

- **Provide an explanation of therapy following an observed or stated frustration or concern.**

"Today we are going to make the letter 'B,' and we get to use glitter," the kindergarten teacher said.

"Yea!" the class yelled in unison.

Six-year-old Scotty threw his hands over his ears. "That's too loud."

Later that afternoon, I smiled at Scotty, introduced myself, and said, "I saw that when everyone yelled today it bothered you." He nodded. "Well, I work with kids and teachers to figure out ways to make school more comfortable. I want to learn what you do that helps. Then we can figure out more ways for you to feel better, especially when the class gets really noisy."

- **Describe therapy in connection to children's needs or interests.**

On Rose's first day in her new school, I joined her second-grade class in the lunch room. I watched Rose frown as her hand shook with tremors, making it difficult to scoop the food onto the spoon. I left and returned with a weighted spoon, a scoop bowl with raised edges, and a sheet of nonslip plastic to keep the bowl from sliding. "Hi, Rose. I'm Dr. Clare. I'm an occupational therapist. I can help make it easier for you to eat."

- **Connect your explanation of therapy to the children's environment.**

"Occupational therapy is about learning ways to help you in school. It's about getting to know your strengths—that means those things you do well. And your strategies—that means all your good ideas. We'll use activities to help your eyes and hands work together and make writing easier. I work with your teachers and parents too to find out what helps you learn the best."

"I don't write good," 7-year-old Stefan said.

"Well, together we'll figure out how to make it better."

Incorporate Books or Stories to Describe Therapy

Many children appreciate and better understand a description of therapy if it is presented in a book. Children are accustomed to books. Often caregivers read stories to children that contain a message. For instance, the lesson of numerous fairy tales is how good prevails over evil. At school, older children are used to learning math, history, and science through textbooks.

Books are an ordinary part of children's school lives and a familiar way of learning. One benefit of using them

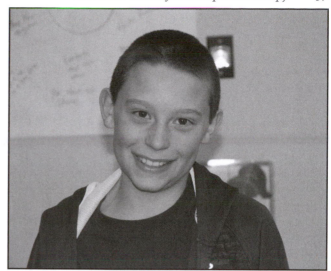

Figure 4-1. Explain therapy using words children understand.

is that it is easier for children to visualize what will happen when you match pictures to your description of therapy. Illustrations are especially helpful for those who are visual learners or limited in their understanding of words. For younger children you may want to design a book or a PowerPoint presentation showing photographs of you, the therapy space, and various activities. You can then send it to caregivers to show children before they come to see you. You also may create a booklet with drawings of various children to correspond to the words used. Depending on their reading level, some may want to read it themselves or you may read to them.

Another way to capture children's interest and attention is to put together your own story about therapy and encourage the children to participate. You may adjust the details in the story to the children's own circumstances. This adaptation makes it relevant to their lives. By talking about children in general, you also may convey that others have similar feelings or experiences. For example, how it is common for most children to be afraid when in a hospital.

A creative twist is to present your description through the use of a cartoon character. Draw your own figure and use this imaginary person to explain therapy. Even if you question your drawing ability, you can always sketch a simple face. When children chuckle at your drawing, use the opportunity to mention how you tried your best, acknowledge the funny-looking character, and then laugh at yourself.

In addition, children can make their own books. Have a description of therapy on one page and ask children to draw themselves. Many children like drawing and especially like talking about themselves. This allows them to be the star of the story and implies that they are special. You could then add more pages in future therapy sessions.

Fabulous Five: Use Books to Explain Therapy

- **Give caregivers a book of photographs and descriptions of therapy to show children before the first session.**

I wrote a note to 3-year-old Ian's caregiver and attached it to the book for him. "Sometimes it's hard for children to meet someone new. To make it easier for Ian, I am sending this book. It would be helpful if you could read it to him before he comes to the clinic."

On the first page underneath my photo were the words, "Hi. My name is Dr. Clare. I am an occupational therapist." On the second page was a picture of the clinic. "Here is our room where we do fun activities. Kids call it OT." The third page contained photos of puzzles, toys, and construction materials. "You get to play with toys and games. You will learn how to do things all by yourself."

- **Develop a booklet to give to children explaining therapy.**

On 6-year-old Janessa's first day in the children's psychiatric unit, she was given our booklet explaining the unit. She turned the pages and looked at the pictures as the nurse read her the following page about therapy:

You will have occupational therapy to learn ways to help yourself. Occupations are activities such as playing, learning, making friends, talking with others, and taking care of yourself. In occupational therapy, you will be involved in activities to learn ways and behaviors to help you be the best you can be.

- **Write and read a story about children coming to therapy.**

When 4-year-old Lacey came from her hospital room into the therapy room, I said, "I know this is your first day here so I want to tell you a story.

"Once upon a time there were boys and girls who came to a place called occupational therapy. Some kids called it OT. One girl's name was…

"What should her name be?"

"Susie," she replied.

"On the first day, Susie was scared because she had to meet someone new and she did not know what to do. The therapist's name was Dr. Clare, just like mine. 'I am happy to meet you,' Dr. Clare said to Susie. 'Here in OT, you get to play special games so that you will get stronger and be able to do more. It always helps me to know what you are good at and what you like. I also want to hear what you are thinking and feeling.' Dr. Clare showed Susie a game.

"'This looks hard,' Susie said. 'I don't know if I can do it.'

"'Just try. I will help you,' Dr. Clare said.

"Susie tried. 'I did it. OT is fun.' The end."

Lacey grinned and relaxed.

- **Create a cartoon book about therapy.**

On the first page of the book, I read the captions of my smiling cartoon character: "Hi! Welcome to occupational therapy. I am an occupational therapist and my name is Dr. Clare. This is a place where you can use activities to learn about yourself. First, I am going to talk with you to find out what you like to do and what is important to you. Okay, tell me what you are good at doing?"

Eight-year-old Greg, who was starting to experience muscle weakness, drew himself on the corresponding blank page and wrote, "Playing soccer."

"What is going well for you?" the character asked.

"In school, they are going to give me a motor scooter."

"Oh, that should help you get around school. I know toward the end of the day you get tired," I said and then pointed back to the figure.

On the following pages, the cartoon character asked the questions: "What do you like to do for fun? What's easy for you? What helps you learn? What do you wish was easier or better?" Then, on the last page, the figure said, "Thanks for telling me about you. Now we can decide what do together."

- **Have children make their own therapy book.**

"You get to make your own book. Let me read the words at the top of the page." I tapped the first piece of paper. "In occupational therapy I will learn ways to help myself." I looked at 7-year-old Stewart and added, "Draw a picture of yourself at the bottom of the page." After he finished drawing, I turned to the next page with the word "Strengths" on top. "Strengths mean what you are good at or something good about you." I pointed to myself. "For example, I am a good swimmer and I am kind. Write five things about you that are good."

"Hmm." He drummed his index and middle fingers on his lips. "Oh, I know," he said and started writing. "I am good at telling the truth. I am nice. I am good at taking care of my dog, using my brain, and showing respect for others."

Later, we completed a page containing a list of strategies, and on the last day he drew himself leaving therapy.

Use Alternative Formats for Explaining Therapy

There are other possible adaptations, in addition to the use of books, to describe therapy. One consideration is to identify the children's learning style and then match your approach to their best mode of learning. To make this determination, use the information you have already obtained about the children, as well as your observations in the beginning moments. Although many children understand verbal explanations of therapy, others will comprehend better with visual aids such as picture symbols.

Another factor you may change is who provides the explanation. Sometimes it is easier for children to listen to their peers. The children may trust their friends or classmates more than you, a complete stranger. When you have peers describe therapy, they will be more likely to use language or terms the children understand. You also will discover how peers are viewing therapy and their rationale for attending.

An additional way to alter the format is to explain therapy to caregivers in the children's presence. You would choose this step with the assumption that the children are listening to what you say. For this reason, make sure to use words that children understand. This adaptation is especially helpful with children who show trepidation.

To facilitate comprehension use props, toys, or even a playful metaphor. Be creative and transform the simple act of explaining into a fun time. When you use complementary methods in addition to talking, you are shifting to the children's natural ways of expressing themselves. It is easier for children to convey their thoughts and feelings through play. With younger children, you may facilitate understanding by the use of props, puppets, objects, or pictures.

Whatever method you choose, talk with children and relay the gist of therapy in simple terms. Children will value your efforts to include them and help them understand what is going to happen. By providing this important piece of information in child-friendly terms, you will contribute to the development of a collaborative frame.

Fabulous Five: Incorporate Alternative Formats to Explain Therapy

- **Use picture symbols to explain therapy.**

Six-year-old Edward walked into the room flicking his fingers. I introduced myself and asked him to sit down. He slid into the chair and kept his eyes downcast on the table. I moved a Velcro board within his line of vision. It had a row of three picture symbols representing therapy. I pointed to the first picture of a hand writing on paper. "Here in occupational therapy, we will work together to help you with your writing." Then I touched the second picture in the row showing a computer. "Next, we can find ways to make writing on the computer easier. There are new computer programs you can try and see if you like them." Then I pointed to the last picture of two hands using sign language to say "all done." "Every time you come, we will do writing, work on the computer, and then you'll be all done."

- **Have other children explain what you do.**

I went into the third-grade classroom and asked to see Alexis, a student recently referred for therapy. Melissa, who was in one of my groups, saw me. She turned to Alexis and said, "She's fun."

"Tell Alexis what we do," I said.

"We do games to make our hand muscles strong and make writing easier."

- **Describe therapy to caregivers in the presence of children and make sure the children understand the words used.**

Six-year-old Frank and his mother came into the therapy room in the pediatric oncology clinic. I sensed that he was leery of me, so I waved my hand at the various activities on the floor and encouraged Frank to choose. He encircled the magnetic blocks with his arms, pulled them close, and began building a robot. I gave his mother a handout describing therapy and read her the following:

"My name is Clare, and I am an occupational therapist. I will assist your child, Frank, in developing and maintaining normal occupations. This means what your child does in daily life such as playing, being with friends, learning in school, and being involved with your family. As an occupational therapist, I am concerned with how your child is doing in everyday activities including how your child spends time, as well as how your child feels about him- or herself.

"During clinic time, the purpose of therapy will be to provide a place for your child to use activities to express feelings and to help with coping...." I assumed Frank was listening, so I turned toward him and translated, "Coping means helping you get through tough times."

I continued reading, "...To be with other children, who are having a similar experience, and to become more aware of or develop new skills and strengths...." Looking at Frank, I added, "Strengths are things you are good at or do well."

I turned back to his mother. "...To explore new interests and, if needed, to discover ways of maintaining or adapting activities done during the day. Also in occupational therapy, parents often talk with other families. This can be an informal way of meeting and supporting each other. Let me know if I can help you as well as your child at this time." Then I discussed contact information.

Turning my head, I looked at Frank and said, "I know it's not easy to be here in clinic. With me, you will get to meet other kids. We will do different activities to help you when you are here, and together figure out ways to help you at home and at school. I know sometimes kids get tired and can't do all the things they like. We try to find new things they like and can do. If you have any questions just let me know. I'm glad I got to meet you."

He smiled at me and seemed reassured.

- **Incorporate puppets or props to explain therapy.**

"Pick a puppet," I said, pointing to an array of animal and people puppets. Jeremy touched the brown bear. I slipped the puppet on my hand and moved the mouth. "Hello, Jeremy. The reason you are here with Dr. Clare is to learn about all the good things you do and to help you with cutting and making your letters."

"Okay, Mr. Bear," the 4 year old replied.

- **Use a metaphor to describe therapy.**

"We are like detectives," I said, peeking through a magnifying glass. "In therapy we are going to look for and discover as many good things about you as we can— like what you are good at, what you think is fun, and what good ideas you have to help yourself." I handed 8-year-old Max the magnifying glass and asked him to pick one of the folded papers, each one containing a question in tiny print. "Please read the question."

He pressed the magnifying glass close to his right eye as he read the words. "Something good about me is...." He tapped his chin as he thought. "I'm super nice. I don't tell anyone I'm not their friend."

Match Your Approach to the Level of Emotional Involvement Desired By Children

Children might be thinking:
I don't know you.
I'm not sure about you.
I don't know if I want to be with you.
Am I going to miss something good or fun if I am with you?

The approach you choose to start an interaction depends upon the degree of involvement children desire. Unless they are shy or have had traumatic experiences, they usually enjoy having complete attention from an adult. Some children who have been abused will, understandably, be leery of new adults in their lives. They may wonder if you will hurt them. Consequently, they try to protect themselves by shying away from close involvement. Younger children also may be hesitant to talk with you until they have an opportunity to get to know you. They may stay close to their caregivers and look for reassurance.

In addition to their experiences with other adults, familiarity is another major factor affecting how children will act with you. If they see you in their class every week, they will be more at ease with you. However, if you are an unfamiliar adult, you need to earn their trust. You have to demonstrate through your actions, nonverbal language, and words that they will be physically and emotionally safe with you.

Respect children's need for physical and emotional closeness by watching their nonverbal cues regarding how involved they wish to become. Then think about what approaches might be successful. If you are a stranger, plan to proceed more cautiously. For children who are apprehensive, include familiar people in the session and give them time to observe you. At the next level, you may choose to be with children without making any requests for them to respond, for instance watching them play.

A greater level of involvement entails a verbal exchange. Using these approaches, you might ask them to respond in a simple manner such as choosing an activity or showing you their favorite toy. Let the children lead by being responsive to their comfort level and then follow their cues of when to increase interaction.

Give Children an Opportunity to Observe You

One approach that involves the most minimal involvement is to have children observe you. This is a wise choice if they look guarded or skeptical. Observation gives them time to judge and decide whether they are interested in being with you. If you force children to interact before they are ready, they may withdraw, or respond but classify you in the "mean" category. Forcing them to respond also may lead to a power struggle, which taints their perception of you. You may be seen as a person who is more interested in controlling than caring.

For children who are the most mistrustful, let them observe you from a distance. This allows them to feel safe as they see for themselves what kind of person you are. Be patient and give them the time and space needed to determine when is it right to initiate interaction.

Fabulous Five: Provide an Opportunity to Observe You

- **Let children watch you interact with their friends or classmates.**

When 5-year-old Travis flashed a hesitant look at me, I decided to sit at his table next to his classmate, Jenna. She was happy for the attention and started telling me about her picture. I smiled and told her, "The colors you chose are very bright." Travis watched and listened to my conversation with Jenna. Next I shifted my attention to Travis and watched him draw. As the concerned look faded from his face, I said in a gentle tone of voice, "I see you're good at drawing. I would love for you to draw a picture for me. Let's go to my room. I also have some toys that are fun. Come with me." He stood and followed me to the room.

- **Have children observe you talking with their caregivers.**

"What are Carlos's strengths—his good points?" I asked his mother while he colored. *I know he is listening and I want him to understand that I am a nice person.*

"He's funny, helpful, smart, loving, and full of energy," she replied.

I turned to the 4 year old and smiled. "Wow, that's a lot of good things about you."

- **Play next to children with your attention on the activity.**

When I saw 3-year-old Carly on the floor, I sat down next to her. Then I pulled a musical top out of my canvas bag and played with it. Her eyes, snapping with curiosity, swung over to the top. "Can me try that?"

"Sure. It's fun. Check it out."

- **Stay still so children can observe you.**

The day before school started, the classroom staff, caregivers, and students met for a picnic. "This is Mickey," his father said, pointing his 4-year-old son hiding behind his leg.

"Hi. My name is Dr. Clare," I replied and smiled. I remained seated on the picnic bench. After a few minutes, Mickey peeked around his father's leg. I waved hello and said, "You are meeting a lot of new people today. I'm glad you are here. We're going to have fun at school."

- **Wait for children to move closer to you.**

As I moved closer to 6-year-old Landon, he stepped back until he was leaning against the wall. In response, I sat down and said in a soft voice, "When you are ready, join me at the table." He wandered around the room, still wearing his leery look. "I see you want to check out the room first. That's okay," I said and smiled. After 4 minutes of exploring, he came to the table.

Interact With Children With a Familiar Person Present

When younger children are doubtful about you, it is common for them to hide or wrap their arms around their caregiver's leg. One helpful approach, especially with preschoolers, is to include familiar people in the session. The presence of a caregiver, sibling, classmate, or friend can provide a sense of security. The support of another person means they are not alone in facing you, a stranger.

An additional option is to go to their place, such as a classroom or home, where they are at ease. Children can then learn about you by observing how others react in your presence. If, for instance, they see their caregivers smiling and relaxed, they are more likely to be open to engaging with you. The amount of time it takes for children to finally warm up varies. Proceed slowly until they indicate an interest in being with you.

Fabulous Five: Incorporate Familiar People When First Meeting Children

- **Encourage caregivers to stay with or close to younger children.**

"Do you want me to stay in the room or leave?" Carey's mother asked.

"Please stay," the occupational therapy student replied, and the mother settled in the rocking chair.

Three-year-old Carey went to the table. She drew a picture, scrunched it in her hand, and then hurried back to her mother. "Look, Mommy. It's me."

- **Use a familiar adult to help children make transitions in the first session.**

At the private school, Trent's second-grade teacher went to get him at the end of snack time so I could do an evaluation. When he saw me, he threw his crackers on the floor, folded his arms, and refused to budge. The teacher asked her assistant to watch the other children and told me she would join us. "I'll go with you, Trent," she said and he followed. She stayed for the first two test items. She left when Trent looked at ease.

- **Incorporate family members in the first session.**

Three-year-old Ashley hugged her mother's leg as her older sister, Laura, stood nearby. I placed three wooden puzzles on the table and said, "Laura, could you please help your sister do one of the puzzles?"

"Come on, Ashley, I'll show you," Laura said. Ashley followed her to the table and then snuggled close as her sister demonstrated.

- **Join children in a familiar setting surrounded by people they know.**

First, I observed Gina on the playground, and she squinted and pursed her lips showing her uncertainty about me. I stood off to the side and smiled. At the end of recess, I followed the kindergartners into the classroom and sat at her table. I smiled as I watched her color and cut a kite for the letter "k." The others held up their pictures for me to see.

"Pass me the red marker," Ruben said.

"I can only eat red stuff that God made," Gina offered.

"Red stuff—you mean like ketchup?" Ruben replied. "That's the wildest thing I've heard in my whole entire life."

"I can eat ketchup. God made that," she replied in a relaxed tone.

- **Have children be with a friend or classmate in the first session.**

I spent 10 minutes in the kindergarten class before asking Jeff to come with me to another table. I told him I wanted to spend some time with him to do cutting and drawing. He puckered his lips and started to cry. His teacher turned to the child sitting next to Jeff and said, "Martin, go with Dr. Clare too."

"Okay," Martin said. Jeff's tears stopped, and he followed his best buddy Martin to the table.

Join Children Without Making a Request for Them to Respond

A next level of involvement is for you to join children in their play or activities without requiring a response from them. At this juncture, you want to become part of the children's world. They are the center of attention and decide what will happen. It is similar to being at a football game. They are the primary players and you are just watching on the sidelines—often making comments or cheering for them.

For some children, especially younger ones, it is best to start without speaking. With a calm and friendly demeanor, move next to them. You may be a quiet presence or assume the role of a helper. Try not to ask any questions or make any requests. To join them you may have to behave in an unusual way, such as crawling under a table to sit by them, or imitating exactly what they do.

For children who appear more comfortable with you, it can be helpful to comment on their actions. You may state what you observe or joke in a playful way. For instance, when pencils have rolled off the table, I have said, "Oh no, the pencils are running away. Come back, pencils. Come back." Be conscientious to only make comments and avoid demands. By doing so, you show that they get to determine whether and when they would like to engage with you.

Fabulous Five: Be With the Children

- **Sit next to younger children and watch with full attention without talking.**

I sat next to 3-year-old Karen and watched her paint. First, she plopped a yellow blob of paint on the paper. Then she swirled her brush in the water and dabbed the green paint. She made one long vertical stroke for a stem and two short strokes for leaves. I kept my eyes on her creation, and periodically glanced at her face and smiled. Three boys zoomed around us, but my gaze remained on Karen. She shifted her eyes sideways to see if I was still looking and smiled when she saw I was.

- **Join children's play without using words.**

Four-year-old Cole snapped four Lego pieces together. I sat on the floor next to him, smiled, and crossed my legs like him. When he started to hunt for blue pieces, I searched as well. Without saying a word, I handed him five. Cole clicked them together. "It's a cannon—in case bad guys come."

- **Imitate children's actions.**

I slid onto the preschool chair next to 3-year-old Maxine, who was paralyzed on her right side. She pounded her left fist on the table three times. I responded by pounding my fist three times on the table using the same rhythm. She turned her head to the side, glanced at me, and grinned. She hit the table twice, and I imitated her. "Ah–ah," she sang with delight.

- **Comment on children's actions.**

I went into the kindergarten classroom and joined 5-year-old Latoya at her table. "I want to make a bumble bee. I need yellow," she said while searching for the pencil in her box.

"It's hiding from you," I said. She snagged the tip of the pencil but it slipped from her fingers and slid back in the box. "Sometimes they're hard to get out," I commented. She grappled with what to do but then tipped the box so all the pencils dropped on the table. "That makes it easier," I said.

She covered the black body with yellow stripes. "He's so cute."

- **Move next to children instead of asking them to come to you.**

Four-year-old Jimmy crawled under the classroom table. He adjusted his clipboard and drew a circle. I smiled, waved hello, and scooted beneath the table to join him. "I want orange," he said as he fingered the crayons. When he finished coloring, he showed me the picture, "All done. Look what I've made. It's a pumpkin."

Ask Children to Respond in an Easy Way

The highest level of involvement is to interact with children, expecting them to respond either verbally or nonverbally. Follow their lead for when this is appropriate. Even at this point, you want to make it easy for them to be with you. You may start simply by asking children to show you something they value or demonstrate how a toy works.

You also can engage children by having them select an activity or game. For some, it is easier to talk about the activity first and then, as they relax, gradually ease into talking about themselves. For others, you may ask easy-to-answer questions that are related to the activity.

Fabulous Five: Ask Children to Respond in a Way That Is Easy for Them

- **Ask children to show you their favorite toy.**

When I entered 3-year-old Tina's house, I smiled and moved slowly toward her. "Show me your favorite toy or stuffed animal—the one you really, really like." She walked over to the couch and hugged a purple dragon.

"Does your dragon have a name?"

"DeDe."

I sat on the floor, pulled wind-up toys out of my bag, and motioned to Tina. "Bring DeDe with you and sit here. I want to show you some fun toys."

- **Have children choose an activity to start the interaction.**

"What would you like to do?" I asked 7-year-old Jeremy and pointed to a display shelf. He shrugged his shoulders. "There are wood kits, leather wrist bands, or painting," I said and placed models on the table. "Or if you want to do something else that's okay too. Just let me know." Jeremy pondered his choices and then pointed to the car wood kit. "Sand it first," I said as I demonstrated the step. He slid the sandpaper back and forth while I watched without saying a word.

- **Ask children to demonstrate how a toy works to begin the interaction.**

"How do you get that car to move?" I asked 3-year-old Carson.

"It's easy. Look." He pulled the car back and let it go. The toy zipped across the room.

"Wow, that car went really far. I'm glad you were here to show me how it works."

- **Involve children in an activity, discuss the activity, and wait for them to initiate conversation about themselves.**

I handed 5-year-old Adam a hunk of clay. He wrapped his hands around it and squeezed.

"How does it feel?" I asked.

"Wet. I like it."

The clay squished through his fingers and he began to chat. "My dad not at home. He at work. He works downtown. Sometimes he go to North Dakota. He has to go on an airplane."

"I bet you miss him when he's gone." He nodded. "Who else is in your family?"

"My mom and my two sisters."

- **Ask questions related to children's current activities.**

As the occupational therapy student watched 3-year-old Gabriella play with family figurines in the dollhouse, he asked, "Do you have any brothers or sisters?"

She nodded. "My mom has two babies. One baby is in her stomach. It's a girl baby."

Create an Interactive Dialogue When Caregivers Are Present

> **Children might be thinking:**
> *Do I want to stay with you?*
> *Oh, I get to talk too.*
> *I'm glad you're talking to me.*

After greeting, explaining therapy, and approaching children, choose whether to start the initial conversation with them or their caregivers. Because children communicate their desire for involvement nonverbally, watch for subtle signs of willingness. As always, consider the cultural context of the nonverbal messages. Notice how their bodies change once they see you. Do they move closer to their caregivers or friends as if hiding? Do they assume a protective stance like crossing their arms and tucking their chins

to their chests? Or do they stay relaxed? Also observe if they flash an "I'm curious and am willing to talk" look or if they stare at the floor. Use these cues to help you determine how to respond.

Another consideration is whether it is better to talk to children and caregivers separately. It may be best to talk to each party in private when children have concerns about the caregivers or if the caregivers want to focus on the children's difficulties. In situations where children are present when caregivers start talking predominately about problems, acknowledge the caregivers' concerns and then shift to talking about children's strengths or neutral topics. Make arrangements to meet alone with the caregivers. If you talk with children and caregivers separately, make it a practice to summarize to each the key helpful points the other person made. Of course, helpful comments means not sharing information the other person would find hurtful or destructive.

Overall, you want to promote a free-flowing conversation that mingles the voices of the children, caregivers, and you. Sometimes it is a balancing act to make sure all voices are heard. If you find that caregivers answer all the questions without giving children a chance, acknowledge your appreciation for their help. Emphasize how you wish to hear from everyone. Throughout the conversation, you may have to encourage children to speak. Be cognizant about dividing your attention, and consider whether your actions are paving the way for an interactive dialogue.

Let Children Know They Are to Be Partners in the Conversations

It is usually best to ask children the first question to indicate that you are interested in talking with them. Many children enjoy having the attention of an adult even if it is a stranger. They may be pleased to have a primary role in the conversation. However, if they appear reticent, which may be from shyness or distrust, start the conversation with caregivers. This allows children an opportunity to observe you. When they become more comfortable, you may then ask them questions.

> **Fabulous Five: Engage Children in the Conversation.**
> - **Start the first conversation by asking children questions.**
>
> "What are you good at doing?" I asked 7-year-old Kevin.
>
> "Football," he replied.
>
> "Anything else?"
>
> "That's all I know right now. My dad knows more, not me."
>
> "Kevin likes to shoot baskets and ride his bike," his father said. "He's very helpful."

Kevin nodded and added, "It's my job to take out the trash without him asking me."

- **Ask caregivers questions in the first conversation until children feel comfortable to speak.**

When I saw the apprehensive look on 6-year-old Nicole's face, I turned to her mother and started the conversation by asking, "What does Nicole like?"

"She likes teddy bears, butterflies, and ponies. She loves to draw and likes to read."

Nicole smiled at me and said, "She forgot something. I like monkeys."

- **Use information from caregivers to ask children questions.**

"Last week, Kurt had an endoscopy to check his throat," his mother said.

I turned to the 5 year old and asked, "How was it for you?"

"It was okay. They gave me sleeping gas."

- **Divide your attention in the first conversation between caregivers and children.**

"Tell me something you like," I said to 7-year-old Stewart.

"I like to eat."

Then I turned to his mother and she responded, "He also likes to spend time with me. Sometimes we go to the park and he loves to swing."

"What do you like at school?" I asked, pivoting my attention back to Stewart.

"Gym."

"What's easy for you at school?"

"Kickball."

"Stewart is getting good at reading," his mother added. "We read books every night."

"What's hard at school?" I asked as I shifted my gaze back to him.

"Math."

"Spelling too," his mother said. "Second grade is hard."

- **Ask children if they have any questions during or after the first conversation.**

After I introduced myself as Dr. Clare and explained therapy, I said, "Do you have any questions?"

"Why are you called doctor?" 6-year-old Dan asked.

"There are two kinds of doctors. One you go to when you get sick and sometimes that doctor gives pills and shots. I'm another kind of doctor. I went to school for a long time, passed a very hard test, and wrote a book."

His mouth opened in awe. "Oh," he said. "You're just like Dr. Seuss. He wrote a book."

Recognize Children's Presence

While you are talking with caregivers, it is crucial to continually acknowledge the child's presence. This recognition may be conveyed in various ways. Sometimes you only have to glance at him or her and make eye contact. This brief connection gives the message that you are thinking about them. When you periodically look at children, you also are more likely to be aware of what they are doing and be attuned to their feelings. For some it is boring to wait, especially if there is nothing to do. If you plan to ask caregivers more than a couple of questions, involve children in an enticing activity and monitor their interest.

As caregivers relay information, listen for their concerns because this will help you meet their needs. Their worries also provide clues about how the children feel about themselves and their lives. Encourage caregivers to describe their hopes for their children's future. During the discussion, consider children's feelings and perspectives, and then offer an empathetic remark.

Another tactic to involve children in the interaction is to make positive statements. Listen as caregivers talk for any mention of children's strengths or talents and then seize the opportunity to compliment the children. Your positive comments will often capture their interest and foster a desire to stay with you.

When conversing in front of children, continue to assume that all are listening even if they do not look like they are paying attention. Once I was at a meeting where the child sat at a computer at the other side of the room while the adults talked about his problems in school. After a few minutes, I checked with him and saw that he had not even turned on the computer—he was staring at a blank screen and listening to the conversation. I asked him if he wanted to join us or did he prefer to go to another room. He moved to the table with us.

You may use these methods to acknowledge children and to indicate the need for their involvement even at a nonverbal level. Your actions clarify that therapy is a situation in which you expect them to participate. Your recognition of their presence lets them know they are to be a primary partner.

Fabulous Five: Acknowledge Children on a Continual Basis

- **Have frequent eye contact with children while talking to caregivers.**

"Allie has a voice of her own," her grandmother said. "She's good at telling me what she wants."

I turned my head to the 3 year old and smiled.

Her grandmother continued, "She likes to do things by herself. She tells me, 'I can do my own self.'"

I looked at Allie, raised my eyebrows, and made my mouth into an "o" shape to indicate I was impressed.

- **Engage children in an activity while talking with caregivers.**

Four-year-old Brianna entered the occupational therapy clinic and wandered around the room. "Come to the table and try these fun toys," the occupational therapy student said with a smile. Then she turned away to talk with the mother.

Brianna sauntered over in slow motion and sat. She ignored the toys and looked bored. A few seconds later, she jumped out of her seat and grabbed her pink coat. She tugged on her mother's arm and said, "Mommy, I go now."

The occupational therapy student turned her attention back and said, "Let me find something you would like."

- **Make empathetic comments to children while conversing with caregivers.**

"We just moved to a new house," John's father commented. "He keeps asking if we can go back to the old house."

"I bet you were sad to leave your old house," I said to the 5 year old, and he nodded.

- **Say positive statements to children based on caregivers' conversations.**

"What does Nina do well?"

"She's good at keeping the peace," her mother replied. "She tries to make sure everyone is happy. If her brother or sister is crying about a toy, she gives it them."

I looked at the 6 year old and said, "Sounds like they're lucky to have you as a sister."

- **Recognize that children listen to all conversations.**

A doctor and five medical students stood in the doorway, reviewing Amber's case history as I sat by her bedside. The 10 year old locked her eyes on them and listened as the doctor revealed the details.

As they spoke, I asked her, "Is it strange to hear people talk about you, but not to you?"

She nodded her bald head and replied, "Yeah."

Use Nonverbal Language to Convey You Are a Nice Person

> **Children might be thinking:**
> *You look nice.*
> *Maybe you care; I can trust you.*
> *You're nice.*
> *I like being with you.*

While you are greeting children and explaining therapy, you are also speaking to them through nonverbal language. This powerful avenue of communication is crucial for showing your good intentions and for creating the conditions needed to build a connection. Through the use of your body, present yourself as being warm, friendly, and approachable.

Children are experts at reading nonverbal language. They scrutinize all your expressions and actions as they try to determine the kind of person you are. They tend to rely on the gestalt of your cues to ascertain your character. Their perception also is influenced by the degree of congruence between your verbal and nonverbal language. If, for instance, you greet them in a gruff manner, they will give more credence to how it was said than the actual words spoken.

Your nonverbal language is mostly unconscious and is strongly shaped by your culture. Create a routine of mindfully scanning and reflecting on your body language. Although it is challenging, make your unconscious conscious, especially in situations where you are uncomfortable or are with someone with a different cultural background. Think about what children see when they look at you and how they may interpret your unspoken language. For instance, are your arms crossed? Are you standing and towering over the children? Continually be conscious that various cultures ascribe different meanings to nonverbal language.

Children will make judgments about you based upon their appraisal of the configuration of your nonverbal language. Tickle-Degnen and Gavett (2003) found that the nonverbal process of building rapport involves learning about each other by showing friendliness and the intent to work together, providing full attention, and coordinating the level of involvement through the matching of nonverbal cues. The following ideas presented in this section are reflective of a Western culture.

Demonstrate Cooperative Intent and Friendliness

Because children are attentive to how you present yourself nonverbally, it is important to demonstrate friendliness and cooperative intent, considering not only the words you say, but also all types of nonverbal language. Your facial expressions are strong indicators of who you are and of your intentions. A smile is a signal of friendliness. Children will scrutinize the appropriateness of your facial movements and look for signs of whether you are nice or mean.

Your hand gestures can add or detract from the interaction. Sometimes gesturing aids their understanding, shows your excitement to be with them, or suggests that you are a lively person. There are times when too much gesturing can be overwhelming, and children appreciate your being still. Also, learn what gestures are considered offensive in other cultures.

The amount and intensity of what is considered appropriate eye contact varies. You want to look at children enough to demonstrate your interest and attention, yet at the same time being sensitive to what is comfortable to them. Too much eye contact may be viewed as staring or being imposing. Too little suggests you are indifferent or uncaring.

Norms regarding touching also differ. Of course, all touch must be nonsexual in nature. For many countries, touch is a normal part of interaction. When my friend, a Brazilian occupational therapist, went to Canada for a year, she had to consciously limit her amount of touching, which in Brazil was considered normal. In the United States, it is more acceptable to have physical contact with younger children than older ones. You also will need to touch children who require physical assistance such as getting in and out of a wheelchair. When holding them, use a secure but gentle grip, which can convey warmth in a way words cannot.

Consider your body position. When you are standing, you are looking down on them. You may, especially if you are tall, present as being overpowering and overbearing. A different message is given, however, if you squat or sit so you are closer to their eye level. You also can show openness by keeping your arms uncrossed, leaning forward, and staying relaxed.

The range of personal space or the distance maintained between each other depends on the comfort level of you and the children. Learn their cultural, physical, and emotional boundaries of what is comfortable. Watch for and respond to signs of distress, such as backing away, grimacing, or turning their heads to the side. There are times when moving closer becomes a show of support. Younger children often equate sitting closer with the thought that you like them, whereas older ones may desire more distance between you.

Your tone of voice is another crucial aspect. Children want you to use a respectful and caring tone of voice. They find it especially demeaning if you talk to them in the same tone you talk to a baby. A harsh tone of voice implies you are controlling or intimidating. On the other hand, the use of a caring and concerned tone of voice conveys cooperative intent.

Fabulous Five: Show Friendliness and Caring Through Your Nonverbal Language

- **Smile and present yourself in a friendly manner.**

I smiled as I introduced myself to 6-year-old Bobby. He grinned back. We started walking to the therapy room and I asked, "What do you like to do for fun?"

He grabbed and tightly gripped my hand. "I'm a master at Candyland."

I responded, "Wow, that's great."

- **Maintain a relaxed and open body position.**

On my first day at the specialized program, I stood in the doorway surveying the classroom. Twelve-year-old Lynette marched over to me, put her face 3 inches from mine, and raised the right side of her lip as if snarling.

"Hi. My name is Dr. Clare," I said softly. I kept my arms loosely by my side and told myself to stay calm.

Lynette squinted at me and then walked away. Later I heard she had a history of hitting and eye-poking.

- **Move to children's eye level if possible.**

"Carl is in the special education room. He has been having a lot of problems," the school psychologist said. "The kids are making fun of his buck teeth."

When I entered the classroom, I asked his teacher which student was Carl. Then I approached the third grader at his desk. I squatted below his eye level, smiled, and said in a soft, soothing voice, "Are you Carl?"

"Yeah."

"Hi. My name is Dr. Clare, and I am an occupational therapist. I know you had occupational therapy at your old school." He nodded. "It says in your records that we are to meet 30 minutes once a month."

"A month, that's good. I use to go once a week and before that every day."

"That means you have done well," I said, and he smiled. "So next Tuesday, we will meet and you can let me know what's important to you. Then we can decide how we want to spend our time together. I look forward to seeing you then." He nodded in agreement.

- **Use a caring tone of voice rather than demanding and controlling intonations.**

As I headed to Carl's class, the school psychologist told me, "Carl's father died yesterday."

"Oh no. That's so sad," I responded. When I reached his classroom, I reintroduced myself. "Remember we met last week. My name is Dr. Clare and I am an occupational therapist. It's our time together now."

"My name is Carl Brown and my dad is dead."

"I'm so sorry," I said in a gentle and serious tone of voice. We went into a quiet room and I handed him putty.

As he manipulated the putty, he talked about his father. "My dad had bone cancer. He couldn't walk because both of his legs were amputated. They're going to cremate him. The army will shoot off rounds and I'll get a flag."

- **Move close to children to show support.**

"That's not the way to make a 'g.' It goes like this," the school volunteer told 5-year-old Jared, and he began to cry.

I moved close to him and whispered, "I can see that upset you. Let's go over to that table." Because he saw me every week in his class working with other children, he followed me to the empty table. "How come you're crying?"

"Because I was trying my best but the teacher thinks I wasn't."

Maintain Full Attention

To build a rapport with children, it is necessary to provide them with your full attention. Before meeting, it is good to clear your mind of other distractions. Then when you are together, position your body toward them so you can closely watch and listen. Maintain your focus and nonverbally give your utmost and complete attention, for example, leaning forward, changing facial expressions, nodding, and/or maintaining eye contact. You also show your intention to be totally focused and present by waiting for them to interact or respond on their own terms. Your actions and nonverbal language let children know that you value what they say and do.

Fabulous Five: Provide Your Full Attention

- **Position your body toward the children.**

I walked into the green hospital room and sat on an empty bed with my arms relaxed by my side. Ten-year-old Yolanda sat upright on the other bed with her back propped against two fluffy pillows. I shifted my body so I faced her as I introduced myself. "How come you're in the hospital?" I asked in a gentle tone of voice.

"I get headaches and the doctors don't know why."

- **Maintain comfortable eye contact.**

When I introduced myself to 12-year-old Tim in his classroom, his eyes focused on the floor.

"Let's go to another room so we can talk." He stood and followed me into a quiet section of the library. Then he dropped his chin to his chest, pulled a deck of picture cards out of his pocket, and began thumbing through them. "How is school going?" I asked as I snatched a quick glimpse of his face. Then I focused on his hands, following his lead by not making eye contact.

"Mainly I've been getting As and Bs here," he replied as he continued to stare at the rotating cards.

"How are you doing with writing assignments?"

"Okay, I guess. I'm not very good at typing. I can do ten words a minute with two fingers. I need to get better."

- **Lean forward to show attentiveness.**

"My dog PJ ran away. Someone kidnapped her. PJ was a good dog. She never bit a living soul in her life. All she bites is her bones."

As 7-year-old Pam talked, I leaned forward and responded by lowering my eyebrows and making a sad face. "I bet you miss her."

- **Nod your head to indicate you are listening.**

"My mom's friend died. She's sad," 5-year-old Shelley said. I nodded my head in understanding and maintained my focus on her face. She continued, "That's why I give her lots of hugs."

- **Demonstrate attentiveness by being patient and giving children time to respond.**

"I would like to talk to you for a minute," I said to the second grader. Gabriel responded by covering his eyes with a blank piece of paper. I waited a few seconds and he lowered it. "What are you good at?" His eyes met mine for an instant but then he turned his back to me. I slowly swiveled so I could still see his eyes and quietly waited for a response.

"I'm good at playing games."

Coordinate Your Nonverbal Language With That of the Children

You also connect with children when you adjust your nonverbal language to their current emotional state or need. To do this, you have to assume a responsive versus a controlling stance. Observe what puts them at ease and at the same time learn the nuances of their nonverbal language. Adapt your tone of voice to match the children's. For instance, if they are talking in a serious tone, you would respond likewise. For some, you may need to monitor the loudness and pitch of your voice—a loud, booming tone may be overwhelming, especially for younger children. Watch their pace and then either slow down or increase your own until you are moving at the same speed. Also be aware of the intensity and amount of your movements as well as your energy level.

In the beginning, try to use slow motion with limited arm movements, particularly when children are over-stimulated or highly sensitive to excessive movement. Continually adjust your nonverbal language to match theirs. You may provide a mirror reflection by subtly copying the children's body language. If they lean forward with their hands on the table, you would do the same. To be effective, your imitation must not be exaggerated. Get in synchrony with the children by following their lead and adapting your nonverbal language.

Fabulous Five: Adjust Your Nonverbal Language

- **Modify your tone of voice to match children's comfort level.**

I waited in the school doorway to greet 8-year-old Lori and her mother and guide them to the therapy room for testing. When they arrived, I saw the tops of Lori's eyes covered by her blue hood and tufts of shoulder-length blonde hair whipping around in the wind. "Loud noises and the wind bother her," Lori's mother said. She turned to her daughter and added, "You can put your hood down now."

I smiled at Lori and said in a soft, soothing voice that was almost a whisper, "Welcome. I'm glad I get to be with you."

- **Adjust to children's pace.**

Six-year-old Abby strolled down the hallway and stopped every 5 feet to examine whatever she saw. I initially thought, *It's going to take a long time to get to the room. I wish she would hurry up.* Then I told myself, *Slow down. Move at her speed.* We moved in unison and when she stopped to stare at the sunlight on the floor, I commented, "I see you looking at your shadow." She grinned in return and we continued at her pace.

- **Adapt your movement or energy level.**

After the fire drill, 11-year-old Joseph went to the corner of the classroom and faced the blank walls. He repeatedly flicked his shirt with his left hand as he jumped in place. I grabbed his weighted vest from his desk. Because he was already overstimulated, I slowly approached him from the side. "That fire drill was really loud. Here's your vest. It may help you get calm again." He slid on the blue vest and then stood still.

- **Match children's emotional tone.**

As we walked to the therapy room, 5-year-old Matt's voice dropped. "I saw a man get hanged. It's only pretend," he said as if he was trying to convince himself.

"That would be scary," I replied with a serious expression. "Where did you see it? TV? Movie?"

"Movie. It's only pretend."

"Yes. It is not real."

- **Mirror children's body language.**

"Draw about a time when you were really happy. This will help me get to know you."

"Really happy," 9-year-old Nicholas whispered to himself and leaned toward the table. "How can I do that? I don't really draw."

I sat on the other side of the table and, as if looking in a mirror, I leaned with the same angle, matched his serious expression, and whispered back, "It doesn't have to be a perfect picture."

His voice grew louder as he sketched and said, "Probably the day I could ride my bike and then, when it got too cold, I went home and played computer games."

Give the Message That a Partnership Is Desired

One message in creating a collaborative frame is to let children know that you desire a partnership. Through your words and actions, you help develop the mindset that they will have a voice in this relationship. Convey that you are more interested in helping them than controlling them.

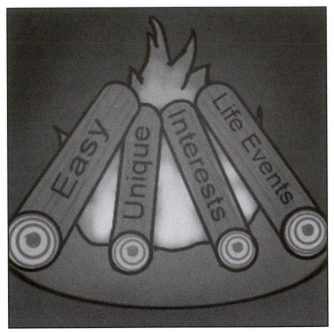

Figure 4-2. Use conversation starters.

Use Conversation Starters

> **Children might be thinking:**
> *It's easy to talk to you.*
> *Hey, I know that answer.*

Experienced therapists must have a repertoire of conversation starters (Figure 4-2). It is helpful to have a variety of topics in your knowledge bank in order to quickly match the first question to the children's circumstances. Casual conversation following your greeting is another opportunity to create a reassuring situation and minimize their anxiety about being with a stranger. This first conversation can put them at ease and breaks the ice so they may get to know you. The way you start an interaction gives children clues about how to act with you. When, for example, you start by asking questions about their lives, you are indicating that you want to hear from them. Your agenda at this time is to make it easy to talk with you. This enables you to learn about their meaningful occupations.

Although most people think of a conversation as an exchange of words, you also may need to create a conversation using nonverbal or alternative communication. Some children teach you about themselves through communication devices, picture symbols, gestures, sign language, or even facial expressions. Another means of starting a conversation is to ask caregivers to bring a photo album of the children. This allows you to ask questions while the children look at the photos. Use of these various types of communication can encourage children to express themselves and begin a meaningful exchange.

As children respond to your questions, listen carefully for any nuggets of information about their character and strengths. Their responses also give you information regarding their developmental level. Language and cognitive abilities are reflected by the words they use and type of answers given. This information helps you adjust your conversation to their level of understanding and match upcoming activities to their abilities.

What seems like a simple conversation can be very beneficial. You are starting the process of having children teach you about their daily occupations. The simplest answers, even from one question, can be useful to engage the children. Furthermore, create a sense of flow by weaving all the tidbits of information gained into future conversations and activities.

Start With Easy Topics

When you first meet, select a topic that would be comfortable to discuss. When you ask easy-to-answer questions, children are pleased because they know the answer. This helps them feel competent and allows for successful conversation. Another factor influencing your choice of the initial question is your location. If you are walking down a school hallway, you may choose casual and light topics such as their interests. However, if you meet children in a hospital room, you may start with a more serious topic to show your awareness of their difficult situation.

Open-ended questions such as, "How is school going?" tend to elicit the most information and give children an opportunity to add what they think is important. Some children, however, prefer to start by answering questions that have a definite answer, such as, "Do you have any brothers or sisters?" Later, switch to open-ended questions.

Fabulous Five: Ask Easy-to-Answer Questions

- **Ask children how old they are.**

"How old are you?" I asked Tammy.

"Four," she said and held up the corresponding number of fingers. "A long, long time ago when I was 3, I went to the zoo."

Seeing the smile on her face, I responded, "I bet you had fun. Tell me about it."

"The elephant pooped." We both laughed.

- **Inquire about children's families.**

"Lukas, do you have any brothers or sisters?" I asked the kindergartner.

"One brother. He born the same day. I born first."

"Oh, you're twins."

"Our birthday is the same day."

- **Ask children what they like.**

Five-year-old Felicity ran into the room. I signed for her to sit and pointed to a chair by the table. She sat down and patted the other chair, indicating where she wanted me to sit. I sat there and pointed to the five picture symbols spread apart on the table. "What do you like?" I asked, moving my index finger over all of the cards. Then I tapped each card. "Do you like puzzles, cut, draw, or play on the computer? If you don't like these, point to the 'more' card." I rested my finger on a picture of two hands signing the word "more."

She picked up the puzzle card and squished it in her palm. "Oh, you like puzzles," I responded. "I'm glad to know that." I proceeded to pull animal and fish puzzles out of the cupboard.

In the second session I mentioned, "I remember you told me you liked puzzles so I made sure to bring more."

- **Inquire if the children have any pets.**

"Do you have any pets?" the occupational therapy student asked 6-year-old Phillip.

"We got a puppy. Puppies are little. They grow up. My dog is black. Her name is Denali. I pet her and we have a purple leash."

- **Ask children questions related to the season or weather.**

"Did you have a good summer?" I asked 5-year-old Dale during the first week of school.

"Yeah. I got a large ice cream cone. I almost ate the whole thing but there was a hole in the cone and I didn't want to get it all over me. That's why I threw it away."

Acknowledge Children's Individuality

For the first conversation, another realm of questions centers on children's uniqueness. This cluster of conversation starters shows that you are paying attention to the constellation of characteristics that makes them individuals. These types of questions also may be used to emphasize how they are special, particularly if you are commenting about their personal appearances or assets.

Children's names are frequently symbolic of a family history or tradition. Some are named after a cherished relative. Others may be the second or third generation to have the honored name. Often, there is a story behind the name. By making this a topic of conversation, you provide them with an opening to tell family stories.

Clothes tend to be a reflection of their interests and a window into their world. One 3-year-old girl wore her beloved butterfly shirt until there were holes in it, and her interest was always piqued by any mention of or pictures of butterflies. Others have worn football jerseys or T-shirts covered with their favorite animals. The reference to clothes can be an easy way to capture their attention and engage them in conversation.

The other method to accentuate their uniqueness is to highlight their strengths and abilities. This requires close observation and a focus on their positive attributes. When you start a conversation in this manner, you convey your awareness that they are individuals with specific likes and talents. This recognition is helpful for developing a positive relationship.

Fabulous Five: Recognize Children's Uniqueness

- **Comment on children's names.**

"What's your name?" I asked the 6 year old.

"Anne Frances."

"Oh, that's a pretty name."

"I was named after my aunt."

- **Mention a detail about the children's appearance.**

"You have gorgeous red hair," I told 11-year-old Gina.

She grinned and replied, "People with red hair bring good luck."

"Well, it's my lucky day because I get to be with you."

- **Comment on children's clothes.**

Seven-year-old Penny, wearing a lavender dress covered with white flowers, swished down the hall. "That's a beautiful dress," I commented.

"My grandmother gave it to me. She lives in New York. We fly on a plane and get to see her in the summer."

- **State an observed strength.**

While helping in the second-grade classroom, I overheard two students talking as they drew pictures of spring. "I need a peach-colored pencil," Winston said out loud to himself.

"I have one you can use," Alex offered, handing it to him.

The next week, I met with Alex. "The last time I was in your class," I said, "I noticed that you were nice to Winston by sharing your pencils with him."

"He used to think I was dumb, but we're good friends now."

- **Comment about children's abilities.**

Five-year-old Ernie raced across the playground with swift strides, and I rushed to stay with him.

"You're a fast runner."

He patted his chest and said with a smile, "I'm getting big."

Inquire About Interests

Another wonderful way to begin a conversation is to inquire about children's interests and favorite things. This line of questioning quickly leads to the discovery of their valued occupations. When you ask them about their favorite activities, you learn what is special and important to them. This information may help you further the conversation by talking about a topic they enjoy.

Information regarding their favorite activities also may be used to explore later whether they are able to participate in them. You might find, for example, that some children with a severe illness are no longer able to be involved in their hobbies. They may need to develop new interests or require adaptations to their old ones. This information can be vital for defining the purpose of therapy.

You also may incorporate their interests into therapy. If, for instance, you find that children love baseball, you may design activities that have a baseball theme or ask them about their experiences with sports. After you learn their favorite color, some children appreciate it if you make a special effort to bring materials with that color. Discovering and using children's interests makes the conversation and ensuing activities fun and engaging.

Fabulous Five: Discover Children's Favorites

- **Ask children about their favorite colors.**

"What's your favorite color?"

"Pink," 6-year-old Hannah replied.

I looked at her shoes and said, "I noticed your pink sneakers have glitter on them."

She nodded. "At home I have pink pillows and pink PJs. I just love pink."

- **Inquire about favorite activities.**

Before the first session, I asked Bruce's father to program the communication device to include the activities his son enjoyed. Then, in our first meeting, I asked the ten year old, "What is your favorite thing to do? What do you like to do the best?"

His father pressed the touch screen until he reached the activities page. "Listen to books, play my keyboards, watch movies, play with my dog," the device said as it scanned the row. Bruce's wobbly fingers touched the switch and the words "play with my dog" appeared on the screen.

- **Ask what is the children's favorite food or drink.**

I joined 5-year-old Carol in the lunch room, introduced myself and informed her that we would do testing the next day. I sat for a few minutes and watched her eat. "Your sandwich looks good. What's your favorite thing to eat or drink?"

"I love pickles. I eat so many I could turn green."

- **Probe about favorite places.**

"Where's your favorite place to go?" I asked 8-year-old Whitney as we walked down the school hallway.

"I love to go camping in Nebraska—just me, my mom, and my dad."

"What do you like about it?"

"It has a big lake and you can swim in it all the time. Last year we almost got hit by a tornado. Sand was blowing, rain was blowing, and hail started to come down. I was scared. I thought I was going to die. I'm too young to die. But the tornado went away."

- **Inquire about children's favorite movie or television show.**

I went into the occupational therapy clinic's waiting room and saw 7-year-old Sean staring at his device. "What are you watching?" I asked.

He replied in his baritone robot-like voice, "A mo-vie."

"What's your favorite movie?"

"Spi-der-Man."

Ask About Life Events

An additional set of useful conversation starters is an inquiry about recent events in children's lives. Their answers to these questions are helpful because it is essential for you to learn what is happening to them and their families. When the conversation centers on children's day-to-day experiences, you get a glimpse into their routines, habits, and daily occupations. Their responses also convey what has made an impression on them and the importance they ascribed to different events.

Children are perceptive and have a keen awareness of their surroundings. Questions about life events are avenues for learning how they understand and interpret their world. Obtaining their perspectives gives you insight into what life is like for them. In addition, creating a conversation about their current circumstances allows you an opportunity to address any fears or misunderstandings. For instance, if you discover children have questions about why they are in the hospital, you can help them get accurate information. When you begin a conversation by asking about their lives, you can gain an appreciation of what they are experiencing.

Fabulous Five: Discuss Recent Life Events
- **Inquire what happened over the weekend.**

"What did you do this weekend?"

Eleven-year-old Evan pressed the switch attached to his communication device. "Movie. Dog. Smart. Excited."

Knowing the latest children's movies, I replied, "Oh, it was exciting for you to see the new movie about the lost dogs who found their way home."

- **Ask about the children's day or week.**

I met 7-year-old Will on a Friday morning, and as we walked, I asked, "How has your week been?"

"Guess what? A real fireman came in my house! There was a real fire! My dad was cooking some food—roasted bologna—and he accidentally overcooked it. My food was

---

all burnt black. It turned to crumbs in my stomach. But I survived!"

"I'm glad you're okay."

- **Inquire about school.**

"How is school going for you?"

Nine-year-old Nick touched different screens on his communication device until he came to the page of feeling words. He tapped the face with the word "boring."

"Is the work too hard?"

He scrolled through the rows and a minute later pressed "no."

"Is the work too easy?"

"Yes" appeared on the screen, and he nodded for emphasis.

- **Ask about current circumstances or situations.**

"How come you are here in the hospital?" I asked 9-year-old Nina.

"Because I vomit every time I cry and get upset."

"Oh, that must be difficult for you."

- **Inquire about recent events in children's lives.**

"I heard your class went to the fire station. Did you like it?"

Three-year-old Robin nodded and said, "Stop, drop, and roll."

"You're right. That's what you do if your clothes are on fire—you stop, drop, and roll."

Create a Common Language

Children might be thinking:
I'm trying to tell you…
Do you understand what I'm saying?
I want…

To have a partnership, every member has to be able to communicate and understand each other. As you begin working together, you develop a common language in which each person uses words the other is likely to comprehend. In addition, everyone tends to develop a shared language after learning each other's style of communication, especially the meaning of nonverbal cues. At times, you as a therapist also may act as a translator converting nonverbal language into words.

You also have to learn children's own ways of speaking and pronunciation. I often have been called Dr. Clay, Care, Air, and Mrs. Doctor Clare. I have learned that reading their lips and watching their facial expressions helps. Expect children to get right to the point and often relay their message in a few words. Recognize that some are more quiet natured than others. There are many meanings behind silence. Be sure to use words they understand. Avoid babbling.

It is important to remember that children's individual communication styles are reflective of their culture. Learn as much as you can about their ways. For instance, to show respect for you as an adult, some children may not make eye contact. Nonverbal language has great potential for cultural misunderstandings. Therefore, understand and respect their cultural norms and values and be open to learning more.

Having a common language provides an avenue for everyone to have a voice and be heard. Children are pleased to discover that you are willing to make every effort to understand them, even if it is not easy, and that you choose to pursue clarification instead of ignoring them. You also connect with them when you listen to all that is relayed and communicate in a way that they easily understand.

Learn Children's Specific Nonverbal Cues

In the beginning, you have to learn children's typical and distinctive nonverbal cues. This allows you to quickly read and interpret the messages children convey without words. When they are nonverbal, it is especially critical to learn their individual ways of communicating. To gain an understanding, talk with caregivers and/or use the environment or situation to identify the meaning of the cues. One time a student signed the word for "where" and then mumbled the word "arf." At first I was confused. Then I saw the therapy dog come into the room, and his question made sense to me.

Often you just have to make your best guess about a possible message. You can let children know what you see. Translate their nonverbal language into words, and then check with them if you are correct. If not, try again.

Fabulous Five: Use Caregivers or the Situation to Identify the Meaning of Children's Nonverbal Language

- **Ask caregivers the meaning of children's nonverbal responses.**

"In October, Peter had surgery to release his tight muscles and was home recovering for a month," his mother said. "He went back to school for one week and then got pneumonia."

I turned to the 11 year old. "Wow, you've been through a lot. Are you feeling better?" Twenty seconds later he moved and his head dropped forward. "What does that mean?" I asked his mother.

"He drops his head for yes and turns his head to the side to say no."

"I'm glad to know that about you, Peter, and I'm happy you're starting to feel better."

- **Suggest caregivers write down how their children, who are nonverbal, communicate.**

"Since you know the common meanings of Henry's sounds, facial expressions, and gestures, it would really help if you could write those down," I said to his father prior to meeting his son. "For example, some children make happy sounds or others have a certain look that means they are upset. Everyone is different. How does Henry show yes and no? How else does he let people know what he is thinking or feeling?"

On the first day, I read the list about the 10 year old. "Henry says yes by smiling or looking at what he wants. Henry says no by pushing things away or looking away."

- **Watch nonverbal language in the first meeting.**

I squatted next to Logan's chair so I would be at his eye level. "Hi, my name is Dr. Clare," I said to the 5 year old. In response, Logan placed his right palm over his eyes. *Maybe he's telling me that he is leery of strangers*, I thought, so I responded, "You don't have to look at me. I just wanted you to know that next Monday I will be spending some time with you. We'll be doing some drawing, cutting, and things like that." He spread his middle and index fingers and his left eye peeked through the v-shaped space. I smiled and added, "I'm looking forward to being with you next Monday."

- **Incorporate information gathered from caregivers to determine how to respond to nonverbal cues.**

Lynette circled around the sixth-grade classroom, flapping her hands. "Happy to you," she repeated four times until she spotted me. Like a race walker, she zoomed over until she was only inches from my face. She tilted her head, narrowed her eyes, and stared down at my Irish-knit cardigan sweater.

I had learned from the staff that Lynette had hurt others but did like order, so I said, "Oh, I think you want me to button my sweater," and then I did so.

She lifted her head upright and flashed me a wide grin.

- **Use the situation to identify possible meanings of children's nonverbal cues.**

Dewy's classmate punched a staff member and screamed as he was escorted to a quiet room. During the commotion, 10-year-old Dewy jumped out of his chair, flapped his hands against his ears, and then pounded his chest with his closed fists.

"You look upset and it's really noisy in here," I said. I showed him two corresponding picture symbols: one of a musical note and the other of a person walking. "Would you like to listen to music on headphones or go for a walk?"

Dewy signed his desire for a walk by moving his outstretched hand in a forward and wavy motion.

Discover Children's Communication Style

To ensure children's dignity and respect, it is critical to learn how they typically communicate their basic wishes and needs. Key messages are *yes, no, stop, more, I need help, I need a break, I am mad,* and *I am frustrated.* For those who are nonverbal, you may have to discern subtle movements, facial expressions, and sounds. Look for any type of response when they are in pleasurable and/or frustrating situations. For instance, watch what happens when they are unsuccessful at a task. Do they make a certain type of grimace, a particular pitch of sound, or repetitive movements like hand flapping? Although many expressions, such as frowning for displeasure, are typical, some children develop their own mannerisms.

It is imperative that all children have at least one way to say yes or no. They must be able to indicate their preferences or desires for them to be active participants in therapy. If you are unsure of what they are telling you, try different types of simple communication systems, such as telling them to touch your hand if they are saying yes.

When working with children, it also is vital to recognize that silence is a form of communication. When they remain silent, they are giving a message. They may be expressing their discomfort, distrust, or dislike of you. Others may stay quiet to allow themselves time to determine if you are "mean" or "nice."

Once you learn children's unique communication styles, you can rapidly respond to their key messages. This quick exchange of meaning then becomes part of the common language, shared by both. In addition, when you understand what children are trying to convey, you can better meet their needs and desires.

Fabulous Five: Learn Basic Communication Messages

- **Learn "yes or no" and "I want…" cues.**

To get to know 7-year-old Carrie, I observed her in class. "Carrie, you haven't had a chance to do the lunch job. Do you want to do it? Make some noise if you do," her teacher said and demonstrated by clicking her tongue. Carrie remained silent and expressionless. Wanting confirmation, her teacher continued, "I don't see a mad or happy face and I want to be sure of your choice."

Her teacher reached for two cards: one containing a smiling face with the word "yes" and one with a frowning face and the word "no." She held the cards two feet apart at Carrie's eye level. "Please let us know—yes or no." Thirty seconds later, Carrie's eyes shifted to the "yes" card. "Yes, you do. You were just being quiet about it."

- **Notice and respect "stop" or "get away from me" cues.**

After a messy painting activity, the paraprofessional used a damp cloth to clean 12-year-old Alfonso's arms and hands. "This would be a good time to push a little harder and give him firm pressure as you wipe his arms," I said, knowing that was a calming sensation for him. The paraprofessional applied the wet cloth with more pressure, and Alfonso sat quietly looking content.

Then the paraprofessional lightly splayed his fingers on Alfonso's knee. "I do this sometimes. He likes it." Alfonso responded by pushing his hand away.

When the paraprofessional tried again, I said, "He's telling you to stop. Respect his cues."

- **Discover the specific ways children ask for help nonverbally.**

During lunch, 8-year-old Flora fiddled with the opening of a milk container. She successfully pulled the flaps apart but then quit. She tapped my arm to get my attention. I turned to her. She gripped my sleeve and pulled it toward her.

"I see you need help. Let me show you how," I said and placed my hands over hers to finish opening the spout.

- **Learn and respect "I need a break" or "I'm frustrated" cues.**

"Sort these shoes," the teacher said to the fifth-grade class during the pre-vocational time.

"Eeeee," Tristan squealed in a piercing high pitch.

Carl responded to the noise by pounding on the desk with his palms, sounding like a drummer. The beat intensified until he flung the desk to the floor. He bounded out of his seat and began clapping, again building to a crescendo. "You are showing us that you need a break. Let's go for a walk where it's quiet," the teacher said and led Carl out of the room.

- **Recognize that children may use silence as a message.**

"Here's some paper. I would like to see your writing. Please write a sentence for me. You could tell me something you like." Seven-year-old Adrian printed "I like…." Then he raised his head and stared at the wall. I waited a minute before asking, "What do you like to eat?" His eyes stayed glued on the wall and he did not respond. Sensing that he was getting uncomfortable, I said, "That's okay. Let's do something else." The next time we met, he jabbered as he played with magnets. "I'm so glad you're talking to me," I said. "Last time you were so quiet."

"That's because I didn't know you," he replied.

Convert Children's Actions Into Words

Once you have learned children's nonverbal cues and overall ways of communicating, you assume the role of a translator. When you see any indication of communication—such as changes in movements, sounds, or facial expressions—interpret what it means. Ask yourself, "What is this child trying to tell me?" Next, convert what you observe into words reflecting the possible meaning of their nonverbal language.

It is good practice to assume that "bad" behavior is also a message. Children often are trying to tell you they are frustrated, angry, or bored. Usually it is helpful to teach children to "use your words" in letting people know what they want or feel. Explain that it is easier to understand words than to guess at what they are thinking or feeling.

When you work with children who do not talk, you must become especially skilled at identifying the subtlest signals conveyed by their body language and deciphering the message. When you do this, you give them a voice, especially for anyone who is oblivious to what they are trying to communicate. Verbalize your thinking as you try to figure out what they are saying so they know you are trying. You may say, "I see you are…. I think you're telling me…." Also let them know when you just cannot understand and say that you really want to know. Sometimes you can ask them to tell or show you in another way like pointing. Make it a habit to use your radar, constantly surveying for what might be their effort to communicate.

Fabulous Five: Translate Nonverbal Cues Into Words

- **Convert eye gaze into words.**

"Who is one of your friends here in class?" the certified occupational therapy assistant asked the 11 year old.

Peter's carrot-topped head turned to the left and his eyes settled in the direction of Liam.

"I see you looking at Liam. Are you are telling me it's him? Is that right? Yes or no?"

Forty seconds later, Peter dropped his head to indicate yes.

- **Interpret body movement or positioning.**

On her way from the cafeteria to her classroom, 11-year-old Louise stopped by the door to music therapy and slid to the floor. "Go back to class," the paraprofessional prompted her, but she did not budge.

"I think you're telling us you want to go to music therapy," I said and presented her with two picture symbols, one showing a hand with a pencil and the second a musical note. "First, you write in class. Then you go to music." In response, Louise reached for my hand and continued down the hall.

- **Convert pointing into words.**

When the occupational therapy student walked into the classroom, 8-year-old Terrance marched over to her. "Ah, ah, ah," he yelled and pointed to the cupboards.

"I see you want something, but I don't know what it is. Show me what you want." Terrance pulled her arm and led her to the top cupboard. She opened it and he gestured to the fish puzzle. "Oh, you want the puzzle. I'll get it for you."

- **Translate children's facial expressions into feeling words.**

Five-year-old Mandy walked down the hall with a droopy mouth. "You look upset. Is something wrong?"

"Daddy left on an airplane. He went to a class for five days. I'm sad."

- **Say, "I see you are/have…. I think you are trying to tell me/us…."**

The preschool class sat at the table and drew circles when the music played. They lifted their markers each time the teacher stopped the music. Four-year-old Xavier made one mark that did not look like that of his classmates. He crossed his arms and put his chin on his chest with a pouting expression. His teacher encouraged him to continue, but he did not move.

"I see you've stopped," I said in a soft, caring voice. "I think you are trying to let us know you need some help." I held a marker in front of him and he reached for it. I gently guided his hand to make the circles and then let him try on his own. "Oh, look, you're doing it," I said as he drew a shape resembling a circle.

Discover Children's Distinct Way of Speaking

For you to develop a common language with children, you also have to be cognizant about their typical ways of speaking. There are some general tendencies. Younger children often talk using a few words or short phrases to get their message across to you. It is common for them to repeat words they have heard adults use. Children also tend to get right to the point and can encapsulate the meaning of their message with minimal words.

Children have accents that vary according to where they were born and other regions where they may have lived. For those whose parents are immigrants, the children may speak combining their native and their new languages. Some children may mix the order of their words. As you spend time with them, you also learn their unique pronunciation that is affected by their language development and their ability to articulate words. Some may leave off the endings of words or substitute sounds for ones they cannot say. Others have unique expressions. One child, instead of saying, "no," always said, "I don't think so."

Initially, you may have to guess at what is being said. You can get clarification by repeating what you thought they said and asking if that is correct. It can help to restate the words you did understand and inquire about the rest of the sentence or message. You may repeat the unrecognized word and ask questions regarding its meaning. These actions will indicate that you appreciate, respect, and want to learn their natural way of communication.

Fabulous Five: Seek an Understanding of the Words Each Child Uses

- **Learn children's idiosyncratic language.**

"Aa, be, be, be," 11-year-old Brian repeated as he paced.

"Go to the bathroom," his teacher responded and made the sign for toilet. She turned to me and said, "That's his way of saying, 'I need to pee.'"

- **Piece words and phrases together.**

"Super Bowl. My birthday," 4-year-old Blair said.

"Your birthday is on the day of the Super Bowl?" I guessed.

He nodded and said, "I'm an oldie. I be 5."

- **Inquire about specific words or phrases you do not understand.**

"Tell me about school."

"I am in the first grade. Our teacher's name is Miss Casanova. It means new house. That's what it means in Spanish. We get to go to Spanish and we get owt class," 6-year-old Eileen replied.

"What's owt class?" I asked, wondering if she was referring to physical education.

"It's where you do some owts—like paint."

"Oh, art class."

- **Repeat the word or phrase you understood and then ask what else was said.**

Four-year-old Deanna drew a picture of her house surrounded by flowers. She started to tell me about her picture but I only understood the last two words, "flew away." So I repeated them, "What flew away?"

"A lady bug. Me and a bunch of lady bugs spend time together."

- **Ask for children's help to clarify words.**

Five-year-old Erin drew a picture of herself by making a circle and adding only a nose, eyes, and two legs. "That looks like a baby."

A few minutes later, I asked her, "What's easy for you at school?"

"Drawing thistles."

"Thistles? Could you help me out? I'm not sure what thistles are." She tapped her self-portrait. "Oh, pictures," I said. "It's easy for you to draw pictures. Thanks for helping me."

Use Kid Language

Because children are your partners in therapy, you have to learn what words the children know and understand. Then you have to be conscientious about either speaking at their level or translating adult words into "kid language." One way to become fluent in this is to listen to children's vocabulary. Increase your awareness of the types of words and phrases that are typically spoken. Count how many

words they use in a sentence. Also listen for their unique ways of expressing their thoughts and feelings. For example, my 3-year-old second cousin in California conveyed how she felt scared by saying, "That earthquake hurt my feelings."

Also think about the effect of children's culture and life experiences on their language. Consider whether they have a mental picture of the words used. I saw a child from a rural area who came to the city; he was amazed to ride on an escalator. Prior to this, "escalator" was not part of his everyday language or experience.

In general, as an adult, it is helpful if you tend to use simple words and shorter sentences. Try to be concise and eliminate extraneous words. Match the children's length of sentences and avoid using pronouns with younger children. If you use big words, make it a habit to check the children's understanding and give an explanation by using kid language to translate the terms.

Fabulous Five: Use Words Children Understand

- **Talk and explain in "kid language."**

"My grandma had a stroke," 6-year-old George said.

"Is she okay?"

"Yeah." Five seconds later, he asked, "What is a stroke?"

I explained, "One reason people have strokes is that in the brain you have arteries and veins that carry blood. They are like tubes that carry blood. When a person has a stroke there is a hole in the artery or vein and blood goes into the brain. After that some people are okay, but some people have a hard time talking or walking. Can your grandma walk and talk?"

"Yeah, but she needs a cane."

- **Avoid using professional jargon unless you translate the words into language the children can understand.**

"It's been difficult for Bert to learn how to ride a bike. He's still using his training wheels," his mother informed me when we first met.

During the session, I observed the 9 year old looking perplexed as he struggled to maneuver his body through an obstacle course. At the end of the session I commented, "I can see that you tried your best, but it seemed like it was hard to get your body to do what you wanted." I looked at his mother. "It's called motor planning."

Then I shifted my attention back to Bert. "When you try something new, like riding a bike, you have to plan how to move and adjust your body to do it. That's hard for some kids. But once you learn it—like bike riding—you just do it and you don't have to think about it. There are some ways to make bike riding easier to learn. Together we can figure out what will work for you." Bert nodded and showed a slight smile in response.

- **Use familiar words or phrases.**

On their weekly community trip, the class walked single-file to their destination. At each street crossing, the teacher said as she signed, "And stop. Look both ways. And go."

The next week I met with 6-year-old Keenan. I showed him a picture of a circle, pointed to him, and then tapped the paper. "You draw a circle." He started with a circular motion, which quickly turned into scribbling. "Keenan, look," I said and waited until he raised his head. "Let me show you how." I demonstrated using the words he knew, "Make a circle. Go around AND STOP."

- **Use children's own wording or explanations.**

"I hurted myself so bad," 4-year-old Jane said. "There's a hole in my foot and it was bleeding."

"Are you okay? Did the hole stop bleeding?" I asked, and she nodded.

- **Say words adults use and then reword with simple words.**

We walked to an office at the end of a hallway and saw a "do not disturb" sign on the doorknob. "I guess we'll have to go somewhere else. They must be testing in that room. 'Do not disturb' means do not go in."

Five-year-old Maddox pivoted and followed me to another room. "I read a book last night. It was easy. There were no words."

"Oh, so you were good at figuring out the story from the pictures?" He nodded and smiled.

Key Points to Remember

- Tell children your name and who you are.
- Explain therapy to children in a way they can understand.
- Match your approach to the level of emotional involvement desired by children.
- Create an interactive dialogue with all involved including children.
- Acknowledge children's presence when talking to others.
- Start conversations with children using easy-to-answer questions.

- Be friendly, attentive, and responsive.
- Create a common language by using words that are understood by all.

Review Questions

1. You do not need to introduce yourself if the children are nonverbal and seem unaware of your presence. True or false.

2. You have been asked by Johnny's second-grade teacher to figure out ways to help him stop having meltdowns when he is in sensory overload. He is especially sensitive to loud and constant noise. What words could you use to introduce yourself to him and the purpose of therapy?

3. If children are hiding behind their parents, name three possible approaches.

4. If children are not looking at you, you can assume they are not listening. True or false.

5. Into what two categories do children tend to classify adults?

6. Name four types of conversation starters.

7. When you first meet a second grader, she avoids eye contact with you. You should require her to look at you before you continue talking. True or false.

8. Name six possible ways children can nonverbally tell you their choices.

9. When you asked a 6 year old to draw a picture, he turned his back to you. What could you say using this phrase: "I see you have…. I think you are telling me…."?

10. You see a 10 year old holding the pen in her fist and moving her arm as she writes each letter. Explain in kid language why that is inefficient.

Reference

Tickle-Degnen, L., & Gavett, E. (2003). Changes in nonverbal behavior during the development of therapeutic relationships. In P. Philippot, R. S. Feldman, & E. J. Coats (Eds.), *Nonverbal behavior in clinical settings* (pp. 75-110). Oxford, UK: University Press.

Establish a Collaborative Frame

CHAPTER OVERVIEW

At the same time you introduce yourself and explain occupational therapy to children, you give the message that collaboration is desired. You establish a collaborative frame. Your words and actions convey that occupational therapy is a safe place, the relationship will be a partnership, their strengths will be emphasized, and they will be co-creators of their educational experiences. The purpose of this chapter is to provide an overview of these four dimensions of the collaborative frame.

CHILDREN'S DESCRIPTIONS OF WHAT THEY THINK YOU SHOULD KNOW

Dr. Clare: "What makes you feel safe when you are with an adult like a teacher or therapist?"

Sara (age 11): "I feel safe around adults if when I get hurt or feel scared they can help me."

Paul (age 12): "I feel safe if I know they will protect me."

Katie (age 11): "I will feel safe if I don't feel like they are going to hurt me."

Cara (age 12): "I don't feel threatened if I know what they are doing."

Dr. Clare: "What can adults like therapists or teachers do so you know you can trust them? How do they act?"

Ashley (age 10): "I would feel trust if they wouldn't try to make me feel uncomfortable. And if I do feel uncomfortable, I would tell them and they would try and fix that."

Jackson (age 10): "They are really trustworthy."

Dan (age 11): "They go above and beyond for people."

Dr. Clare: "How does it make you feel when a therapist talks about your strengths or says nice things about you? Why do you like it?"

Paul (age 12): "It makes me feel confident in myself that I can do more. I like it because it makes me motivated."

Cara (age 12): "It makes me feel good because they are isolating the good things I did and they are trying to make me feel better. I like it because it doesn't make me feel like any other kid. It makes me feel more self-confident."

Ashley (age 10): "It makes me feel good because then I would know what to do or not do."

A COLLABORATIVE FRAME

As you build an initial connection with children, you create a collaborative frame that shapes their thoughts and feelings. A frame is a way you make sense of what is seen, heard, and experienced. It is how you organize your thoughts and feelings and interpret what is happening around you. For instance, if you see two boys shoving each other and

Curtin, C.
Strategies for Collaborating With Children: Creating Partnerships in Occupational Therapy and Research (pp. 77-97).
© 2017 SLACK Incorporated.

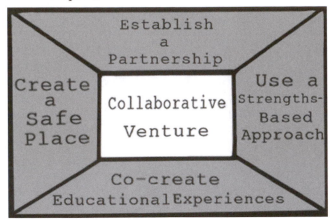

Figure 5-1. Establish a collaborative frame.

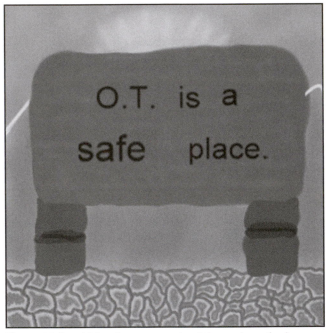

Figure 5-2. Let children know occupational therapy is a safe place.

smirking, you may wonder if they are playing or fighting. If, however, they drop to the ground, wrestle for a few minutes, and end with laughter, you would probably think, *Oh, they're just goofing around.* You would interpret their actions as playful. By doing so, you have developed a play frame. In a similar way, you help children develop a collaborative frame or mentality that promotes a partnership.

There are four essential and interdependent dimensions (Figure 5-1). With the first dimension, you treat children in a manner that fosters the perception of occupational therapy as a safe place. You dispel any doubts, alleviate anxiety, and let them know what to expect. They discover that therapy offers a safe emotional climate, in which you are a supportive adult who is empathetic and cares about them.

The second one is to establish ground rules for the relationship. You define your role as a helper and an advocate who believes in their potential and the range of possibilities

regarding their ability to grow. They discover they are to be in a partnership where they have a say on what happens in the session. A major task in the beginning is to interact with children in a way that encourages their interest, receptivity, and a willingness to engage in therapy. There is an exchange in which you learn about each other. You teach about the nature of occupational therapy and its relevance to them. The children teach you about their lives, meaningful occupations, and dreams for the future. You develop an emotional connection and start to speak a common language, in which the words used are understood by all. The notion of partnership also is established by approaching them on their terms, displaying positive nonverbal language, and being responsive.

The third dimension is having a strengths-based focus. Your actions demonstrate an emphasis on children's competencies and their repertoire of successful strategies. They quickly learn you accept them as they are.

The fourth dimension is to co-create educational experiences. Together you and children use occupations to develop learning experiences that are challenging and fun. They learn that facing challenges promotes growth, enjoyment, and a sense of accomplishment.

The process of creating this frame is vital since collaboration is a joint venture. It is necessary for them to feel comfortable and safe to participate. They have to know what to expect and how to act with you. The establishment of the frame cultivates the development of trust and mutual respect that they need to explore and expand their potential.

Establish That Occupational Therapy Is a Safe Place

For children to take risks and challenge themselves in therapy, they need to feel safe and secure. Therefore, one essential message is that occupational therapy is a safe place (Figure 5-2). Your goal is to establish a supportive emotional climate and maintain physical safety. You want children to be relaxed and feel like they belong. Then they can feel at ease and be open to new experiences.

Prepare the Environment to Be Safe and Prevent Problems

> **Children might be thinking:**
> *I won't get hurt here.*
> *It's safe here.*
> *You want to protect me.*
> *You move stuff out of the way that could be a problem.*

Appreciate children's ingenuity; they have a talent for discovering multiple ways of using tools and supplies—some conventional, some not. It is as if they are on a mission to challenge themselves to explore every tantalizing aspect of an object or a situation. You may think that a simple object will be used only one way. You will quickly learn that you have limited your thinking when you see the amazing and creative abilities of children to study and extend all possible uses.

To keep children safe, you need to expand your adult and conventional way of thinking. Like these young innovators, open your mind to envisioning new and exciting purposes. As you join this mission of discovery, it is critical to also identify any possibility of harm. Recognize that the children's lure to explore often becomes an irresistible temptation even if it is unsafe.

As you analyze, ask yourself questions such as: How can this be used to hurt oneself? Can you cut with this? Does it have sharp edges? Can it pinch? Can it be swallowed? Is it toxic if eaten? Develop the foresight of likely scenarios given the situation, age, and personality of the children. Another consideration is that in group settings, it is impossible to maintain constant attention to everyone for every minute. Taking into account all factors, you may then choose to eliminate the object, substitute a safer one for it, or maintain a watchful eye as they use it.

You also may use the environment to prevent safety issues. For example, you can devise systems and establish a routine that protects them from harm. You also may want to create a self-calming area that gives them a place they can go to regroup. Be sure to give the calming place a positive name. One teacher called her area a "cozy corner." In addition, environmental cues such as a stop sign can be effective.

Fabulous Five: Set Up the Environment to Ensure Safety

- **Create systems for safety.**

My first week working on the psychiatric unit, I devised a system allowing me to quickly check tools. I placed the metal leather stamps in the 30 holes of a plastic container and drew outlines of the hammers and screwdrivers on the inside of the locked cabinet. One quick look and I could see that an empty hole or outlined shape meant one was missing. After my first group, I conducted my scan and was dismayed to find stamping tools gone.

I went up to the classroom and talked to the group of fifth and sixth graders. "The tools were here when your class came but are now missing. It's important to find them, and I would appreciate your help. We need to keep looking until they are found."

Two girls, looking sheepish, reached into their desks. They retrieved the metal stamps and handed them to me. "We wanted to tattoo ourselves," they said and told of their plan to heat them and burn the image into their skin. I was relieved that my system had prevented this.

- **Have a self-calming area.**

During the last period when there was unstructured time, 12-year-old Mitch ran across the room flapping his hands by his shoulders. He paced back and forth, found a strap, and repeatedly waved it.

"Mitch, you look like you need a break. Go sit in the quiet space," I said calmly.

He went to the corner in the classroom filled with heavy pillows and surrounded by a heavy blue mat. After sitting quietly for 3 minutes, he returned looking calmer.

- **Create a routine requiring safety.**

Every week, the class went on a community outing. The group waited until every child was standing in line. When 7-year-old Kirk stepped off the sidewalk into the street, his teacher used sign language and said, "Not safe. Get in line." Kirk stepped back. "Good," the teacher responded. "We are all walking in a straight line. That's safe."

At the end of the school year, Kirk's mother joined the group. When she started walking in the street, Kirk tugged her arm and motioned for her to get on the sidewalk.

- **Use an environmental support to maintain safety.**

During the first week of school, 8-year-old Jana frequently jumped up and flew out of the room with a staff member in hot pursuit. To change Jana's habit of running, the teacher taped a communication device next to the door. From then on, every time Jana left the room, she stopped at the door, pushed the red button, and the recorded message played, "Goodbye."

- **Analyze how equipment or materials can be harmful.**

The occupational therapy student brought a glue gun to attach wiggly eyes on the sock puppets. "You are not supposed to touch this glue gun. It's very hot. I am the only one allowed to use it because you could get burned," she told the group.

Knowing that 6-year-old Hector liked to finger everything, I looked at him and had a gut feeling that he was going to touch it. Our hands went toward the glue gun at the exact same second. I intercepted his finger an inch away from the gun.

Foster a Sense of Safety and Security

Children might be thinking:
Are you going to hurt me?
Are you going to put me to sleep?
Am I in trouble?
Will you embarrass me?

A basic need of children (and adults) is to feel safe. They need to know that you will not harm them physically or verbally. They want to make sure that you are not critical, judgmental, overpowering, or intimidating. Until they determine you are a safe person, they will stay on guard and be cautious about what they say and do.

Therefore, it is important for you to convey that you will keep them safe and support them in all their efforts. Show them by your facial expressions, words, and actions your acceptance and openness to who they are as individuals. You gain their trust when they see that you are an emotionally safe and empathetic person who protects them from harm. They will become more comfortable and likely to assume an active role in therapy. They also will feel they can be themselves.

Recognize Children's Worries About Meeting a Stranger

When children first see you, it is common for them to worry about who you are and what you are going to do. Their initial anxiety may be high if they have not been given any information or have had bad experiences with other adults in that setting. For instance, hospitalized children learn that most doctors, nurses, and medical technologists conduct painful procedures. It is quite usual to have an unannounced stranger come to take blood or to give shots. Because children often do not know when this will happen, they tend to be suspicious of any new adult entering their hospital room.

In a school setting, children discover that an unexpected visitor could be an authority figure who is there to take a troublemaker to the principal's office. The overwhelming concern when their name is called is that something bad is going to happen. They will wonder what they did wrong. Older children also may worry about being embarrassed in front of their peers.

Because these unspoken fears are common, it is best to directly address these feelings within the first few moments. By doing so, your actions and words demonstrate that you are attuned to what they are experiencing. You also alleviate discomfort by offering reassurance that you are a different kind of adult who is there to help.

Fabulous Five: Address Children's Anxiety Regarding You

- **Acknowledge you are a new person in their lives.**

  I introduced myself and asked the first grader, "How old are you?"

  Scott stared straight ahead.

  "Are you 6 or 7?" I guessed, but again no response. "That's okay. You don't have to talk. I know you are just getting to know me." I smiled and remained silent until we sat at the table in the therapy room. "Just draw a picture of yourself. When you're done, it's up to you if you want to tell me about it."

- **Tell hospitalized children you will not hurt them.**

  As I entered the hospital room, 7-year-old Stacy ducked her head under the blanket.

  I introduced myself and said, "I want you to know that I don't give shots or take blood or do anything that hurts. I know being in the hospital can be hard so I brought some activities for you." Stacy slid upright, peeked at me, and then chose to paint a small wooden box.

- **Mention how you feel meeting new people.**

  Six-year-old Erin lingered at the clinic doorway with her eyes fixed on the floor. In a soft tone of voice, I told her, "Sometimes I get scared when I go somewhere and I don't know the people or what I'm supposed to do. I get nervous if I don't know what to expect." She shifted her eyes and nodded in response.

- **Let children know they are not in trouble when taking them from a classroom.**

  "Pearl, come here," the teacher said, gesturing toward the front of the classroom. Eight-year-old Pearl pressed her arms close to her body as an expression of worry covered her face.

  I moved next to her desk and reassured her in a soft voice, "It's nothing bad. You're not in trouble. I'm going to have you come with me. We're going to do some games to see how fast you can move your hands. You will get to cut and draw through mazes—things like that. Most kids think it's fun." Pearl's arms relaxed and she moved out of her seat.

- **Acknowledge if being with you is stressful.**

  I joined 5-year-old Cole in his hospital room. After I asked a few neutral questions, Cole's eyes clouded with concern and he cringed. I stopped and said, "You look upset. I know it's hard to be in the hospital. I don't want to make things harder for you. If you would like to talk to me, I want to hear what you have to say. We'll stop and just play now." I placed three toys on the table, and he chose the bag of blocks.

Be Empathetic to Children's Situation or Experience

When you assume the children's perspective and focus on what they are feeling, you begin to convey your commitment to understanding their experience. Your perceptiveness and sensitivity, along with acceptance, teach children that you care about them. The recognition of what they are going through also may provide validation and comfort.

To be empathetic means you have to continually think about what it is like for them in their particular situation. To do this, first learn what typically scares or upsets children. For instance, the first day of preschool is often very scary because they have to leave their caregivers and stay with strangers in a new place. Second, reflect on your own childhood. Think about what frightened you. When I was a young child in St. Louis, I saw the aftermath of a tornado. To this day, I can still picture the demolished gas station and the white stone church standing without a roof. A third way to identify what it is like for them is to ask yourself how you would feel if you were in those circumstances. If you work in a hospital, think about how you would feel if you were the patient waiting for surgery or a medical procedure. What would be your prevalent thoughts and feelings? You may worry about how much it will hurt. How will it turn out afterward? Will you be able to do the things you like?

After figuring out your best guess at what the children are going through, check with them to see if you are right. They will appreciate your attempt to understand what the experience means to them. In some cases, you may say what you think they are feeling. Then watch to see if there is a response in their facial expressions or actions.

Fabulous Five: Recognize What Children Are Experiencing

- **Assume the children's perspective and comfort them.**

Before preschool started, the teacher and I wrote the following story and attached corresponding pictures:

My name is….
I go to T. C. Preschool.
My teachers are Dr. M and Miss Mary.
Our classroom helper (volunteer) is Dr. Clare.
I will play in centers.
I will play outside.
School is fun!

At the open house just before school started, the teacher asked caregivers to attach their child's photo next to the name and read the story before the first day. Then they were to bring the story back to school.

The next day in class, 4-year-old Mara cried after her dad dropped her off. "I miss my daddy."

The teacher brought over the story with her picture. "You're sad to say goodbye to your dad. I understand. I have the story your daddy read to you. Here you are. See, you're here at school. " As she read the story and pointed to each picture, Mara stopped crying.

- **Voice your awareness of the children's current experience.**

When I entered 7-year-old Amanda's hospital room, I saw the intravenous (IV) pole with the chemotherapy drip. For a few minutes, we chatted about her life and her interests. Then I looked at her IV bag and said, "I know you're here to get chemo, and that's not easy. You're going through a lot. I would like to do some activities with you

to help you get through this tough time. Is that all right?" She nodded with a look of interest. "But if you feel too sick to do anything, just tell me. That's okay too."

- **Show you understand the children's situation by putting words to their feelings or actions.**

"I'm sorry I have to go. I love you," Debbie's mother said as she left her 3-year-old daughter at the children's hospital.

Debbie ran to the corner of the clinic and dragged a 3-foot-tall teddy bear to the rocking chair. After sliding into the chair, she tugged the bear onto her lap. Then she circled her arms around the stuffed animal and held tightly.

After a few minutes of silence, I said what I thought Debbie was feeling: "I'm so sad my mom left. I miss my mom. It's hard to be here by myself."

Debbie's eyes softened and she relaxed her grip on the bear. After a few minutes of rocking, she went to the table and began coloring.

- **Acknowledge children's stressful times.**

"How is your day going?" I asked 8-year-old Genevieve as we walked down the school hallway.

"Not good."

"What happened?"

"My dad won't send money to us."

"So what is your mom going to do?"

"I don't know."

"It's just hard to see her worrying?"

"Yeah," she said and sighed.

- **Explain what is happening around the children.**

As 5-year-old Justin and I walked down the school hall, we heard a blood-curdling scream. We saw a young boy on the floor hanging onto his mother's leg while the principal talked to him.

Because I thought the incident might be scaring Justin, I turned to him to comfort him by saying, "He's all right. No one is hurting him. He's at a new school and is upset his mom is leaving. The principal is trying to help him."

Develop the Idea of Therapy as Being "Our Place"

Children might be thinking:
Is it safe to be here?
Thanks for making it more comfortable.
Thanks for checking.
Thanks for letting me have a say.
This is a good place.
I like being here.

Children must feel safe on an emotional level to be able to collaborate with you. This means you have to create a place where they are secure enough to freely voice their wants and needs. It is also important to establish a sense of togetherness and belonging to help the children become partners.

Define Therapy as a Safe Place

As children get to know you, they will wonder if you are trustworthy. They will examine everything you do and say to make their determination that you are a safe person. With younger ones, you see that they have made that decision when they are willing to leave their caregivers and come join you.

To help them feel secure with you, use phrases such as, "I will keep you safe," or, "this is a safe place to…." Describe therapy as being a safe place by referring more to your relationship and time spent together than just location. Another way to cultivate the notion of therapy as a safe place is to use a metaphor to describe your supportive nature.

Your intention at this point is to set up both the social and physical environment in a way that children feel accepted as themselves. They do not have to worry about being teased or criticized and their feelings will not be minimized. Instead, they can explore, take risks, and make mistakes. They can feel free to talk and make decisions. They see that you will protect them and be respectful. It is a place for them to flourish.

Fabulous Five: Say or Show That It Is Safe to Be With You

- **Promise children that they are safe with you.**

On his first day, 4-year-old Jamal explored the hospital clinic. He peeked in the carpeted barrel and ran up the scooter board ramp but stopped and hesitated at the platform swing. I held the swing still and said, "I promise I will not let you fall. Try it." He situated himself with his legs crossed and his fingers tightly gripping the ropes. I held both sides of the wooden swing and gently moved the swing back and forth in a straight line to help Jamal keep his balance. "See how safe you are."

- **Tell children, "This is a safe place."**

The group of three fifth graders met the first week of school. Because Tony was new to our group, I told him, "This is a safe place to try things."

"Yeah. No one makes fun of you," Laralyn said with a lisp.

"It's a no-bully zone," Bethany added.

- **Use a metaphor to convey that occupational therapy is a safe place.**

"These look hard," Matt said, looking at two woodworking kits.

"Pick one and try it," I said to the 7 year old. "I can help you if you need it. This is a place where it's okay to make mistakes. Here we just vacuum up the mistakes and start over."

- **Set up the room with items or materials children may touch.**

When I talked with Bob's mother, I discovered that the 3 year old was active and curious. So before our appointment, I scanned the room for items I did not want him to touch. I placed my ceramic coffee mug and the scissors in my desk drawer. I moved games with small pieces to the top shelf.

Bob stormed into the room and circled like a tornado, fingering every item in sight. I smiled as he explored and I did not have to tell him stop. After surveying the room, he crawled in a carpeted barrel. I followed his lead and slowly rocked the barrel.

- **Show children you respect them by preparing before moving them.**

"Now I'm going to take your brakes off and we're going to move. We're going to OT. Brakes off," I cued 10-year-old Jason. He pushed the lever of his wheelchair with his palm on the right brake and I adjusted the left side. When we reached the therapy room, I said, "Open the door. Use your foot rest to open it." He pushed the door with the metal attachment and it swung open. Then he wheeled over to the table.

"You have to put your brakes on before I can help you out of your chair," I said and he locked the wheels. "When you're ready for me to help you stand and move to the chair, scoot up and tell me."

Twenty seconds passed. Then Jason moved forward on his seat and placed his hand on my shoulder, indicating his readiness to move.

Create a Sense of Belonging

To foster the feeling of therapy being a safe place that supports collaboration, you also help children develop a sense of belonging. They become insiders with ownership of their environment. To start with, the room needs to be warm and inviting. Have child-size furniture if possible and if not adapt the adult chairs such as giving them a footrest. The materials in the room need to match their age level and not look too babyish. Always refer to the space as "our room" to convey joint ownership. Encourage children to add their own touch such as making a drawing and hanging it on the wall. If the room is shared with other professionals, you can always take the pictures down at the end of the day and put them back the next time you come. For children who are unable to draw, you may want to make a group picture by having them color or scribble and then placing an outline of a cutout shape on top of it. Then they can view their artwork.

When you are in a permanent location, such as a hospital clinic, give them a tour so they can see what you have and where supplies are located. Depending on your setting, you may want to give children their own storage area like a bin or even just a folder. When there is a sense of belonging, children tend to feel more at ease and view therapy as a place they want to be.

Fabulous Five: Develop a Feeling of Belonging

- **Place a welcome sign on the door of the therapy room.**

I wrote "Welcome to occupational therapy!" on the poster, using a different color for each letter and drawing a character with a smiling face. I taped it on the door at the children's eye level. On Carter's first day, I pointed to the sign. "Welcome! I'm glad I get to meet you. Let's go in our room. I'll explain what's going to happen here, and then we'll do something fun."

- **Refer to the therapy space as "our room" or "our place."**

"Guess what?" Gus said.

"What?"

"I got a new shirt." He pointed to his chest. "The dinosaurs glow in the dark."

"Wow, that's exciting. Head down the hall and go past the drinking fountain. Our room is on the right."

- **Give a tour of the therapy room.**

"Let me show you around," I told Barbara. As we circled the hospital clinic, I opened each cabinet to show her the supplies. "Let me know what you want to do."

Her eyes widened when she saw a black velveteen poster of a butterfly. "This one."

- **Encourage children to personalize the therapy space.**

"It would be wonderful to have a picture made by you for our room. I have brand new markers and colored pencils."

"I'm going to make a beautiful picture," 4-year-old Janna said as she drew on the blue paper. "I'm standing on a pony. I'm going to fall. I landed on my feet."

"Hang it wherever you would like." Her eyes searched the therapy room in the oncology clinic for the perfect spot, and then she pinned her artwork on the wall. "Your picture looks great in our room."

- **Establish the children's own space or storage.**

On Kira's first day, I wrote her name on tape and handed the label to her. "Here, put your name on your very own special bin to use in here. You can keep all your things in it." Kira printed each letter and drew a heart instead of a dot over the letter "i."

Let Children Have a Say Regarding Their Environment

Another aspect of giving children a voice is letting them have a say regarding their environment. If it is an option, let them decide where they want to be for therapy. For instance, if they are hospitalized, ask if they want to stay in their room or go to the therapy clinic. Also be open to adapting the space or moving if children request it or show discomfort. For children who are unable to manipulate their own wheelchairs, consider their surveillance zone when you move them. Watch and respond to children's nonverbal signs of unease. If they react to the sound level, temperature, or smell in the room, make it a point to check in and ask what they would like done. Being respectful of their needs emphasizes the partnership aspect of therapy.

Fabulous Five: Involve Children in Making Decisions About Their Environment

- **Give options of where to have therapy, if possible.**

On 8-year-old Jolene's third day of hospitalization for chemotherapy, I went into her room. Seeing her pale face, I said, "Do you want me to stay or do you want to rest?"

"Stay."

"Yesterday you started a heart-shaped box. Would you like me to bring it here or do you want to go down the hall to the OT clinic?"

"OT clinic."

"Okay. I can get you a wheelchair if you are feeling weak."

"No, that's okay. I can walk."

- **Offer to adapt the space or move.**

Midway through the session, 7-year-old Trenton heard three teachers talking loudly in the room and said, "There are too many people in here."

"Should we move to another room?" I replied. "We can if you want."

Trenton nodded, and we went to the room next door.

- **Be sensitive to the temperature in the room.**

I met 5-year-old Noah after recess and saw his red cheeks. Sweat poured down his face. "I think I'm melting," he said.

When we arrived at the therapy room, I said, "It's hot in here. Would you like me to turn on a fan?" He nodded.

- **Maintain a comfortable sound level.**

Three-year-old Julie pressed her finger against her lips and said, "Sh, sh."

"Julie wants us to talk softer," I said to the group.

"Why?"

"Because it hurts her ears when we're too loud."

- **Be aware that some smells are bothersome to children.**

  "I wonder what that smell is," I said because I thought it might be bothering 7-year-old Art.

  "It smells awful."

  "It may be burnt popcorn. Let me open a window so we can get some fresh air."

Establish That Therapy Is a Safe Place to Talk and You Will Listen

Children might be thinking:

Thanks for asking how I am.

I've been through a lot.

I like talking. I'm glad I get to tell you.

I like drawing. Drawing makes me feel better.

Thanks for listening.

As a protective measure, children learn to keep many of their thoughts to themselves. If, however, they find that you are interested in their perspective and truly willing to listen, they tend to share their thoughts and feelings. Create a culture where talking is the norm. Provide opportunities that encourage them to share what they are thinking or feeling. Show that you will listen to both their words and nonverbal messages. Convey your desire to understand what they are saying and to take their concerns seriously.

Make Casual Conversation Part of the Routine

When you make casual conversation part of your routine, you create an opportunity for children to talk about their thoughts and feelings. This shows you are interested in how they are. Talking casually helps in getting to know each other and creating a bond.

By continually checking in with them and being a good listener, you give the message that it is okay to talk and that you want to hear their perspective. It is during this type of conversation that children will often mention their concerns. At the same time, because it is casual conversation, there is no pressure for them to reveal their worries. They get to decide whether they want to talk and how much they say.

Fabulous Five: Engage in Casual Conversation

- **Ask, "How are you doing?"**

  "How are you doing?"

  "I'm tired because my mom and stepdad were fighting in front of me in the living room," 8-year-old Alice replied. "My mom said she was sorry. My mom is getting married."

"Are you in the wedding?"

"I'll be a snow girl. I get to throw snowflakes. My dress is blue."

- **Check how the children's day is going.**

  "How's your day going?"

  "I drank hot cocoa," 6-year-old Logan said. "It burnt my tongue. It burnt my face off."

  "That really hurts when that happens."

- **Inquire about what has happened since you last saw them.**

  "Did you have a good Thanksgiving?"

  "No, not really," 9-year-old Andre replied.

  "How come?"

  "I had a basketball tournament and it didn't go well."

  "No? What happened?"

  "We won but our coach was kind of mad. He was yelling at the other team's coach."

  "So that took the fun away—seeing him yell? Were you afraid he was going to yell at you too?"

  Andre nodded.

- **Ask children what is new with them.**

  "What's new with you?" I asked 5-year-old Kaylin.

  "I want to tell you something. In a couple of days I'm going to move to another house."

  "Will you change schools?"

  "No. And I have a new sister. Her name is Isabelle. My grandma calls her Poopy-do. I love my mom and my sissy. I love all my family."

- **Inquire about any changes in the children's lives.**

  Because I knew Mary had switched to a different second-grade classroom, I asked, "How is it going in your new class?"

  "I like it."

  "What do you like about it?"

  "My new teacher gives me more chances."

Provide Ways for Children to Share Their Thoughts, Feelings, and Experiences

Children appreciate being given the opportunity to express their thoughts, feelings, and experiences. You can provide ways for them to share and allow them to choose whether to proceed. Drawing and play materials are natural means of self-expression. Writing about their experiences can also be beneficial. Another way is to encourage a group to talk with each other about what is happening in their lives.

Fabulous Five: Provide Ways for Children to Share Thoughts, Feelings, and Experiences

- **Let children know that drawing is an option for sharing their experiences.**

"I have paper. You can draw a picture if you want," I said.

"I'm going to draw my dad," 5-year-old Dugan said. "He has a broken leg."

"What happened?"

"He fell down at work." Dugan then drew a smaller figure. "This is me. I was spinning around the swing and I got smacked on my face. I got a bruise. Now I is done."

"That must have hurt. Are you okay now?"

He nodded.

- **Encourage children to draw a picture about their experiences.**

Hearing that 5-year-old Hailey had just returned home, I asked her, "I heard you were in the hospital. What was it like for you? I brought some paper and markers in case you want to draw."

She reached for the paper, drew a picture of her in a hospital bed, and said, "That's me. Sometimes I have trouble breathing. We have to go to the doctor. There's a machine that helps me breathe. When I was in the hospital, I got to color. They talked to me about animals. When I woke up I got a chocolate bear."

"That must be scary when you can't breathe."

She nodded.

"I'm glad you are feeling better now."

- **Provide play materials to act out experiences.**

When I went to get 3-year-old Brett, the head nurse said, "He had a horrible night. A young intern fumbled as he put in a nasogastric tube. It took him many attempts before he was successful."

As Brett and I walked to the occupational therapy clinic, he was quiet and subdued. He sat on a platform swing, and I brought over some toys, a stuffed bear, and plastic tubing. He took the tubing and tried to stick it down the bear's nose. "Oh, that hurts," I said, pretending to be the bear.

"And would you cry?" he said in a soft voice.

Nodding, I said, "Yes, I would."

"I did too," he whispered.

- **Encourage children to write about their experiences.**

In the oncology clinic, 12-year-old John wrote in a group newspaper entitled, *The Occupational Therapy Tribune.* The following story was about his hospital experiences:

My Story

Once upon time about 3 month ago I was in the hospital here and I was here because I got cancer and I needed to stay. It was fun. But I didn't like all those needles in my arm legs feet and my family came to see me a lot. But they need to get more new cooks because the food was not that good.

About My Feelings

When I was in the hospital, I felt really bad at the time because I didn't know what was going on at the time. I didn't know what kind of medicine that was going in my body and when I was going to radiation they was trying to explain to me. But I didn't understand because the kind of words that they was using.

What I Learn in the Hospital

When I was at the hospital, I learn a little bit about medicine. I know about certain kinds of pills. I know how to put in IVs in people. I know how to give medicine throw the IVs. I know how to get blood from people and I met kind people when I was there. I met kind doctors and nurses.

- **Have the group share their experiences with one another.**

As the group of third graders played with putty, I asked, "What do you find annoying?"

"I really hate when my dad yells at me. I don't like people pushing me on the swing. I can push myself."

"I get annoyed when someone laughs at me because I can't say it right. I keep saying, 'That's not nice.'"

"My baby brother hits me a lot. My mom asks questions about stuff I don't really want to talk about. My dad doesn't annoy me because he's mostly at work."

Provide a Running Commentary to Children's Nonverbal "Talking"

Show children, especially those who are young or nonverbal, that you will listen to the messages conveyed by their actions. You can do this by giving them your full attention and providing a running commentary regarding what you see them doing. In addition, you are helping them learn the meanings of different words.

As you watch children, comment on which toys or activities they gravitate toward. Guess what you think they want if you see them searching or looking at a closed cupboard. During activities, describe any actions they take. For instance, say, "You are making the car go fast." Also state any decisions you see them make. Closely observe their facial expressions and nonverbal language and identify possible feelings they may have.

Be sensitive to their reactions when you speak. Limit the amount of talking if children appear to be in sensory overload, especially if there is a lot of noise and commotion in their classroom. Even if children are nonverbal, with your help they can still have a voice.

Fabulous Five: Provide a Running Commentary About Children's Actions

- **Say what decisions you see children making.**

"Aa-ee," 4-year-old Nolan said as he walked on his toes and flapped his ears with his hands. He headed for the pumpkin on the table and began pounding golf tees into it. After hammering a few in, he dropped the mallet on the table and looked around the room.

"You're done," I said. "You want to do something else."

He flitted across the room to the easel, which had a sample picture of an autumn tree with falling leaves. I followed him and said, "You want to paint. Let me get paper for you."

After I clipped it onto the easel, Nolan grabbed a thick paintbrush and dabbed yellow, orange, and red colors on the paper. Later when the painting was dry, his teacher had him glue a cutout tree on top of his painting. He then pointed to where he wanted it placed on the bulletin board.

- **Say aloud what you think children want as indicated by their actions.**

In the specialized classroom, 5-year-old Isabella walked over to me with her index finger pressed against the inside of her cheek. She took her finger out and tapped my sleeve. Then she pointed to a wind-up toy a classmate had.

"You want a turn," I said to her. I retrieved another toy and said to the classmate, "Could Isabella have a turn? I brought a car that you like."

He reached for the car and handed her the toy.

- **State a possible feeling children might be indicating by their actions.**

Five-year-old Keith held his hands over his ears and continued crying after his class returned from a fire drill. I went up to him and said, "That fire alarm scared you. It was really loud and hurt your ears. Let's go get a drink of water so you'll feel better."

He reached for my hand and calmed as we slowly walked to the drinking fountain in the quiet hallway.

- **Describe the action you see children doing.**

As 3-year-old Madeline participated in a play-based assessment, her father watched and chatted with another staff member. Upon hearing her father's voice, Madeline dropped the blocks and turned toward him.

"You heard your daddy's voice," I said. "He's talking to Ms. G. and telling her things you like to do at home. Check out this toy."

Madeline shifted her attention back to a musical toy.

- **State what you see children enjoying or liking.**

During free time, 3-year-old Owen went to the bookcase and grabbed a book on marine animals. He roamed the room aimlessly with the book under his arm.

I approached him and said, "You have your favorite book. I know you like to look at sharks, dolphins, and whales. Let's look at them."

He sat down and opened the book.

"Where's the shark?" I asked, and he pointed. "Turn the page please. Where's the whale?"

He flipped the page and smiled as he tapped the picture of the humpback whale.

Establish Roles in the Relationship

When you delineate the roles, it makes it clearer on how to act with each other. This eliminates the need to guess and facilitates a level of comfort. Discussing the expectations also is important because it may be a new experience for them to be in a partnership with an adult.

Clarify Children's Role in the Partnership

> **Children might be thinking:**
> *What do I do?*
> *It's okay to ask questions?*

For children, it is better if you explicitly say or show them what their role is to be. You begin by defining the ground rules for the relationship. As a partner, they have a say in what happens in the session. Their ideas are wanted and welcomed. They can lead or direct you; they do not have to be followers. You also hope they will tell you what they are thinking and feeling and not hesitate to ask questions. In addition, their views are to be considered equally important to yours.

As members of the partnership, they need to teach you about their lives including their occupations and daily experiences. You want to get to know them and discover what they value. There needs to be an air of openness in hearing different viewpoints and customs. Expect each to learn from the other.

Fabulous Five: Facilitate Children Having a Say or Voice

- **Tell children their ideas are welcomed.**

"What would you like to do today? Do you have any ideas? I would love to hear them," I told the preschoolers.

"I have a good idea," 4-year-old Cammie said to the group. "I'm going to get the flashlights from the cupboard. Everybody turn on your flashlight so you can see." Four streams of light appeared.

"What do you want us to do?" I asked.

She made circular motions on the ceiling, and the group followed. "Everyone make a big one." Swirling circles danced on the ceiling. "I made this game up," she said and smiled.

"It's a fun one. Hey, do you want to play tag with the flashlights too?" I asked.

"Yeah!"

"See if your light can catch mine."

"Got ya," she laughed.

- **Encourage children to say what they are thinking.**

"How are you?" I asked 7-year-old David when I saw the frown on his face.

He shrugged and then said, "Okay."

"You don't look okay. What are you thinking?"

"My dad doesn't believe men should cry, so when he gets mad he punches the door and throws the phone on the floor."

"What do you do when that happens?"

"I run to my room and get under my blanket."

"I think it's pretty scary when someone is that mad."

"I'm not as scared of my dad as I used to be."

"Do you talk to your mom about it?" He nodded. "It sounds like you are doing a good thing by going to your room when your dad is mad and giving him space to cool down."

"It happened today. My dad watches TV and sits like a slug on the couch. He only works 5 minutes a day. He makes my mom buy a new phone."

- **Show children that it is all right to ask questions.**

Five-year-old Andrew colored his picture but then stopped and asked, "How do they get babies out of moms?"

"You don't want to ask THAT question," his classmate said.

"It's okay to ask questions," I replied. "When babies get big enough, they just come out."

Andrew nodded and resumed coloring.

- **Have children teach you about their lives.**

"Tell me about your school day. What time do you get up?"

"I get up at six. I watch TV, play, and eat breakfast. I go to school at seven," 7-year-old Cara replied.

"What do you do after school?"

"I change my clothes, do homework—spelling and reading—and then I do whatever I want. When Dad gets home, we eat dinner. Then I play or watch TV. I go to bed at eight. Then I fall asleep and wake up and start all over again."

- **Let children have an opportunity to direct you.**

"Do you want to draw a picture?" I asked the first grader. Bruce nodded. "Would you like a big or small chalkboard?"

"Big."

I handed him the oversized board and small pieces of chalk. When he handed me a piece of chalk, I said, "Do you want me to draw too?" He nodded, so I drew a picture of him flexing his biceps. He smiled, then erased my picture. "Oh, I guess we were ready for that picture to be gone."

Define Your Role as a Helper, an Informant, and an Advocate

> **Children might be thinking:**
> *Oh good, you will help me.*
> *You can help me anytime.*

In addition to identifying the children's role, you also need to outline yours. Let children know you are there to help and support them. The type of relationship desired continues to be relayed through your words, actions, and the experiences you help create. Your main role is being a helper, especially helping the children blossom. This can involve actions like providing assistance, intervening, or, on a grander scale, advocating for them with adults.

To help create the notion of a partnership, use words reflecting collaboration, such as *we, together,* or *team.* Also, demonstrate that you are attentive to their wishes and willing to take their side. You also view their concerns seriously and will pursue the necessary avenues to get their needs met.

Fabulous Five: State and Show That You Will Be a Helper

- **Tell children your job is to be there for them and help them if they want assistance.**

As I gave 10-year-old Miranda a tour around the hospital clinic, I told her, "We have all kinds of fun things to do. Some are easy, some are harder. If you pick something hard, you can always let me know if you want help. My job is to be here for you. Also, be sure and tell me if I'm doing too much and you want to do it yourself. I want to know." Miranda nodded, showing her understanding.

- **Talk about working together as a team.**

"Look around the room and see what you might like to do."

Eleven-year-old Louella's eyes settled on a cross-stitch plaque with the word *welcome.* "I think that would be too hard for me to do."

"Go ahead and try it. I can help you if you need it. That's why I'm here. We'll work together. It can be a team effort."

- **Demonstrate to children that you will advocate for them.**

"Jessie went to the dentist yesterday and had two fillings put in," her second-grade teacher said as our group walked out of the classroom on the way to the therapy room.

Once in the room, everyone colored for a few minutes. "Can I go to clinic? I don't feel good," Jessie asked. I nodded, and she left but quickly returned. "Miss M. is mean."

"How is she mean?" I replied.

"She told me to go back to class." Jessie resumed coloring but then said, "My teeth hurt real bad. I want to call my mom. I feel sick. I need my mom."

"Wait a couple minutes until group is over, and then I will go with you. Let's talk to your teacher first." Then I accompanied her back to class.

"Will you talk to my teacher?"

"Sure," I responded, and after a chat with the teacher, I went with Jessie to the clinic.

"Will you talk with Miss M.?" Jessie asked.

"I will."

As soon as the clinic aide saw us, she barked, "Jessie has been here two times already. I gave her pain medicine 2 hours ago and I can't give her anything else."

"Well, she's still in pain and wants to call her mother," I replied.

"I will call her mother," the clinic aide said with a huff. She phoned the mother, who came 10 minutes later to take her daughter back to the dentist.

- **Ask children to tell you if they want assistance with an activity.**

At the beginning of the session, I said, "If you need help, let me know."

After working independently for 5 minutes, 5-year-old Tasha said, "You can help me."

"What kind of help would you like?"

"You could stamp too," she replied, turning her head toward the other dinosaur stamps.

"You're really good with the stamps. Would you like me to hold the paper for you instead?"

"That'd be good."

- **Ask children if they want you to intervene.**

Seven-year-old Walt walked in the room with his shoulders slumped. He sat down and turned his head away from me.

"I'm worried about you because you seem sad today," the certified occupational therapy assistant said.

He turned and said, "School is so hard. I'm having trouble getting my homework done."

"Have you talked to your teacher?"

"No," he said, sounding hesitant to do so.

"Would you like me to talk to her?"

"That would be good."

"I'll talk to her and see if she has some ideas."

Provide Essential Information to Children

> **Children might be thinking:**
> *Thanks for telling me.*
> *That's good to know.*

Another crucial aspect of being in a partnership is to keep each other well informed. There are times when adults forget or do not think it is necessary to give children information. This omission can lead to children misunderstanding or feeling confused or baffled. They are very perceptive and will develop their own theories regarding what and why things are happening. Let children know you will keep them informed by talking with them, discovering their concerns, clarifying any questions, and providing your perspective on the situation.

Fabulous Five: Keep Children Informed

- **Explain what you are thinking with ongoing actions.**

"I noticed that when you write, you keep your head really close to the paper. I know that would make my back hurt if I did that for a long time. What have you tried that helps you write?"

"I don't know."

"I have one idea that might make writing easier for you. Could I show it to you?" Nine-year-old Brandon nodded, so I slid a slant board under his paper. "Try writing now." He sat upright as he wrote. "This makes it easier for you to see. What do you think? Does it help?"

"It's good. I like it."

- **Keep children informed regarding what is happening with their bodies or current situation.**

After a parent meeting, I told 5-year-old Lewis, "We met with your mom yesterday and told her how good you are doing in school. We told her you try everything, and you do not give up. She was very happy."

- **Explain information that affects the children.**

"Judy, I saw that your fingers are wrapped around the pencil. When you hold your pencil that way, you are using all of your hand muscles to write. You're using a lot of muscles." I demonstrated writing with large movements. "Now watch me," I said and wrote with a tripod pencil grasp, moving only my thumb, index, and middle fingers. "See, I'm only moving my fingers. I can write more this way without getting tired. So, if you want, we can try different pencil grips and you can decide if any of them help you just move your fingers." The third grader nodded in agreement.

- **Teach concepts children need to know.**

Because I knew 6-year-old Victor would experience more fatigue as his disease progressed, I said, "I hear you're getting more tired in the afternoon. Something that is good for you to know is called 'energy conservation.' Those big words mean that you save your energy for the good things like learning and playing. If you use all your energy up, you get tired."

"And if you eat junk food, you have no energy. If you eat vegetables, you get strong," he added.

"You're right. So you want to use your energy wisely. What you can do is to think before you move. Watch me. I have to get paper, a ruler, and a book. Look how much energy I use if I go back to my chair each time." I demonstrated getting up three times. "Instead, I could think, 'I need to get three things. I should get them all in one trip.'" Then I showed Victor getting all the items one after another and then sitting. "So tell yourself, 'Think before I move.'"

- **Tell children you can help them get information.**

"I see you have a substitute teacher," I said. Five-year-old Ross lowered his brown eyes, focusing on the table. "What you are thinking?"

"I don't like this teacher."

"How come?"

"She said if we can't remember her name, we can't ask questions."

"Does she have a hard name?"

"I don't know what her name is."

"Would you like me to find out for you, or do you want to ask someone in your class?"

"I'll ask my friend Brian," he said, as much to himself as to me.

Use a Strengths-Based Approach

The third message given to children to develop the collaborative frame is that you use a strengths-based approach. Your emphasis is on their competencies and potential. In addition, you convey your appreciation for their expertise and foster the expression of their creativity.

Highlight Competencies

> **Children might be thinking:**
> *You say nice things.*
> *Thank you for the compliment.*
> *I feel comfortable around you.*

When you consistently identify and discuss children's strengths, you build a solid foundation for your relationship. Your positive statements reflect your intention to

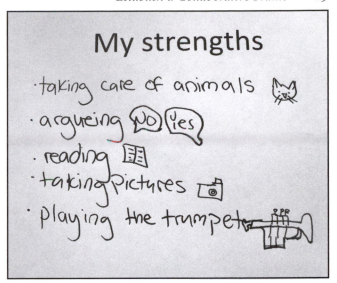

Figure 5-3. Elicit and recognize children's strengths.

search for and discover their various assets. They usually appreciate hearing nice comments about themselves, which makes them want to spend more time with you.

For some children it is beneficial to name or describe their strengths as a way to call attention to them. You may recognize a competence that they are unaware of having. By openly discussing these strengths, you can then use them in the development of future strategies.

Be sensitive, however, to the children's culture. For some, talking about strengths may be viewed as bragging, which is discouraged. In other cultures, some believe that without taking action to counteract the spirits or the "evil eye," compliments can cause illness (Drewes, 2005, p. 79). Hence, continue to learn about the children's culture and, again, respect their values and beliefs.

Recognize Strengths

Children's strengths are there to be discovered. Like hunting for treasures in the attic, some of their strengths are visible and others are hidden. One crucial aspect of therapy is to explore for all kinds of competencies. Within the first few moments, make it a habit to mention at least one obvious strength. You can always comment on their actions, their effort, or their ideas. This positive stance sets a pleasant tone for the session.

At the same time, begin actively looking for slightly hidden competencies. Listen carefully to their conversations as well as what caregivers say for any inkling of strengths. Also watch what they do and make positive comments. When you see actions that you may consider negative, train yourself to view them in a constructive way. For instance, if you see children running around the room, comment on their curiosity. Props such as cards with pictures of strengths or having children draw pictures are additional avenues for finding their "treasures" (Figure 5-3).

Whether you provide compliments or make positive statements, be sure to be honest and real. Children can easily detect if you are being fake. Your tone of voice affects the perceived sincerity. It also is better to include details in your comments versus only making vague statements. As you search for strengths, make the hunt for buried treasure a fun adventure.

Fabulous Five: Identify Strengths

- **Listen to children's conversation for strengths.**

"I strong," 3-year-old Leon said as he carried the game box across the room.

"I see your muscles. You are strong," I replied. "Let's do that game so you get to use your strong muscles."

- **Discover and mention at least one strength of the children's within the first 5 minutes.**

Four-year-old Sherrie stretched a large red rubber band around the nails on a wooden board. "Isn't it amazing? I have to show my mom. It's a square. I made it myself."

"It is amazing. I see you have wonderful ideas."

- **Mention strengths caregivers have stated.**

"What are Jon's strengths?" I asked his kindergarten teacher.

"He's quick-witted, has good sense of humor, is empathetic and caring, wants to please, and knows what he likes."

When I saw Jon the next day, I said, "I talked with your teacher and she said a lot of good things about you. She told me you really care about people—like you're the first one to get a Band-Aid if someone gets hurt or to offer to walk with them to the clinic."

He smiled and nodded. "I've taken people to the nurse all my life."

- **Identify strengths based upon your observations of the children.**

"I'm making a bird."

"I see you are good with clay," I said.

"Yeah, I'm a good artist," 6-year-old Ron replied. "I was the goodest in my neighborhood."

"You were the best?"

"Yeah." He fashioned a hooked beak and rolled the clay into eyes. "The eyes need to be the same size."

"You have a good imagination. Do you know what that means?"

"Yeah. It means you have brains."

"Yes. It means you come up with great ideas."

- **Have children sort cards reflecting different strengths.**

"As a way to get to know you, I have these cards that show different strengths. Strengths are something you are good at or something that is good about you. Go through the cards and pick the top three or four—the best ones about you."

Six-year-old Erin sorted through the picture cards and placed four on the table. "I'm easy to get along with," she said and added, "I get along with my friends at school and some of my friends are in the second grade." Then she looked at the next card. "I care about other people's feelings. This is my favorite one." She pointed to the next card. "I work hard. Well, when I was in kindergarten, Mrs. C. wanted to see if we can tie our shoes. I tied my shoes and got a cookie." For the last card, she lifted it and said, "I have good manners." She smiled. "In Brownies, I say, 'Thank you.'"

Emphasize Children's Expertise

As you hunt for children's strengths, also zero in on their unique expertise or resourcefulness. By doing so, you continue to recognize who they are and all they can do. When you encourage them to teach what they can do, you are opening an avenue of creativity in future sessions. Also acknowledge any expertise the children have that differ from yours. For instance, I am not mechanical minded. So when I need a toy or game assembled, I know which children can put it together easily. I am always grateful for their talent, and they are pleased to help me.

Fabulous Five: Focus on the Children's Expertise

- **Tell children you are glad they are there to fix a problem.**

"This toy came apart. Thank goodness you're here to fix it," I said.

Seven-year-old Grant played with the pieces for 3 minutes and snapped the parts into place. "I also fixed the radio and clock in my dad's car," he said, flashing a proud grin.

- **Ask children to "show me how you did that."**

When I walked in the room, I saw a pyramid made out of cups. "Show me how you did that."

"It's easy." Eleven-year-old Denny disassembled the tower by slipping the cups into each other. Then, like magic, the cups slid out of his hand as he stacked them into a perfect inverted "v."

- **Acknowledge children's original ideas.**

"I have an idea. A super good idea," 7-year-old Spencer said. He snapped six yellow pieces together to form a box and then attached red, purple, and blue gear wheels so they interlocked. He spun one wheel, and the other wheels on the box turned, creating a blur of colors.

"You are the first person to do that. It was a super good idea. I'll have to show your idea to other children."

> • **Emphasize children's expertise.**
>
> I fiddled with a maze that required turning and pushing knobs to move a silver ball through a course, but I was unsuccessful in the first section. "Frank, I need your help. I'm not sure how this works. Could you figure it out for me?"
>
> Ten-year-old Frank played with the knob for ten seconds and analyzed what was needed. "Here, I'll show you. You have to turn the knob when the ball is in the middle of the track."
>
> "Thanks so much!"
>
> • **Highlight creativity or cleverness.**
>
> After the group at the day treatment program made a collage on feelings, I said, "David, help us clean up. Please get the scraps of paper that are on the floor and throw them in the trash can."
>
> "Hey, look," the 6-year-old said, using his glue-covered index finger to lift the pieces. "It's a glue finger!"
>
> "What a clever idea," I replied, and we both grinned.

Promote Self-Reflection on Positives

When you promote children's self-reflections on their own competencies, you learn how they see themselves. This is important to know because their self-perceptions can affect their participation in occupations. In addition, the children may reveal strengths they use in other settings that may not be observed when they are with you. For instance, it could be unknown to you that they supervise their siblings.

Although it may be easy for you to identify their assets, some children have a difficult time viewing themselves in a positive light. They may think they are bad or stupid and cannot believe any compliments. In therapy, you want to help them focus on what they did right and their successful strategies.

> ### *Fabulous Five: Strive to Teach Children to Reflect on Their Strengths*
> • **Encourage children to reflect on their own actions and competencies.**
>
> "How am I doing?" 9-year-old Tyson asked as he adjusted the glasses hanging on the tip of his nose.
>
> I looked at the picture he had colored and replied, "How do you think you're doing?"
>
> "I'm doing awesome," he said with a wide grin.
>
> I smiled and nodded in agreement.
>
> • **Ask children how they feel after experiencing success.**
>
> Krista demonstrated a crab walk with her stomach in the air and her hands on the floor. "Watch, I'm like

a table. I learned how to do that myself. I'm a walking table."

"How does that make you feel when you do that?" I asked.

"Happy."

"It is a good feeling to learn something new, especially when you teach yourself."

> • **Teach children in the first session to focus on what they did right.**
>
> "I was very wrong when I made that 8," 6-year-old Laura said glumly as she printed the date.
>
> "After you have your name and the date on the page, the second step is to color the bee," I instructed the group.
>
> "Bees are scary."
>
> I nodded. Maria and Maureen reached for the long black crayons, leaving only the broken ones. "There are no long crayons left."
>
> Laura asked, "Do you have any other black crayons?"
>
> "You did a good thing. I am glad you asked me. You found a way to fix a problem, and by talking about it I was able to help you."
>
> • **Comment about children's competencies and ask probing questions.**
>
> "I noticed you did the mazes so well. Do you do something like them at home or school?"
>
> "Yeah, I love to do puzzle books. I do my cousin's. They're really hard. I'm good at playing games too."
>
> • **Encourage children to talk about their accomplishments.**
>
> "I'm on a wrestling team. I won my last meet," 11-year-old Doug said.
>
> "Tell me more about it," I replied, and he described his wrestling feats.
>
> Three months later, he walked into the therapy room wearing a gray long-sleeved T-shirt with "State Championship" printed on the chest.
>
> "I came in fourth in the state. There were over 3,000 kids, though not all of them were in my category. I brought my trophy to show you."
>
> "Congratulations! You must be really proud. It takes a lot of hard work to get that far."
>
> He nodded and beamed.

Observe, Listen for, and Discuss Children's, Caregivers', and Educational Staff Members' Current Strategies

> **Children might be thinking:**
> *I have good ideas.*
> *My mom and dad know what helps me too.*

In addition to asking children explicit questions, you can learn their strategies by close observation and talking with caregivers and teachers. When conversing with children, pay attention to how they successfully handled situations. You also may need to help others recognize children's current strategies. Learn what children bring to the situation and build on and emphasize their strengths.

Fabulous Five: Learn Children's, Caregivers', and Teachers' Current Strategies

- **Observe what children do that is an effective strategy.**

"Andy, I remember that in the fall it was hard for you to pay attention to your teacher. But today I noticed you kept your eyes on your teacher when she was giving directions. What did you discover that helps you pay attention?"

The 9 year old replied, "I clear my mind of distractions in the room and I tell myself, 'Focus.'"

- **Learn from caregivers and teachers what strategies and approaches help the children.**

"What strategies have you found that help your child?" I asked the mother of 9-year-old John.

"I give him choices and remove myself from the situation. For example, last night he started whining that he didn't want to do his homework. I told him, 'You can choose to do your homework or you can miss bowling'— and he really loves bowling.

"'But, Mom,' he said, 'I don't want to do my homework.'

"'It's your choice,' I told him. 'I love you and I am going to do the dishes.' I walked away and he started his math."

"So it sounds like John does better when he is given choices," I said, and his mother nodded.

- **Discuss with caregivers and educational staff the possible meanings of children's actions.**

When we met with 3-year-old Kurt's father, I said, "In class I have seen him rub his earlobes. I'm not sure if his ears are bothering him or if he finds that soothing."

"Yeah, at home he rubs his ear for calming."

"What else does he do to calm himself?"

"He likes to wrap himself in his blanket."

- **Listen for strategies as children talk.**

"I was throwing a fit because we didn't see the wolves at the zoo and we were leaving," Angelina said. "But then I went home and drew a picture of the wolves and I felt like I was at the zoo."

"Whose idea was that?" I asked.

The 8-year-old pointed to herself and said with a smile, "Mine."

- **Reframe what others consider a problem as being the children's strategy.**

I watched 3-year-old Doug and noticed that after getting upset, he would jump up and run to the children's drinking fountain in the corner of the classroom. "I'm sick. I need a drink," he said and came back to the group looking calmer. I noticed that this became a pattern.

"Doug keeps leaving the group," his teacher said, sounding frustrated with him.

"What I see is that he uses the drinking fountain for self-calming," I replied. "If you want to give him another option, you could give him a water bottle with a straw. You could see if he finds that soothing. Then he could stay with the group."

Co-Create Educational Experiences

Developing the collaborative frame entails giving children the fourth message that together you will be co-creating educational experiences. You both will collaborate to design experiences that help the children learn about themselves. They will make decisions and have a say in what is done.

Establish the Criteria of Challenge and Fun in the Beginning Sessions

> **Children might be thinking:**
> *I wonder if I can do this.*
> *Wow, I get to do what I want.*
> *This will be fun.*
> *We're going to have a fun time together.*

There are two critical factors of an educational experience in therapy. First, to grow, children have to be challenged outside their current realm of functioning. Second, they experience fun. It may be a sense of enjoyment in the moment or even pleasure following an accomplishment. Facing challenges promotes learning. Having fun is motivating for them to start and stay with the challenge. The interplay of these two factors helps children move forward into new experiences.

Incorporate the Fun Factor in the First Session

You capture most children's attention when you talk about having fun. They will immediately wonder, "What is it?" or, "What are we going to do?" Children are motivated to participate if they view the activity as pleasurable. Your intention also is to have them create a mindset where they associate therapy with fun. It is vital that in the first session you collaborate with the children in designing a fun experience. For example, you may offer an activity that matches their interests or that you know other children have enjoyed.

Fabulous Five: Weave in Fun

- **Talk about being fun or having fun things to do when you introduce yourself.**

I squatted to Bob's eye level, introduced myself, and added, "I brought fun things for us to do. Come with me, I think you'll like it." The 5 year old with ruffled black hair gave me a long evaluating look, then followed me down the hallway. I smiled at him, and his face relaxed.

"Guess what? I'm good at swinging. I stick my feet up and I fly."

"Now that you're good at swinging, I bet it's a lot of fun," I said, and he nodded.

- **Tell children, "I think you are going to like this."**

"I think you're going to like this," I said.

"What is it?" 3-year-old Cliff replied.

I pulled a barber Play-Doh set out of my canvas bag. "You get to be a barber. Give this boy a haircut." I squished the putty into the top of the figure, and blue spaghetti-strand hair popped out of the plastic head.

Enthralled, Cliff snipped at the hair with scissors.

- **Make the first activity enticing.**

"I have markers that do magic tricks," I said to 5-year-old Megan. "First, write your name."

Megan printed her first name using a yellow marker and then, with a curious glint in her eye, said, "Now what?"

"Take this other marker and trace your name. See what color it makes it. It's magic."

"Whoa, it turned purple."

- **Connect the first activity to children's interests.**

Six-year-old Donovan strolled into the room with a book tucked under his arm. "Would you like to see all the fish?"

"Sure," I replied and thumbed through the pages. I handed it back to him. "Would you like to draw a picture?"

He nodded and began to sketch the outline of a trout. "I'm drawing a fish."

"You have a real talent for drawing."

"Do I have to color the whole thing?"

"It might be good to add a little color to it." Donovan proceeded to color the entire body, and when he was done, I said, "Because you like fishing, I have a game you probably will like. You catch fish with a fishing rod and magnet. Then you write whatever letter is on the fish."

"Yeah, I love to fish."

- **Show children that therapy can be fun.**

"I've brought some fun stuff," I told the kindergartners in their first session, pulling out putty. "Do you want me to bury these dinosaur erasers?" Three heads nodded. I squashed the erasers until they disappeared in the putty. "Dig these out."

"I'm going to pretend I'm digging for dinosaur bones," Dean said. "I found one. Look, I found something."

"You found one already, you're quick," I replied. "Get more out."

Susan retrieved four and then placed them upright. "They're sleeping and nothing bad happened to them."

"Oh good," I said. "We have 3 minutes left, and then it will be time for recess. I enjoyed being with you, and I will see you next week."

Dean pressed the putty into the container and, as he walked out of the room, said, "This is a fun place."

Introduce the Notion of the Just-Right Challenge

In addition to having fun, you want children to equate therapy with being challenged and as a place to try something new. You need to let them know that the challenge has to be meaningful to them and be at the just-right level. You do not want them to feel overwhelmed, panicked, or anxious. On the other hand, it should not be so easy that it is boring. Ask children to let you know or watch their facial expressions to determine the just-right level. In the beginning, you may need to model how to increase the level of difficulty or cue them to do it themselves.

Fabulous Five: Create Challenges

- **Tell children that occupational therapy is a place to try new things.**

In the first session, 5-year-old Jeff looked at the lacing activity on the table and said, "I can't do that."

"In this room, give yourself a chance to try new things. It doesn't help if you say, 'I can't,'" the certified occupational therapy assistant replied.

"I try," his friend cued him with the words to say.

"That's right. Jeff, tell yourself, 'I will try this even if it's new or looks hard.' That's all I ask—that in this room you just try. I will always be here to help you if you need it."

- **Ask children if the activity is too hard, too easy, or just right.**

"This is easy," 6-year-old Sammie said. He pinched the red tongs to pluck the 1-inch erasers and then dropped them in a bowl. Sammie tapped the ends of the tongs together. "These are like chopsticks."

I nodded and replaced the large erasers with half-inch heart-shaped ones.

Sammie struggled to get a grip on one. "This is hard."

"Is it too hard or a just-right challenge?" I asked.

"It's okay," he replied and persisted with the task.

- **Cue children to independently increase the level of difficulty if the activity becomes too easy.**

"If this game gets too easy, make it harder," I said.

Neal balanced on a one-legged stool and threw the yellow tennis ball into a box. All three throws were successful. "How about I make it even trickier?" Neal said. He stood, smiled, and grabbed a smaller box. "This is making it real tricky."

- **Give an idea on how to make an activity harder and allow children to decide.**

"Throw the beanbags into the clown target," I said.

Seven-year-old Jose stood 6 inches away and lightly tossed the yellow beanbag into the clown's mouth. "Yes," he yelled.

"You might want to challenge yourself. If this is too easy, you could just move back. It's up to you if you want to do that."

Jose moved two steps back and resumed throwing.

- **Ask, "How can you make this harder?" especially if the children say, "This is too easy."**

Rick created his own game by using masking tape to make a target on the carpet. Then he took poker chips and threw them by the handful toward the target. Three chips landed on the bullseye. "This is easy," he said, pleased with his success.

"How can you make it harder?" I asked.

"Hmm, I don't have any ideas."

"Try throwing one chip." I moved the chips off the target and added, "Outside the target is water. What is the target? An island or a boat?"

"An island." Rick threw one chip at a time, missing the first three. "This is harder than I thought. Oh, I finally got one." He threw another into the center circle. "YES, I got it!"

Engage Children in Creating Experiences in the Initial Sessions

Children might be thinking:
Wow. I can do this.
I get to say what I want.
You're good to be around.
This fun. I want to do it again.

You want children to become partners. To motivate them to participate, you need to create successful experiences for them. In the process, they will find that they get to make decisions and have a say. Together, you collaborate to develop learning experiences that involve the just-right challenge and fun.

Provide a Successful Beginning Experience

To create experiences that are challenging and fun, the children have to be engaged in the process. Facing a challenge involves the risk of failing. Before children can even entertain the idea of trying, there has to be the belief that success is possible. The challenge has to be just right and attainable in their eyes. They also have to believe that they have the needed ability. Your goal is for them to succeed.

Many children who are seen in therapy have unfortunately had many failures. They discover that when they try a new venture, they often struggle without positive results. At the same time, they see their peers completing the same task effortlessly. Consequently, you often see them respond to any new or difficult-looking task by saying, "I can't do this," or, "This is too hard." Or they may hesitantly attempt one step but declare after the first mistake, "I'm stupid."

To entice the children to take risks, you have to help nurture and develop their own beliefs about their competence. One way to break the cycle of failure followed by self-doubt is to adjust the task so they can be successful. Change the nature of the activity to an achievable level.

There is a range of ways to tweak an activity to ensure success. You may start with an action or activity they already do and slightly modify it. Or you may look and note what is currently in their repertoire. For example, if a child is good at releasing objects, you may design a game that only requires releasing an object into a target. The amount of assistance you provide can be altered to whatever is needed to succeed.

The type of activity also can be varied. One with a clear end product can become a symbol of accomplishment. On the other hand, an activity with no defined ending is harder to fail. When children experience success in their first session, they will tend to feel safe knowing that you are building on their assets. When you acknowledge their efforts, you show your recognition that facing a challenge is difficult for them. They will be pleased to have you as a witness to their accomplishments.

Fabulous Five: Start With Success
- **Take children thorough the motion to ensure success.**

Nine-year-old James gripped a yellow wheel game piece. He slid it back and forth on his desk and then dropped it on the floor. "Let me show you. I'm going to put my hand on yours," I said as I provided hand-over-hand assistance to guide the piece to the hole. "Push down." He patted it with his palm. "Look, now you can spin it," I said and gave the wheel a twirl.

- **Use an activity children cannot fail.**

I handed 3-year-old Jonah a book and said, "Pick a picture. This is really fun to do." He thumbed through three pages and pointed to a dog. "Okay," I said. "Paint this picture—get water on your brush and paint the dog. The water makes the colors magically appear."

He dipped the brush in a cup of water and splashed a few drips on the page. He grinned when the brown dog began to emerge.

- **Start with an action or activity you know the children can do.**

As I watched Eddie in class, I saw that all objects placed on his desk were quickly dumped on the floor. I thought, *He's good at grasping things and releasing them.* I went into my office and grabbed an empty box and beanbags that made sounds when they hit the ground. I put the beanbags on his desk and said, "Throw these into the box." As predicted, he scrunched the beanbags in his palm and dropped them. I moved the box to catch each one. "Good throw!" I said.

- **Begin with an activity with a clear ending so children can see the successful result.**

"These are sun catchers," I said to 7-year-old Josie, pointing to five plastic circles, each with raised edges outlining different designs. "You paint them and then hang them in a window so the sun can shine through them. Pick one."

Josie lifted the hummingbird design. "This one." She reached for her brush and tapped it to her lips while deciding on her colors. Then she painted the bird a bright yellow surrounded by blue sky.

"Hold it up to the lamp," I suggested. The colors glistened as the light shone through it. "What are you going to do with it?"

"I'm giving it to my dad," she replied with a proud smile.

- **Try an unstructured activity with no clear ending.**

"Here's some clay. Go ahead and play with it," the occupational therapy student said. "You can make something if you want."

Eight-year-old Jamal rolled the clay first with his right palm and then switched to his left because he was unable to coordinate both hands together. "I'm making a cat."

"I see the cat's body. Here's more clay for the head," she replied, handing him a round ball of clay.

He poked in two eyes and attached it to the body. Then he rolled a tail and added it to his animal. "I'm done."

"What a cool cat."

Ensure That Children Make Decisions

For children to be true partners, it is paramount that they get to make decisions and have the right to say no. Show them that they have a say in what occurs in the session. Give them choices and respect their answers. If they appear overwhelmed with too many choices, narrow the selection down to two or three. Allow time for them to choose and wait even if you feel impatient. Watch their response to determine their choice and if needed ask them to communicate in a different manner, such as looking at it. If you suggest an idea, still check if they are interested or want to modify it.

Listen to children when they say no. It may be that they do not like the activity or just do not feel like doing it that day. If, however, you sense children are saying no because they do not believe they can do it, then ask what they are thinking about it. That gives you an opportunity to address their fears and either adapt the activity or suggest other choices.

Fabulous Five: Give Choices and Respect "No" Regarding Activity Decisions

- **Provide choices regarding initial activities and let children decide.**

On the table, there was a magnetic building set, painting supplies, and a puzzle. "What should we start with?" I asked the 8 year old with a pixie haircut.

"The magnets."

"You can make all kinds of cool stuff with them." To demonstrate, I placed a rectangle piece upright and then balanced a circle on top. It resembled the vague outline of a person.

Rebecca picked up two triangles and turned them sideways so the two tips touched each other. "Look. It's an angel."

- **Encourage children to make their own decisions.**

For his first activity, 7-year-old Jorge decided to make a racecar pop-up book. "What color should I do the car?" he asked.

"It's up to you. It's your book," I responded.

"I'll use red." He colored the body of the car and said, "This car should have smoke."

"Here's paper. You could make smoke and glue it on."

"No."

"Okay. It's your book. You decide."

- **Respect when children say no regarding activity decisions.**

Four-year-old Berry barreled over to the upright easel and scribbled a picture, looking like a loose ball of yarn. "Do you want me to draw a road for you? We could make it a game and see if you can stay on the road," I suggested.

"No. Not yet," he responded and continued to swerve the marker in all directions.

"Okay," I responded.

"Now I want you to draw a road. I want you to draw some water and a shark."

I sketched a windy path surrounded by waves and three sharks and suggested he draw through the maze. "Stay on the road. You don't want the sharks to bite you."

- **Clarify unclear responses when children are making decisions.**

"Trevor, do you want a book or music?" I asked after placing the two objects in front of him.

"Ah, ah," the 9 year old replied and reached with both hands, touching the book with his left hand and the device with his right.

"I'm not sure which one you want." I gently placed my palm on his nondominant left hand and said, "Pick the one you want."

He then reached with his right hand and rested on the book about the Halloween frog.

- **Ask for feedback whenever you suggest a treatment idea.**

"I have a gingerbread man or a Christmas tree. If you don't want to do these, it's okay. Just tell me. We can do something else."

"He's all mixed up," 4-year-old Gina said and reached for the gingerbread man, letting me know she was interested.

"You're right. It's a puzzle. You have to cut out all the pieces and put them together to make the picture. You have to fix him."

Adapt the Activity to Create the Just-Right Challenge

To grade an activity means to analyze and adapt it to the level at which children experience the perfect challenge. The first step is to become aware of the basic skills or requirements needed. One way to do this is to try the activity yourself. As you attempt it, consider what supplies you need, how many steps are involved, what might be difficult, what strategies would help, and what ways could you make it easier or harder. Adapting an activity also requires knowledge of what children can usually do. You need a repertoire of creative ways to adjust or fine-tune activities if children have limitations. For example, if you work with children who are blind, you would identify ways to use touch or sound to complete the task. This becomes easier the more experienced you are.

There are many ways to adapt and create the ideal match. You may shorten the duration of the activity or make it one easy step. The materials or the game rules may be changed. The amount of assistance you provide is another factor that you can tailor to their abilities. You also can look at toys as being on a continuum from easy to being harder to manipulate. At first, make your best guess at what activities the children can do. Then with observation and their feedback, including nonverbal responses, you can achieve the just-right level.

Fabulous Five: Grade the Activity to the Children's Current Level of Competence and Comfort

- **Make the first activity one easy step.**

"Aaa," Joni chanted as she waddled around the room and then sat at the table. The 7 year old reached for the wooden puzzle of four various size apples. She wrapped her pudgy fingers around the largest apple. To ensure success, I covered three holes and then pointed to the largest hole. "Put it in."

Joni slammed it down sideways and grimaced when her effort was thwarted. "Turn it," I said as I demonstrated a rotating motion.

She pivoted the piece, and the apple plopped into place.

- **Adjust the activity to the exact step where children feel comfortable trying.**

Five-year-old Jay wandered aimlessly around the classroom, mumbling, "Wake up. We go to the store. Go to store. Oranges. Oranges. Oranges. Start the bus. Pick up the house. Pick up the mess."

"Check your schedule," the paraprofessional said, pointing to the wall of pictures for each activity in his routine.

Jay pulled the visual symbol of a table with the word "sensory" off the Velcro strip, went into the hall, and sat at a small table. The paraprofessional squirted shaving cream onto a tin baking sheet. Jay flapped his hands at his side and said, "Messy, messy. It's a mess."

"Please touch it," the paraprofessional cued him and demonstrated by drawing a face.

"Touch it," Jay repeated. "It's messy. Touch this mess." He poked his index finger in the tray for only a second and then pulled back. "Get off." He alternated between placing his open palms just above the cream and withdrawing his hands.

I put shaving cream on my finger and held it close to Jay's hands. I smiled and waited.

He lightly tapped my finger and then rubbed his hands until the cream disappeared. After three times of touching the shaving cream on my finger and rubbing it off his fingers, he slowly placed his palms in the shaving cream and began making circular motions.

- **Simplify an activity that is too hard.**

Six-year-old Jeri pushed the tail of the plastic frog to make it pop into the target. Her frog left the ground but only went 2 inches. She stood and started to wander away from the group.

"Jeri," I called to her.

"It's too hard to do," she said from a distance.

I made a larger target using tape. "Jeri, try again. I made it easier."

"You made it easier," she repeated to herself and returned. She pressed and the frog flew into the target. "I got one in," she said with a smile.

- **Provide assistance and gradually withdraw the help.**

When the preschool class at the Sight Center headed to the playground, Hannah ran to a scooter that she could straddle with her legs and push with her feet. She cruised up and down the pathways used to teach mobility training. After a few minutes, I brought over a small tricycle. "Hannah, check this bike out." She hesitated but stepped off the scooter.

"Here, try sitting on the bike. I'll hold it still." She stood at the tricycle for a minute. "First put your hand on the handlebar," I said and gently guided her right hand. "Then swing your leg around." I helped her get situated on the seat with her feet off the ground. "When you get used to having your feet on the pedals and learn how to ride, it will be so much fun."

She gripped the handlebars tightly for 5 seconds, pushed the pedals one time, and then put her feet back on solid ground. For the next few weeks, I helped her get started. Once her balance improved, she became more confident and began riding without help.

- **Change the materials or game to match the children's abilities.**

"Maria has low vision but wants to do whatever her classmates are doing," the special education teacher who worked in the preschool classroom told me.

I talked with Maria's preschool teacher and obtained one of their cutting activities. I darkened the line, made it thicker, and brought it back to class.

Maria held the paper a couple of inches from her eyes and started cutting with her classmates. "This is easy," she said with a grin.

KEY POINTS TO REMEMBER

- Alleviate children's anxiety about meeting you, especially when you are a stranger.
- Recognize and acknowledge children's current situation and associated feelings.
- Create a safe environment and climate of caring.
- Give the message that occupational therapy is a safe place.
- Create a sense of belonging.

- Define the relationship as a partnership in which children have a voice and their views are equally valued.
- Define your role as a helper, informant, and advocate.
- Convey through your nonverbal language, words, and actions that you desire collaboration.
- Elicit, recognize, and emphasize children's strengths and strategies in the first session.
- Engage children in co-creating educational experiences that are challenging and fun in the initial sessions.

REVIEW QUESTIONS

1. Occupational therapists use the term *safe place* to refer to just the location where therapy happens. True or false.
2. You enter a hospital room for the first time and see that a child is getting a shot or having an IV put in (or any other painful medical procedure). Tears are running down the child's cheeks. What can you say to convey empathy?
3. You should prepare children for what you are going to do before moving them. True or false.
4. Convert the following into strengths:
   - Passive
   - Distractible
   - Opinionated
5. What possible feelings may arise when you ask children about their strengths?
6. If children are unable to answer your question about their strengths, you should move on to another topic. True or false.
7. What are signs that children think the activity is fun?
8. What is a just-right challenge?
9. It is important for children to experience success the first time they are with you. True or false.
10. What are some of the different ways to grade an activity?

REFERENCE

Drewes, A. A. (2005). Suggestions and research on multicultural play therapy. In E. Gil & A. A. Drewes (Eds.), *Cultural issues in play therapy* (pp. 72-95). New York, NY: Guilford Press.

6

Learn About Children and Their Worlds Through Interviews

CHAPTER OVERVIEW

To make therapy meaningful, you need to learn about the children and their worlds. Interviews are an avenue for discovering children's perspectives on their life as well as their hopes and dreams. This chapter outlines methods for conducting a child-friendly interview from start to finish. Included are ways to word and reword questions in "kid language." This chapter also shows how much information can be obtained by talking with children.

CHILDREN'S DESCRIPTIONS OF WHAT THEY THINK YOU SHOULD KNOW

Dr. Clare: "Why is it important for therapists to ask children what they are thinking and feeling?"

Ned (age 8): "Because the kids would like it."

Martin (age 12): "If they don't, then they don't know what the kids are thinking."

Tony (age 10): "So they can help us feel happy."

Sean (age 9): "Then they can learn what kids do and what they like."

Bill (age 10): "The kid may know something the adult doesn't."

CREATE MEANINGFUL CONVERSATIONS

Ongoing conversations are required to foster the development of a partnership. An interview is a way to let children know you are serious about hearing what they have to say about their lives. It is an opportunity to gain in-depth information in a short time.

Introduce the Interview and Decide on the Format

The first purpose of an interview is to invite children to talk about their lives, including their valued occupations. Your topics and corresponding questions define the area of interest as occupational functioning. Let children know you want to learn about their everyday experiences at home, at school, with friends, and at play. The interview questions often promote self-reflection and increase awareness of their already effective strategies and strengths. Assume the stance that they are the experts on their lives and you are a learner who is open to getting to know them.

A second purpose of the interview is to discover not only what is happening in their lives, but also their perceptions of these events and their explanations about why things occur. This is important because their reality is based on

Curtin, C.
Strategies for Collaborating With Children: Creating Partnerships in Occupational Therapy and Research (pp. 99-120).
© 2017 SLACK Incorporated.

their perceptions and this knowledge helps you enter their world and their way of seeing people and situations.

Introduce the Interview

> **Children might be thinking:**
> *What are we going to talk about?*
> *Why do you want to talk to me?*
> *I am not sure I want to talk to you.*
> *Will you ask hard questions?*
> *Is this a test? Can I fail?*
> *Will I get in trouble if I tell you something bad?*
> *Are you going to tell anyone what I said?*

Before you start the interview, pick a place that is quiet. It is essential that you be able to hear the children, especially soft-spoken ones. Limit the amount of distractions in the room. You may want to cover or put away extra toys or supplies. Also sit at the same level as the children. It is a good idea to always have a variety of materials to facilitate the interview. Basic supplies would be paper, markers, colored pencils, scissors, glue, puppets, small toys, and putty. Have these available but out of sight.

Another good habit is to create your own recording system. This allows you to quickly write down direct quotes from children and permits you to more accurately represent their voices in reports and meetings. When possible, try to use abbreviations or symbols for words. For example, instead of writing, "I don't know" as a response, you could just print "IDK." You have to be fast when writing so you do not disrupt the flow of the interview. Maintain eye contact as much as possible and avoid only looking at your paper. If they ask what you are writing, be truthful. I usually say, "I am writing down what you tell me. It helps me to remember." If children ask, also be honest about who you will share the information with and let them know you cannot keep secrets.

Before starting the interview, you need to determine your time constraints. If you know you only have a few minutes, carefully select priority questions. You may want to learn about their perceptions of themselves, their occupations, and their lives so you may ask questions about their interests, competencies, and dreams for the future. In a school setting, some key questions are, "What are you good at doing?" "What is easy for you at school?" "What is hard?" "What do you like to do?" "What helps you learn best?" and, "What do you want to get better at?" This pertinent information can be obtained in as little as 5 minutes. In situations where you have more time, it is helpful to develop a list of questions for different domain of life and design a semi-structured interview guide.

For children who are nonverbal, provide ways for them to respond without speaking. You can ask yes/no questions and they can answer using their eyes, facial expressions, or sign language. Some can reply using their communication devices that vocalize for them. You need to adapt to their way of communicating.

Initiate the Interview

When you talk with children, begin by introducing the purpose of your conversation. You may do this simply by saying that you want to get to know them. You can emphasize your desire to learn: what they like, what they do during the week, and what is important to them. By clearly stating your agenda, they will have a better understanding of your intentions. This is helpful because some children may worry about why you are talking to them and what you are going to do with the information.

Start the interview with questions that they can answer easily and that draw out positive responses. This sets a pleasant tone and conveys that you are interested in learning about their strengths as well as their difficulties. Avoid starting with questions that might entail painful feelings or require acknowledging any difficulties. Open-ended questions such as, "Tell me about…." allow them to express what they consider vital and tend to elicit more information. Some children respond better to closed-ended questions that have a definite answer (e.g., "Do you have any pets?"). You would then gradually shift to open-ended type questions.

> ### *Fabulous Five: Start the Interview*
>
> - **Let children know the purpose of the interview is to get to know them.**
>
> When I headed to the third-grade classroom to get Kassi, I discovered her curled on the hallway floor crying. "What's the matter?" I asked.
>
> Between sobs, she said, "I don't feel good."
>
> "Did you go to the clinic?"
>
> "Yes, I took an aspirin."
>
> "Oh, it's hard to be at school when you feel sick." I paused, then continued in a soft voice, "Actually I came to see you. Why don't you come with me to my room and we can talk. Would that be okay with you?" She nodded and followed me. Once in the room, I said, "If you want to stop, just let me know, because I know you're not feeling well. I want to get to know you better. So tell me about your day at school when you're not sick."
>
> She stopped sniffling and started talking about her routine.
>
> - **Emphasize how they will benefit from doing the interview.**
>
> "I want to talk to you so I can find out what's important to you. When I know what you think is fun, it will be easier for me to bring activities that you like. What is your favorite thing to do?" I asked 10-year-old Harriet.

"I love horses. My bedroom is covered with posters of ponies."

The next day, I brought a velveteen picture of a horse and a copper tooling model of a stallion to her hospital room. "Which one would you like to make?" I asked, and she pointed to the picture.

- **Start the interview with open-ended questions.**

I looked at the 8 year old with his tousled brown hair and green-striped T-shirt. Smiling, I asked him, "Who lives at your house?"

"There are five of us, including me," Ruppert replied.

"Who are they?"

"My mom, dad, uncle, and my older sister."

"What does your family like to do together?"

"Go to restaurants. Go to the park. And watch TV."

- **Begin the interview with closed questions to define topics and allow for easy answers, and then move to open-ended questions.**

"Do you have any brothers or sisters?"

Five-year-old John nodded. "I have two sisters."

"Tell me about them."

"Well, my sisters are as big as my mom and dad. They paint their nails. Sometimes they scratch me."

- **Start the interview on a positive note.**

"What are you really good at or what do you know how to do well?" I asked 6-year-old Marty as the first question.

"Memory games. I always beat my mom," he said and smiled a toothless grin.

Identify Rules for Responding

As you start the interview, children try to determine what you want to know. They may wonder if your line of questioning is like school, where their teachers already know the answers to the questions asked. This can lead to the children's perception that there are correct answers. They also may worry that your questions are a test, which implies the possibility of failure if they do not respond correctly. It is important in the beginning to state explicitly the purpose of your questions and say there are no wrong answers.

Most children want to be good respondents and please you. It creates a dilemma for them if they do not understand what you are asking, cannot remember a situation, or do not know the answer. Although some will not hesitate to tell you they do not know, others will make up an answer. Again, it is helpful to clarify the interview "rules." Tell them to let you know if they do not understand the question, and then you can say it in another way. Convey your acceptance and comfort with any difficulties they might have with remembering or just not knowing.

Fabulous Five: Cue Children on How to Respond to Interview Questions

- **Let children know there are no wrong answers.**

"What do you like about your family?"

"They help me and make sure I never fall in the water," 5-year-old Matthew replied.

"What do you dislike or not like about your family?"

"Nothing," he said in a hesitant voice, giving me the impression that he wondered if that was an okay answer.

"That's all right. There are no wrong answers."

- **Reassure children that the interview is not a test.**

"Do loud noises ever bother you?"

"Is this a test I can fail?"

"No. This is not a test," I reassured 9-year-old Nick. "These are questions that help me learn about you and get to know how things are going for you. I also want to find out what helps you."

- **Ask children to tell you if they do not understand your questions or what you are saying.**

"Who do you admire?" I asked 7-year-old Rose.

She pressed her index finger against her lips, assuming the pose of a thinker, and then crinkled her mouth as if to say, "I don't know."

"If you don't understand my question, it's okay to just tell me or say, 'I don't know.' Who do you look up to or want to be like?"

"My sister because she's so nice."

- **Tell children it is all right if they do not know an answer.**

"What activities do you like to do with your friends?" I asked.

Six-year-old Samuel stared at me in silence and then shrugged his shoulders. "I don't know."

"That's okay. What do you like to do?"

"I like to check my e-mail and play computer games," he replied with a grin.

- **Let children know it is okay if they cannot remember the answer to the question.**

"What are you good at doing?"

"I'm good at drawing and art," 7-year-old Darren replied.

"What is easy for you at school?"

"Math."

"Tell me about your happiest day."

"I don't remember."

Sensing his discomfort, I replied, "That's okay. Tell me about your family."

"I have a mom and four sisters. They all love me. I used to have five sisters but one died."

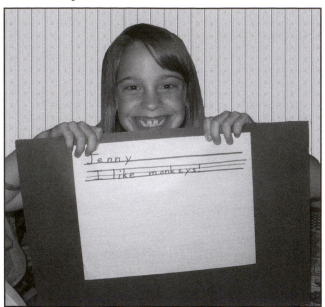

Figure 6-1. Children enjoy telling you their interests.

Clarify the Topic

When asking questions, be clear about the topic. Be direct and define the aspect of their lives that you want children to discuss (Figure 6-1). The "Tell me…" phrase is straightforward and consequently well defined. Some will respond, "Okay," and proceed to talk. Others may not like a direct approach. To them it may sound like a command. They would do better with more subtle phrases like, "I am wondering…" or, "It would help me to know…." Then, by responding, they may view themselves as a helper. An interested and inquiring tone of voice makes a difference for all children.

> ### *Fabulous Five: State the Topic*
>
> - **Say, "Tell me about…."**
>
>   "Tell me about your family," I asked 6-year-old Zach.
>
>   "I live with my dad and my little sister. She's a big pain. Every time I ask her to play, she yells, 'Go away.'"
>
> - **Tell children, "It would help me to know…."**
>
>   "It would help me to know whether writing is easy or hard for you."
>
>   "Sometimes it's hard, especially when I have to write a lot. I'm doing a little better with cursive. I want to get faster because I'm turning into an adult," 10-year-old Trent answered.
>
> - **Say, "Tell me everything you can about…."**
>
>   "Tell me everything you can about your friends."
>
>   "Stephanie's not bossing me anymore," 5-year-old Iris replied. "I usually play with Ashley. Ashley taught me how to do the monkey bars. Someday a friend is going to invite me to a slumber party."

- **Comment, "I would like to know…."**

  "I would like to know what you enjoy doing with your family."

  "I like to go grocery shopping. We go every day and we get food and something to drink. I like to eat with my family and go to the movies with them." Nine-year-old Nate smiled and added, "My dad likes playing with me too."

- **Say, "I'm wondering how…."**

  "I'm wondering how things are going with your friends?" the occupational therapy student asked the second grader.

  "Oh, good. My friend Bob—he just talks and talks and talks. He never gives up. He's funny."

Match Interview Format to the Children

> **Children might be thinking:**
> *I like to draw.*
> *I like to play.*
> *I like toys and puppets.*
> *It's fun to talk to you.*
> *You're really fun.*

There is more than one way to converse with children. A variety of creative and playful approaches can be used as alternatives to just talking. Some children like to talk while they draw, engage in games, play with puppets, or take photos. Younger children often like to chat while participating in an activity. The use of props or toys can be enticing. You want to match the format to the children's comfort and developmental levels. At times, you may choose to start the interview with a play activity to get them started. A playful approach also is a good backup plan if you see children becoming restless. Switching to an activity can eliminate the pressure to talk, and the children can then choose when they want to speak. Given the right format, you will discover that most children can articulate what they are thinking.

Incorporate Drawing as Part of the Interview

Drawing is a medium that children naturally use to express themselves (Figure 6-2). It is often easier, especially for younger ones, to create a picture first and then talk. You may start the interview by asking them to make a picture. When given the freedom to draw what they choose, children often depict scenes from a recent and/or prominent experience that has made a lasting impression on them. The second option is for you to define a theme and then ask them to draw about it. You may ask them to make a picture of themselves or their family and then encourage them to talk about it. Another theme is to have them draw

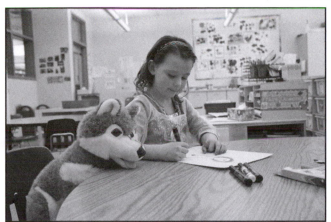

Figure 6-2. Make drawing an option when conducting an interview.

their room, house, or neighborhood. These pictures provide clues to their identity, interests, and daily occupations. For instance, as they describe their bedroom, they may tell you what is hanging on their walls, such as awards or favorite family photographs. The picture of their room can also be used to gather more details about their routine. If you suspect a child might have been abused, you would ask them to draw a playroom instead of a bedroom. The third way to use drawing is to have them create a picture in response to your question and then discuss it. They can depend less on words with this approach, and the children can choose how much they want to say.

Fabulous Five: Have Children Draw to Start the Interview or to Answer the Questions

- **Ask children to draw a picture.**

"Please make a picture for me."

Six-year-old Cecilia started to draw curved lines with different colors. "My favorite holiday is St. Patrick's Day because some people say there is a rainbow and a pot of gold. Last spring I saw a pretty rainbow, but when I went to tell my family, it disappeared and never came back. I don't think it's returned."

- **Request that children make a picture of themselves.**

"Here's some paper. Please make a picture of yourself."

Four-year-old Alex drew a circle for his body and then added body parts. "That's me." He pointed first to his left and then his right foot. "This foot doesn't work good, and this foot works. That's just the way God made me."

- **Have children draw their room, house, or neighborhood to gain information about their lives.**

"I would like to learn more about your life. Here's some paper. Please draw a picture of your bedroom."

"I don't have a bedroom. I usually sleep on the floor at my dad's house, and I sleep on the couch at my mom's house," 10-year-old Colton replied.

"Where do you keep your clothes and toys?"

"In the basement. My house is kinda strange."

"I know you just switched schools. Did you move?"

"I didn't really move when I came here."

"So you're still living in the same place; you only changed schools. Did your parents want you to go to another school?"

"No, I wanted to go to another school."

"It must make you feel good that they listened to you. What do you think of this school?"

"I like it."

"Oh, good. I'm glad it's better for you."

- **Ask children to draw their family.**

"Here's some paper. Please draw a picture of your family," the occupational therapy student told 6-year-old Deanna. He handed her paper and a box of crayons containing different skin colors.

She chose a cocoa color and drew her family. "Here's my mom. Here's my dad. I almost left my sister out. I better draw her too. My uncle Eric is going to take me to Mexico for 3 days. I'm too afraid of the plane. I know it'll be okay. I get to look out the window. I know it'll be fun."

- **Request that children draw the answers to your questions.**

"Here's some paper. Draw your favorite thing to do. Favorite means what you really, really like doing the best," I said to 4-year-old Frances.

She drew a figure with four legs. "I like to ride on a real pony. I rode one at the fair named Buddy. I like Buddy. I want a pony. I can't get one until I live by myself and get a job."

Use Props or Games in the Interview

Children respond well to adults who use play-based approaches. Therefore, another interview format is to integrate questions into a game or an activity. For some, playing a game with an adult is considered special and fun. Games are usually enticing and associated with happy feelings, especially if they win. Children know that they get choices when playing and can change the rules if everyone agrees. For example, if they pick up a card with a question they do not want to answer, they can ask to select another one. A spinner with picture symbols provides the element of surprise because they do not know where the arrow will land. Toys and puppets also are engaging. For younger children, it may be easier to talk to a puppet than participate in a formal interview. To them, a puppet represents a pretend friend or animal who is nonjudgmental. Because the use of games and props is familiar and a normal part of their routine, this type of format can be beneficial, especially with hesitant or younger children.

Fabulous Five: Incorporate Games or Props

- **Create a game with embedded questions.**

Five-year-old Haley swung the magnetic fishing rod and hooked a fish with a question written on it. I pulled the fish off the magnet and read out loud, "How is school?"

"Good. We get to do things like paint and read books. We get to play and listen to music."

She fished again, and I read the next question. "What do you think about your teacher?"

"She's good. She's old but we love her. I like all the stuff she does. We get free time to play."

- **Adapt a board game to include interview questions.**

I unfolded the Candyland game on the table. Six-year-old Craig picked a card with a blue circle and moved his piece to the corresponding spot on the board. I picked the top card from a pile of questions I had written. "What will you do this summer?"

"I go to Kiddie Land. Teacups is me and my brother's favorite ride. We like it. It's fun, fun."

- **Make a spinner of different topics.**

I created a laminated spinner with surrounding pictures representing friends, family, school, and play. Five-year-old Elaine flicked the spinner, and the arrow landed on a picture of a school.

"What do you like about school?" I asked her.

"It's fun. Tomorrow is zoo day. If you have a family, you get to split up and go with your family. We have to go where Mrs. A. goes."

"So you have to stay with your teacher?"

She nodded. "If we get lost we have to freeze so they can find us."

- **Use toys for asking questions.**

"You are a star—like a movie star—and I want to get to know you." I handed a toy microphone to the 5 year old. "So, Ariel, what do you love to do?"

"I love to play dress-up. I like to be a princess or a fairy."

- **Manipulate puppets to ask questions.**

Holding an owl puppet and flapping his wings, I said, "Whooo do you live with?"

"I live with my grandma and grandpa because I can't be with my mom or dad," 4-year-old Gabby replied.

Incorporate Visuals as Part of an Interview

In addition to using drawing and games, another interview format is to incorporate visual cues and prompts. When children see the facial expressions of animals or people that reflect different feelings, they are more likely to recall memories related to a feeling. This link to feelings makes it easier for them to discuss their experiences. In a similar way, responding to a cartoon character is more natural and playful. Together you can draw a visual representation through a genogram to help you clarify whom children define as their family. This drawing of lines connecting family members also promotes the telling of stories about family members.

Fabulous Five: Use Visual Characters or Diagram

- **Draw a face and fill in a thought bubble.**

I handed 8-year-old Serena a blank page with a thought bubble on it. "Draw your face and tell me about a time you were happy."

"Here's me. I'm happy because a friend came over to my house," she replied, and then wrote in the bubble: *I'm happy when my friend plays with me.*

"What's your friend's name?"

"Gina."

"When Gina comes over, what kinds of things do you do?"

"We play dress-up."

- **Incorporate puzzles of animals or people with different facial expressions.**

"The bear's face is missing. Pick one," I said, waving my hand over eight faces, each with a different facial expression. Four-year-old Jenna chose a frowning face and slipped it into place. "How does the bear feel?" I asked.

"Scared."

"Tell me what scares you."

"I scared of lots of things—like ghosts, snakes, monsters, and bugs. Know what I don't like?"

"What?"

"Crickets. I scared when they hop. I scream really loud when I see them hop. If one goes on me, I'll really scream. I can scream louder than anybody. I'm scared of big black spiders. My mom swatted one."

"Spiders scare me too."

- **Use pictures of faces to facilitate answers.**

I pointed to five facial expressions. "This child is happy. This child is sad. This child is excited. This one is mad. This one is scared. Pick one and tell me about a time you felt that way." Six-year-old Vicky pointed to the happy face, and I wrote the words *I feel happy when…*

Vicky added, "I feel happy when I play with my bear. One day in school, I made a perfect 'B.' It was like a grown-up did it."

- **Have children respond to a cartoon character.**

I opened a simple cartoon book I had created, pointed to the figure, and read the first page. He says, "What do you like to do?"

"Cook," 6-year-old Quinn replied.

"What do you cook?"

"Pancakes. I just have to flip the pancakes at 6 minutes."

- **Do a genogram and then talk about family.**

As we started drawing lines connecting the various family members, 7-year-old Louis said, "I have a new brother. He's 3."

"Is he adopted?" I asked.

"Yeah—like me. I had another brother. He went with my birth dad. He lives in Utah. When we're 13, we can go see him and figure out who he is."

Connect Questions to a Place, Context, or Activity

Younger children often do better answering questions when they have a visual reference. For instance, it is easier for them to talk about their favorite place at school while they are looking around or giving you a tour. When you connect your questions to their current activity, it is also easier for them to respond. The use of photographs is another productive method. Children can be given a camera and asked to take photos as a means for you to learn more about them. In addition, you may use pictures, such as family or school scenes, as prompts to initiate conversation. Picture symbols are another way to facilitate children's ability to respond, especially those who are nonverbal.

Fabulous Five: Incorporate a Visual Reference When Questioning

- **Point to different places or activities and ask children to show you the answer to your question.**

"What is your favorite center?" I asked 3-year-old Jessica, pointing to the five areas in the class. When she did not response, I said, "Show me."

Jessica walked past three play areas and went to dramatic play. She opened and closed the curtains on the stage for puppets.

"What do you like to do here?" I asked.

She grabbed the tray of dinosaur puppets, put one on her hand, and smiled.

- **Weave in questions during and related to a play activity.**

I watched 3-year-old Taylor paint with watercolors. "Who are you making your picture for?"

"My mom. My dad is mean. My dad is big."

"What did your dad say?"

"The cops said, 'Bad daddy.' My dad's in jail. My nana is at home."

"So you are safe with your grandma now. I'm glad you are talking about it."

- **Link questions to photographs of the children's family, home, or school.**

Looking at his family photograph on the classroom wall, I asked 4-year-old Fabian, "What makes you happy at home?"

"I am happy when I play with my brother. My brother runs fast. I can't catch him."

- **Ask a question and then have children take photographs as a response.**

"I have a camera for you. Take three pictures. First, what is your favorite thing to play with in this room? Take a picture of it."

Three-year-old Andy marched over, focused on the wolf costume, and pushed the camera button.

"Next, what is your favorite center?"

He walked sideways to the next center and took a photograph of the cardboard castle. "I like to be a prince," he said. "I like to play persons."

"You like to be different people when you are in the castle?" I asked, and he nodded. "Now you decide what you want to take a picture of."

He moved toward two classmates. "These are my friends," he said as he snapped the picture.

"That's good to know about you, especially who your friends are."

- **Use picture symbols when asking questions.**

"What did you do this weekend?" I asked and showed 4-year-old Cole a communication device containing four picture symbols. "Did you watch TV, play with toys, see a movie, or read books?"

He pressed the button underneath toys, and the pre-programmed message said, "I played with toys."

"Your mom told me you love to play with trucks. Did you get to play with your trucks?"

He nodded and said, "T-rucks."

Be Cognizant About Your Role in the Interview

Because an interview is an interactive dialogue, you play a major role in guiding the process. This means that if children are struggling, you have to examine how *you* are conducting the interview. An alternative to possibly blaming children or thinking they are incompetent would be take responsibility for your role and alter the wording of your questions and responses.

Reflect on Your Role During the Interview

> **Children might be thinking:**
> *What?*
> *What are you asking?*
> *Is this a yes/no question?*
> *I don't get it.*
> *How much longer do I have to answer these questions?*
> *Now I get it.*
> *It's okay to talk with you.*
> *Can I tell you more?*

An interview is a shared event, and each person has a role in making it successful. One aspect of your role is to ask questions that are easy for children to comprehend and that promote detailed answers. If they are having a difficult time answering questions, examine your role in the interaction. Recognize that it is more your issue than theirs and make changes. Once children begin talking, convey your acceptance by assuming a neutral and nonjudgmental stance.

Be Clear in Your Questions

When wording your questions, use kid language. Make sure you only ask one question at a time. For instance, asking, "How do you get along with your family and friends?" entails two questions. You may simplify by saying, "How do you get along with your family?" Then, after their response, ask about their relationship with their friends.

Carefully consider how you form your questions. Initially use easy ones about the present. Try to follow any yes/no questions with more open-ended ones. Avoid leading questions such as, "You like school, don't you?" Also refrain from asking a barrage of questions to the point that it feels like an interrogation. Rather, use a variety of responses that promote further conversation by the children. Be prepared for short answers but realize that they often get right to the point and can convey their message in very few words.

If children hesitate or look confused, reword the questions or give examples. Do not repeat the exact wording twice. Throughout the interview, pay attention to your role and change your wording and the type of questions as needed.

> ### *Fabulous Five: Ask Questions That Are Clear and Elicit More In-Depth Responses*
>
> - **Word questions in a way that children can understand.**
>
>   "Your teacher told me that you tend to move around a lot. Where do you move around the most?" I asked 9-year-old Clark.
>
>   "Gym and playing basketball with my friends."
>
>   Realizing that I worded the question wrong, I said, "Where in school is it the hardest to sit still?"
>
>   "Music."
>
> - **Vary questions that can be answered with a yes or no with questions requiring the use of other words.**
>
>   "Do you have a best friend?" I asked 8-year-old Donnie.
>
>   "Yes."
>
>   "What's your friend's name?"
>
>   He looked at the ceiling and whispered to himself, "What is his name?"
>
> - **Ask the children only one question at a time.**
>
>   "How are things going with the kids in your class? Do you feel like you can play and talk with them without any problems? Can you speak up for yourself when you're with them?"
>
>   "Hmm," 10-year-old Ron replied.
>
>   I recognized that I had asked too many questions, so I said, "Tell me about the kids in your class."
>
>   "Some are good and a lot of the others are bad."
>
>   "What's happening with the ones that are bad?"
>
>   "They talk too much or they like to fight."
>
>   "With you or just in general?"
>
>   "With other kids."
>
>   "Do they give you a hard time?"
>
>   "Sometimes. They have a little gang where if you want to join they have to punch you in the chest real hard. They asked me if I wanted to join and I told them no."
>
> - **Reword the questions or add more explanation if children give a different kind of answer than expected.**
>
>   "What are you good at?"
>
>   "Root beer. I like root beer," 6-year-old Jareth replied.
>
>   "What are you good at doing?"
>
>   "Coloring animals."
>
> - **Give examples if children look confused about the question.**
>
>   "What strategies have you found that helped you?" I asked 10-year-old Mark. He crinkled his lips, looking confused. "A strategy is a plan you decide to use to make things better—like if you are tapping your ruler and your teacher asks you to stop. Some kids might tell themselves, 'It'll be easier for me if I just put my ruler in my desk.' That's an example of a strategy."
>
>   "Sometimes I put my folder up to help me think about my work and not look around."

Be Neutral and Nonjudgmental in Your Responses

The way you respond to children's comments indicates what they are supposed to do next. The use of a neutral phrase is like a green light to signal "go" and continue. Interruptions, on the other hand, are similar to yellow or red signals. They can slow or stop the flow of conversation.

Being a good listener means you have to be open to hearing whatever is said. To do this, you have to be aware of your values and frame of reference in order not to judge the children. If, for instance, you hear children describe situations where they have caused trouble, it does not help to tell them that was a bad thing to do. Instead, encourage them to talk about how they handled it or what they learned from the experience. This can be another great opportunity to discover their strengths and effective strategies. Of course, if they are gloating about hurting someone or destroying property, then you can shift the conversation by asking questions such as, "How did the other person feel or act when you did that?" Listen and acknowledge any positive action taken or lessons learned. Avoid forming hasty judgments based on your personal stereotypes and expectations.

Fabulous Five: Convey Acceptance

- **Use neutral words or statements as your response.**

"What do you do after school?" I asked the second grader.

"I go to my grandma's and I play with my cousins."

"I see."

"My mom and dad got divorced. I went to court. I spend Saturdays with my dad for 24 hours. My mom cleans on Sundays, and I help her."

"I bet she likes that."

- **Avoid critical or blaming responses.**

"What's good about school?"

"Playing with my friends," 5-year-old Jessica answered.

"Tell me about your friends."

"Jake and Kinsey are my friends. Jake tries to keep me from being Kinsey's friend. He tells me to say bad things to her."

"So what do you do?"

"I listen to him."

"What does Kinsey do when you do what Jake says?"

"It makes her real mad. She tries to pull my hair. She scratched me. Jake and Kinsey don't get along with each other. Not at all. When I'm not Jake's friend, I'm her friend. I go back and forth."

"That must be hard for you to be in the middle."

"It is hard. Sometimes they both take my arms and pull me. They yell, 'Play with me first.' Then I yell, 'Stop.' And they stop. I say, 'Okay, let's have a deal. Jake first, then Kinsey.'"

- **Limit interrupting when children are talking.**

"What have you done that you're really proud of?"

"I've had my birthday. I'm 8 years old. I'm 4 foot 2 inches."

As he talked, I wondered if he understood the question. I wanted to interrupt but decided to wait.

"I like helping my dad build stuff."

"So you're proud of what you've made with your dad?" I said, and he nodded with a smile.

- **Support children's attempts to answer the questions.**

"What do you do when you get upset?"

"What does upset mean?" 12-year-old Trevor asked. "Is it like when someone gets hurt or dies?"

"You're right. You may feel upset when something bad happens to you or when something bothers you."

- **Recognize strengths or effective strategies in the children's responses.**

"How are you getting along with everyone in your class?"

"Lisa doesn't hate me anymore," 7-year-old Pablo said and shook his head. "She doesn't like people calling her 'pizza.'"

"So was she upset because you called her a name?"

"She told me to stop, so I never did it again."

"Sounds like you listened to your friend."

Choose the Wording of Your Questions

> **Children might be thinking:**
> *What do you want to know?*
> *I'm glad you asked.*
> *That's a good question.*

To best understand children, ask different types of questions about their daily lives. In addition to learning about their occupations, you also want children to talk about their feelings, experiences, and life events. To get this information, you have to ask questions that let children know it is all right to talk about their personal views and experiences.

Use the Classic Questions

The basic questions of a newspaper reporter are simple ways to obtain a variety of information. These questions—Who? What? Where? and When?—may elicit diverse responses. Younger children do better with "who," "what," or "where" questions. Asking "when" and "why" questions is more difficult and requires children to reflect on abstract information. Another problem with "why" questions is that many adults ask children to explain their behavior by saying, "Why did you do that?" Consequently, some children associate a "why" question with being in trouble. In the interview, use a variety of questions and monitor for children's understanding.

Fabulous Five: Use the Classic Questions

- **Ask, "Who…?"**

"Who is your best friend?" I asked the 5 year old.

"Gabriella. She's half Chinese. Her mom speaks Chinese, Spanish, and English."

- **Inquire, "What…?"**

"What do you want to be when you grow up?"

"When I grow up I want to be an orthopedic surgeon and fix bones," 7-year-old Alice replied. "I'll make a movie called 'Alice's Dreams Come True.' It'll be a 7-hour movie about all my dreams."

- **Ask, "Where…?"**

"Where do you like to go for fun?"

"I love to go to the park. I don't want to go to the ocean," 7-year-old Saul answered.

"How come?"

"I don't want to get ate-ten."

"You don't want to get eaten?"

"Yeah, by piranhas and sharks."

- **Inquire, "When…?"**

"When was a time you were scared?" I asked 6-year-old Lori.

"My grandma lifted me to feed the llama. I was scared. I thought it would bite me."

- **Ask, "How…?"**

"How was school today?"

"I did all my work," 7-year-old Jacqueline replied. "I did my journal. We write about monkeys and Jane Goodall. I wish I could go to Africa. I have to be more old. We saw a gorilla. I like going to grandma's zoo. It's a bunch of fun. There was a merry-go-round. I roded on it."

- **Ask, "What is it like for you?"**

"What is it like to get chemo?"

"It's really weird," 12-year-old Liz answered. "You get this metal taste. It's like having pennies in your mouth."

- **Ask, "How come you…?"**

"How old are you?"

"I'm 7."

"How come you are here at the hospital?"

"I got diabetes. I got sugar. I believe it was high. Sometimes I get sick because I eat the wrong things."

- **Inquire, "How is it going…?"**

"How is it going in school?" the certified occupational therapy assistant asked.

"My teacher is mean a little bit when she yells at us," 6-year-old Martin replied. "I like recess and I like to count. These kids named Cody and Ryan are mean to me. They make fun of me."

- **Say, "Tell me how you feel…."**

"Tell me how you feel about your friends."

"I feel bad about Carlos beating me in soccer," 6-year-old Griffen replied. "When I use my words, he doesn't listen. I don't like it when he does that. I like Kenny because he's nice and a true friend."

Alter the Type of Questions

Children might be thinking:
Are we done yet?
How much longer?
I don't want to talk about that.

Inquire About Experiences

When you use questions such as, "What is it like for you?" you cue children to talk about their experiences and what they mean to them. Children are often grateful to be given an open invitation to describe their thoughts and feelings. These types of phrases or short questions are open-ended, which allows them to highlight pressing issues or concerns. It also becomes validating to have another person really listen to, acknowledge, and empathize with them.

Fabulous Five: Use Phrases or Short Questions to Elicit Children's Experience

- **Inquire, "What do you think about…?"**

"What do you think about school?" I asked the first grader.

"I like my teacher and the fun things we do. I'm going to be a teacher when I grow up. I like babies, kids, and shopping."

Throughout the interview, you have to make a number of choices, especially about how many questions to ask and what topics to cover. Although most children enjoy talking with adults when they start the interview, they may become restless or disinterested later. They may think their information is none of your business and that you are prying into their lives. You can either stop or ask them if it is all right to ask a small number of quick questions. Some may become impatient if you take too long to write their answers in your notes.

At times, children are uncomfortable talking about certain topics, such as family strife or a lack of friends. They may remain silent, say "I don't know," or become upset. You can acknowledge that you have asked about a difficult topic. Then you can choose to change to an easier subject or stop. Some children also hesitate to describe what they think is bad about them or their family. You can help them save face by stating that all children have similar feelings or experiences. The implication is that it is all right to talk and you will not think less of them for what they have to say. As children speak, be sensitive and responsive to their comfort level.

Fabulous Five: Alter Questions

- **Adjust the number of questions to the children's needs.**

"Today I want to talk to you about how school is going."

"If you ask too many questions, I'll explode," Gordon replied.

"If it is all right with you, I just have three quick questions." He nodded, so I continued. "What are you good at?"

"I'm good at keeping my eye on my sisters. I'm allowed to babysit them, and I'm only 11."

"What do you like to do?"

"Play computer games. My mom says it's good for my eye-hand coordination."

"What do you wish was easier?"

"Writing in cursive."

"Thanks for answering the questions. That helps me get to know you."

- **Ask questions in a way that allows children to save face.**

"Tell me about a time you were frustrated or upset," I asked 8-year-old Emily.

"That's hard because I'm always happy."

"Everyone has a time where they get upset or frustrated."

"Well, my brother makes me mad and frustrated."

"What does he say or do?"

"When I was doing my homework at the kitchen table, he was annoying me—singing out loud when I needed quiet to work."

- **Shift the pace of asking questions.**

For 10 minutes, our conversation wove around 9-year-old Delany's family, friends, and school life. Then she drummed her fingers on the table. "Are we almost done yet?"

"Just one more." I quickened my speed in writing the answers. "When you are angry, what do you do that helps you?"

"I just splash some water on my face. That helps me calm down."

- **Stop or change topics based on the children's responses.**

"What do you like about your family?" I asked 8-year-old Leila.

"I don't know," she replied in a whispery voice.

"What do you like best about yourself?"

"Nothing really," she said. She stared at the blue wall and then became teary-eyed.

"I know these are hard questions. We can stop. I did notice that when I was in your class, I saw you help your friends. It seems like you're a good friend."

- **Change to a positive topic.**

"What do you like about school?"

"I like math."

"What don't you like about school?"

"I don't like getting in trouble because if I do I have to tell my mom."

"What do you think about your teacher?"

"My teacher is kinda mean sometimes. She's mean when she says I'm being bad," 7-year-old Annette said and grimaced.

In response to her look, I asked, "What are you good at?"

"Math and work. Being helpful to my friends."

Gain a Rich Understanding of Children's Perspectives

Because the purpose of an interview is to learn about children's lives and perspectives, you want to elicit as much information as possible. Throughout the interview, check your understanding of children's responses and encourage them to continue telling you more. Then respond in a way that shows your empathy and grasp of what their lives are like.

Gain an Understanding of Children's Nonverbal and Verbal Responses

---

Children might be thinking:
I can't wait for it to be over.
I'm bored.
You are listening to me.
You really want to know what I have to say.

There is an art to reading and understanding their non-verbal responses during a conversation. Sometimes children are very clear about what they are saying and it is easy to comprehend their message. With others, it is a challenge to decipher what is being said. Many nonverbal messages have multiple meanings. For example, sighing can mean tiredness, boredom, or sadness. Similarly, some phrases, such as "I don't know," can be ambiguous. Inquire about the meaning or the message and show children that you are willing to devote time to truly understand.

Explore When There Are Multiple Meanings of Nonverbal Cues

As you listen to children's words, also read their nonverbal language. Cues such as yawning, sighing, or fidgeting have meaning, and it is your job to discover what they are meaning by them. It can be a guessing game, which may be solved by looking at the situation. Have the children been sitting for a long time? Are they tired? Are they getting stressed? Are your questions about touchy topics? Identify what you see, and check with them about what it means. Then respond and respect what they are telling you.

Children's silence or long pauses also are indicators of a message. They may be saying something as simple as, "I need time to think." It might mean they are reluctant to talk about certain topics or to say anything bad. They may also be uncomfortable with you or may not understand the question. Pay attention to this often subtle cue.

Fabulous Five: Respond to Nonverbal Answers to Questions

- **Consider the meaning of sighs.**

"What do you want to be when you grow up?"

Eight-year-old Colin sighed and replied, "I don't know quite yet." Because he looked pensive, I waited. "I want to be a police officer. I can tell them if I want a car or motorcycle. Motorcycles are cool."

- **Respond to yawns and check if the children are tired or bored or if the room is too hot.**

When 10-year-old Tasha yawned, I asked, "Are you tired?"

"Yeah, I feel tired because I woke up very, very early and it was so dark. And I didn't get to take a shower this morning."

"I know it's hard to stay awake if you don't get enough sleep."

- **Check the meaning of long pauses.**

"Do you belong to any groups?"

Seven-year-old Barbara paused for 30 seconds with a slight squint of her eyes.

"Do you know what 'belong' means?"

She shook her head.

"Are you with any clubs or going to any groups like Girl Scouts or 4-H?"

"I'm in Girl Scouts. I'm an official Brownie."

- **Respond to fidgeting.**

"What are you good at doing?" I asked 6-year-old Marcus.

"I'm good at drawing, math, science, and reading. I'm good at climbing trees and building stuff," he replied, but then started to squirm in his seat. He put his hands between his legs and looked around the room.

"Do you have to go to the bathroom?"

He nodded, popped out of his chair, and dashed down the hall.

- **Clarify what children's silence means during an interview.**

"What do you like to do for fun?"

Nine-year-old Nate shrugged his shoulders.

"What's easy for you at school?"

Nate shifted his head and stared at the ceiling.

"What are you thinking? You're so quiet," I said.

"I wish I could be smarter."

Check Your Understanding of What Children Said

When you cannot comprehend what is being said, ask children to give you more information. As they talk, their words or ideas may become clearer. With more details, you also have a better chance at deciphering their message. Convey your intention to listen until they are understood. For soft-spoken children, it helps if you watch their faces and, if possible, read their lips as they whisper. You may have to ask them to speak louder, but refer to it as a problem with your own hearing. This can help them save face instead of pressuring them or indicating something is wrong. This approach also makes them think they are doing you a favor.

Fabulous Five: Check Your Understanding of What Children Said

- **Let children know when you do not understand the gist or general meaning of what they are saying.**

"I'm the police," 12-year-old Nathan said in the middle of the interview.

"Are you going to ride along with the police?" I guessed.

"No."

"I don't understand. What do you mean?"

He pulled out a notebook with crime scene tape plastered across it. "I have to figure out this mystery using clues. It's to teach me logic."

- **Attribute your difficulty understanding or hearing as being your problem.**

"What do you want to be when you grow up?"

Three-year-old Benny mumbled.

"Can you say it louder?" I asked, tugging on my ear. "Sometimes my ears don't work so good."

"I want to be a choo-choo driver. I want to help people get on the train."

- **Tell children you can understand them better when they look at you, if it is culturally appropriate.**

"What do you like best about school?"

"I need to think," 6-year-old Haley said. She turned her brown curly head to the side and murmured a few words.

"It will help me understand if you look at me," I said in a gentle tone of voice.

Her eyes met mine, and I read her lips as she whispered, "I like to try new things."

- **Tell the children you really want to know what they are saying.**

"What do you like about school?"

"I like to play on the slide and play chase."

"What don't you like about school?"

Six-year-old Carl whispered back.

"I'm sorry," I said. "I couldn't understand what you said, and I really want to know what you're trying to tell me."

"I said I don't like to hit. Don't hit. I like my teacher to be happy so I don't hit."

- **Ask for more information.**

"Do you have any pets?" I asked 5-year-old Natasha.

"I have dog. His name is Bo. He's been barfing, barfing, barfing."

"Is your dog sick?"

"No, all dogs barf when there's a full moon."

"Oh, he's been barking all the time."

Check on Ambiguous Words or Sayings

At times, children may respond to interview questions with vague wording, use their own invented words, or say words with their own meaning (e.g., their personal slang). Others may repeat the same answer multiple times. This may leave you baffled. Again, make an effort to discover the meaning. Pursue any discrepancies that you observe between the children's words and their nonverbal cues. Mention any conflicting responses and ask for clarification.

Fabulous Five: Clarify Vague Words or Responses

- **Check the meaning of "I guess."**

"Do you get along with everyone in your class?" I asked.

"I guess," 8-year-old Christy said, and her eyes settled on the floor.

"Not always?" I said in a soft voice.

"Well, sometimes I have a problem with immature little boys. They call me 'big butt.'"

- **Clarify the meaning of general or vague words.**

"What do you wish was easier in school?" I asked 5-year-old Helena after the first week of school.

"The hard work. She makes us do hard work."

"What's hard work?"

"You have to make letters and circle them with red, yellow, and blue."

- **Consider the meaning of "I don't know."**

"What do you like about school?"

"I don't know," 9-year-old Bill said.

"What's easy for you in school?"

"I don't know."

"What do you dislike or not like about school?"

"I forgot." His eyes shifted to the table.

Sensing that his responses reflected his being uncomfortable with talking, I said, "That's okay. These are hard questions. Let's do a game now"

- **Clarify conflicting responses.**

"What are you good at or do well?" I asked the 11 year old.

"Drawing."

"What do you want to be when you grow up?"

"A cartoon maker."

"What do you want to get better at?"

"Drawing."

"I'm confused because you said you were good at drawing."

"Yeah, but I want to draw as good as the real cartoon makers."

- **Watch if children's tone of voice matches the words said.**

"How do you get along with other kids?"

"They always call me names," 7-year-old Sean said. His voice dropped. "But they don't bother me."

Hearing the sadness in his voice, I responded, "That can be upsetting for many kids."

Obtain More Information

Children might be thinking:
Oh, you want to hear more.
You're really paying attention.
You're considerate.
You respect what I am saying.
It's okay to keep talking.

Children will try to determine how simple or complicated an answer you want. They will watch for hints about how long they should talk and how much detail they should provide. They also may wonder if it is all right to discuss information not related to your questions.

There are multiple ways to provide continuation cues. First, you can allow ample time for children to answer before saying the next question. Second, you need to use open-ended questions, which let children decide what is important to tell you. You may use nonverbal signals or short phrases as indicators that you wish for them to proceed. A nod or short phrase, such as, "Go on," can often provide just enough encouragement to continue. Asking short questions related to the children's conversations also cues them to reflect on their thoughts and expand their answers. These neutral prompts give children time to finish their thoughts and, if they so desire, change the course of the conversation.

Give Nonverbal Encouragement

A nonverbal gesture or facial expression can demonstrate to children that you are listening to every word. Because children are experts at reading nonverbal language, subtle signs such as leaning forward, staying quiet, or giving complete attention to their faces can be powerful continuation cues. These silent signals also are the least likely to disrupt the flow of the conversation.

Fabulous Five: Show Nonverbal Encouragement

- **Stay quiet and allow time for children to reflect and continue.**

"What are you good at?" I asked 10-year-old Dean.

"My ability in sports and my drawing."

I sat still and waited in silence as Dean cocked his head in thought.

Then he continued, "Kids in my class say I'm a good artist. I guess I am."

- **Lean forward to prompt more conversation.**

"Tell me about your friends," I said to 6-year-old Carter.

"I have three friends: Amanda, Taylor, and Justin."

I smiled and leaned a little closer.

Then he added, "Friends are like the best thing you have in your whole life."

- **Respond with head nodding.**

"What is your favorite class?" I asked 8-year-old Ellen, whose blue eyes were magnified by her wire-rim glasses.

"Art. I like to paint, draw, mix colors, and play with clay."

"What is hard at school?"

"Writing. Playground equipment." I nodded and Ellen continued, "Swings are easy. The balance beam is hard. It's kind of hard to shoot at the high basketball hoop."

"What part of writing is hard?"

"If I have to copy something. It's hard to read the directions from the board. It's hard for my vision. It makes me feel tired and frustrated."

- **Maintain eye contact to encourage further conversation.**

"Do you have many friends?" I asked 10-year-old Tara.

"Not really."

I remained silent as I looked at her.

"I feel invisible with my friend Kayla. She hardly even notices me. Sometimes I ask if she wants to sit with me at lunch. Sometimes she wants to sit with other friends, and I feel left out."

- **Give a questioning or serious look mixed with interest to gain more information.**

"I had my tonsils taken out," 6-year-old Seth said.

I tilted my head, made a serious expression, and looked in his eyes to encourage him to continue.

"I was breathing through a mask. They put the mask on my mouth. I was sleeping the whole time. I didn't feel nothing."

Use Phrases to Suggest That Children Add More

One- to three-word phrases can be used to communicate your desire to hear more. Simple questions like, "Anything more?" or "What else?" imply that you will wait patiently as they delve deeper into their thoughts. Saying, "Tell me more," in an empathetic tone of voice is also a clear message that children may continue talking if they want.

Fabulous Five: Integrate Short Questions or Phrases for Additional Information

- **Say, "Tell me more."**

"What do you like about school?" I asked 11-year-old Erik.

"Nothing."

"What don't you like about school?"

"Everything."

"Tell me more."

"All the kids pick on me. The teachers send me to the office every single day. The work is too hard."

- **Ask, "What else?"**

"What do you want to be when you grow up?"

"I'm going to be a vet," 5-year-old Peggy said. "I have to hold a pig down and wrestle crocodiles. I'm going to hold his mouth shut so he won't bite me."

"Why do you want to be one?"

"I like kittens."

"What else?"

"I saw on TV—you get to check on the pony. Her tail is kinda ripped because she was having a baby foal."

- **Add, "And?"**

"What do you think about your teacher?"

"She is fun and nice," 9-year-old Laura replied. "She lets us make clay brains."

"And?"

"And she lets us sit on balls. She tells us stories like Indian folklore and stuff about the Eskimos."

- **Ask, "Anything more?"**

"What are you proud of?" I asked 8-year-old Ethan.

"Can I be proud of when I was a baby and I was cute?"

"Sure."

"Yeah, I was really cute."

"Anything more?"

"I'm proud that I'm an artist. Hmm. And I cook well. I bake well. I help my mom cook everything."

- **Tell children, "Go on," or "Keep talking."**

"What grade are you in?"

"First."

"Tell me about school."

"I like school but I get tired of sitting all the time."

"Go on. I'm listening."

"I'm kinda bored in my class."

Use Clarifying Questions

Another way to acknowledge that you are listening is to use pertinent follow-up questions. Seeking more information helps clarify and deepen your understanding. Your questions also let children know about what part of the conversation you would like to have more information.

Fabulous Five: Clarify to Obtain More Information

- **Ask, "What happened?"**

"On one side of your paper draw your happiest day, and on the other side draw the worst day of your life."

"I don't want to draw. I want to write."

"That's fine."

"I'm going to write with my favorite color—red."

"I see you have a runny nose."

Seven-year-old Kerry nodded. "I had a worster sick. I had pneumonia. That was my worst day."

"What happened?"

"They had to take an x-ray of my lungs. That was my first entire x-ray. I was in the hospital for 4 days. I felt sick." He paused for a moment. "I was kinda happy cuz I had a whole lot of TV and movies."

- **Ask, "Where does…?"**

"Billy Joe's been mean and calls me names," the kindergartner said.

"Where does that happen?"

"On the playground. He won't play with me."

- **Ask, "When does…?"**

"What do you like about school?" the occupational therapy student asked the second grader.

"That I get to learn."

"What don't you like about school?"

"That I get tired."

"When does that happen?"

"It happens a lot after recess. I get tired and want to sleep."

- **Comment, "You said…. Tell me more about that."**

"You said things are good with your friends. Tell me more about that."

"My friend Rebecca plays nice with me," 6-year-old Reba replied. "She helps me on the monkey bars and she pushes my feet. She always sits by me."

- **Inquire, "Then?" or "Then what?"**

"I've never been to your school. What's it like?" I asked 5-year-old Chelsea.

"Our teachers are all girls. We learn history—a little bit. We have four centers: playhouse, two shelves are math lessons, blocks and drawing, and we have a computer center. We sit on the rug and we read a book. The teacher says put your books down and we do the pledge. Then it's rest time."

"What's rest time?"

"You lay your head down and your eyes are closed. Sometimes I'm a little wiggly. Then somebody who is really good is the cozy superstar. The superstar turns on the lights."

"Then what?"

"The teacher reads a book. You finish your work on your desk. If you're done, you get free time. We get candy if we finish our work. She's a nice teacher."

Incorporate Probing Questions

When children's answers are vague or unclear, it can be beneficial to ask probing questions. It is similar to when you greet another and ask, "How are you?" and they give the usual reply, "Fine." Then if you ask a probing question, they will provide more detail and may even describe how they are not fine. The probing questions cue the children that you want to go beyond a vague or general answer.

Fabulous Five: Ask Probing Questions

- **Ask a short question to encourage children to expand their thoughts.**

"What do you dislike or not like about school?" I asked the second grader.

"When Sammy scribbles."

"So that bothers you?"

"He used to be my best friend. Sometimes he tries to force me to play with him. I have a new best friend now."

- **Repeat children's last word or phrase as a question to elicit more information.**

"How's school going?"

"Good," 5-year-old Gwen replied.

"What's good about it?"

"It's not so hard for me now."

- **Follow a general question with a more detailed question.**

"What do you like to do for fun?" I asked the 10 year old.

"I like all kinds of things."

"Tell me one thing."

"How about two?"

"Sure. That would be great. Tell me as many as you like."

"No, I'll tell one. I like skateboarding."

- **Cue children to finish their thoughts.**

"What do you wish was better at school?"

"I wish there would be politeness in my class. The fourth graders—lazy Dora, dumb Dan."

"What about the fourth graders in your class?"

"They just think I'm stupid."

- **Say, "Tell me about a time…."**

"I'm good at helping people," 6-year-old Chad said.

"Oh, tell me about a time you helped someone."

"I told the teacher one of my friends was hurt."

Inquire About Children's Perspectives

Another type of continuation cue is to inquire about the children's perspectives on the topic. Ask them how they feel or what they think about the life events they are describing. This helps you better comprehend how they see their world. Some children may provide a partial answer but then hesitate, wondering if they should continue. Acknowledge that you want to hear their thoughts and concerns.

Fabulous Five: Ask More About Their Perspective

- **Ask, "How do you feel about…?"**

"How are things going with your family?"

"My mom has to work Saturday," 6-year-old Monica said, "and I have to stay with my grandma."

"How do you feel about that?"

"I'm sad. I miss my mom. My grandma is not good at games. She's 55 years old. It's hard for her to play."

- **Ask, "What were you thinking when…?"**

"My mom and dad got separated, and I live with my dad. Everything is going cuckoo. Someone called and said give me the money or you have to live someplace else."

"What were you thinking when that happened?" I asked the 7 year old.

"That my dad only gets paid on Tuesday. How can he pay rent if he has no money?"

- **Inquire, "Are you feeling…?" or "Were you feeling…?"**

"I miss being 4," Stephanie said on the last day of school.

"How come?"

"Because my Tinkerbell pajamas are getting too small and I don't want to go to kindergarten."

I knew she liked her preschool teacher, so I asked, "Are you feeling sad to leave Mrs. V.?"

Stephanie nodded. "She's funny."

- **Ask, "In what way?"**

"Are you a good friend?"

"Yes," 8-year-old April answered.

"In what way?"

"I don't tell on my friends."

- **Ask, "How come?"**

"What do you want to be when you grow up?" I asked 9-year-old Neill.

"A cop."

"How come?"

"Because they are good at saving people and putting bad guys in jail."

Convey Your Understanding of Children's Answers

Children might be thinking:
You're really listening.
You understand.
You get it.

There are different levels of responses you may provide. The simplest one is to restate the words you heard or paraphrase the sentence. Rewording what children have said indicates that you are listening to their words. Another level is to reply with an empathetic remark showing that you understand and that you care about them. When you acknowledge their feelings, you connect on an emotional level. The hardest level is to search for the deeper meaning of the children's message and express your interpretation of what is being said.

To provide a sincere response you must maintain the mindset that you are open to learning from them. Then listen and consider the words spoken, the nonverbal language, their feelings displayed, and the situation. Also hear what is not said and watch for the incongruity among the factors. Your interpretation is a best guess of their message. The children can then determine if you are right or even close. It is essential to check with them to see if your thoughts are similar to theirs and whether your thinking makes any sense. Providing an interpretation does run the risk of being wrong. Children may think, *You don't get it*, and wonder if it is worth trying again. They will look for signs that you sincerely desire to understand their perspective rather than impose your own way of thinking on them. The process of reflecting back to children gives them an opportunity to correct you and clarify the meaning of their message.

Reflect Back With Sensory Responses

During the conversation, use your senses to help identify children's emotions as part of your response. Listen to their vocal intonation, their hesitations, and the intensity of the words spoken. A phrase such as, "I hear [name of the feeling] in your voice," is one way to show empathy and promote more discussion. In a similar manner, you can describe what you observe on their faces. This description opens the door for you to offer a possible interpretation, such as, "The way you look makes me wonder...," gives children an opportunity to add more detail. Interpretations also may be presented using the introductory phrases of "I hear you saying..." or "Sounds like...." Children can then confirm whether you are accurate.

Fabulous Five: Use the Senses in Your Response

- **Respond, "Sounds like...."**

"I left my old school because some kids were being mean to me," 7-year-old Keith said. "All my friends are nice to me at this school."

"Sounds like you're happy to be here and have new friends who treat you nice."

- **Tell children, "I hear...."**

"My family stresses a lot about bills they have to pay," 11-year-old Scott said.

"I hear the worry in your voice."

"Yeah, I just wish somebody would pay off the bills and my mom would be a little happier."

- **Say, "I can see...."**

"What do you like to do with your friends?"

"I don't have no friends," 8-year-old Vicki replied as her eyes became teary.

"I can see how upsetting that is for you."

- **Respond, "You look..." or "It looks like...."**

"I fell on the gym floor because somebody tripped me. It hurt my leg," 5-year-old Flora said with a frown.

"It looks like that upset you."

She nodded. "It made me mad."

- **Tell children, "The way you look make makes me wonder...."**

"How is school going?"

"Good," 6-year-old Geoffrey replied with a grimace.

"The way you look when you said that makes me wonder if there's something about school that is not good."

"Well, school is really hard."

"What's hard for you?"

"Math, social studies, spelling, writing, and art."

Use Empathetic Responses

When children are sharing their feelings or describing difficult experiences, you will want to use an empathetic response. Acknowledge their emotions in a caring tone of voice. For some, it is helpful to let them know their feelings are normal reactions to a difficult situation and that other children feel the same way. Show compassion by your words and nonverbal language.

Fabulous Five: Give Empathetic Responses

- **Respond, "That must have been hard for you."**

"I'm glad you moved back and I get to see you again. What was it like in California?"

"Kinda ugly and stuff."

"How was it ugly?" I asked the third grader.

"My dad was being mean to us."

"How was your school there?"

"Mean. People were saying cuss words and stuff. My mom said I never have to go back there again. I don't want to go back."

"That must have been hard for you."

- **Repeat the feeling words the children have said.**

"How are things going at school?"

"I'm upset," 4-year-old Billy replied. "My tooth came out yesterday and my sister lost it at school."

"That would be upsetting."

- **Say, "I know that's [state feeling word] for other children too."**

"We had a lockdown at school. No one could go out. The policemen had their guns pulled out. It made me scared," 6-year-old Shannon said.

"I know that's scary for other children too," the occupational therapy student replied.

- **Tell children, "You've been through a lot...."**

I met 12-year-old Carl his first week at our school. We talked for a few minutes, and then I asked, "Who do you live with?"

"My guardian. He's my dad's friend for 65 years."

"How long have you lived there?"

"Two weeks."

"New home. New school. You've been through a lot of changes."

- **Respond, "I'm sorry that happened."**

"How are things at home?"

Tears trickled down her cheeks. Six-year-old Brenda said between gulps, "Do you know why I'm crying? My dog was hit by a car. We had to put her to sleep."

"Oh, that's so sad. I'm sorry that happened."

Search for the Deeper Meaning

As children talk, listen to the words said while you search for the underlying message. Follow the children's conversation and, at the same time, dig for the deeper meaning of what is being said. For instance, children might say they are bored but then go on to discuss their difficult schoolwork. On the surface, you could acknowledge the feeling of boredom. At a deeper level, you could recognize and reflect back that school can be boring when you do not understand what to do and the work is too hard. You also could consider the possibility that the word *boring* may be their way of describing their frustration, embarrassment, or worries about being thought stupid.

To discover the deeper meaning, you need to make connections between ideas and look for possible messages. Present your thoughts as being tentative and not definite by using phrases such as, "I wonder..." or "So you feel... because...?" This allows children to correct you and say, "No, I feel...." You also may identify what you think the children are feeling but reference other children in your description.

At times children, as well as adults, are not consciously aware of the deeper message. As a neutral listener, you can reflect back the possible significance of what you hear and then look at the children for signs of confirmation. This can be an opportunity for the children to learn about themselves and for you to gain an understanding about their experiences.

Fabulous Five: Reflect Back the Underlying Meaning

- **Say, "I wonder if...."**

"I'm real busy today," 7-year-old Madeline said. "I'm going to a party with my dad. My mom is coming with me in case he yells, screams, or gets real mad."

"I wonder if you have mixed feelings about being with your dad. You want to be with him but sometimes he scares you when he's mad."

She nodded.

- **Refer to children in general when stating one possible meaning.**

"When I get mad, I tell everyone to stay out of my way," 10-year-old Trey said. "One time I hit my mom. She called the cops. I wish I hadn't done that."

"I know some children feel upset when they lose control, and it scares them. They wish they knew something else to do when they get mad so they don't hurt others."

- **Guess at the children's underlying meaning of their responses.**

"What's good about school?"

"Lunch and recess," 11-year-old Evan replied.

"What's not so good about school?"

"Everything."

"Is it hard?" I guessed.

"It's stupid," he replied, indicating that he did not see the value of the work.

- **Respond, "You feel...because...?"**

"How are you getting along with your friends?" I asked 6-year-old Sondra.

"I wish Brooke would be nice to me again. She's not talking to me. She says that I'm not listening. I say, 'Please stop that.' I keep getting madder and madder."

"So you feel mad and hurt because your friend is not talking with you?"

"Brooke doesn't play with me outside. I'm all alone playing. It makes me really sad that she doesn't want to be my friend anymore."

- **State what the children have implied but left unspoken.**

"Over Thanksgiving, I'm staying with my dad. I don't get to spend any time with my mom."

"How is it at your dad's house?"

"It's fun sometimes but...." 8-year-old Shelly said, then stopped.

"But sometimes it's not?"

"What I'm worried about is that if he makes me watch scary movies, I have to tell my mom and we have to go back to court. One time, he made me watch a scary movie and I had nightmares."

Promote Seamless Transitions Between Topics and Provide Closure

Part of the art of conducting an interview is helping children easily transition from one topic to another. Creating a sense of flow keeps them engaged. At the end, it is important to provide closure by summarizing what they said and what you learned.

Create Smooth Transitions to Make the Interview Flow

> **Children might be thinking:**
> *What next?*
> *What am I supposed to be talking about now?*

An interview can flow like a river when there is a natural rhythm to the conversation. You create this sense of flow through smooth transitions, especially when you shift to new topics. When you use words or statements to ease the change, children are more likely to follow and maintain their attention. Some children will find it jarring if you abruptly change the subject.

Transitional statements also prepare children for a different line of conversation (Figure 6-3). Make such a statement if you are changing topics by acknowledging that you heard children's responses and then make a statement leading to the next one. The use of summaries is another method for transitioning. Connect the important parts of what the children said by condensing two or three of the children's thoughts on one subject into a summary. After you do so, you then can move on to a different theme.

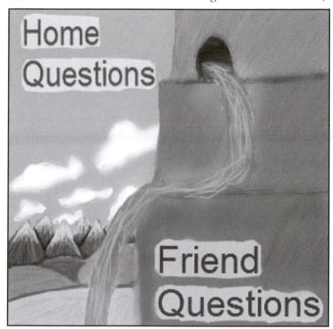

Figure 6-3. Transitional statements make an interview flow.

Fabulous Five: Use Transitional Statements to Shift Topics

- **Tell the children you appreciate them telling you about something, then change to a different topic.**

Seven-year-old Ricky continued on about his adventures with his bike. To shift the conversation, I said, "I appreciate your telling me all about the exciting times you had with your bike. I also would like to hear about your family."

"Somebody took our house away from us. They made me really mad. Now we live in an apartment."

- **Acknowledge what was said and then say, "I am wondering about...."**

"What do you like to do with your friends?" I asked 7-year-old Joel.

"Play football and make jokes. That's always fun."

We talked for a few more minutes about his friends, and then I said, "You've told me about your friends. I'm wondering about your family. Who is in your family?"

"My two brothers, me, and Mom and Dad."

"What do you and your family do together?"

"I go shopping with my mom. I don't do nothing with my dad."

- **Shift to different questions within the same topic.**

"Do you have a best friend?"

"I have a girlfriend. Her name is Lila," 6-year-old Larry replied. "I want to get married with her. Her and me grew up together. We know each other since we're born."

"What do you like about her?'

"She's nice. It takes a long time to get to her state. Two long roads."

"So you have Lila as a close friend. What about friends at school?"

"Mark is my friend here."

- **Cue children about a change by saying, "Now I would like to know...."**

"This is my house. That's my windows. This is my street," 5-year-old Jacob said as he drew. "When I was little I was still a baby. This is my old house that got destroyed. I was feeling sad. They got a gun and shot my house. Now I got a new house."

"What happened to your old house?"

"They knocked it down."

"Who lives with you in your new house?"

"My mom and sister. I wish they would not fight no more. My dad and brother live in Minnesota. I don't really know a lot about my brother."

"Now I would like to know about your friends."

"I don't have any friends at home—only at school."

- **Summarize discussion on one subject before moving on to the next topic.**

"I'm wondering how school is going for you."

"Good. I'm in the first grade, and we get to go to Spanish. The Spanish teacher told us how to talk in

Spanish, but I forgot how. The work is really easy. Some is first-grade work, some is kindergarten work. My arm hurts if I color too much. Hmm. My teacher is good. She helps us. We have homework every day. I'm not kidding."

"I believe you. So, you like your teacher. Some work is easy and some work, like Spanish and doing a lot of coloring, is sometimes harder. Now tell me about your friends."

End the Interview

> **Children might be thinking:**
> *Are we done?*
> *Is it really over?*
> *Oh, it's time to stop.*
> *Do we have to stop?*
> *I liked talking to you.*
> *You really listened to me.*

As the interview comes to an end, you need to provide closure. You start to do this by reviewing, connecting, and summarizing the key points you heard. It only takes a few minutes to do this. You also signal the end by saying you are asking the last question, eliciting any missed information the children want to relay, and revisiting the purpose of talking together.

Review Important Points Made by the Children

The use of summaries is one way to wrap up the conversation and confirm to children that you heard what they had to say. Tie together the essential bits of information discussed throughout the interview. You may start with phrases such as, "What I hear you saying…," or "Let me see if I have it right…" to convey your perception of what they said. This type of wording implies that you want to be corrected if you misunderstood them.

Fabulous Five: Connect the Various Responses

- **Refer to information children had previously mentioned.**

"What's your favorite thing to do?"
"Draw."
"What do you like about your family?"
"They are funny. They're creative. They know what I like."
"You said you like to draw. I would love to see you draw yourself."

Ten-year-old David sketched his spiky hair and added jagged lines for his body, resulting in a cartoon-like figure.

"Wow! You said your family is creative. I see that you're creative too—especially with drawing."

- **Tell children, "What I hear you saying…."**

"Who do you want to be like when you grow up?"
"My uncle, my dad, and my mom. They've lived good lives, and when I'm older, I want to live a good life too," 11-year-old Colin replied.
"What do you like about your family?"
"They're really nice to me and they help me out with homework or with any problems I have."
"What I hear you saying is that you admire your family and appreciate what they do for you."

- **Pull together different parts of the entire conversation.**

"What are you good at?"
"Karate. I'm a brown belt," 8-year-old Rochelle said.
I was impressed and flashed a smile. "What else?"
"Swimming, jumping rope, helping others. I like to help other kids. I think that's it."
For the next 5 minutes, we talked about her family, friends, and school. "What's your favorite class?" I asked.
"P.E.," she replied, referring to physical education.
"I know you said you were good at karate, swimming, and jumping rope. You have to be coordinated to do that. I bet you're good in P.E. too."
She nodded and smiled.

- **Say, "Let me see if I have it right," and then summarize what was said.**

"What do you like about your family?"
"We go to the park," 6-year-old Marc replied. "My mom buys me stuff. We went out to eat at a restaurant—just her and me."
"What don't you like about your family?"
"I don't like kisses. I don't like mom's lipstick on me—it's too much ink. Sometimes my mom and dad fight. My mom says, 'It's embarrassing. Please go back to work.' I fight with my little brother. He steals a lot of stuff from me, and I don't like it. He keeps it in his clothes drawer."
"Let me see if I have it right. So there are times when you're happy to be with your family—like when your mom buys you something or takes you out. And there are times when it's upsetting to hear your parents fight or when your brother takes your things."

- **Summarize the main points of the children's conversation.**

"What do you like about school?" I asked 5-year-old Lyndie.
"I like to learn."

"What is hard for you at school?"

"I have memory loss. I keep forgetting things."

"I would like to know more about your family. Who lives with you at home?"

"My mom, my dad, and Vanessa. She's my aunt. She's a big person with big hair, makeup, and spray. I don't like it when people go away. Vanessa is going to the train station."

"It is sad when people leave," I replied.

"Yeah, but she'll visit."

"What's your favorite thing to do?"

"I like to color with different kinds of colors. I like to ride my bike. I fall down. My eyesight is not very good because I was riding my bike really fast and I flipped and hit my stomach. Good thing I landed in the grass. I still have the mark. It doesn't hurt anymore. I'm still riding my bike and I'm not falling as much now."

"So you enjoy learning, coloring, and riding your bike. You're also getting better at balancing on your bike. At times, remembering things at school can be hard for you. And then it sounds like you are going to miss your aunt."

Lyndie nodded.

Provide Closure to the Interview

Another way you may finish the interview is to reflect back to children the overall emotional content, highlighting the underlying feelings expressed. Then give them a cue that you are nearing the end by making statements such as, "This is the last question." The next step is to ask if there is anything else they want to tell you or anything else they think is important for you to know. Make it an open-ended request so they are free to provide any information they desire. When they are finished talking, mention something you learned about them that you did not know. Emphasize their uniqueness and competencies. Finally, acknowledge your appreciation for their talking with you.

Fabulous Five: Put Closure on the Interview

- **Reflect back the overall tone or underlying feelings of the conversation.**

"What do you like about school?"

"Nothing. Leaving. Hmm. Recess and gym."

"What do you think about your teacher?" I asked 12-year-old Tony.

"I don't like her. I told her I would hit her if she didn't get away from me."

"How are things going with your classmates?"

"I'm getting a headache from Jed cuz he's never quiet. He doesn't have any manners. He just says, 'Move.' He tells me, 'You're annoying.' And I say, 'Leave me alone.'"

"So overall, school is very stressful and at times upsetting."

- **Tell children when you are asking the last question.**

"Tell me about a time you were happy?"

"When I rode a horse," 6-year-old Nancy replied. "His name was Noah. He was a cute pony. He's my best friend. I got to go in a circle. It's pretty easy to steer him."

We talked for a few more minutes, and then I said, "This is the last question. Who do you look up to or admire?"

"My mom. She's the one mostly at home and she really cares about me."

- **Ask children if there is anything else they think you should know.**

"Is there anything else you think I should know?" I asked 7-year-old Bradley.

"I fight with my brother a lot."

"What has helped you when that happens?"

"I tell my mom or dad."

- **Mention one thing you were glad to learn from talking with the children.**

"What are you good at?"

"Painting."

"What do you like best about school?"

"Painting."

"What is your favorite thing to do?"

"Painting."

"What do you like best about yourself?"

"Painting," 8-year-old Pedro said with a wide smile.

Sensing that Pedro was emphasizing his love and pride of painting, I smiled and responded, "So you're really good at painting and enjoy it. That's good to know about you."

- **Restate the purpose of the interview and what you will do with the information provided.**

At the end of the interview, I asked 10-year-old Elizabeth, "What do you want to change about yourself?"

"To not be mean."

"With whom?"

"With the people I don't like. Like some boys who tease me on the playground."

"What have you found helps when they are mean to you?"

"Sometimes I walk away and that helps. Or sometimes I ignore them."

"Those sound like good ideas. You also can talk to the adults on the playground and they can help too. Well, Elizabeth, I really appreciate that you talked with me. That helped me get to know you and find out what's important to you. If you would like, I could talk to your teacher and share with him your good ideas as well as your concerns." She nodded in agreement.

Key Points to Remember

- Use an interview to invite children to talk about their lives, including their meaningful occupations.

- Give the message that you assume they are competent to speak and you want to hear what they have to say.

- State that the purpose of the interview is to get to know them.

- Tell children there are no right or wrong answers.

- Decide on the interview's format.

- Connect questions with younger children to a visual reference such as a place, activity, or context.

- Be mindful of your role by asking clear questions, using nonjudgmental responses, and carefully choosing your wording.

- Respond to children's cues regarding sensitive topics and the length of the interview.

- Explore the meaning of children's nonverbal responses such as silence, sighing, fidgeting, pausing, or yawning.

- Check on vague responses and ask children to tell you more.

- Prompt children to clarify and give more information.

- Reflect back your understanding of children's responses and possible underlying messages.

- Use transitional statements between topics to create a sense of flow.

- End the interview by reviewing key points stated by the children.

Review Questions

1. Children will often wonder if the interview is a test. True or false.

2. You should never use yes/no questions in the interview. True or false.

3. Name five prompts you can use to ask children to talk about a certain topic (e.g., their family or friends).

4. All younger children like drawing as a way to provide answers to your questions. True or false.

5. Name at least three creative ways to ask questions in an interview.

6. You cannot interview children who are nonverbal. True or false.

7. If children cannot answer your questions, assume the interview is too difficult for them. True or false.

8. When asking questions, you have to observe children's nonverbal responses as well as listen to their words. True or false.

9. It is not enough to just nod your head to let children know you are listening. True or false.

10. Why is it paramount to put closure on the interview by summarizing the important points the children made?

7

Observe and Promote
Stress-Free Testing

CHAPTER OVERVIEW

In addition to interviewing, you can learn about children and their worlds through observations and testing. Observations allow you to see what happens around the children and how their environments affect their participation in occupations. Testing is one way to ascertain what they can and cannot do. This chapter highlights ways to be an unobtrusive observer and make testing a pleasant rather than stressful situation.

CHILDREN'S DESCRIPTIONS OF WHAT THEY THINK YOU SHOULD KNOW

Dr. Clare: "What is important for therapists to do when they observe or visit you in class?"

Cody (age 12): "Tell the teacher that you are there. Tell kids they're not in trouble. Make them feel comfortable. Say you are just there to watch. If they do something really good, you can compliment them, and if they make any mistakes, help them."

Dr. Clare: "Where should therapists be when watching you?"

Brady (age 11): "Off to the side. The most important thing you shouldn't do is introduce yourself in front of the whole class because it would embarrass the kid. He would slump down."

Dr. Clare: "Did that happen to you?"

Brady: "Yes. She walked in front of the class and said, 'I'm here to see Brady.' It was very embarrassing."

LEARN ABOUT CHILDREN'S WORLDS AND COMPETENCIES

When you observe children, you have an opportunity to see their lives and natural ways of being. It is a window into their world seen through your own filters as you make sense of what you see and hear. Your view is only one interpretation, which means you need to be open to other explanations. Testing is an opportunity to gain more information regarding children's competencies and challenges.

Observe Children and Their Environments

Like a camera lens, you observe by zooming in and out. Start with an examination of the big picture and then move into smaller details and subtle nuances. Typical questions you might ask yourself include the following:

- What in the environment is helping or supporting the children?
- What are the children's abilities and strengths?
- Is there a good match between the children and their social and physical environments?
- How are the children alike and different from others their age?

Curtin, C.
*Strategies for Collaborating With Children: Creating Partnerships
in Occupational Therapy and Research* (pp. 121-140).
© 2017 SLACK Incorporated.

- Does their developmental level match their chronological age?
- What helps or hinders their occupational functioning?
- What do you like and enjoy about them?

To help you make sense of what you see, it is important to learn what children generally do at each age. Understand that there is always a range of what is considered "normal." Also, check with caregivers and teachers to determine if what you saw was typical. When I first started working, I watched children everywhere I went. I studied how they moved, what they said, and how they acted. Then I would guess how old they were. In the school setting, I took time to examine all the posted artwork and writing samples from different grades hanging in the hallway. I also strolled around the classroom looking and admiring children's work.

Be a Good Observer

> **Children might be thinking:**
> *Who are you?*
> *Are you a teacher or a parent?*

After getting the big picture, you can ask yourself more specific questions. Doing so defines what you are going to watch closely. For instance, if you are interested in children's fine motor skills, you might ask the following questions: How are they sitting? Are they using whole-arm versus finger movement? How are they holding the pencil? Do they stabilize the paper with their other hand? How is their motor control? These questions give you a focus.

When writing your observations, jot down what you see or hear. Use concrete language and separate your interpretations from the observations. In my notes, I use brackets to record my interpretations and impressions. Then look for themes or patterns that are emerging. For example, after seeing a child in different situation, you may notice that he or she shows displeasure every time he or she is touched unexpectedly.

Another consideration is that children act differently in various contexts. The environment is a major influence on what they do. You must be careful to always consider the role of the environment and avoid blaming the children. For example, watching a child in a room with boring toys, you could make the mistake of labeling the child as passive. The real problem could be the lack of enticing play objects. If possible, observe them in as many settings as you can. Some children do fine in a structured setting like a classroom yet struggle with free time at recess, whereas others may barely contain themselves in a structured setting but abound with joy when left to their own devices in playtime. Additionally, watch children in different groups as well as by themselves.

Fabulous Five: Be a Good Observer

- **Define your questions before you observe.**

"Bobby constantly moves in large group," his preschool teacher told me. "He rarely sits still. He rolls and often bumps into the children sitting next to him. Could you observe him and see what you think?"

I agreed and formulated the questions to guide my observations. Is Bobby seeking movement to stay alert? Does he seek or avoid other sensations? How does he react to sensations, such as loud noises, in the classroom?

- **Use concrete language when writing observations describing what you saw and heard.**

Justin's preschool teacher told our special education team that he was having difficulty with his classmates. "He threw sand in one girl's face because he said she was in his way."

When I was in his class the next day, I watched for how he reacted to sensations, his body awareness, and the kind of interaction he had with his peers. I wrote in my notebook:

As Justin's class lined up for recess, he ran over and squeezed his body between Kellen and Alyssa. Alyssa frowned.

Justin asked Kellen, "Can I play with you?"

Kellen said, "Only if you play nice and don't hurt me."

- **Separate your interpretations from the observations.**

Five-year-old Glenn sat at a table with his teacher and four classmates while they played a memory game. As they played, he stood, put his palms on the table, and pushed down. Keeping his eyes on the game, he then put his head in his hands with his elbows on the table. He answered his teacher's question correctly. Then, keeping his elbows on the table, he lifted his feet and placed them on top of the chair. I wrote down exactly what I saw. Then, using brackets, I wrote my interpretation:

[Glenn appears to be seeking deep pressure sensation by weight bearing on his hands and elbows while staying focused on the activity.]

- **Look for patterns or themes.**

When 3-year-old Troy was observed in class, the following was noted:

The group was told to sit on the rug, and he was the last one to sit down. His clapping for the calendar started after the class clapped five times. He only answered the teacher's last question about the weather. Stood still during the movement activity. With the songs, he was about 10 seconds behind in doing the finger movements.

Later, we talked as a team and discussed the observations. We agreed that although Troy looked like he was off-task, it seemed that he just needed more time to process what to do.

- **Observe children at different times and places.**

As his second-grade teacher gave directions, Ken rotated his pencil like a baton with his eyes glued to it. Then he slipped the pencil into the hole of the paper and swung the paper. After about 20 rotations, he dropped the pencil on the floor and then slapped his cheeks with alternating hands. A few minutes later, he rolled his head and then rested his chin on his desk. Finally, he started the writing task.

At recess, Ken swung on the monkey bars like a circus performer. Next, he ran smoothly through a maze as two boys tried to keep up with him. His friend threw a football and he smiled as they played catch.

Be Sensitive to How Children Feel About Being Observed

Children might be thinking:
Why are you here?
Why are you in the room with me?
Why are you looking at me?
Am I in trouble?
Is something wrong?
What are you writing down?

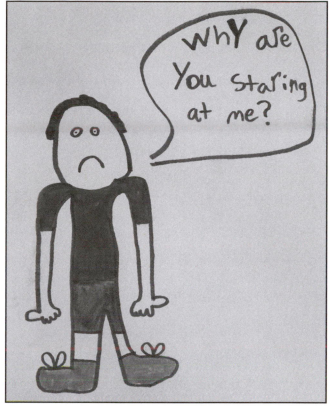

Figure 7-1. Avoid looking too intently at only one child.

Be aware that your presence influences and changes the situation. People act differently if they know they are being watched. Try to blend into the setting by finding a place where you can observe and at the same time be the least noticeable and disruptive. It is common for children to wonder who you are, why are you observing, and if you are judging them. The more familiar they are with you, the more likely they are to act like themselves. Smile and use body language that conveys that you are accepting and not judgmental. Try to avoid watching too intently because children interpret this as staring, which might stigmatize them and/or make them feel uncomfortable (Figure 7-1). This type of attention implies something is wrong with them.

Children may wonder if you are there because they are in trouble. It helps to give a general explanation when they ask why you are there, such as, "I'm here to visit so I can see what your class is like." They also may wonder why and what you are writing. You can tell them that you are writing what you see so you can remember. With younger children, you can tell them you are writing down all the good things they are doing. That usually pleases them, and they are likely to go back to what they were doing.

Fabulous Five: Observe the Children's Worlds
- **Observe all the children in the setting so they do not feel like you are staring.**

I went into the fourth-grade class to observe Max, who was experiencing muscle fatigue in the afternoon. The teacher knew I was coming and nodded at me. I sat on the side of the classroom, where I continually scanned the room as the children wrote, but I also watched Max. I saw that his feet dangled in the air and he tended to slump over the desk, keeping his nose to the paper. Later, I talked with Max and his teacher. Together we explored the possible suggestions of using a footrest, getting a gel pen for less resistance when writing, and turning a three-ring binder sideways to create an inconspicuous slant board.

- **Be aware that your presence is noticed and influences what happens.**

Twelve-year-old Lynette jumped in place as she flapped her hands. She glared at me as I took notes at the side of the class. Then she marched over to me and said in a gruff voice, "I see you."

I said softly, "I see you too." I smiled and added, "It's nice to see you." She stared at me and then stomped back to the other side of the room.

- **Be unobtrusive.**

Before going into Debbie's first-grade classroom, I removed my coat, opened my notebook to a blank page, and took my pen out of my purse. I walked quietly into the classroom, smiled, and whispered to the teacher, "Which one is Debbie?"

The teacher walked around the room. and when she passed the child with wavy red hair, she said, "Debbie, be sure to put your folder in your desk when you are done."

- **Tell children you are taking notes to help you remember.**

As I observed 6-year-old Jacob on a playground, he raced up the stairs without hesitation and flung himself down the slide. Then he climbed the tower, held on to the outside rails, and hung over the edge. I began writing down what I observed. With furrowed brow, Jacob ran over to me, looked at my notepad, and said, "What are you doing?"

"I'm writing down that you are a really good climber. Writing helps me remember that."

- **Tell young children you are writing down all the good things you see them doing.**

Four-year-old Eva ran over to me when she saw me writing observations in my notebook. "What are you writing?"

"I'm writing down all the good things I see children doing," I replied.

She smiled and said, "Oh," and returned to her center to play.

Make Strengths-Based Observations

Children might be thinking:
Are you writing bad things about me?
Are you going to report me?

As you observe, apply a strengths-based perspective by watching for what promotes and supports children's development and functioning. Look for positives about them, including their personal qualities, abilities, and actions. Be vigilant in noting the ways their caregivers and educational staff support them. When documenting concerns, be sure to describe the context as well as the observable behavior. Refrain from using negative labels when describing them, such as calling them disruptive, noncompliant, or aggressive.

Fabulous Five: Make Strengths-Based Observations

- **Observe for children's personal qualities that assist them in being resilient.**

When I went into the classroom to see Rebecca, the preschool teacher told me, "She's a really cute and very determined little girl. She has cerebral palsy and wears ankle-foot orthoses on her ankles."

I sat at her table and talked to all the children around me. Then they lined up to wash their hands, and Rebecca walked over, keeping her legs stiff. When the paraprofessional reached for the faucet knobs, Rebecca pushed her hand away and said, "I do it." As the group ate their snacks, she opened her own containers, although it took her 3 to 4 minutes to do so. She declined all offers of assistance.

After writing what I saw, I added my interpretation: *[Rebecca shows a lot of determination to do things by herself, and her persistence even with hard tasks is a real strength.]*

Later, I noted these strengths in her Individualized Education Program.

- **Note abilities that are children's strengths.**

I watched the teacher put blue and green crayons on Peyton's lapboard connected to his wheelchair. "We are doing a coloring project. What color do you want to use?" she asked and waited for 2 minutes.

Peyton, who had limited movement, did not respond.

Then she held up a crayon in each hand and said, "Look at the one you want. Do you want the blue or green one?"

Peyton shifted his eyes to the green crayon.

"Okay. I'm not surprised. I know you like green."

I recorded the interaction in my notes and added that one of his strengths was his ability to indicate his choices through eye movements. I wrote down that by allowing him additional time to make choices, he could give a meaningful response.

- **Watch for children's actions and solutions that supports their functioning.**

"Kelsey is very sensitive to noise," her preschool teacher said in our meeting. "Last year she wore headphones the first month of school. This year she wears an earplug in one ear, and that has helped."

The next day I watched as she played with the dollhouse and three boys in the block center built a 3-foot tower. A few minutes later, they yelled as they pushed the wooden blocks down.

Kelsey turned to them and said, "No screaming, guys." They quieted down.

She is good at telling her peers when it is too loud for her, I thought. *That is a nice strength.*

- **Identify caregivers' and/or educational staff's actions that support children.**

"Ross has trouble with changes. I have a hard time getting him to school," his mother told me the first week of class.

I observed him moving slowly to the coat cupboard with his name on it. "If your name is in red, go to the table with a red square on it," his preschool teacher told him. "That's going to be your table." When all the children were seated, she pointed to a visual schedule and reviewed the daily activities. Next, she said, "It's time to look at the calendar and weather. Red table, please go to the rug and sit down." Ross followed his classmates, looking relaxed.

I put in my notes: *[His teacher's organization and use of a visual schedule is making transitions easier for Ross.]*

- **State the context when recording concerns.**

After conducting follow-up observations, I wrote:

Sam's fine motor skills are strengths for him, and he shows delight when drawing. He has shown progress in his processing of some sensory information, such as being better able to tolerate some touch sensations (like getting a haircut). Sam is beginning to self-initiate the use of sensory self-regulation strategies for calming, such as requesting to take a quiet break or using the weighted lapbag. He has had to learn many new routines and rules in kindergarten, which has been a major transition for him.

When an event, activity, or interaction does not go the way Sam expects or wants, many times he has been seen saying, "No, no, no," raising his voice, and sometimes crying. At times this works for him (e.g., a peer will give him a toy he wants), but at other times it does not, especially in situations where he does not have control, like when a peer chooses not to do what he asks. It is in these situations that he is sometimes seen reacting by grabbing or hitting another child. He does better when an adult prompts him on what to do before he becomes upset. The use of Social Stories has also helped Sam learn positive ways to get what he wants.

CHILDREN'S DESCRIPTIONS OF WHAT THEY THINK YOU SHOULD KNOW

Dr. Clare: "What should therapists know when they give tests to kids?"

Craig (age 9): "Tell them what the test is about."

Kerry (age 10): "Be really clear about what we're supposed to do."

Nicole (age 9): "Tell them instructions in a nice, happy, and caring way. If kids need them repeated, you shouldn't say it in a mean way."

Sara (age 9): "Say, 'Good luck.'"

Promote Stress-Free Testing

Another way for you to learn about children is with tests. The ultimate goal is to capture the essence of what they can do and how they learn. To start, gather information to identify strengths and determine concerns by observing children in various settings and conducting interviews. Then decide which tests will be the most beneficial.

Also, decide whether to use standardized tests, informal assessments, or a play-based assessment. Standardized tests give you certain information on how children perform or function, which is then compared with their same-age peers or defined criteria for that particular test. Informal assessments, such as examining children's quality of movement, are important as well. Younger children often do better within a play-based assessment, in which the environment is set up with enticing play activities. You then observe their skill levels as they play.

Because testing often tends to be a more rigid situation, you will glean how the children tend to respond to structured and sometimes stressful circumstances. The children's responses and approaches also give you information regarding their cognitive, language, social, and coping abilities. For instance, notice the following:

- Do they enjoy mastering difficult tasks or do they withdraw?

- What do they do when faced with frustration?

- When following test directions, what is their style of interaction, especially when they do not have control of the situation?

- What are their beliefs and perceptions that are expressed through self-talk (e.g., "I can do this" or "This is too hard")?

- Are they concerned with achieving perfection and feel that any mistake is unacceptable?

Compare and contrast the information from testing with what you have observed and learned from interviews.

If the test does not require a certain sequence, then you must decide in which order to do different items. Before meeting with the children, decide what information is the most important to obtain and think about what might be the most discouraging or difficult aspects of the test. You may want to start with easy items so children experience success and want to continue. However, some children do better if you give them the hardest one first while you have their full cooperation and attention and then shift to easier items. Understand, then, that there is the possible risk that they may quit if they think all test items will be hard.

Plan and Prepare Before Testing

Children might be thinking:
Will this test be hard?
Why do I have to do this?
I don't know what to do.
Will I get in trouble if I don't do good?

The more prepared you are, the better. You can make the process more comfortable if you are well versed in giving the tests. If a test is new to you, practice beforehand so you can proceed quickly. Try to memorize the directions and scoring. Or you may want to create a "cheat sheet" that organizes the items in a way that helps you. Children find waiting to be boring. With down time, they are more likely to become distracted. Some children who have to wait may get anxious as they wonder how hard the test will be. Be considerate of their time and feelings.

It is vital that you notify and prepare children before testing, especially if they do not know you. If you cannot see them ahead of time, ask caregivers to let them know about your meeting. When children are aware of what is going to happen, there is less anxiety.

Another important component of testing is to establish an optimal environment that promotes concentration. If you have a choice, select a room that is quiet with good lighting and as few visual and auditory distractions as possible. Prepare the room and test materials ahead of time. Try to place only the required materials on the table. Children may feel overwhelmed if they see several test items on a cluttered table. For example, they may think, *Do I have to do all these?* or *This is too much.* You can always store extra items on a chair next to you. It also helps to get in the habit of clearing off the table as you go and moving items out of sight once completed. Another essential element is to always have backup supplies that you can use if the testing is too hard or upsetting for the children. The goal is to create a testing environment that is conducive to gathering the most information while facilitating the children's comfort to ensure accurate results.

Fabulous Five: Prepare for Testing

- **Prepare the room for testing before children arrive.**

Five-year-old Bobby started the eye-hand coordination test without any problems. However, I forgot about the hanging Halloween spider that made spooky sounds when activated by movement. A staff member walked into the room and the spider echoed, "OOOOH." Bobby spun toward the spider and grinned. After the spider stopped, I tried another test item. Bobby held the pencil loosely, looked at the wall, and barely touched the paper. "Bobby, are you still thinking about that spider?"

"Uh huh."

"Scare him once and then we'll move him into the next room so he can rest. When you are finished, you can scare him again."

"BOO," he shouted, laughing when "OOOOH" filled the room. Then we carried the spider to the office.

I tried the next test item, but no luck. Bobby's eyes drifted around the room. "Let's take a break. Try spinning these spider tops." He perked up and began playing.

"It's hard to think about this test when you are still thinking about that spider. Let's try just a few more. Which one do you want to do next?" I said as I pointed at the test cards and then a pegboard. He completed two more tasks, but it was obvious that it was hard for him to concentrate on the testing. We stopped, scared the spider again, and finished the test the next day.

- **Have all test items ready, organized, and within your reach before starting.**

A teacher brought 7-year-old Jeremy to the room before I was ready. I scurried to organize the testing materials on the table. Then I started to slip most of the items onto a chair next to me so they would be within easy reach but out of sight. When Jeremy started wandering around the room, I handed him a set of test cards. "Could you please shuffle these for me? Thanks." He focused on the cards, and I finished the test preparation.

- **Have supplies for backup activities.**

Cody stared at the circle to be cut and said, "I can't." Then he crossed his arms, lowered his eyes, and studied the floor.

The occupational therapy student drew a smiling face inside the circle. She pulled out brightly colored paper and scented markers. Then she drew a square on yellow neon paper. "Smell this marker. It's blueberry."

Cody took a whiff as she placed the marker under his nose.

"Let's make a picture. Cut out his head and body. Cut on the dark line."

Cody raised his eyes, reached for the paper, and began snipping.

"What should his name be?"

"Louie. He's a superhero."

- **Keep extra test items out of the children's view.**

The occupational therapy student placed cards, scissors, beads, a pegboard, and a test booklet on the table.

Six-year-old Libby strolled to the room, stopped in the doorway, and stared at the covered table. "Let's not do ALL that stuff, okay?"

"All right," the occupational therapy student agreed. "We'll just do a few." She then moved the unneeded items out of view.

- **Select a test that matches the children's level of functioning.**

To help a therapist who was ill, I was asked to do an evaluation of a 5-year-old boy in a specialized program. Because I did not know the student or the general range of his abilities, I brought two fine motor tests: one for younger students and one for older children. First, I talked with his teacher about her concerns. "It's hard for him to hold the pencil. He struggles with writing but he's getting better at copying his name."

Then I observed him in class and saw that he easily matched colored cubes to a design card. He looked at his name strip as a model and printed his name while his teacher cued him on how to make the letters. Still unsure of what he could do, I started by having him cut out a simple thick-line square and circle. He accurately cut the square but grunted as he struggled with the larger circle, cueing me to choose the easier test.

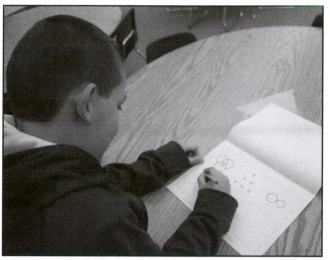

Figure 7-2. Tell children to just try their best on the test.

Create an Optimal and Engaging Testing Atmosphere

> **Children might be thinking:**
> *Why are you giving me a test?*
> *I don't want to take a test.*
> *I hate tests.*
> *Am I going to fail?*
> *I'm not good at tests.*

To engage children in testing, you want to create a pleasant atmosphere that is different from traditional school tests. You can do this by using a gentle and lighthearted tone of voice and adding the element of fun by using toys or puppets. It also helps to encourage children to challenge themselves and eliminate fears about getting a failing grade.

Set a Positive Tone for Testing

When testing, it is helpful to have a beginning, middle, and end. Start by describing the purpose, what it entails, and what is to be gained from the process. Stress to the children that this is a chance to discover and learn more about themselves. Prepare them that some parts of the test may be hard and they just need to try their best (Figure 7-2). The purpose is not to judge them and is not to determine if they are good or bad. Creating this mindset of being a voyage of discovery makes it safer for them to try, knowing that they may experience failure. You also can make the testing a more positive experience by smiling and using a light and playful tone of voice. Show some animation and excitement to be spending time with them while encouraging and commenting on their effort. Be certain to make the situation a time where children enjoy being with you, even if the test is hard.

Fabulous Five: Create a Positive Atmosphere

- **Explain the purpose of testing.**

"Your teacher told me you are really good at math and you are trying your best but that sometimes writing can be hard for you."

"Yeah, it is," 8-year-old Jessie said, nodding.

"So today I am going to have you do different things to see if we can discover what you are doing well and what is working for you, as well as to figure out what is making writing so hard."

- **Use a light and playful tone of voice when testing younger children.**

"We are going to play some games and do some drawing and cutting," I said in a light and carefree tone of voice. "I'm glad I get to be with you. I want to see what you can do. I bet you can do a lot." I smiled and pointed to the testing room.

"I'm good at puzzles," 3-year-old Morgan replied.

- **Prepare children that some parts of the test may be hard.**

"On this test, some parts are easy. Some are hard. I just need you to try your best."

"These mazes are easy for me," 7-year-old Austin said with a smile. He started the first maze and veered outside the line. "It's small. Do you have a magnifying glass?"

- **Make positive and encouraging statements throughout the testing.**

Four-year-old Dale raised his arms and flexed his biceps like a body builder. I felt his muscles to check his muscle tone and said, "Wow, you're strong."

He smiled. "I'm so strong I can carry the cat food. Know why I'm strong? It's because I eat oatmeal."

- **Praise effort rather than accuracy during testing.**

Five-year-old Brenda started to build a block pyramid like the one she had just been shown. The blue block slipped from her fingers and clunked on the table. "I messed up." She tucked her loose black hair behind her ears, grasped the block again, and tried to balance it on another block.

"It's great that you are not giving up."

Incorporate Toys and Puppets When Testing

Toys and puppets are an essential part of any test kit and can be used for various purposes. They are enticing and are an easy way to engage young children in the testing. They can be used as a warm-up activity, a captivating method to give directions, or as a celebration after each item. With older children, you can incorporate puppets and toys to take a break, to aid during transition between test items, or to finish in a fun way. It is better to have toys available but kept out of sight because they can be become distracting.

It is all right to be playful and even goofy between test items. You will find your demeanor and tone of voice often change when you are not overly serious. Caregivers are pleased to see their children having fun and laughing while you are gathering information. Children also appreciate it when you help them relax and make testing a more positive experience.

Fabulous Five: Integrate Puppets and Toys Into the Testing

- **Use toys as a warm-up activity before testing.**

"Come with me. I have something I want to show you, and then we'll do some games," I told 3-year-old Jim. He jumped up and followed me to the next room, where I had all the test items arranged. "Look at this horse. If you push here, he moves his head and legs," I said as I pressed a button under the toy.

Jim snatched it out of my hands and made the horse nod his head up and down for a few minutes.

"Next I want to show you a catching game," I said, referring to the test. "Have the horse rest while you catch this ball."

Jim left the toy on the table and ran over to me, holding his pudgy arms out, ready to play.

- **Use puppets to give directions to the test.**

"Hi! My name is Casey the cow, and we are going to have fun today," the occupational therapy student said as she moved the puppet's head and arms.

Three-year-old Annie waved back. The occupational therapy student gave directions while manipulating the puppet, and Annie followed them. "I did it, Mom," she yelled with her success.

"Great job. Do some more," her mother replied.

"Casey is having fun with you. Are you having fun?" Annie nodded.

"Casey has another fun game for us," the occupational therapy student said and stated the next the direction. At the end, she said, "Can Casey give you a hug?"

"Yeah," Annie said and smiled.

The cow puppet hugged her. "Thank you for playing with me."

- **Incorporate toys to celebrate the completion of each test item.**

"Today we get to have special time together. I'm glad I get to be with you. We're going to do all kinds of fun things," I said, and 3-year-old Jade smiled back. "First is to build with blocks." I dropped 10 blocks on the table and had her make a tower. When she finished, I pulled out a wind-up toy that was a grey horse with a pink mane. I turned the knob and the horse danced.

"Hors-ey," Jade said and grinned.

When it stopped, I demonstrated the next block design for her to copy. For the rest of the test, the horse pranced after the completion of each item. Then at the end, the horse said, "Bye-bye, Jade."

"Bye-bye, hors-ey," Jade replied.

- **Have toys available for transitions between test items.**

Five-year-old Connor completed a step block design and cut different shapes. He started to fidget, so I handed him a small toy dog whose body opened and closed like an accordion. He played for 2 minutes while I cleared off the table and put out paper and a pencil. "Have the puppy watch you as you draw yourself," I suggested.

He placed the dog on the edge of the paper. Then he drew a picture of himself and added an animal figure. "I saw a dead squirrel. He be dead. He never see his mom and dad again."

"That is sad."

- **Use toys at the end of testing.**

"We're done," I said as I pulled out a small bag of toys. "Would you like to play with these for a few minutes?"

"Sure," 10-year-old Terry replied.

"I have some easy and hard tops. This one is the trickiest. If you spin it just right, it flips over and spins upright, looking like a mushroom."

"I want to try that one."

Assist Children Throughout Testing

You will often need to provide support to help children get through testing. Be prepared to address various feelings such as fear or anxiety that may hinder participation. Incorporate strategies for promoting alertness and attention to the test. You also may have to alter your approach with children who are hesitant or refuse to participate. Be flexible and guide children throughout the process.

Address Children's Feelings About Testing

> **Children might be thinking:**
> *I'm nervous.*
> *I'm not good at this.*
> *I might goof up.*
> *I want to be right.*
> *What will happen if I make a mistake?*
> *I'm no good.*

Tests are often emotionally laden events associated with the possibility of failure. So it is common for children to be worried or afraid about failing, and most of all fearful of the possibility of seeming stupid. It is important to help children become comfortable with you before starting and to create an atmosphere where trying feels safe. Make it a habit to keep a watchful eye on how the children are feeling throughout the testing.

Address Initial Anxiety Regarding Taking Tests

When you see children becoming anxious, re-emphasize that the purpose of testing is to learn about them. Mention that when you know what they can do, you are better able to help them. Then it will be easier for you to discuss with them, what they would like to do to change their lives. For those who look like they might not start the test, pick a task that is easy to do and fail proof. You also may want to address children's self-talk. Some may say, "Oh, this looks easy," as a way to convince themselves to do the test. Others may tell themselves that they cannot do it. For these children, ask them to try and give themselves a chance to see what they can do. Stress the value of effort more than performance. In other words, emphasize that you want them to try their best—not necessarily get a perfect score.

> ### Fabulous Five: Attend to Children's Initial Anxiety Regarding Tests
> - **Tell children their efforts on the test let you know what they can do.**
>
> "First, put your name on the paper," I directed 5-year-old Haley.
>
> "I not know how to write my name."
>
> "That's okay. Just write the letters you do know. That helps me know what you can do."
>
> She printed "HA" and then stopped.
>
> "Thanks for showing me what you know."

> - **Reframe children's worry about failing the test into an opportunity to make their lives better.**
>
> "I don't do very good on tests," 10-year-old Kathryn said.
>
> "This is not like a test you take in school. Other kids have said they thought it was fun. I just want to see what you know and what you can do. This helps me learn about your strengths and what areas are difficult for you. Then we can work together to figure out how to make things easier for you."
>
> - **Start the testing with a task in which children can succeed.**
>
> Seeing 5-year-old Savannah's fearful look, I told her, "Draw a picture of you."
>
> She started to relax as she began her portrait and drew 10 body parts. Then she added lines under her eyes. "Look, I'm crying."
>
> "Oh dear, are you sad?"
>
> She nodded. "I'm choking when the candy was going down my throat."
>
> "I bet that was scary. How did you get it out?"
>
> "My mom hit my back."
>
> "I'm glad you're okay," I replied.
>
> She smiled, and then I shifted to the standardized test.
>
> - **Be aware that when children look at a test and say, "These are easy," they may be trying to reassure or convince themselves.**
>
> Eight-year-old Josephine studied the figure of three intertwined circles that she was supposed to copy and announced, "This is easy." Then she crinkled her eyebrows and muttered to herself, "I don't know how to do this."
>
> I responded to her doubts by saying, "Just try and do the best that you can."
>
> - **Tell children who hesitate to give themselves a chance to try.**
>
> Seven-year-old Tricia looked at the circle she had to copy. "I'm good at drawing." She drew the next two shapes, but when she saw the picture of overlapping pencils, she curled her lip and said, "Is it time to go? I'm getting so tired."
>
> "These are challenging," I replied in a gentle tone of voice. "Give yourself a chance to try them."

Deal With Ongoing Feelings About Testing

As the testing continues, check with children about how they are feeling. Use open-ended questions such as, "How are you doing?" Respond to any expressed concerns or any nonverbal messages of distress. Some possible signs are sighing, chewing on fingers or clothes, or restless movement. Provide encouragement, and focus more on effort.

You can help them overcome their reluctance by saying that the test is hard for all children. If necessary, break the testing into a number of short sessions.

Fabulous Five: Assist With Ongoing Feelings About Testing

- **Ask children how they are feeling throughout the testing.**

"I'll bring Susan to your room," the special education teacher at the private school said. When he brought her, I heard him say on the other side of my door, "Take some deep breaths."

She then walked in the room, and I greeted the 10 year old in a friendly manner. After a few minutes of testing, I asked, "How are you doing?"

"Okay. This is easier than I thought it'd be."

- **Acknowledge that taking a test can be frustrating.**

During the motor testing, 5-year-old Cameron held the button strip in his left hand. He fingered the white button and then tried pushing it against the hole. He continued for around 10 seconds and then threw the strip across the table. "I can't. It doesn't work."

"I saw that you tried," I responded. "This test is hard and can be frustrating. Let's take a break."

- **Address nonverbal signs of anxiety or frustration while testing.**

Five-year-old Rae repeatedly pushed her blue glasses on the bridge of her nose. As the test continued, she started to suck her left thumb and twist her auburn hair in her right hand.

"Let's take a break," I suggested. We went for a walk and stopped at the drinking fountain. When we returned, I switched to an easier test item, making sure to build in success.

- **Acknowledge that the test is hard for other children.**

"Whew," 7-year-old Walt said after he completed each test item and then started to gnaw on his fingernails.

After two test items, I said, "This test is hard for older kids too. You're doing a great job of trying everything."

Seemingly feeling a little better, he sighed and put his hands on the table for the next item.

- **Divide the testing into short sessions if children appear overwhelmed or fatigued.**

The wiry 6 year old completed cutting and drawing test items. Then we walked to a balance beam, and Christian gazed at it. "This is scary," he said with a quiver in his voice. "I could fall off and break my head."

"I promise I will not let you fall. I will be right next to you," I assured him.

He darted to an indoor play gym and hid behind the slide.

"That's okay," I said. "We do not have to do this today. I know it looks hard. You did a lot already so I think this is a good time to stop. I will come back tomorrow."

Then he followed me to his classroom.

I returned the next day and started with the easiest test items, leaving the balance beam for the end. I hovered over him as he tried to walk on the beam and steadied him as soon as he started to lose his balance. "See, I am keeping you safe. I will not let you fall." He tried one more time, and the cloud of unease lifted as he walked across the beam.

Recognize Signs That Children Have Given Up During Testing

As you are testing, watch for signs that the children are giving up because they perceive the test to be too hard. They may get restless and start to look around the room. They might ask to do something else. Others may not say anything but attempt the test item only halfheartedly. Some children will race through the item, going as fast as they can just to get it over with. Another sign is when children say, "I can't do this," before even making an attempt. Others will say they are bored or tired when they think the test is too difficult.

Try giving words of encouragement or suggest taking a break. Let them know that you just want them to try their best. Some will do better if they think their parents will see their work. You also may want to tell them how many test items are left or what they can do once they are finished. If children are adamant about stopping, respect their wishes. You want accurate and valid test results that require children's full effort. You can try again on another day or write about the information you have, including their request to stop.

Fabulous Five: Recognize Signs That the Children Have Given Up During Testing

- **Encourage children to slow down if they are rushing during a test.**

Using a marker, I drew a circle with a thick black line. Inside the circle, I added eyes and a smile. Holding it up, I said in a funny tone of voice to 4-year-old Justin, "He says, 'Help, help. Cut me out.'"

Justin smiled, reached for it, and began cutting on the line. But he started going so fast that the paper wrinkled and he went off the line.

"Stop for a minute. Slow down. You are going too fast."

When he resumed at a slower speed, he was able to stay on the line.

- **Recognize that children may say they are bored or tired if the test seems too hard.**

"I'm bored," 6-year-old Lisa said as she looked at the diamond figure she was to copy.

"I know it looks hard," I responded.

"I don't know how to draw a diamond. Can you draw it for me?"

"Not this time. Just try your best. It's okay if it's not perfect."

- **State how many test items are left.**

Three-fourths of the way through a test, 3-year-old Max pushed his chair away from the table and said, "Can I play with that fire truck?"

"Yes, you will get to play with it. We just have four more things to do and then you can play with the truck. You are almost done. Keep going."

Max moved his chair back to the table. After he finished, I brought over the toy fire engine.

- **Suggest taking a break and redoing a test item if allowed.**

"How many more to do?" 5-year-old Cameron asked as he carelessly drew an incomplete circle.

Thinking he could do better, I said, "Let's take a break and get a drink of water." When we came back, I had him try again, and he drew a nicely formed circle.

- **Tell children you want to show their parents their very best after the test.**

"Please draw a picture of yourself," I said to 4-year-old Sean.

He started to draw an airplane but then scribbled all over it.

"Please stop," I said. I gave him another piece of paper. "Draw you. Do your best. I want to show this to your parents."

He then drew himself, appearing to take his time.

Assist Children in Maintaining Attention to the Test

Children might be thinking:

What is that noise?

Why is there so much noise?

What is that over there?

This test is hard.

I don't feel like doing this anymore.

How much longer do I have to do this?

A crucial aspect of test taking is to get children's attention and then help them maintain their focus on the task. Attention is needed to listen to the directions and keep their

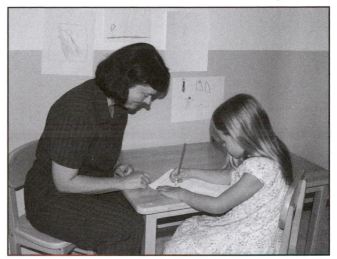

Figure 7-3. Cue children to stay focused on the test.

mind on what to do. Many children are easily distracted by what is happening around them, what is in the room, or any noises they hear. Some tend to move constantly, which makes concentrating more challenging. Others may become tired and stop thinking about the test. Watch for these issues and change what you are doing to gain and maintain children's attention.

Help Children Gain and Maintain Attention on the Test

At first, you have to get children's attention before starting the test. If they are looking around the room, say their name and wait until they are looking at you or the test item. Once you have eye contact, you can give the directions. For some, you may want to capture their attention by using mystery or showing your excitement about what they can do. Others may grab any object in sight. For instance, they may impulsively snatch scissors off the table and start cutting before you have given the directions. To help them focus on the directions, keep your hand on the test supplies and make a stopping gesture. After they look at you, say the directions.

The next challenge is keep their focus on the task (Figure 7-3). Maintaining attention is the best. It is vital that you are quick, especially between test items. To regain attention, provide a verbal cue such as, "Think about…," or tap the test object.

Fabulous Five: Help Children Gain and Maintain Attention to the Test

- **Say children's names and have them look at you before giving directions for the test.**

Five-year-old Eleni wandered around the room opening the teacher's cabinets. "Eleni," I said, and when she looked at me, I gestured. "Come sit at the table."

"I think my stomach will fall asleep soon. I have to give it some water."

"Okay. Get a drink and then sit down."

She went to the water fountain, took a few sips, and returned to the table. She started to look at the shelves, so I said, "Eyes on me, please." When she made eye contact, I gave the first direction.

- **Get children's attention by making intriguing requests.**

I watched 5-year-old Jamal's head bob as he drew a picture with his classmates. To check his scissors skills, I handed him a piece of paper with a line on it. Then I said, "Here, cut this paper in half so I can write you a secret message."

He snipped across the paper and waited anxiously for the surprise.

I wrote, "I like you," folded it three times, and slipped it into his palm. Gingerly, he unfolded the message, and when I read it to him, he grinned.

- **Keep one hand on the test materials and make a stopping gesture with the other hand if children are impulsive.**

As soon as 7-year-old Scott sat down, he grabbed a handful of pennies that were on the testing mat and threw them into the box.

"Wait a minute," I said. "I have to give you the directions." I put the pennies back on the mat and kept my left hand over them. I raised my right hand to indicate "stop" and read the test instructions.

- **Encourage children to keep their minds on the test item by saying, "Think about [name test item]."**

Six-year-old Kristen slipped the scissors on her fingers and began cutting with her thumb down toward the ground. "I don't know how good I'll do, but I'll try my best." She started cutting a thin black circle that would later be measured as part of the test, and then stopped. "We're learning about bones."

"Kristen, think about cutting right now." When she was finished, I asked, "So what did you learn about bones?"

- **Tap or point to where you want children to focus on the test.**

"Ready, set, go," I said and pressed the button on the stopwatch.

Seven-year-old Mack began the timed test. But before I said stop, he lifted his head and stared at the stopwatch in my palm.

I pointed to and tapped the test booklet and said, "You have to keep your eyes on the paper. I will show you the watch when we are done."

Use Movement to Maintain Alertness

To get the most valid results, children must be able to concentrate on the test. For some children, it is a challenge to keep their bodies in a calm and alert state. There are ones who use movement to organize themselves. For instance, I once observed a child who rocked in his chair for 20 seconds and then stopped and sat perfectly still while he printed his name. For those who do better with subtle movement, provide alternative seating, such as a therapy ball or a T-stool. Similarly, watch to determine if children's performance is enhanced when in a different body position besides sitting.

Be sensitive to any signs of withdrawal or fading. If you find that children are becoming lethargic or fatigued, take a break and involve them in movement activities. Fast motions, such as running, swinging, or jumping, are the most alerting. On the other hand, when children are constantly moving and not able to stay still, move the test items to the floor. Children often settle down when they sit on the ground. Find the right balance, where you use the just-right amount of movement needed for children to focus on the test.

Fabulous Five: Incorporate Movement if Needed to Maintain Alertness

- **Allow children to change positions during testing especially if they are restless.**

Six-year-old Carlos rocked and then tipped his chair until it teetered on two legs. He balanced in midair, then landed with a thud.

"Would it help you to stand?" I asked Carlos with a soft tone of voice.

He nodded, stood, and placed his left palm on the table. "What's next?"

- **Change the type of seating during testing.**

We walked in the room, and 9-year-old Ruth ran to the board. "Draw a picture, and then let's go to the table," I said.

She sketched a fairy. When at the table, she sat on the edge of her chair and rocked it back and forth.

I handed her a T-stool and said, "Here, try this."

She shifted subtly left to right but kept her eyes on the table.

- **Take breaks from testing when nonverbal cues suggest fatigue.**

Five-year-old Bob completed 10 items on the fine motor test. Then he started to yawn, and his eyelids began to droop. "Let's take a break. Would you like to get some water?" I asked. He nodded. As we headed to another building, I said, "Let me see how fast you can run to the water fountain." He sprinted at full speed. When we returned to the testing room, he was alert and ready to continue.

- **Have children move fast if they are lethargic during testing.**

Halfway through the testing, 7-year-old Lenny propped his head in his right hand. Then he laid his head on the table and yawned.

"You look sleepy. Let's do a game. Stand up. How many jumping jacks can you do?"

"A lot," he responded. After we counted 10 jumps, he returned to the table for the pencil-and-paper test items more alert and awake.

- **Test on the floor if children are restless.**

Seven-year-old Kevin roamed around the special education room and then stopped. "Know what I like?"

"What?"

"I like motorcycles." As he talked, I moved the test items to the floor and put the test booklet on a clipboard.

Then I held my hands like I was shifting gears on a motorcycle and said, "Kevin, zoom over here."

He pretended to rev his engine, zipped across the room, and sat next to me. We started the test, and his body stayed still as if his motorcycle was parked.

Engage Children Who Want to Be in Control While Testing

Children might be thinking:
I don't like tests.
I'm not good at tests.
I'm not ready.
Am I going to get a bad grade or do bad?
I don't want to do this.
I don't want to do it today—maybe another day.
This looks too hard.
I don't do good on tests.
I don't want to do this test, so I won't.
You can't make me do this.

At times when you are testing, you may be with children who need to be in control. This becomes evident when they start to tell you what they will or will not do. They may also express their desire for control through their actions. When you give test directions, you might see them react by staring at the wall, folding their arms, or even turning their backs to you. They may only follow the directions halfheartedly. This need for control may be seen more when you are giving a test because it is a structured situation, which involves telling them what to do. Unlike an interview or completing an activity, there is usually less leeway for adapting test administration or for allowing the children to take the lead.

The important step at this juncture is to consciously think about why the children have the need for control. There are a multitude of reasons children might balk at testing. Although it is easy to think of them as being "bad," this type of thinking can be judgmental. It is common to feel frustrated and wonder what you can do. If you take an authoritarian approach and try to force children by saying they have to do the testing, you may easily slip into a full-blown power struggle. Then, even if the children comply with your demands, there are no guarantees they will put forth their best effort, and your testing will be invalid.

What is most helpful is to assume an open-minded and understanding approach. Children have to feel safe with you before they can begin the test. It is not easy to take a test, especially because we usually examine areas in which the children are delayed, so there is a higher risk of failure.

Some children fail miserably on tests and they know it. As a consequence, they may not want to try test items in which they already know they are not proficient. They may take one peek at the test and decide it looks too hard. It then becomes easier to not attempt a test, rather than risk another experience of failure. It is not worth continuing the test if it is going to damage your relationship or become a stressful and negative experience for the children. If you cannot encourage them to finish the test, you may always describe the situation in your report. The way children respond is important information. It is beneficial to describe the strategies you attempt, even if unsuccessful.

Explore Possible Reasons for Refusing to Take the Test

Using an understanding approach, delve deeper into the reasons children refuse to participate in the testing. Consider the possibility that they do not feel well. They may be ill. They may be upset or preoccupied about a situation unrelated to you. Or, like adults, they might be having a bad day. Check to see if they are missing something fun because they are with you. Some may not believe that they have the ability to do the test and decide that it is better not to try. Provide encouragement to continue by conveying your belief in them, or stop if the test becomes too hard.

Fabulous Five: Investigate Reasons for Refusing to Take the Test

- **Make sure children are not missing something fun while testing.**

When I tried to engage 6-year-old Ricky in fine motor testing, he backed into a corner and tucked his head. "Did you know I was coming?" I asked.

"Yes."

"I know it's hard when you are getting to know someone new." Ricky did not move or look up. "Let's play with some toys first."

"I don't want to play with toys."

"What's bothering you?"

His eyes became teary as he said, "I'm missing recess."

"Oh, I'm so glad you told me. Let's go to recess, and we will start when it's over."

He ran out of the room as fast as he could. When the bell rang at the end of recess, he came over and followed me to the testing room without hesitation.

- **Check if children are having a hard day or not feeling well on the day of the test.**

Seven-year-old Jane dragged herself down the stairs and pouted as she walked into the room. She did the first test item but then stopped.

"Are you having a rough morning?" I said.

"No."

"How was your weekend?" She stared at the floor. "Is it just the Monday blues? You don't look right. Is something wrong?"

"My stomach hurts. I threw up last night."

"I'm sorry you don't feel good. We can do this next week. I hope you get better."

- **Encourage children to attempt testing by saying you believe in them.**

"I can't do this," 8-year-old Nate said when his eyes settled on the testing booklet.

"Just do your best," I encouraged him, and he drew the first design. Then I placed the cutting task on the table.

"I'm not good at cutting."

"I really believe you can do this. Remember, you didn't think you could draw and you did it. Just try. You can do this too. That's all I ask."

- **Watch to see if the test is too hard.**

"RJ spends most of his time hiding under the table. It's hard to know what he can really do," his kindergarten teacher told me.

I started the motor skills test and asked the 5 year old to copy different shapes. Instead, he took the pencil and traced over the shapes. Then I asked him to sort cards by color. He took the pack of cards and turned the whole pack over.

"How come you don't want to do the cards?"

"I don't like cards," he said, pushed his chair back, and began walking around the room.

"I have another game. See if you can beat me," I said.

He returned to the table and sat across from me. "I want to sit here."

"That's fine." I quickly moved the pegboard over to him. He stared at it and then followed the directions but moved slowly. After that, he refused to do any other items. "I'll do it tomorrow," became his refrain.

I switched to an easy draw-and-cut activity. As I watched, I saw that his skills were like a young 3 year old. *That test was too hard for him*, I thought. *And he knew it.*

- **Check if children are upset over another incident or situation if they are hesitant or refuse to start the test.**

Nine-year-old Jim came to the table and settled in the chair. He pushed his lips together and mumbled, "I'm not going to cut. I don't want to do this. This is dumb."

"You look upset. Did something happen?" I asked.

He nodded. "Carol picked on me." Jim's breathing slowed as he told me about the incident at recess.

"I'm glad you told me about it. Are you ready to cut?"

He nodded and grabbed the scissors.

Use Nonconfrontational Approaches During Testing

For a power struggle to occur, both you and the children have to be engaged in it. One way to diffuse a brewing struggle is to use nonconfrontational approaches. For instance, a struggle cannot continue if you remain silent or agree with the children. Incorporating humor as a response can also be effective. Other tactics are making the test into a game or suggesting turn taking.

Fabulous Five: Avoid Confrontations During Testing

- **Give test directions and stay quiet.**

When I went to test Ken at the day treatment, his second-grade teacher said, "Ken, you need to go with Dr. Clare. You'll be playing some games."

He followed me to the testing room but then ran to the corner of the room. He plopped onto a red pillow and shouted, "I don't want to play."

"Mm. You don't know me, and you don't know what I brought. I'm wondering how come you don't want to play."

"I don't want to play," he yelled back. He put his chin down, folded his arms, and huffed.

"You don't like to play?" I replied. "Okay then, come sit here." I pointed to a chair next to me.

"I don't want to," he said, flailing his arms. Abruptly he jumped off the pillow, ran to a chair at the other end of the table, and threw himself into the seat with as much force as he could muster.

I quickly moved the scissors and paper over to his end of the table. "I won't do any games," he said.

"Okay. No games. This is just cutting. Cut this circle on the heaviest black line." I backed away 3 feet and sat quietly in the chair.

Ken stabbed the middle of the paper circle but then started cutting on the line. One by one, I placed the test items in front of him and gave the directions. "I'm not doin' it," he shouted each time.

I sat quietly in the chair and did not respond. Although he continually protested, he followed the directions and completed the entire test.

- **Go with the children's stance.**

"Write your name on the paper," I told the 7 year old. He printed "ore," and I gave him a puzzled look. "I thought your name was Jacob."

"Ore is my real name. Jacob is my nickname."

"Well then, write your nickname on the paper."

- **Use humor during testing.**

"Draw a picture of yourself," I said to 6-year-old Russ.

Within 3 seconds, he made a stick figure with a head and four lines for arms and legs. "There. Done."

"Oh, you are much cuter that," I said with a smile. "Here is another piece of paper. Make a better picture of you."

He grumbled but began drawing a more detailed picture.

- **Suggest taking turns to help children start a test.**

As soon as 5-year-old Victor saw the blocks, he started building. After a few minutes, I said his name to get his attention. He kept his eyes downcast and started building another structure. "It looks like you like to build," I said. He smiled. "Go ahead. It's your turn. Do one more, and I will copy it. Then it's my turn," I said. When he finished, I demonstrated as I gave the test directions for making a bridge out of blocks.

- **Make the test into a game.**

After completing a cutting task, 5-year-old Tony dropped the scissors on the table and said, "I'm too tired."

"Keep going," I encouraged him. "I want to see how fast you can move your hand. Pick up the pennies one at a time and put them into the box as fast as you can."

He loosely scooped three pennies in his palm and dropped them in the box in slow motion.

I repeated the directions but added, "If you follow the directions just right, you get a point. If you don't, I get a point."

"Okay," he said in his husky voice and picked up one penny as I timed him. "I win," he shouted after finishing each test item.

At the end of the test, I shook his hand and said, "Congratulations. You won. You beat me."

A smile spread across his face.

Change the Focus When Giving Test Directions

Another way you may avoid or move out of a power struggle is to alter the focus of your requests. When you give directions for a test, some children may think they sound like a harsh command, even if you used a neutral tone of voice. If children balk, you need to shift to a softer approach. You may do this by requesting help or giving choices. Some children do better if you reassure them that the task will not take long. Others will start to participate if you incorporate counting and make the test into a contest where they can beat you or their own record. Another approach to get out of a struggle is to subtly shift your requests and avoid demanding compliance. Remember to document any related changes and the results.

Fabulous Five: Shift the Focus When Giving Test Directions

- **Ask children to help you.**

The 3 year old ignored my requests as she wandered around the room looking at all the supplies. "Heather, come here. I need your help," I said and waited.

She meandered over and sat next to me.

"Please unbutton this for me," I said as I handed her a button strip.

Her chubby fingers finagled all three buttons until they were loose.

"That's great. Thanks so much."

- **Let children decide which test item to do next if the test allows it.**

"It's making my eyes water," 7-year-old Cecilia complained, but she continued drawing a line within the maze.

"We just have two things left. Which one do you want to do next?"

Cecilia's eyes scanned the test materials. Then she fingered the pegboard and the cards. "The cards."

- **Use counting as encouragement to try a test item.**

"I don't want to do this," 4-year-old Gregg griped.

"Let's see how many you can do. I'll count," I said as if challenging him to a contest. I counted as he stacked the blocks making a tower. "Wow, you did 10."

- **Tell children the test item or task will not take long.**

To get a handwriting sample, I said, "Please write a sentence about what you like to do at home."

"I don't like writing," 8-year-old Jude replied.

"It's very short. You only have to write one sentence. It won't take long."

"That's all?"

"Yes," I said, and he picked up his pencil to write.

- **Make subtle changes to the test directions to avoid a power struggle.**

When I started the motor test, 10-year-old Marty did the opposite of what I asked. "Stand on your right foot," I said.

He stood on his left and smirked.

Then I switched and said, "Stand on one foot."

He automatically stood on his dominant right foot.

Make Adaptations to the Test

> **Children might be thinking:**
> *What's this?*
> *What?*
> *This is hard.*
> *I don't know.*
> *I don't know what to do.*

Many children are unable to complete standardized tests for a multitude of reasons. Some have difficulty understanding the test directions. Some lack the motor control needed to complete items. Others may have limited or no vision. Whatever the reason, you may need to make adaptations to a test to get accurate information on what the children are capable of doing. Because you are changing the administration of the test, it is not valid to use the norms of the particular test. However, you can still collect valuable information by making adjustments. One possible way is to change the test materials, such as making a thicker line to cut so children can see it better. You may provide extra cues to make sure children understand. For instance, using hand over hand assistance, you can take them through the motions and then see if they understand. Doing such adaptations may enable you to separate children's comprehension of the directions from their ability to do the task. For some, you may need to simplify the task into one easy step. Providing adaptive equipment is another option.

Fabulous Five: Make Adaptations to the Test

- **Adapt the test materials.**

I needed to test 7-year-old Brooke, who had limited vision. Before the session, I used a black marker to darken and enlarge the cutting lines. I obtained a slant board and raised-line paper to get a handwriting sample. In addition, I made sure I had black paper to put under the lightly colored test items to create contrast. The day of the test, Brooke lowered her head a few inches from the items and followed all the directions.

- **Simplify the test item to one step or action.**

"A-ee," 3-year-old Mitch babbled as he ran around the room. I guided him to the table and pulled the wooden circle out of the form board containing three different shapes. Next, I tapped the piece against the table to get his attention. When he looked, I said, "Put the circle in," and demonstrated. Then I gave him the wooden piece and gently pushed his elbow so his hand was near the form board. "Put the circle in," I repeated.

He briefly looked at the puzzle but then dropped the piece on the floor.

- **Start the motion and then see if the children can continue the test item.**

I drew a half-inch line across the middle of a piece of paper and gave 8-year-old Eli the scissors.

His hand went limp, and he dropped the scissors.

"I'm going to put my hand on yours," I said. Placing my hand over his, I helped him wrap his fingers around the flex-loop scissors. I squeezed his hand and released, making the first cut on the line. I slightly lifted my fingers, waiting to see if Eli would continue.

After three more trials, Eli began cutting on his own and continued across the paper.

- **Provide extra cues when giving test directions.**

Six-year-old Sabrina shook her head side to side and flicked a puzzle piece against the table. She then flapped the bottom of her right ear as she tapped her feet. I joined her at the table, bringing paper and a marker. Instead of following the test instructions of showing her a picture of a circle and asking her to copy it, I provided extra cues with the directions. First, when she was looking at the paper, I drew a circle. Then, letting her know I was going to touch her, I placed my hand over her hand and helped her trace the circle. Next, I pointed to the space under the shape and said, "Draw a circle."

Sabrina made a complete circle and then scribbled over it.

- **Provide adaptive equipment for an alternative assessment of ability or function.**

When I observed 7-year-old Barbara Ann in class, I saw the hand tremors. The next day, I had her print her name. She made a 3-inch "B" with such faint pressure it was barely visible.

"That's all I can do," she said.

"That's all right," I replied. Thinking that she did not have the motor control needed to do the test, I switched to checking what she could do when provided adaptive equipment. "I noticed that your hand shakes, which makes it hard to write. I brought a few things for you to try. Try writing a 'B' with them and let me know what you think."

"Okay." First, she tried a 1-pound wrist weight and a large pencil grip. Next, she tried a weighted pencil.

"What do you think?" I asked.

"I like these," she said, pointing to the wrist weight and pencil grip.

"Let's try both of these with a slant board."

She printed the "B" with heavier and smoother lines. "Oh, that looks good," I said, and she nodded in agreement.

End Testing and Share Results

When all the test items are completed, put closure on the experience. This entails spending a couple of minutes talking about your time together and ending on a positive note. Later, after scoring test items and compiling the information, share the results with all involved, including the children.

End Testing Session in a Positive Way

> **Children might be thinking:**
> *Oh, we're done.*
> *That was hard.*
> *I'm glad that's done.*
> *That wasn't so hard.*
> *That was fun.*
> *I did better than I thought.*
> *You're caring for spending time to help me learn.*

When testing is completed, end the session on a pleasant note. For some children, it is important to make the last task into a successful one if they have not been doing well. Check what the experience was like for them. Ask them what they liked about it and inquire about any unanswered questions. Mention one thing you learned from the testing and one possible idea that would help them. Also state at least one competency or strength you observed. Then let them know you enjoyed getting to know them better and will get back to them regarding the results.

> ### *Fabulous Five: End Testing Session in a Positive Way*
>
> - **End the test with success.**
>
> There was one task left on the motor test. "Catch the ball," I said, tossing it 5 feet.
>
> "I missed," 4-year-old Jack said with the next three attempts.
>
> I marked his score on the test booklet. Seeing his frown, I said, "This tennis ball is small. I have a bigger one." I pulled out a soft playground ball, moved closer to Jack, and threw it.
>
> He curled his arms around the ball and hugged it tightly. "I did it," he yelled with a smile.
>
> - **Ask children what they liked the best about the testing.**
>
> To observe 5-year-old Eve's equilibrium reactions, I said, "Come try this rocking boat," and helped her onto a balance board. She stood with her legs a foot apart and tried to maintain her balance.
>
> "Hey," she giggled as I tipped the board left and right and she teetered on the edge.

"Stay on the boat. Don't fall in the water and get nipped by the fish," I said, pretending she was in the ocean. Then we moved to the table and started a test booklet. At the end of the session, I asked, "What did you like best?"

"The boat."

- **State at least one thing you noticed that the testing showed and what you can do to help.**

"I noticed that when you hold a pencil, you are using your whole hand to write," I said to 7-year-old Hannah. Then I demonstrated her grip and the difference when writing with just the thumb, index, and middle fingers.

"Yeah, I squeeze the pencil too hard, and when I take my fingers off, it hurts."

"I have some rubber pencil grips you can try to see if you like them. We can also work on your hand muscles to make it easier to write." Hannah nodded in agreement.

- **Ask if they have any questions and elicit their thoughts about the testing.**

"We're done. Do you have any questions?"

"When can I try those pencil grips?" 7-year-old Hannah asked.

"I can stop by your school tomorrow. I have lots of different kinds. You can try them and see if one works best for you. How was it taking this test? Fun or not fun? Interesting, not interesting? Easy, frustrating? I know it is different for all kids. I'm wondering what it was like for you."

"It was fun. I liked doing all the games."

- **State what went well during the testing and let children know you enjoyed being with them.**

At the end of testing, I stood and said to Margo, "We're finished. What I saw was that you did a nice job of trying everything. I noticed that some of those shapes were hard to copy, and you didn't give up. You did awesome. It was so nice to spend time with you and learn more about you. After I score the test, I will get back to you about how you did, and we can talk about what to do next."

Share Test Results With Children and Caregivers

> **Children might be thinking:**
> *I think I did okay.*
> *That test was hard/easy.*
> *I wonder how I did on that test.*
> *Thanks for telling me.*

After scoring the test and reflecting on your observations, it is important to share the results with children and their caregivers. You will want to present information in a way that children can understand what you are saying. One way to do that is to emphasize how testing is an opportunity to learn about themselves and not to find their faults. Being sensitive and tactful will also show your respect.

Normalize Findings From Testing Results

Although it is common to share the test results with caregivers, again, remember to convey this information to children too. Comment on how everyone has strengths and everyone has some difficulties. Let them know that other children have struggled in the same area. Presenting the information in this manner also lets children know that learning about themselves is a lifelong process. This approach contrasts with taking a deficit-focused and fault-finding one. It is very different from saying, "The problem with you is…." which implies blame, weakness, or character flaws. Telling them that they are still learning implies that change is possible. At the same time, address their worries about whether their day-to-day life will get better.

Fabulous Five: Normalize Findings From the Test Results

- **Present test results as being information to learn about themselves.**

"The last time you were with me, you did a test of your motor skills," I said to 7-year-old Valerie. "The test is one way to learn more about yourself—what's easy and what's hard for you. You did really well drawing different shapes and had good coordination when moving your fingers. For example, you were really good at sorting cards, moving pegs, and stringing beads. On the test, the areas that were harder for you were catching a ball and keeping your balance."

Valerie nodded in agreement.

"If you want, we can do different activities to make those easier for you."

She nodded again.

- **Comment on how everyone is good at some things and everyone has a hard time with others as you talk about test results.**

While explaining the test results, I said, "Everyone is good at some things and has a hard time with others."

"I know," 8-year-old Karla said. "I'm a good reader, but when I am writing, I'm kind of slow. I'm a slow poke."

- **Say other children have struggled in that area when explaining test results.**

"This is getting really hard, especially because I don't have good control of my hand," the third grader said as he drew shapes during the test. "I don't write so clear in my notebook. It's better if I go slow, but then it takes longer. And it might not be done when my teacher wants it done."

Later, when talking about the testing, I told him, "I've worked with other children who had a hard time writing neatly and fast enough. Together we were able to figure out ways to help."

- **Talk about how the children are still learning when discussing test results.**

When 6-year-old Nathan tried to print his name, he ended up erasing every letter. "Ugh," he said as rubbed the paper. Three times he tried to print a sentence, but each time he missed one letter, he erased the entire word. Then he was asked to draw a picture of himself. "I can't. I can't draw." With encouragement, he did begin to draw.

In the next session, I said, "I saw how hard it was for you to write and draw and that it was upsetting for you when it was not right. I know you are still learning how to write and draw. If you want, we can work together to figure out ways to make it easier to learn."

- **Address children's possible worry that they cannot get better.**

During testing, 7-year-old Cassie made the following comments: "I'm not a good cutter. I can't concentrate on this maze. I don't know how to draw these shapes. I'm too tired to write a sentence."

Afterward, I thought about the statements she made about herself. When I met with her the next time, I said, "I noticed that test was hard for you. I'm glad you tried everything. And you told me that in class, writing and cutting are harder for you than for your friends. I can help make cutting and writing easier so you can catch up."

Present Testing Information in a Tactful Manner

Explain the test results in a way that shows your utmost respect for children. Start by highlighting their strengths illuminated by the testing. Give details on and emphasize what they did well. Use gentle and kind language that is easy to understand. Children easily comprehend words or phrases such as "harder," "more difficult," or "not easy." Remember, they often worry that someone will call them stupid or dumb. Keep your explanation simple. Be honest about what was learned, and make connections regarding the possible impact on their life.

Fabulous Five: Present Testing Information in a Tactful Manner

- **Give details on what they did well on the test.**

"Your teacher wanted me to check to see how you are doing with drawing, cutting, and holding the marker," I said to 4-year-old Cooper at the beginning of the test. Afterward, I said, "You did really well. You drew a great picture of yourself with lots of details, like your face, body, hair, arms, and legs. You held the marker like big kids do, and you were good at cutting out a circle and square. You cut right on the line. Let's go tell your teacher how you tried everything and did well."

Cooper smiled and grabbed my hand as we walked back to his class.

- **Use gentle language to explain test results.**

After doing a test for motor skills, I told the 9 year old, "You are very good at moving your hands quickly when doing activities. What is harder for you is your eye-hand coordination—using your eyes and hands together—which can make things like writing neatly more difficult."

- **Describe delays or difficulties using words or phrases such as "harder," "more difficult," or "not easy."**

"Riley has hemiparesis on her right side, which makes her right hand weaker," her mother told the special education team. "However, you will see that she tries everything and is very persistent."

After doing a typing test with the 5 year old, I told her, "I know you told me you want to get better at using the computer. You are good at using all your fingers on the keys except for your ring and baby fingers on your right hand. I saw that you had to move your hand off the keyboard to press down with those fingers."

"Yeah, that's hard for me."

"You have some choices. For example, you can learn to type on the school computers with just one hand, you can use a keyboard made for one hand, or you can use a computer program where you talk and it prints what you say."

"I want to be able to type on the same computers my friends use in class."

- **Explain what information was learned from testing.**

"Your parents and teacher filled out a sensory profile, which tells us what you were okay with and what sensations bother you. For instance, do noise, people touching you, or certain clothes or foods bother you? Also, are there times when you get on sensory overload—where there's too much happening around you and you want to go someplace quiet?"

"Yeah, I don't like kids bumping me in line," 6-year-old River said. "And I can't think if there's too much noise."

"Your parents and teachers noticed that too. They said that you are very sensitive and can get distracted by noise or people moving around you. They also notice that you don't like to get things like glue or markers on your hand. And when you do, you go to the sink and wash your hands."

"Yeah, I do that."

"Well, we can all work together to figure out some ideas to help you feel more comfortable. Is that okay?"

"Yeah, that's okay."

- **Relate test results to impact on life.**

"I saw on the test that keeping your balance was really hard for you. I know that makes it difficult to do everything in P.E. that your teachers ask you to do. I know you are trying. It's not that you don't want to do everything in P.E.; it's just that it's hard."

Seven-year-old Justin nodded with a look of relief.

"You and I can work on your balance. Let's go talk to your teacher about the results too."

KEY POINTS TO REMEMBER

- Be like a camera lens: first observe children's social and physical environments and then zoom in using a specific question to guide you.
- Try to blend in and avoid looking at only one child.
- Know the test, be quick in the administration of it, and minimize wait time between items.
- Set up the test environment to promote comfort and concentration.
- Tell children that the purpose of testing is to learn about themselves, not to judge them.
- Make testing a fun experience by being playful and using toys or puppets.
- Be supportive, especially if children are anxious or worried.
- Add movement if children's alertness is fading.
- Try to discover why children are refusing to take the test.
- Find ways to give them some control of the testing.
- Make adaptations to determine what children can do when they are unable to complete formalized testing.
- End the testing on a positive note and share results with the children and caregivers.

REVIEW QUESTIONS

1. Does the following sentence describe an observation or an interpretation?

   "This preschooler is poking at children because he wants their attention and wants to play with them."

2. After completing your observations, check with caregivers and teachers if what you saw was typical. True or false.

3. Name four ways small toys or puppets can be used during testing.

4. Why do children dislike waiting when taking a test?

5. Why is it stressful for children to take tests?

6. Before testing, examine what distractions are in the room, then guide children to sit in the chair with the fewest distractions in their view. True or false.

7. It helps to emphasize accuracy over effort. True or false.

8. You asked 4-year-old Sam to cut on the thick black line of a circle. He responded by cutting the circle in half. What can you do to check if he understood the verbal directions?

9. What can you do if children are not sitting still during testing?

10. Seven-year-old Miles comes to your room but shakes his head when you asked him to try the first test item. Name at least four questions to ask yourself about why he might be refusing.

8

Collaborate to Determine the Purpose of Therapy

CHAPTER OVERVIEW

To make a meaningful difference in children's lives, you need to discover their and their caregivers' visions of a good life. This chapter explores ways to elicit their desired changes, share your expertise, and reach an agreement regarding the purpose of therapy. Also discussed is strengths-based treatment planning, which differs from a problem-solving approach.

CHILDREN'S DESCRIPTIONS OF WHAT THEY THINK YOU SHOULD KNOW

Dr. Clare: "Why is important for children to help determine the purpose for our time together?"

Kris (age 11): "So the child understands more. It makes it more fun because then the child would be more involved and he would like to come back again instead of getting out of it."

Caleb (age 9): "It's important so the kids don't feel left out."

Kent (age 11): "I think if they know what the kid is thinking, it makes the kid feel more stable and safer."

Dr. Clare: "What should therapists know or do when they work with children who cannot talk or need a lot of extra help?"

Blanca (age 11): "Be kind. Be nice because they're like us. They hear everything. They're like us but they don't know how to talk."

Suzanne (age 10): "They should learn sign language."

Rachel (age 11): "If they work with someone who can't talk, they have to be very understanding and they have to give them respect and lots of attention."

Tina (age 11): "They should say words slow, not too fast."

Sara (age 10): "Don't be mean because a lot of them have fear over things."

TRAVEL DOWN THE SAME ROAD

Deciding on the purpose of therapy and planning what to do is like taking a road trip. Together with the children, caregivers, and teachers, you will create a plan for moving forward away from their current day-to-day lives. When going on a vacation, everyone has to agree on the purpose of the trip. For example, are they seeking relaxation, physical challenges, or educational opportunities? Their decision would determine if they go to a beach, climb a mountain, or visit a historical site. Similarly, you, the children, caregivers, and teachers have to determine *why* you will spend time together and what your destination is. Together you will decide what you want to accomplish and how as you start the journey headed in the agreed direction. And, like any trip, be open to bumps in the road or unexpected detours.

- 141 -

Curtin, C.
Strategies for Collaborating With Children: Creating Partnerships in Occupational Therapy and Research (pp. 141-165).
© 2017 SLACK Incorporated.

STRENGTHS-BASED TREATMENT PLANNING

Traditionally, treatment planning has often been presented in the following sequence: (1) identify problem areas, (2) create goals to alleviate problems, and (3) develop treatment activities as a way to achieve the goals. Therapists were encouraged to develop rapport, engage clients, and collaborate.

To move to a strengths-based approach, Fanger (1993, p. 86) suggested that instead of focusing on, "What is wrong and why?" you focus on, "What is wanted and how?" The word *problems* tends to have a negative connotation, which implies fixing children and often leads to blame. In a strengths-based process, the emphasis is on identifying strengths, strategies, dreams, desires, and concerns. The impact of the environment is also considered. Instead of trying to fix problems, children are encouraged to build on their current strengths, create personal challenges, and explore new possibilities and solutions. This positive focus promotes a desire to learn and develops a sense of competence and mastery.

With this approach, treatment planning involves a partnership. The process entails the co-development of a plan by (a) learning about each other; (b) eliciting strengths, desires, and concerns; (c) clarifying what is their vision of a good life; and (d) discussing, negotiating, and summarizing the purpose for being together and the plan.

The first stage of treatment planning is to learn about each other. Children and caregivers need to learn about you and what participation in occupational therapy involves. You would establish a collaborative frame, described in Chapter 5. Applying an ecological perspective, you would seek information about the children and their different environments. It would be necessary to learn about their culture, their town and neighborhood, their home and school setting, as well as their families and educational staff. You could then discover what resources and available occupations exist; what limitations are present (e.g., poverty); social, emotional, or physical barriers; and the perspectives and expectations of the influential and important people in the children's lives.

At the same time, children's, caregivers', and teachers' strengths, desires, and concerns would be elicited. Much of this information would be learned through observations, interviews, reports, and testing. Another vital part of the process is clarifying what they consider as a good life. You guide the process to assist them in defining what kind of life they desire. Caregivers and teachers will talk about what they wish for the children as well as themselves. With guidance, children can tell you how they would like their life to change so that it is a good life. Commonly, children will tell you their desire to have friends, be successful in school, get along with their family, participate in sports, and be able to do self-care tasks independently. Through thoughtful questioning, help them identify what is their vision of a good life with meaningful occupations.

Treatment planning also requires discussion and negotiation. Together, you would pinpoint resources, environmental supports and the hindrances that need to change. Together, you would build on current strengths and strategies, identify personal challenges, and explore future possibilities and solutions. Lastly, you would summarize the plan, by emphasizing children's strengths, and restating: (a) children's, caregivers', and teachers' desired changes; (b) the required environmental modifications; (c) the agreed-upon goals; and (d) the methods for creating the change.

Although the process may appear time intensive, it can be simplified—often into a few questions and responses. In this chapter, there are multiple ways and wording you can use to discover what children, their caregivers, and teachers want to change. You may rely on just a few key questions and methods. For children who are nonverbal, you can still include them by discovering what is important to them. You might find that children are more concerned about changing their present experience then thinking about the future. Keep in mind that by starting with the children's goals of change, their present experience will also affect their future.

Another consideration is where children are in their desire to change. Some have never been asked or never thought about different possibilities. They may be unaware of the impact of their actions or not realize that change is possible. Others may not be interested, especially if they think a discussion is going to emphasize their failures and make them look bad. Some children want their lives to be different but are not sure what to do. Others may have tried but found that they need more support and resources.

Find What Is Meaningful to Children Who Are Young or Unable to Communicate

> **Children might be thinking:**
> *I want to do that.*
> *I like doing....*
> *I want to do it by myself.*

If children are young or cannot use a communication system, give them a voice by finding out what is meaningful to them. Use a powerful first step in collaboration by watching closely for their interests and find out what is important to them (Figure 8-1). Gaining more information from caregivers and educational staff also will help.

Next, tell children, often in one sentence, what you will be helping them do. It is best to state a goal at the same time they are doing the activity. You will find that the following are some common desires:

- Do more of what they like
- Be like their friends
- Play with their friends
- Make things easier for them
- Do things by themselves

As you write goals that focus on increasing participation in occupations, be thoughtful and try to include a goal that is meaningful to the children too.

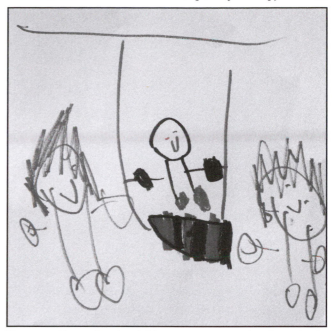

Figure 8-1. Observe for what children enjoy or want to do independently.

Fabulous Five: Observe Children Who Are Young or Nonverbal to Identify What Is Important to Them

- **State the goal as being able to increase participation in a favorite activity.**

In the specialized class, I watched 5-year-old AJ every day repeatedly snipping strips of paper into small scraps. A few days later, I said, "I see that you like to cut. You're really good at opening and closing the scissors. I have some really fun pictures and can help you cut different shapes."

He looked up and allowed me to help him cut out three long strips of a car puzzle.

After he aligned and glued the strips in the right order to make a picture of a car, he happily put it in his cubby to take home.

- **Make the goal to be able to do things by themselves.**

"I do," 6-year-old Kerry said any time an adult tried to give assistance.

"You want to do it yourself," I said. "I'm going to help you do lots of things by yourself." The next day I brought a strip of picture symbols showing how to wash hands. I taped it to the wall and pointed to each picture as she followed the steps. "Turn the knob," I said and made a twisting motion.

"Now add soap. Push.

"Rub your hands.

"More water."

She rinsed.

"Turn the knob off."

Kerry stopped the water.

"All clean. All better. You did it all by yourself!"

She smiled in return. Throughout the school year, we continued working on becoming independent in self-care tasks.

- **State the goal as making it easier in one area in which the children struggle.**

"Toni had a stroke when she was a baby," the preschool teacher told me. "She's weak on her left side."

As I watched her at the table with her classmates, she tried but struggled to color and cut a paper butterfly. She pulled her hand away when the teacher offered help. The butterfly ended up in pieces.

"I see that you want to color and cut all by yourself," I said to her. "I'm going to help make coloring and cutting pictures easier for you." The next time I came, I brought a slant board, thicker crayons, and adaptive scissors. As she relaxed, she let me give her a little help. Her motor control improved as the year progressed.

- **Describe the goal as being able to do what friends are doing.**

Four-year-old Jessa waddled over to the steps of the slide, looked at the children on top, and grunted.

"I see you want to go up on the slide and be with your friends," I said. "I will keep helping you until you can do it by yourself." I guided her hand to the rail and held her other hand. Slowly she stepped up the ladder to the top and squealed as she slid down the slide. To facilitate her new progress, I brought a balance board into her classroom and used it during different activities to improve her balance.

- **State a goal regarding playing with friends.**

Whenever 3-year-old Karen saw a group of children, she walked over to join them. She would then grab toys out of their hands and hit them if they tried to retrieve them. Sometimes the children would hit her back. As she headed for a group, I walked over to her and said, "I see you want to play with your friends and have a turn playing with the toys. Let me help you get a turn and play nicely with friends."

She approached the group and I told her, "Say 'please' and point to what you want."

She used sign language for "please" by making a circle on her chest and pointed to a red bear.

Johnny handed it to her, and she grinned. We continued practicing as the year went on.

Decide on the Format of Collaboration Based on Children's Level of Comfort and Understanding

Children might be thinking:
I like doing something while we talk.
I like to fiddle with something in my hands while we talk.

One of your responsibilities as a therapist is to guide the collaboration process. When you first meet children, you have to look for cues regarding their comfort level. Before starting the conversation about defining the purpose of therapy, determine your approach based on those cues. For instance, if children appear shy or timid, you could start by involving them in an activity. This allows them more time to get to know you and to decide whether they want to talk.

As we know, one approach does not fit all. Tailor what you do based on the children's desired level of interaction. Conversations during an activity tend to be more casual and there is less pressure to converse. Some children have a better understanding of what therapy entails after a few sessions. When they feel more comfortable they may tell you what they want help with changing. Other children enjoy adult attention and like participating in an interview.

Fabulous Five: Determine the Format of Collaborative Goal Setting

- **Do an activity and casually talk.**

As 6-year-old Krista colored a picture, she talked about her family pet. "I have a baby dog. She's a little girl. She's starting to bark."

A few minutes later, I asked, "How is school going?"

"I've made some new friends. I want to get better at soccer and the monkey bars so I can play with my friends."

- **Provide experiences in therapy and then talk when children feel comfortable.**

On 7-year-old Maurice's first day in the occupational therapy sensory integration clinic, he responded to my questions by nodding or shaking his head. Sensing his

discomfort, I said, "This is a place where you can play and do activities that will make it easier for you to move and help you get stronger."

At the end of the second session, I asked him, "What is your favorite thing to do here?"

"Fishing," he replied, referring to catching fish while on a platform swing.

"At home or at school, what are you good at?"
"Math."
"At home or at school, what do you wish was easier?"
"Gym."
"Doing what?"
"I want to get better at running in a race. I want to go faster."

- **Conduct an interview, involve in an activity, and then talk about goals.**

"What is easy for you?" I asked the fourth grader.

"Math, making new friends, helping my friends, and writing."

"What do you need to work on?"

"Reading and listening. I daydream a lot. It's hard for me to pay attention."

"When does this happen?"

"At home and school. Sometimes when my mom is talking, I daydream. But it's easy for me to pay attention to TV and computer games."

As Clark played with building materials, he was in constant motion. Within 5 minutes, he went from kneeling on his chair to shifting side to side to standing. He also alternated between clicking his tongue repeatedly and putting one hand in his mouth.

Afterward, we talked. "I noticed that while you were building, you needed to move a lot. Does that happen in class too?"

"Yeah."

"So you told me you are good at math and writing and you are a good friend. That's great! Those are nice strengths. You said you want to get better at reading and listening. Is there anything else?"

"My teacher yells at me to stop making noises. I need to stay in my seat."

We talked about how some children need extra sensations such as movement. I added, "If it's okay with you, together we can figure out some sensory strategies. You can use them in class and not get in trouble." He agreed.

- **Do an interview and then use alternative methods to elicit goals.**

"What's the best part of school?" I asked 5-year-old Elsie.

"The best part of kindergarten is choice time, swinging on the swings, getting to be a helper, coloring, writing, and making books."

I waved a toy magic wand and said, "In school, I wish…." Then I handed it to her.

"In school I wish I could color even better than before."

- **Sit and talk with children about their lives and desired goals.**

After doing an interview with 8-year-old Joel, I asked, "What would you like to get better at?"

"I want to write better so I can make books. I want to type better, clean my desk, and make one new friend."

Elicit Children's Perspectives on Their Occupational Functioning

To make therapy meaningful, it is vital to obtain children's perspectives about their lives and dreams for the future. Put them at ease and show in your demeanor that you are open to hearing whatever they have to say. Ask questions about their functioning, what they value, and what they desire. In addition to doing interviews, you can make the process fun by using games, props, or prompts. Help them feel as comfortable to talk as they do when they are in their homes airing their concerns while they play.

In this section, there are multiple questions and methods you can use to learn about children's lives and what they want for the future. Choose the ones that best match the children's level of understanding and your setting. When there are time constraints, prioritize and ask a question about their strengths, interests, what is easy and hard for them, what they want to get better at, or what they wish would be easier. Not every child will be able to answer every question, but they will appreciate that you asked. You also can ask more questions during activities in future sessions.

Identify Children's Strengths

> **Children might be thinking:**
> *I'm good at….*
> *I like talking about what I can do.*
> *Thank you for saying those nice things.*

Ask Children to Identify Their Strengths, Personal Qualities, and Competencies

When defining the purpose of therapy, it is important to include children's strengths. You can do this by observing them, asking their caregivers and teachers, and directly asking them. It is imperative to let children know that you see their competencies and will not just focus on their difficulties. Having a balanced perspective also gives the message that you believe in their ability to grow and do not believe they are the problem and need to be fixed. By not blaming them, this approach allows for discussing other factors that might be contributing to their concerns, such as a lack of support by adults. Help children create change in their lives by identifying and building on their competencies. It will be easier for them to use their strengths and strategies that are already in their repertoires.

> ### *Fabulous Five: Pinpoint Children's Strengths*
>
> - **Ask, "What are your strengths?"**
>
>   "What are your strengths?"
>
>   "I'm a good friend," 12-year-old Jessica replied.
>
>   "In what way?"
>
>   "Everyone comes to me for advice. My one friend calls himself a loser. I told him, 'You need to stop thinking bad about yourself. You're not that. You're better than that.' I think everyone likes me. I compliment them. If I don't like someone, I try not to show it."
>
> - **Ask, "What are your good points?"**
>
>   "What are your good points?"
>
>   "That I walk away from fights," 10-year-old Jason replied. "When people bully my friends, I tell them not to."
>
> - **Ask, "What do you like best about yourself?"**
>
>   "What do you like best about yourself?" I asked 8-year-old Carson.
>
>   "I can build almost anything."
>
> - **Say, "Tell me something good about you."**
>
>   "Tell me something good about yourself."
>
>   "I'm nice," 7-year-old Sydney replied.
>
>   "How are you nice?"
>
>   "I don't yell at my friends. I don't scream at them. I don't hit them."
>
> - **Ask, "What do you like about yourself?"**
>
>   "What do you like about yourself?"
>
>   "I'm a good friend. Yesterday, I saw my friend crying," 11-year-old Catherine said. "So I went up to her and said, 'What's wrong?' but she didn't answer. At first, she didn't want to talk about it. Then she said, 'It's been a bad day. I can't tell you everything but now I forgot my track stuff and my mom will be mad.' I asked her, 'Do you need a shoulder to cry on?' She said yes and hugged me."

Discover What Children Think They Can Do Well or Find Easy

A second way to learn about children's assets is to ask them direct and open-ended questions about what they do well or find easy. This may be done in the midst of an activity or during an interview. You will find that children often smile as they describe their competencies and look pleased that you want this information. For some, this type of conversation is a new experience. I have had children tell me that they have never thought about what they could do well. With older children, you also might ask them to reflect on what others say is good about them.

Fabulous Five: Ask Questions to Elicit Strengths

- **Inquire, "What are you good at, or what do you do well?"**

"What are you good at, or what do you do well?" I asked the second grader.

"I work hard. I read hard and write hard. I draw hard. I help hard. I hide good at hide and seek. I play good with my cat and dog. I play good with my little brother. I throw hard. Hmm. I have some more."

"Go on."

"I make stuff. I kick hard when I kick balls."

- **Ask, "What is easy for you?"**

"What's easy for you to do?" I asked the 8 year old.

"Jump rope."

"What do you like about yourself?"

"I'm good at writing. I have a really good singing voice. I can play piano, violin, and guitar."

"Wow, you have many talents."

- **Ask, "What are you most proud of doing, or what do you feel really good about doing?"**

I asked 5-year-old Cassidy, "What are you most proud of doing?"

"Being brave at the dentist."

- **Tell children, "All children are good at something. What can you do well?"**

"All children are good at something," I said to 10-year-old Kendall. "What can you do well?"

"Sports."

"Like what?"

"Soccer, football, basketball, softball, and pretty much that's it."

- **Ask, "What might other people, like your teacher or your parents, say is good about you?"**

"What might other people, like your teacher or parents, say is good about you?"

Nine-year-old Ian replied, "My teacher would say that it takes me a long time to figure something out, but it will be right."

Ask Detailed Questions About Competencies

A third approach to glean information about strengths is to inquire about specific instances or accomplishments. Your questions about trophies or metals often elicit stories

about successes and proud moments. Some children do better if you add a time frame to the questions such as asking them to reflect on what they did that week. For others, you may obtain more information by suggesting that they tell you a certain number of strengths. Another avenue to bring out children's assets is to have them tell you details about a time they did something good or were nice to one another. Asking about their happiest day also may provide description about their competencies as well as their values and interests.

Fabulous Five: Request Specific Examples of Strengths or Accomplishments

- **Inquire, "Have you ever gotten a medal or trophy, and if so, for what?"**

"Have you ever gotten a medal or trophy?"

"Yes."

"For what?"

"I won lots of events at my swimming meets. I have 10 medals hanging on my bedroom wall."

- **Say, "Tell me five things about you that are good."**

"Tell me five things about you that are good."

"I'm totally good at jumping rope. I can jump a long time. I'm a good thinker. I'm good at drawing and, um, the monkey bars. And I'm good at reading."

- **Ask, "What is something good you have done this week?"**

"What is something good you have done this week?"

"I helped a friend who got hurt. He fell and hit his head. He was crying. I went with him to the clinic."

- **Say, "Tell me about a time you did something nice."**

"Tell me about a time you did something nice."

"My friend Lily wanted me to tie her shoes and I did it."

- **Say, "Tell me about the best or happiest day of your life."**

"Tell me about the happiest day in your life. You can draw it if you want."

"That'll be easy. There's the basketball. Here's me. I got the ball. The crowd was here. I slammed it on the floor and then I shoot it in the hoop and we won. My coach was very happy with me."

Obtain Children's Perspectives on Their Functioning

Children might be thinking:
I like talking.
Thanks for asking about my life.

It is important to ask children about their daily lives. Doing so gives you the opportunity to get to know them better. Obtaining children's perspectives is important because they may be different from those of their caregivers. Have children tell you about their daily schedule, interests, and values. Also, inquire about their family, friends, and school. This allows you to gain information regarding their participation in occupations and how satisfied they are. Learning about children's lives will help you understand their priorities for change.

Ask About Daily Schedule and Values

To get a more inclusive picture of children's worlds, ask questions about their daily activities and values. Have children describe their daily schedule on a weekday and weekends. Inquire about whether they participate in any groups, organizations, and/or sports. Also, explore if they volunteer, have a job, and/or do chores at home. Listen for examples of the following: What do they think about their involvement? Which activities do they find the most meaningful? How often do they participate? Are they doing too much or too little? What do they enjoy the most?

It is also important to discover what children value. To help children reveal this information, ask them what they want to be when they grow up. They are usually delighted to tell you about their dreams. Also, ask if there is anyone they admire and want to be like. Explore what they emulate about the person. For some children, you can also ask what is something they value—something that is really, really important to them.

Fabulous Five: Inquire About Daily Schedule and Values

- **Ask about a typical weekday and weekend.**

"Tell me about a school day," I said to 12-year-old Lilly.

"I get up at 7 and lie in my bed for about 10 minutes. Then I get dressed, go downstairs, and talk to my brother, and do nothing. I get my backpack, my ID, and go to the car."

"Do you eat breakfast?"

"It depends. When my first hour is gym, no. But my reading class lets us eat."

"After you get home what do you do?"

"I walk home. I take the dogs to the bathroom. I get something to eat, change into something more comfortable, and go on the computer."

"Then what?"

"I wait for my mom to come home. Tuesday, Wednesday, and Friday, I have swim practice. On Monday and Wednesday, my dad takes us sometimes. After swim practice, I do my homework. At 8 o'clock, I eat dinner, and between 9 and 10, I go to bed."

"What do you do on a weekend?"

"On Saturdays, my brother has football and I have swim meets. On Sunday, I go to church and catechism, do

---

my homework, and go to Dad's around 5 o'clock. After we eat there, we all spread out. My stepmother goes on the computer. Dad watches a movie with us. Sometimes my brother plays on his computer, and so do I. At 9 o'clock, I go to bed. Then he takes us to school on Monday."

- **Inquire if children are in any groups, organizations, and/or sports.**

I asked 9-year-old Carey, "Are you in any groups, organizations, or sports?"

"I'm in Girl Scouts."

"What's your favorite thing about Girl Scouts?"

"We get to ride ponies. We rode horses without holding on, and we get new uniforms every 3 years."

- **Ask if children are involved in any volunteer work, jobs, and/or chores.**

"Do you do any volunteer work, jobs, and/or chores?"

"I have to fix my bed and clean my room," the 8 year old replied.

- **Ask what children want to be when they grow up.**

"What do you want to be when you grow up?" I asked 4-year-old Body.

"A monster truck driver."

"I want to be a horse rider," his twin sister added. "I'm going to ride horses!"

- **Inquire, "Is there anyone you look up to or admire? Anyone you would like to be like?"**

"Is there anyone you look up to and admire?"

The 9 year old nodded.

"Who and why?"

"My dad. I've always wanted to do things like him."

Inquire About Children's Favorite Occupations

A major tenet of occupational therapy is that it is crucial to have meaningful occupations in one's life. Therefore, to discover some of the children's valued occupations you need to ask them what they enjoy doing. You want to find out what they like to do by themselves for fun, as well as what they like to do with their families and friends. Discovering their favorite interests will help you get to know them as individuals and provides useful information when planning treatment.

Fabulous Five: Discover Favorite Occupations

- **Ask, "What do you like to do?"**

"What do you like to do at home?" I asked the 4 year old.

"I like to play with my toy cake. It is so big. It has candles. You have to put candles on it. I like the letter game, and when I get bored with that, I make necklaces. And when I'm bored with that, then I play with my stuffed animals. My fairy cat is pink. It wears a fairy dress."

- **Ask, "What is your favorite thing to do?"**

"What is your favorite thing to do?" I asked the 10 year old.

Five-year-old Devin replied, "I like to paint with lots of different colors."

- **Ask, "What is your favorite thing to do with your family?"**

I asked the 11 year old, "What is your favorite thing to do with your family?"

"I like to watch baseball games, ride horses with my mom, talk baseball with my dad and brother, and play with my dog."

- **Inquire, "What is your favorite thing to do with friends?"**

"What is your favorite thing to do with friends?" I asked the 10 year old.

"I like to ride my skates. I gave skates to my best friend. We always skate together and ride bikes. We play taxi where I ride my skates and he rides his bike, and I put my hands on his bike seat."

- **Have children draw or write about their dream day.**

Twelve-year-old Katherine titled her page *My Dream Day*. She then wrote:

When I woke up and my eyes adjusted to the clock, I saw it was 8:59. I walked down the stairs and into my kitchen. I saw the most awesome breakfast ever, PANCAKES. I added some chocolate chips to my pancakes and dug in. After that, I got dressed and went to Mrs. Hannah's. When I got there, I got on her horse Hope until lunch. After we got home, I went out and got Chinese food. For dessert after lunch, I went on the grass. I watched the clouds drift by very slowly. Then after the remainder of my Chinese food was eaten for dinner, I went out for ice cream. This is and always will be the best dream day ever.

Gain Information About Children's Families

To gain a thorough understanding of children's lives, it is important to learn about their family. First of all, ask them who is in their family. For some, their family may consist of people who are not blood relatives. Their description of family members also reflects their culture. Then ask children who lives with them since every living situation varies.

Inquire about the activities they do together and what they do and do not like about their family. Some children may think they are being disloyal if they say anything negative. Reassure them that they do not have to answer that question if they do not want to. As the children talk, listen for indications regarding their standard of living. Are they homeless? Do they live in poverty? Does their family live paycheck to paycheck? Do they go to day care? Do they have a nanny? Also, listen for the type and the amount of support the family provides. Hearing about their family gives you an opportunity to learn more about their culture.

Fabulous Five: Elicit Information About Children's Families

- **Inquire, "Who is in your family?"**

I asked the 8 year old, "Who is in your family?"

"My mom, Robert—my mom's boyfriend. He's my dad. Two brothers and one sister. Sometimes my grandma visits and stays. I always tell my mom and dad to buy new shoes. He doesn't have a lot of money so I don't get the shoes."

- **Ask, "Who lives with you?"**

"Who lives with you?"

"My mom and dad got divorced," the second grader responded. "My dad lives in Minnesota. I have one sister here and one sister in Minnesota. I don't really know a lot about my brother. My horse lives in Minnesota."

- **Inquire, "What activities do you do with your family?"**

"What activities do you do with your family?"

"I play hide-and-seek with my brother and sister," the 7 year old said. "I go grocery shopping. We go every day and get food. I eat with them."

- **Ask, "What do you like about your family?"**

"What do you like about your family?"

"They don't fight. They don't yell at each other," the 5 year old replied. "My dad builds cars that are made out of metal. My dad likes playing with me too. He's my friend too. My sister has two dads."

- **Inquire, "What don't you like about your family?"**

I asked 8-year-old Emily, "What don't you like about your family?"

"Sometimes they are cranky. I'm serious."

"I believe you."

Ask About Friendships

Friendships are an important part of children's lives. Without friends, children may feel lonely or isolated especially at school. Ask children if they have many friends. If they say yes, inquire if they have a best friend and what is that person's name. Check if they think they are a good friend to others. Listen for signs whether they know how to be a friend.

Discover what activities they like to do with friends and whether they are able to participate. Explore how well they get along. As they talk, listen for the following: Do they have fun together? Are their friends supportive and there for them? Do they find themselves in frequent tiffs with them? Learning how to make and keep friends is a major life lesson.

Fabulous Five: Inquire About Friendships

- Ask, "Do you have many friends?"

"Do you have many friends?" I asked 7-year-old Becca. "I don't have no friends."

- Ask, "What do you like to do with your friends?"

The occupational therapy student asked the 9 year old, "What do you like to do with your friends?"

"I like to play sports with them. I like to do basketball and football. One more thing—I like to do back flips on the trampoline."

- Ask, "Do you consider yourself a good friend? In what way?"

I asked 11-year-old Joseph, "Do you consider yourself a good friend?"

"Yes."

"In what way?"

"I try to help them out with their assignments."

- Inquire, "Do you have a best friend? What is your friend's name?"

"Do you have a best friend?"

"Yes," 6-year-old Jacey replied.

"What is her name?"

"Gabby. I went to her birthday party. They had a little tree house with a ladder. We barefooted. She had a little swing set and also she has a thing to stand on. Her brother likes football. They're twins."

- Ask, "How do you get along with your friends?"

"How do you get along with your friends?"

"Very well," 12-year-old Lucy replied.

"In what ways do you get along?"

"We talk a lot. We're friendly to each other. We don't get in fights very often."

Inquire About School Functioning

Children's ability to function in school affects their quality of life. If they are constantly struggling, it can be an unpleasant and distasteful experience. If they are doing well, it can be enjoyable. To discover how children perceive their school experience, ask them what they like and dislike about it. You also can ask them what they feel is easy and what is hard when they are there. These questions tend to elicit what children consider as their strengths and their challenges in that setting.

Discover their perspectives on their teachers. Ask if they have a favorite teacher and if so what they like about that person. Listen for the following: Do they feel their teachers are helpful and supportive? Can they talk to them if they do not understand the lesson or there's a problem? Do they think the teachers are fair?

Fabulous Five: Ask About the School Experience

- Inquire, "What do you like about school?" and "What don't you like about school?"

"What do you like about school?"

"I have friends," the 8 year old replied. "I like to write at school. I like to learn new things a lot."

"What don't you like about school?"

"The homework."

- Ask, "What do you think about your teachers?"

I asked the second grader, "What do you think about your teacher?"

"She's nice and understanding. She always gives us chance. She lets us do things and play games a lot."

- Ask, "Do you have a favorite teacher?"

"Do you have a favorite teacher?"

Six-year-old Nancy nodded and replied, "Mrs. R."

"What do you like about her?"

"She's nice and funny. We get to paint. In art class, she showed us how to make clouds. Every Friday we get a Friday treat, like popcorn, cookies, or some pretzels."

- Inquire, "What is easy about school?" and "What is hard about school?"

"What is easy about school?" I asked 9-year-old Jake.

"Art."

"What is hard about school?"

"Homework."

"What's hard about it?"

"I don't know."

"Is it hard to do or does it take too long?"

"It's hard to do."

- Ask, "What is good about school?" and "What is not so good about school?"

What is good about school?" I asked 8-year-old Ella.

"School is fun. I like music, art, and lunch. I like playing with my friends."

"What is not so good about school?"

"Writing and homework."

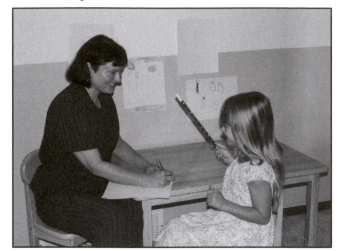

Figure 8-2. Give children the prompt, "In school, I wish…" and ask them to make wishes.

Elicit Children's Dreams, Desires, and Concerns

> **Children might be thinking:**
> *Why are we going to spend time together?*
> *I'm glad you are talking to me about what I want.*
> *I get a chance to talk.*
> *I like making wishes.*
> *That was fun.*

It is crucial for you to find out in which areas children want to continue to grow. What children consider important to change may be different from what caregivers and you think. Some children have never been asked thought-provoking questions about what they want for their future. Others have never been asked in a way that is comfortable and easy to understand and respond to. Like adults, you can directly ask children about their dreams, desires, and concerns. Younger children can tell you more with the use of pictures, games, or visuals. Be creative and make the process fun.

Explore Children's Dreams and Wishes for the Future

Some young children may not understand the notion of goals. However, children do understand wishes, dreams, and wanting to do things by themselves. To find out in what areas they want to grow, learn, or change, you can ask them to make wishes. A fun way to elicit this information is to hand them a toy magic wand and encourage them to wave and wish (Figure 8-2). Using this prop is enticing, playful, and freeing. Another method to gain information is to ask them what they want to learn or what they would like to do more often. Discovering their desired occupations and dreams for the future will give you a better awareness of what they would like their life to be.

Fabulous Five: Elicit Dreams

- **Ask, "If you could have three wishes and you could wish for anything, what would you want?"**

"If you could have three wishes and you could wish for anything, what would you want?"

"To be a rapper star," 7-year-old Sean said. "To be better at school. I want to do neat printing and to walk on the balance beam in P.E."

- **Provide a toy magic wand and ask children to make wishes.**

"Draw yourself," I said to 6-year-old Jake, who had left-side weakness.

He held the pencil loosely, drew four body parts, and then said, "I can't do this. I can't draw."

"Just try your best," I replied in a gentle tone of voice. He added hair and stopped. Then I placed scissors and a circle on the table. Jake took one look and swiveled in his chair so his back was to me. "I think you're telling me you don't want to do this now. We can do it another time. I have something fun I want to show you." Jake peeked over his shoulder.

I pulled out a toy magic wand and made a figure-8 with it. "You get to make pretend wishes." I gave as a prompt, "In school, I wish…."

He grinned, waved the wand, and made the following wishes: "In school I wish I can learn to play games and work at school. I wish that I can learn how to write and learn how to play Go Fish. I wish I can learn to do the monkey bars and do stuff like my uncles. They play lots of games. I wish I could learn how to write my name. I wish I could learn how to play with my friends and cousins."

- **Ask, "What would you like to learn?"**

"What would you like to learn?" I asked the 10 year old, who found new motor movements challenging.

"I really want to accomplish the hand bells in music. I also really want to learn how to do lacrosse and archery."

- **Have children use a toy crystal ball to tell you what they wished was easier.**

"Rub this wishing ball and tell me what you wish was easier in school," I said to 7-year-old Chad.

He curled his fingers around the gel ball and said, "I wish they don't have no more homework. I wish for one million dollars. I would buy a race car. I wish we could have summer forever and no school. I wish working on the computer was more easier. I wish I could have one of these. I wish you would give me all your toys."

I chuckled and said, "I wish I could give you all my toys too, but I need them to work with other children. What we can do is work on making using the computer easier for you."

- **Ask, "What would you like to do more often?"**

I asked 12-year-old Cindy, "What would you like to do more often?"

"At home, something important to me that I want to do more is riding my bike or rollerskating. I'd like to do something outside while the weather is nice. It's good to get fresh air and exercise. At school, I would like more recess time. We're stuck in the classroom for hours. We need more time to let out our energy. I need to move more."

Having heard from her teacher that she often looked distracted, I said, "So should we work on figuring out some ways you can move in class that will help you get your work done?"

"That would be good."

Ask Questions About Children's Concerns and Desired Changes

Another collaborative way to determine the purpose of therapy is to ask children questions about their concerns and desires. Carefully consider the wording of your questions. The wrong wording might imply to the children that you think they are bad or stupid, or that they need to admit something is wrong with them. Instead, phrase your questions in a way that promotes growth and recognizes their competencies. You can ask what they want to get better at, which implies they already have competencies in that area. Another way is to ask an open-ended question regarding what they want to change in themselves. This allows them to talk to you about issues that are important to them.

Fabulous Five: Talk to Children About Their Desired Changes

- **Ask, "What do you wish was different at school/home?"**

"What do you wish was different at school?" I asked the first grader.

"I wish people would play with me."

- **Inquire, "What do you wish was easier at school/home?"**

The occupational therapy student asked, "What do you wish was easier at school?"

"I wish writing was easier," 7-year-old Shania replied. "I wish my printing would get better, faster, and smaller."

- **Ask, "What is good about school? What is not so good about school? Is that something you want to change?"**

"What is good about school?" I asked.

"That I get to play at recess. I also like gym," 8-year-old Bud replied.

"What's not so good about school?"

"I get in trouble a lot. I don't listen to my teacher. Sometimes I act like a crazy monkey. And I don't get my homework done."

"Are those things you want to change?"

"Yeah."

Having seen him react to loud noises and unexpected touches in his class, I said, "Would it be okay if we talked about ways to help stay calm, keep out of trouble, and make your homework easier?"

He nodded.

- **Ask, "What do you want to get better at?"**

I asked the 8 year old, "What do you want to get better at?"

"Art."

"What in art do you want to get better at?"

"Making pictures. Painting pictures like a real artist. There's one more thing. I wish I could be a real artist."

- **Ask children what they want to change about themselves.**

"What do you want to change about yourself?" I asked.

"My attitude," 10-year-old Iris replied. "I want to get along with people more."

"What do you want to get better at?"

"People tease me and say I'm a fat pig. Sometimes it makes me think I don't like myself and don't care about myself."

"So you want to discover what you do like about yourself? And maybe find more ways to get along with others, including how to deal with those acting like bullies?"

"That'd be good."

Have Children Draw or Respond to Prompts Regarding Interests, Desires, and Concerns

Being given a prompt makes it easier for children to know what information you want. A prompt is clear and direct and assists in getting right to the point. For many, it also is easier to finish an incomplete sentence, such as, "In school, I wish…." A prompt is also quick for gaining essential information in a short amount of time.

- **Ask children to draw responding to the prompts: "What are your strengths? What do you want to change about yourself?"**

"Draw about a strength of yours," I said as I read the words on the paper.

Eleven-year-old Kiera drew herself and said, "I am good at arguing. My grandpa says I should be a lawyer."

She turned the paper over and looked at the prompt: What do you want to change about yourself?

Then she wrote: *To not be mean to my friends.*

- **Ask children to draw a picture to the prompt: "I want to learn to do...."**

"Draw a picture of something you would like to learn to do," I said to 9-year-old Vince.

"I have to practice shooting balls," he said, "because I don't know how to do that good." He drew himself throwing a ball into a basketball hoop. "I want to be able to play with my friends."

- **Have the children draw a picture of doing what they want to get better at.**

"Tell me something you want to get better at," I said as I gave Dane a paper with the words *I want to get better at...* at the top. "You can draw a picture if you want."

He began to draw himself. "I look like I'm 6 but I'm 7. I want to try to not get angry at home. Sometimes I get angry but I don't hit people." Then he drew a volcano over his head. "This is to show that I get angry in the head and then cool down. At recess, Carol made fun of me. I'm going to get her back."

"Will that make things better?" I asked.

"No," he replied reluctantly.

"What else could you do when Carol does that?"

"Walk away or tell an adult."

"Those are better ideas of what to do if someone gives you a hard time. Everyone gets angry at times, even at home. You already know some good ideas. Would you like to learn a few more on what you can when you feel mad, especially at home?" He nodded in agreement.

- **Use the writing and drawing prompt: "In school/at home, I wish...."**

When given a page with the words *In school, I wish...* at the top, 7-year-old Kevin said as he wrote: "In school, I wish gym was easier. I'm not very good at gym. I'm not good at jumping down to the ground."

- **Incorporate the prompt: "I am good at.... I want to get better at...."**

I handed 11-year-old Zachary a paper with the words *I am good at...* at the top and *I want to get better at...* in the middle.

He thought for a minute and then wrote: *I am good at playing cards, collecting cards, learning, playing games, and helping people.* Then he went to the next prompt and added: *I want to get better at math, science, getting homework in, and not talking back.*

Use Games or Visuals to Discover What Children Want to Change

In addition to talking with children about their concerns, you can incorporate visuals and games to elicit information. For some children who are younger or nonverbal, you can show them pictures of possible goals and ask them to point to what they want help with. Even if they do not understand the concept of a goal, they do understand the notion of getting help. Another option is to pair smiling or frowning faces with the words, "I feel happy when...," "I feel sad when...," and "I want...." Children can then draw or write their answers. You also can create a comic strip in which your character asked questions about desired changes. They respond by drawing themselves and writing their goals in the thought bubbles.

A fun way to discover goals is to have children create a visual of a football or soccer field and write their goal at the net or goal post. They can then move their ball down the field as they achieve each step closer to their goal. The use of games is another alternative.

- **Point to pictures of possible goals.**

"What do you ask your teacher to help you with?" I said to four-year-old Sean. I showed him a paper with six picture symbols and described each picture. "Do you need help with drawing, cutting, writing your name, jumping, playing with friends, or playing on the playground?"

"Miss J. helps me write."

"What do you want me to help you with?"

He pointed to the picture of drawing.

"You want me to help you when you're drawing your plan for playing in centers?" He nodded.

- **Have children respond to smiling and frowning faces with the words: "I feel happy when.... I feel sad when.... I want...."**

I handed 6-year-old Melinda a paper with a smiling face next to the words *I feel happy when....*

She drew a horse and said, "I felt happy when I rode a horse. His name was Noah. He was a cute pony. He's my best friend. I got to go in a circle. It's pretty easy to steer him."

Next, she looked at a frowning face and the words *I feel sad when….* She drew tears on the face and said, "I feel sad when Rachel did not invite me to her birthday party." On the next page, she saw a smiling face and the words *I want….* She drew herself and added, "I want some friends."

- **Create a visual of a football or soccer field and have the children identify the touchdown goal.**

"You get to make your own football field," I told the five third-grade boys in the day treatment as I handed them file folders and rulers. "First draw your lines and the goal post. Think of what would be a good goal for you."

"I want to learn cursive," 10-year-old Donald replied. He took a ruler and traced the lines. At the end of the paper, he added: *Touchdown!* I wrote the letters to be learned on top of each line. Next, he made a football and attached sticky tape so he could move the ball down the field as he accomplished writing each letter.

- **Have characters in a comic strip ask questions and children respond by drawing themselves and writing their goals in a thought bubble.**

I heard that 8-year-old Greg was quickly losing function of his legs. When I met with him, I brought a comic strip, and on one side I drew a character and wrote questions. On the other side of the page, Greg drew pictures of himself with the answers.

"What are you good at or doing well?"

"Playing soccer."

"What is going well for you?"

"In school, they are going to give me a motor scooter."

"Oh, that should help you get around school. I know toward the end of the day you get tired. What do you wish was easier in school?"

"Running."

"What have you found that makes things easier for you?"

"Not running."

"So I hear that being involved with soccer is really important to you. I know that it's getting harder for you to move around, and that has to be upsetting. What if in therapy we try to figure out ways you can be part of the soccer game without running? Would you like to do that?"

He nodded. Later we explored the possibility of him being a scorekeeper or even doing computer games revolving around soccer because he still had hand function.

- **Use a game to discover strengths and concerns.**

In the second group session at the day treatment, I brought a game I adapted from the *Jeopardy!* TV show. "There are four categories: self, coping, strategies, and situations," I said to the fourth graders. "Pick a category and then go down the column and choose a number. Hidden under the numbers are the questions and the

number of points you will get. Everyone will get a prize. Whoever gets the most points will get first pick."

"What's the prize?" 10-year-old Timmy asked with excitement in his voice.

"The prize is a surprise." I smiled back.

"Do we get to keep it?"

"Yes. Let's start the game."

"I want the category 'Self,' and I pick number two," Nathan said.

I lifted the paper and read, "Say something good about you."

"I'm a nice kid," Nathan responded.

"I'm handsome," Timmy said.

"I'm respectful for other things and people. When I borrow toys, I keep them nice and neat. I don't break them," Ricky added.

The group picked two more, and then it was Timmy's turn. I read his selection: "What do you want to change about yourself?"

"I'm not doing that question," he said, scribbling circles on his paper.

"I'll give you more time to think," I replied, turning to ask Nathan.

"I want to bring in homework when it's due," Nathan replied.

"To control my anger, not be so angry, not be sad so much," Ricky said.

I turned back to Timmy, and to help him save face, I reworded the question. "What do you want to get better at? It can be anything. I know you like to ride dirt bikes. It can even be about that. You have to give an answer to get a prize."

He swirled his paper for 10 seconds, then said, "Stop sucking my thumb."

"All right. Everyone gets a prize. They're special pens." The next time we met, I brought Timmy some sensory ideas that could help him stop.

Interview or Use Questionnaires to Obtain Caregivers' and Teachers' Perspectives and Expectations

Children might be thinking:
I'm glad you are trying to find out how things are going at home.

It's good to talk to my mom and dad because then you can help me if it's bad.

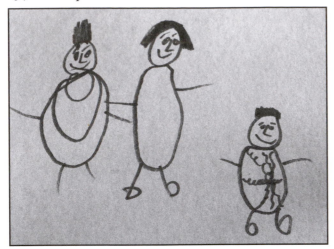

Figure 8-3. It is imperative to obtain caregivers' perspectives and goals.

Another important and essential part of treatment planning is getting caregivers' and teachers' perspectives and expectations for the future (Figure 8-3). Talk to them to discover what they view as the children's strengths, interests, and areas of success. Inquire about their concerns and what they hope for in the future. Ask what they found helps the children.

Caregivers can give you information that you would not have without asking. They are able to provide a picture of the children's worlds, including their cultural values and expectations. This is critical information that is needed for determining the purpose of therapy.

Fabulous Five: Interview or Use Questionnaires to Obtain Caregivers' Perspectives and Expectations

- **Inquire, "What is going well in your child's life?"**

I asked the 9 year old's mother, "What is going well in Melissa's life?"

"Piano lessons, friendships, and drama club."

- **Ask, "What are your child's strengths and interests?"**

"What are Laurie's strengths and interests?" I asked the 8 year old's father.

"She is outgoing, creative, friendly, and energetic. She loves all animals."

- **Ask, "What concerns do you have?"**

"What concerns do you have?" I asked Jeff's third-grade teacher.

"The speed of his work, his handwriting, and his ability to stay focused on the task."

- **Inquire, "What are your hopes and dreams for your child?"**

"What are your hopes and dreams for your child?" I asked the fourth grader's mother.

"First, that she becomes a Christian. Second, that she will be successful enough to go to college if she wishes, and third, that she will be generally happy."

- **Ask, "What have you found that is really helpful for your child?"**

Being the main caregivers, I asked 7-year-old Mark's grandparents, "What have you found that is really helpful for Mark?"

"He does better with frequent short breaks during school and switching activities frequently."

Provide Your Perspective on What Would Help Children Grow

There may be times when it is obvious to everyone—the children, caregivers, and you—that the children are struggling. For some children, this might be difficult for them to acknowledge. If you ignore this, it can be like an elephant in the room—an issue that is not being discussed. When this situation occurs, address the issue but do it in a sensitive and face-saving manner.

Avoid presenting the problem in a way that suggests that you think the children are stupid or bad and that you blame them. Instead, state what you see or hear in a nonjudgmental tone of voice. Express your concern that they are experiencing difficulty and empathize with them. Mention that you have seen other children in the same situation and offer hope. Then talk about how to make things better or easier for them.

Discuss Your Observations, Test Results, and Environmental Demands

---

Children might be thinking:
Wow, you're honest.
That's an idea; maybe I could work on that.

Giving children constructive and tactful feedback can promote change. You or caregivers often may notice their strategies as well as the challenges they are facing. Children may not be aware of what they are doing and the impact it has on others. When determining the purpose of therapy, share what you have seen. If needed, discuss with them any differences in viewpoints. Continue to focus on competencies and promote an increased use of their current strategies. You also can ask them to think about what other people may say about how they are doing. If they are in a dilemma, provide options and have them decide what to do.

Fabulous Five: Provide Your Perspective on What Would Help Children Change

- **Comment on what children are doing well and encourage them to expand their actions to other areas.**

"What are you good at?" I asked the 7 year old.

"Running and the trampoline."

"What do you like to do?"

"Play with my dog, watch scary movies, and play games."

"What do you like about school?"

"P.E."

"What don't you like about school?"

"Art."

"What do you wish was easier?"

"That I can learn a new game and work at school." Next, he started the testing. "I can run real fast. I can move real fast," he said as he completed the fine motor tasks requiring speed.

"I see."

During testing, he said as he turned the paper, "I'm not really a good cutter."

When he was asked to draw shapes, he said, "I don't know how to draw that."

"Just try," I replied.

"I'm never going to get these." He became teary-eyed. "Everyone is better than me." He drew slowly but was successful in copying the shapes.

Afterward, I said, "One thing I noticed was that it was easier for you when you told yourself you could do a hard activity, like the running and speed tests. That's a great strategy. So the challenge now is to use that idea of telling yourself you can do it before starting something hard. Then give yourself a chance to try, like with the drawing. That will help you when learning new games too. Could that be a goal—to use your good idea more?"

He nodded.

- **Mention highlights from observations and/or testing results.**

"I saw that when you used your walker, you became stuck in the corner and were not sure how to move. At times when you get stuck, is it hard for you to figure out what to do?" I asked 8-year-old Mandy.

"Yeah, it is."

"What if we made it a goal that when you get stuck, you will try to think of one idea of what to do before asking for help?"

"Okay, I can do that."

- **Comment on what you observed about the impact of the children's actions.**

"I noticed that when you want a turn, you pulled toys out of kids' hands. I see them get mad, and then they don't want to play with you," I said to 6-year-old Austin. "Can I show you some ways to make friends? What do you think?" He nodded.

The next week, we worked together to write a Social Story on how to ask for a turn. Then he drew pictures to match the words.

- **Ask children what they think another person would say.**

"What are you good at?" I asked 11-year-old Ellen.

"Writing."

"What do you like best about school?"

"Writing."

"What do you wish was easier in school?"

"Math."

Because I knew her teacher had reported difficulties with her written work, I asked, "So what do you think your teacher would say about your class work?"

"Yeah, she's concerned. I need to get better at handwriting. I need to slow down and not be so sloppy."

- **Provide your perspectives and concerns in a respectful way and ask children to decide on the goal.**

Roger, a fifth grader, tested in the gifted range. His teachers were concerned because he stopped both doing written work in class and turning in major assignments. He was a slow printer and said he did not want to learn cursive handwriting or use the computer. He did well on a test of his fine motor skills.

After testing and then interviewing both him and his mother, I said, "It seems like you have yourself stuck. You are very smart and have wonderful ideas, but for teachers to know what you are thinking, it usually has to be written on paper or typed on the computer. Now there is a dilemma. Do you know what that means?"

He nodded.

"You have great ideas, but the teachers do not have a way to know what you know. You're older now, and you need to make a decision which method, writing or using the computer, you want to get better at. This decision is not up to your mom. It's up to you because you are the one who has to do the work. Whatever you pick, keep in mind that you are doing this for you. Which one do you want to get better at—writing or the computer?"

"Computer," he said without hesitation, and his mother nodded. We then talked about word-prediction programs he could use on devices at school and possible speech-recognition programs he could use for his homework at home.

Offer Hope That Change Is Possible

Children might be thinking:
It's nice to know you've helped other kids.
Maybe things will get easier.
Maybe my life will be a lot better.

Offering hope is a critical step in treatment planning. When you convey belief in change, children become more aware of possibilities. You can be influential both in helping them believe in themselves and in beginning to envision a better future. Having hope allows children to leave behind their self-limiting doubts and shift to focusing on what they can do in the future. They become more willing and ready to consider changes and begin to believe that they can succeed. They are motivated to engage in therapy and may start to believe that their dreams are attainable.

Convey That Change Is Possible

Although not usually mentioned in the process of treatment planning, a necessary step is offering hope. You need to convey your belief that either they or how they handle a situation can change. First, let them know you see their potential. Convey your optimism and faith in them. You may want to talk about other children with similar conditions or circumstances where positive change occurred. You may also want to talk about what ideas have helped others. When there is hope, children are more likely to take the first step in adjusting their expectations and creating change.

Fabulous Five: Convey That Change Is Possible

- **Let children know you will not give up on them.**

On the children's psychiatric unit, 8-year-old Jeremy kept refusing to meet with me. So one day when he declined and remained in bed, I changed my approach. To give the message that I would not give up on him, I moseyed to his room, sat by his bedside, and said, "Jeremy, it's our time together. Let's go to the OT room."

He yanked the brown blanket over his head.

"It's our time together, so I'll just sit here and join you. You can decide what you want to do."

After about 4 minutes, he rolled toward me and peeked. "You're not going to go away, are you?"

"No. It's our time together. It would be more fun if we go to the OT room, but it's up to you."

After another minute, he dragged himself out of bed and inched his way to the therapy room.

- **Talk about other children with similar difficulties and how they became better.**

"He tends to wander around the playground and doesn't really play with other children," Mica's first-grade teacher said.

I met with him and started the motor test. He easily lost his balance and struggled with any tasks involving motor planning. When a hopeless look crossed his face, I said, "I can see you are really trying and these are hard for you. I want you to know that I have seen a lot of children who have a hard time like you do. You are not the only one. And you know what?"

"What?"

"I had some ideas that helped them, and after we spent some time together, it was easier for them to try new things." He looked at me with grateful eyes.

- **Use words that imply change is possible and will occur.**

Nine-year-old Jude walked into the room using his forearm crutches and sat down. After talking about his family, friends, and school, I asked him, "What you do like about yourself?"

"That I have a really good friend."

"What don't you like about yourself?"

"When someone is mean to me. Sometimes I get real mad. I don't want to hurt someone, and sometimes I want to but I don't."

"What do you want to change about yourself?"

"Having enemies at school. Kids are mean to me. Sometimes they call me names or cuss at me."

"Have you told anyone about this?"

"I just try to live with it."

"You just try to live with it and ignore them?"

"Yeah."

"Ignoring is one way to deal with those acting like bullies. Getting help from other adults and kids is another way. If ignoring them is not working, would you consider talking to your parents and an adult at school? The situation can get better if you get more help."

He nodded in response.

- **Relate what specific ideas have helped other children.**

Nine-year-old Nicole had tremors that made cutting and writing difficult. So I gave her a wrist weight and said, "Try using this weight when you write or cut. When other children have tried it, it has helped them hold their hand still. Try it and tell me what you think."

She put it on, and as she wrote with a steadier hand, she said, "It's good."

- **Tell about a time you had difficulty but learned what to do.**

"Dr. Clare, has there ever been something you can't do that others can do?" 8-year-old Grace asked.

"Yes. Three years ago, I wanted to do a race called a triathlon in which you swim, run, and bike. But I was a terrible swimmer."

"You didn't know how to swim?" she asked with disbelief.

"Not very good. So I took swimming lessons, learned different strokes, and became a good swimmer. Then I was able to do the race. So I learned to swim when I was way old."

"I can't ride a bike."

"Yet." I paused and added, "Give yourself some time. We can work on improving your balance to make that easier too."

Respond in a Way That Promotes Thinking About Possibilities

When children have multiple experiences of failure, they often lose hope. They may think they will never be good enough. Some end up calling themselves names, such as, "I'm a bad boy." Upon hearing this self-defeating talk, help children separate the results of past actions from future possibilities. Let them know that just because they did not succeed in the past does not mean they cannot do it in the future.

To help change their thoughts, O'Hanlon and Beadle (1997) suggest some helpful techniques. You can respond to children's definitive statements of *never* or *always* with more open-ended words such as *often* or *at times*. You can use the word *yet* in your response to imply that change is possible. Other options are to respond back using a past-tense verb, change a label into action words, or talk about what can be done next time. When children talk about difficulties, you can reword them into possible goals.

Fabulous Five: Respond in a Way That Can Change Children's Thinking

- **Respond back to statements of "never" or "always" with "at times" or "often."**

Seven-year-old Vincent said, "I'm never good in gym."

"So you often find it difficult to do what your classmates are doing in gym?"

He nodded.

- **Use the word *yet* to imply that change is possible.**

"I can't tie my shoes," 6-year-old Donny said as his voice dropped to a whisper.

"Yet," I replied. "I can show you some different ways to make shoe tying easier to learn."

- **Convert a difficulty into a goal.**

"I'm mostly shy," 8-year-old Alyssa said. "I don't have anyone to play with at recess. I hide a lot behind that basketball thing."

"So you would like to have a friend to play with at recess?"

"Yes."

- **Respond back using a past-tense verb.**

"What would you like to change about yourself?" I asked 11-year-old McKenna.

"Not to be mean."

"For example?"

"Like with people I don't like. There's some boys who tease me."

"Here at school?"

"Yeah."

"How are you mean?"

"I say things that are not true about them because they say something not true about me."

"So you're saying you've been mean in the past but now you want to find different ways to get people to stop teasing you."

She nodded.

- **Change a label into action words.**

"I'm a bad boy," the first grader told me.

"It sounds like there have been some times when you have gotten in trouble. I have some ideas that can help you change that."

Suggest Ideas for Possible Goals

Children might be thinking:
Let me think about it.
I could work on that.
Yeah, that's an okay one.

When trying to discover children's concerns or identify areas for change, it may not always be as simple as asking them directly what they want to change. Sometimes you learn about their concerns while they are in the midst of an activity or when it comes up in a conversation. Listen and check with them if they would like therapy to address these concerns.

If children are not sure what they want to change, you may need to offer possible ideas. Your suggestions can be based on your work with children in similar circumstances or your assessment of how their current physical, mental, or social status affects their participation in occupations. If children are nonverbal, offer possibilities and have them respond through eye or body movements. Let children tell you what they value so that the purpose of therapy is meaningful for them.

Fabulous Five: Suggest Ideas for Possible Goals

- **Present ideas based upon the children's concerns expressed during an activity.**

I watched 7-year-old Henry write and noticed that he had a weak thumb joint, which created an awkward pencil grasp. He held the pencil tightly and moved both his hand and arm as he printed each letter. "My hand is getting sore from doing writing every week. My hand goes numb."

"I can help you with that if you want," I replied. "We can try to figure out ways that will prevent your hand from going numb and make writing easier. Do you want to work on that?" Henry nodded. "There are some pencil grips you can check out to see if they help. Sometimes holding the pencil between your index and middle fingers can make a difference. What do you think? Do you want to try these ideas?"

"Sure."

- **Make suggestions for the purpose of therapy based on the concerns or desires expressed in children's conversations.**

"I only have one friend and that's me," 8-year-old Brock said as I sat next to him in art class.

"Is that something you want to change?"

"Yeah, no one plays with me."

"If you want, we can work on what you need to do to make friends."

"Okay."

- **Suggest possibilities and ask children to tell you their choices using nonverbal means.**

I met with 10-year-old Paul and moved his wheelchair to a quiet corner of the class. "We are going to meet with your mom to talk about how well you have done this year. I need to know what you want to work on this year—what you want for goals. I have some ideas. Squeeze my hand or drop your head for yes. Or as you usually do, turn your head for no. Let me tell you my ideas. Do you want to get better at touching the correct screen on your communication device?" I waited for a minute, and he squeezed my hand. We went over three other possibilities, and he chose using a stamp for his signature as a second goal.

- **Suggest possible treatment goals based your experience with children in similar circumstances.**

In the pediatric oncology clinic, I asked 8-year-old Iris what she would like to be able to do, and she shrugged her shoulders. Then I said, "I know other kids going through chemo often feel tired and can't always do the things they like. It has helped them to try new activities that are easy to do at home. Is that something you would want to do?"

"Yeah."

- **Suggest ideas based on your observation of how children's current status impacts their participation in occupations.**

"Janet has just come back from the hospital," her third-grade teacher told me. "She had a stroke resulting in partial paralysis in her right side. Now she's learning how to write with her left hand."

After I introduced myself and we spent a few minutes talking, I asked, "What do you like about school?"

"Reading."

"What have you found that helps you in class?"

"I'm good at stretching my hand," she replied and demonstrated putting her affected hand on the table.

"That's great. That will keep your hand from getting too tight. If you want, I can suggest to your teacher that everyone do this as a stretch break. It's good for other kids too. What do you think?"

"Okay."

"What do you want to get better at in school?"

"I do get tired when I write."

"Do you want to work on getting your left hand stronger now that it's your writing hand?"

She nodded.

"I also have a one-handed typing program or a one-handed keyboard. Are you interested in trying those?"

She nodded again.

"So our goals will be to get your left hand stronger, get so you can use the class computers with one hand either with a one-handed typing program or keyboard, and increase your endurance when writing. We can talk to your teacher about having stretching your right hand be part of the school routine and maybe get the whole class to do stretches. Do those goals sound all right to you? Do I need to change anything?"

"No. Those are good."

Guide the Process

After eliciting children's strengths, strategies, desires, and concerns, assist them in creating personal challenges. If needed, explore any lack of interest or ambivalences. Identify resources and what needs to change in the environment. When there are differences in perspectives, search for underlying needs and explore options. Finally, define the purpose of therapy and co-develop the final plan.

Help Children Make Their Desired Changes Into Challenges

> **Children might be thinking:**
> *I really want….*
> *I'm going to see if I can….*
> *I'm going to… and work on….*

Although children can often tell you what they want to change, they may question how to go about doing so. Emphasize their resourcefulness, help them make their goals achievable, and convert desired changes into personal challenges. When their goals are large or vague, identify the smaller and more detailed steps they can take. As they define their personal challenges, encourage them to build on their current skills or competencies and expand them to other areas. Talk about the resources available, including the support you offer. In the discussion, also pinpoint their priority for change.

Fabulous Five: Convert Children's Desired Changes Into Personal Challenges

- **Break large or vague goals into smaller, detailed steps.**

"Why did you come to the hospital?" I asked 7-year-old Shelley.

"For asthma. I keep getting sick."

"What do you want to change?"

"Quit being sick and get better."

"What is one thing you want to change that you can do to help yourself get and stay better?"

"I want to learn to remind my mother when I need medicine."

"So could one goal be to practice speaking up for yourself, especially in asking for your medicine and for help when you need it?"

"Yeah," she replied with a nod.

We then talked about exploring what activities were better for her and how to pace herself.

- **Build on present skills or competencies.**

"Do you have many friends?" I asked 9-year-old Bruce in the day treatment program.

"I have one friend, Mitch."

"What makes you a good friend?"

"I like to be there for him when he needs me."

"What do you like best about yourself?"

"My baseball skills."

"What do you dislike or not like about yourself?"

"I'm not able to make many friends."

"What do you want to change?"

"My attitude toward other people. I want to be nicer to people."

"You have one friend and would like to make more. You like to be there for Mitch and help him. Those are important aspects of being a friend that you are already good at. So next you want to get better at saying and doing nice things with others so you can make new friends too."

- **Expand current skills or competencies to other areas.**

Twelve-year-old Danielle told me, "I never ask a teacher for help. I only go to a friend. But a couple of days ago Mrs. B. saw me having a hard time with pre-algebra. She asked, 'What's wrong?' and I said, 'I don't get it.' She said I need to tell her if I don't understand, otherwise she wouldn't know that I needed help.

"Then last week I got a fortune cookie: 'You have good ideas and you have to back them up.' Now I'm trying to make that fortune come true."

"Right now you are good at asking friends for help. So the challenge for you is to speak up for yourself and ask teachers for help."

- **Talk about available resources, including your support.**

"What are you good at?" I asked 6-year-old Keaton.

"Games and singing."

"What's hard for you?"

"Sometimes my legs hurt so I stop running and I walk. I don't play basketball anymore. It's too scary for me."

Knowing that his muscles were becoming weaker each year and he easily fatigued, I said, "Would you like to try new things and games now that it is harder to move and you get tired?"

He nodded.

"I can help you find new fun things to do."

"That'd be good."

- **Identify priorities for change.**

I asked the second grader with low muscle tone, "What would you like to get better at?"

Caleb wrote: *Have bedder handwrit cuz in first grade I hade sopi handwrit. I want to be a bedder atlet. I want to be a bedder machine.*

"Do you want to get stronger or faster?"

"Stronger."

"So, you're telling me want to get better at writing neatly, get stronger as an athlete, and be like a strong machine. Which one is the most important to you?"

"Getting strong."

Explore Children's Ambivalences or Lack of Interest in Changing

> **Children might be thinking:**
> *I'm not sure I want to do that.*
> *I don't know.*
> *I'm fine.*
> *I didn't realize I was doing that.*

It is the adults in children's lives who recommend or bring them to therapy. Children may not have a say. Consequently, they may not be interested in exploring what could change. They may believe they are fine the way they are. Some may be unaware that change is possible. For instance, they may not know that with therapy their motor skills or sensory processing can improve, making everyday life easier. Being the focus of conversation may make them uncomfortable, especially if others are discussing their failures. They may want to just play instead of talking. In these situations, emphasize their strengths and avoid pressuring children to admit failure. Instead, talk about therapy being a chance to try new things and learn more about themselves, especially the good things they can do.

Other children may be ambivalent about changing or not know how to do so. Listen for discrepancies in their conversations or actions, especially if they say they want to change but have not tried. Discuss the benefits of changing, and talk about available resources, including your assistance. Often these strategies can sway them. Then have them identify their priorities for change.

Fabulous Five: Explore Children's Ambivalences or Disinterest in Changing

- **Listen for ambivalences in children's conversations.**

"What do you like about yourself?" I asked 9-year-old Tyler.

"I'm a nice person. I try to get along with people. Sometimes I feel like a good person."

"But sometimes you don't?"

"Yeah. Sometimes I get mad and beat up my sister."

- **Talk about the discrepancies between children's desired changes and their actions.**

"I want to get better at typing," the fifth grader told me.

"What is holding you back? " I asked.

"Nothing. It's pretty much my effort. I don't put forth a lot of effort into getting better."

"Sounds like you're saying more effort would help you get better."

- **State that the purpose of therapy is to learn more about themselves.**

"What are you good at?" I asked 7-year-old Stephanie.

"Math, games, making necklaces, anything."

"What do you want to get better at?"

"I don't know."

"What you want to change?"

"Nothing."

"So right now you are good at math, games, and doing lots of things. What we can do is use our time together to give you a chance to try new things and learn more about yourself. It's a chance to learn more good things about who you are. Is that okay?"

She smiled and nodded.

- **Discuss the benefits of changing.**

"What do you like about school?" I asked 9-year-old Paris.

"I like to learn."

"What do you dislike about school?"

"My teacher. She's not very nice."

"What does she do?"

"She raises her voices and tells me to pay attention. I wish I had a different teacher."

"Have you talked to your parents about this?"

"Yeah, my mom met with her."

"Because you are in a tough situation and can't change teachers, would it be okay to talk and figure out what you can do to have a better day at school? That way you can be happier at school."

"Yeah. That'd be good."

- **Give more information on how they can achieve desires.**

In the occupational therapy clinic, I asked 7-year-old Martin, "What's easy for you at school?"

"Math and science."

"What's hard for you at school?"

"It's really hard for me to do the buttons on my jeans. I wait until I get home to use the bathroom because of that." He paused. "It's hard for me to cut my food with a knife too."

"Do you want to get better at those?"

"I guess."

Sensing that he did not believe he could do them by himself, I said, "I'm concerned that at times it must get uncomfortable to have to wait and not be able to use the school bathroom. Also, it must be embarrassing to have trouble with your knife if you are around friends. I can help you so you can do it yourself. There are tricks that I can show you to make it easier. We can figure out ways to manipulate various buttons and a knife and work on coordinating your fingers with your eyes. Would that be okay?"

He nodded, seeming a bit relieved.

Identify What Needs to Change in the Children's Environment During Treatment Planning

> **Children might be thinking:**
> *You're going to make things easier for me.*
> *It will be good if... changes.*

Effective treatment planning requires identifying and addressing what needs to change in the environment. First, determine what factors are the social, emotional, or physical barriers impacting children. Do what you can to eliminate them. Then examine what must be changed in the environment to meet the children's needs. You may end up adding or removing elements or making suggestions that support an individual and benefits the group as well.

Fabulous Five: Identify What Needs to Change in the Environment

- **Identify and address social barriers in the environment.**

"We have a new boy coming," the preschool director told the special education team. "If you touch him, he bleeds under his skin."

When Darius came to visit, I introduced myself and told him, "I'm going to make a book to let your friends know that you like to play but it does hurt when they touch you." He nodded. I took pictures of him as he walked around the classroom and put them in a book. The teacher read the following story to the class for the next couple of days:

Hi. My name is Darius.
I am happy to come to preschool.
If you touch me, it hurts me.
You can wave to me.
You can say hi and talk to me.
I love to play too.

On Darius' first day, Kellen approached him, waved, and said, "Hi, Darius. My name is Kellen. I want to be your friend."

- **Identify and address physical barriers in the environment.**

On 3-year-old Jade's first day of preschool, I spent the morning in her classroom. Her parents pushed her wheelchair in, and Jade insisted on being placed on the floor with her classmates. She lay on her stomach in a frog-like position. Her parents quietly mentioned how a tumor on her foot hindered her from walking and that sitting was often painful.

After introducing myself, I told her, "I'm going to bring some different kinds of chairs and pillows so you can sit with your friends. Let me know if they are comfortable." I left and returned with a beanbag chair and various pillows.

"It hurts," she said as she tried each one.

Then I brought a homemade carpeted cube chair and put an air cushion on the seat. She smiled as she shifted right and left on the air cushion, taking the pressure off her bottom. She put her hands on the side of the chair and lifted her body up and down. As the day went on, she maneuvered herself in and out of the chair. Jade looked over at me and said, "I like it."

- **Eliminate one element of the environment to meet children's needs.**

"Bailey is very sensitive to loud noises," the 3 year old's parents told the special education team. "If there is too much noise, she gets overwhelmed and cries."

On her first day of preschool, I observed that her classmates were more active and noisier than most. During transitions, the noise level increased, and Bailey yelled, "You're hurting my ears."

"It is really loud in here," I said. "It's hurting my ears too. I'm going to talk to your teacher and see if we can figure out some ways to make it quieter."

When the class was out, the teacher and I came up with ideas for how to do quiet transitions.

- **Identify and provide needed additions to the environment.**

"We have a set of twins starting in January. They were preemies," the special education teacher told me. "They just turned 3, and this is their first time in school. They are really tiny and so cute."

On Mike and Joseph's first day, they walked in with pacifiers in their mouths, looking leery. "What do they like to play with?" I asked their mom as we walked down the hall.

"They love cars, trucks, and blocks."

The other staff members help them get settled and put their pacifiers in their backpack. I went to the storeroom and gathered cars, trucks, manipulatives, and cause-and-effect toys. I thought, *I don't think they will like the toys in the centers now. It would probably be hard for them to play with those.*

I carried a bin of the new toys at the beginning of center time and told them, "I brought some toys that I heard you liked." Mike grabbed the shiny blue car, and Joseph reached for the pickup truck. I built a roadway using long blocks, and they added to it.

- **Change the environment to meet an individual's need that also benefits the group.**

"We have a new girl named Whitney who is nonverbal and is diagnosed as having autism," the preschool director told our special education team as she handed us her report. We then met with Whitney's two teachers and talked about helpful strategies.

"Visual strategies using picture symbols," I explained, "are easier to understand than just words. Using them would help the class too."

The team then worked together and created a visual schedule, cue cards with pictures for directions, a choice board, and pictures of different roles children could assume while playing in centers.

Negotiate When There Are Discrepancies or Differences

> **Children might be thinking:**
> *I'm not sure I want to work on that.*
> *I don't know.*
> *I'm glad you listened to both of us.*
> *Sure I can try that.*
> *Thanks for coming up with ideas we both can agree on.*

When you find there are differences in viewpoints, desires, or concerns, start a negotiation process. First, make sure you have elicited caregivers', teachers', and children's perspectives and have shared yours. Be sure to describe what you have learned from supporting research and knowledge gained from your experiences. All perspectives are equally valued.

If there are glaring discrepancies in perspectives and desired goals, look for common elements or themes. One way to do this is to identify the underlying needs expressed in "I want…" statements. For instance, a teacher may want a child's constant movement to not disrupt the class. The child may want to keep moving and not have to sit still. Combining the child's need for movement and the teacher's need for minimal distractions when teaching, the goal could be to identify and implement strategies for the child to move in a way that would not distract the class. Possible options in this scenario would be teaching the child to do chair push-ups, providing a move-and-sit air cushion, or having the child assist the teacher in taking materials to the school office.

In situations when there are differences between what children say and others' observations, be kind, tactful, and candid in your comments. Think outside the box and try to discover ways to address the differences. Keep in mind that within a session, multiple needs often can be addressed even within one activity. When you identify all the underlying needs, it is easier to explore options and solutions. At this point, accept where children are in thinking about change, and start with their priorities.

Fabulous Five: Negotiate When There Are Discrepancies or Differences

- **Elicit all views when negotiating.**

"What are Bryan's strengths?" I asked his mother.

"He's gentle, sensitive, and affectionate. He compliments others and uses good manners at home."

I turned to his second-grade teacher.

"He has a sweet disposition, is inquisitive, and has a good sense of humor."

"What are your concerns?"

"I want him to stand up for himself with other children," his mother replied. "His brother dominates when they play together. I just want him to work up to his potential."

"I would like for him to attend better and participate in tasks without one-to-one assistance," his teacher said. "To accept feedback without crying or tantrums and be able to handle conflict and disagreements without crying." She then described a situation in which he and a classmate decided to take turns. "I would like to see him do that more."

Later, I interviewed Bryan. "What do you think about school?"

"It's boring. I don't get to do anything. I like playing with my friends."

"What are you good at?"

"Running and counting."

"What's easy about school?"

"Math."

"What's hard about school?"

"Sitting and standing still."

"I talked with your mom and your teacher. They told me so many good things about you. They said you were really nice and kind. You have good manners, ask good questions, and have a good sense of humor. Wow, you have so many strengths. That's wonderful!

"What I heard everyone say, including you, was that we all want to figure out ways to make learning easier for you, including helping you with sitting. I also heard from your mom and teacher that it would help if you could get better at speaking up for yourself, especially when your brother keeps telling you what to do, and learn more things you can do if your friends do not agree with you. Your teacher said the other day you and Robert did not agree during science but talked and decided to take turns. You came up with a great idea! So it would be good to keep using your idea and, if you want, to learn some more.

"What do you think? Would it be okay to find ways to help you with sitting, to speak up for yourself, and to learn more ideas of what to do if other people do not agree with you?"

"That's okay with me."

- **Discuss discrepancies between what children say and observations from other adults.**

"I'm good at writing. It's easy for me," 8-year-old Lisa said with a smile.

"I'm curious," I said. "You say you are good at writing. And yet I saw some of your writing in your notebook. On one page, I could read a little of what you wrote, but the rest was hard to read."

"That's my fast writing."

"I see you like writing fast. I hear that if you write too fast, your teacher can't read it and you end up having to do it over again. What if we figure out ideas to help you write both fast and neat so your teacher can read it?"

She nodded.

- **Find common ground.**

"I want to get better at playing computer games because I can't beat anyone in my family," 6-year-old Noah told me.

"Your teacher said it would be good for you to get better at printing your name and to go a little faster when you're doing your work," I said. "What if we work on you being able to move your hands quickly and accurately? That would help you get better at computer games and writing. How does that sound to you? Is that okay?"

"Yeah, I really want to beat my brother."

- **Start where children are at regarding their thinking about change.**

After doing an interview with 10-year-old Megan, I observed how she managed with her walker and involuntary movements while making a snack in the occupational therapy clinic. She made multiple trips to get the food items on the counter. We then sat down to talk. After highlighting what she did well, I said, "When you made your snack, I noticed you kept going back and forth for the food. You didn't plan ahead. Is that something you want to get better at?"

"I think I'm good at that."

"So you're not concerned about that right now?"

"Yeah."

"Is it okay with you that if I see you not planning ahead and jumping into something without thinking, I talk to you about it?"

"Yeah, that's okay."

"Would it be okay to give some suggestions too?"

"Yeah, you can."

- **Discover ways to address different views.**

"Do you have any ideas what you would like to work on?" I asked 7-year-old Selena, who struggled with fluctuating muscle tone.

"Can it be anything?"

"Yes."

"I want to learn how to pull up my own pants and put on my shoes, undershirt, and my own earrings."

"When you made a snack," I said, "I saw that you could get around pretty good." She nodded. "I also talked with your mom and dad about what they wanted you to do to. They said they wanted you to get your underwear and jacket on. What do you think about that?"

"I'm just thinking about getting dressed. I'm not really thinking about my jacket."

"Do you want to work on putting on your clothes first and then maybe later work on the jacket?"

"Yeah."

"Another thing they told me is that it would be important for you to learn how to use a knife and fork."

"I think they are right because I really do want to learn how to cut."

"Can we add that as a goal?"

"Yeah."

Summarize the Plan

> **Children might be thinking:**
> *I'm glad you went over why we are together.*
> *That's a good plan.*

After any discussion or negotiation, it is best to summarize the key points and areas of agreement. Incorporate children's words or phrases in your description. Always start by highlighting the children's strengths and then review the main points. State what children have identified as their personal challenges. Finally, summarize the gist of what was said regarding the purpose for being together and the plan for the future. Taking a few minutes to do this summary lets children know that you were listening and gives everyone an opportunity to clarify any misunderstandings. The result is a plan that all parties, including children, can support.

Fabulous Five: Summarize Plan

- **Use children's words or phrases when describing the plan.**

After talking with 8-year-old David, I summarized our discussion. "So you told me that you are good at gym and one of the fastest runners in your class, especially when your class plays red light, green light. You said that sometimes in class, you lose your focus and wiggle, like tipping your chair back and forth, and then your teacher gets upset with you. If it's okay with you, we can figure out what you can do when you feel like wiggling that will not upset your teacher."

"It's okay."

- **Mention children's competencies or strengths as part of the plan.**

"Casey is an 11 year old who has cerebral palsy," her previous therapist told me.

I met with Casey the next day and asked, "What do you know how to do well or what are you good at?"

"In school I'm good at math. Mmm. I'm good at reading, and I do a lot of computer games."

"Is there anything you did that you felt really good about?"

"Several times I got straight As."

"Wow! That's quite an accomplishment."

After finishing the interview regarding different aspects of her life, I asked, "What would you like to get better at?"

"I can do my pants and top, but I need improvement in doing my own hair and putting on my shoes and socks."

"Can you think of anything else you would like to do or that we can work on together?" I waited 30 seconds as she thought. "Anything you'd like to be doing but is still kind of hard?"

"More typing on the computer."

"What do you want to be doing when typing on the computer?"

"Like writing friends, doing schoolwork. I want to do more schoolwork faster."

"You are already good at putting on your pants and shirt by yourself." I said as I wrote: "So for goals: 1. To do your hair, socks, and shoes by yourself with minimal assistance, very little help. You're also good at computer games but want to get faster with typing. What if we make the second goal: 2. To do schoolwork faster on the computer and get assignments done on time? What do you think?"

"Yeah, those are good." We then discussed her current typing speed and how fast she wanted to be.

- **Review the key points you have heard the children and/or others say.**

"I'm feeling depressed," 11-year-old Brody said. "I feel sad all over."

"Tell me more."

"I feel school depressed. I don't have any friends. I don't have anyone to play with. We have to do a lot of reading and writing and I am not good at writing, and we have to sit for a long time. That's hard for me. I need to move."

"I'm concerned about how sad you are feeling. Have you talked to your parents or teacher about this?"

"Not yet."

"Would you like to tell them or would you like me to?"

"I'll tell my mom."

"Okay. Then when we are together, you and I can figure out some ways to find friends, make writing easier, and be able to move more in class."

- **Talk about goals being challenges.**

When I observed 8-year-old Tracy at recess and in physical education, I noticed that she moved awkwardly. It also was challenging for her to do activities requiring bilateral coordination, when she had to move both sides of her body together.

Later, I asked her, "What do you like about school?"

"Art."

"What is easy for you?"

"Science. That's it."

"What's hard for you?"

"I have no clue."

"What's your favorite activity?"

"When we play tag."

"What do you like about your family?"

"They like to play tetherball. We talk a lot. They're nice and they buy me things when they don't have to get me anything."

"What activities do you do with your family?"

"Play tetherball."

"What do you want to get better at?"

"Beating my cousin at tetherball."

"So the challenge for you is to get better at moving your body quickly and accurately hitting the ball so you can beat your cousin."

She nodded.

- **Summarize the purpose for being together and the plan.**

"What's your favorite activity?" I asked 10-year-old Lauren.

"I like to paint and draw and mix up color and clay."

"What are you good at?"

"Swings are easy for me."

"What's hard for you at school?"

"Writing and playground equipment. The balance beam. It's kind of hard to shoot at the high basketball thing."

"What parts of writing are hard for you?"

"If I have to copy something from the board, it's better if I sit in front. It's hard to read the directions from the board. It's hard on my vision. I can get off from what my class is doing. It makes me feel tired and frustrated. Ever since first grade, I have been a slow poke at everything."

"When you write, do your fingers hurt?"

"Sometimes I get pencil blisters."

"If we could make school easier, what could we do?"

"Try to help me write faster and stay on top of things like my class work."

> "So what I heard you say is that you enjoy art and you are good at swinging all by yourself. At times, it's challenging for you for copy from the board, to keep your mind on your work, and to write as fast as others. You came up with a great strategy of making sure you sit in the front of the class. If you want, we can work together to figure out ways to write faster, keep doing what everyone is doing, and stop getting finger blisters."
>
> "Yeah. That sounds good."

KEY POINTS TO REMEMBER

- A strengths-based approach to treatment planning focuses on what is wanted in the future and how to achieve the desired change.
- An emphasis on problems can lead to blaming the children.
- An emphasis on strengths, strategies, and desires and addressing concerns promotes a sense of competence and mastery.
- Treatment planning entails (a) learning about each other; (b) eliciting strengths, desires, and concerns; (c) clarifying a vision of a good life; and (d) discussing, identifying, and negotiating the purpose of therapy.
- Give children who are young or nonverbal a voice by finding and building on what is important to them.
- Match the format of collaboration to children's level of understanding and comfort.
- Obtain children's perspectives on their strengths and occupational functioning.
- Interview or use questionnaires to obtain caregivers' and teachers' perspectives and expectations for the children.
- Use creative ways to elicit children's desired changes.
- Provide your perspective and offer hope that change is possible.
- Incorporate all perspectives and negotiate to define the purpose of therapy.
- Convert children's desired changes into personal challenges.

- Identify resources and what needs to change in the environment to support children.
- Summarize the plan.

REVIEW QUESTIONS

1. Treatment planning is best thought of as a problem-solving process. True or false.
2. Children who are nonverbal or young can show you what is important to them. True or false.
3. Children are usually unaware of what is going right or wrong in their lives. True or false.
4. You need to obtain the children's perspectives to ensure therapy is meaningful. True or false.
5. Asking children, "What do you want for goals?" is the best way to include them. True or false.
6. The use of creative participation methods engages children and makes it easier for them to communicate their concerns. True or false.
7. It is easier for children to build on the successful strategies in their repertoire than to learn something new. True or false.
8. Children's, caregivers', teachers', and your perspectives are equally important. True or false.
9. Identifying and prioritizing the goals for therapy is a straightforward process. True or false.
10. What do you need to include when you summarize the plan for treatment?

REFERENCES

Fanger, M. T. (1993). After the shift: Time-effective treatment in the possibility frame. In S. Friedman (Ed.), *The new language of change: Constructive collaboration in psychotherapy* (pp. 85-91). New York, NY: Guilford.

O'Hanlon, B., & Beadle, S. (1997). *A guide to possibility land: Fifty-one methods for doing, brief, respectful therapy.* New York, NY: W. W. Norton & Company.

9

Teach Children Self-Advocacy

CHAPTER OVERVIEW

After defining the purpose of therapy, the process continues by assisting children to further increase their self-awareness and confidence. As partners, their right to dissent is respected, and they are encouraged to be assertive to get their needs met. In this chapter, there is a continued focus on guiding children to (a) identify their successful strategies and solutions, (b) address their concerns, and (c) expand their repertoire.

CHILDREN'S DESCRIPTIONS OF WHAT THEY THINK YOU SHOULD KNOW

Dr. Clare: "Why is it important to speak up for yourself, such as saying what you think, asking questions if you don't understand, or requesting what you need?"

Logan (age 12): "You should be sticking up for yourself because you might not end up doing what you wanted to do."

Debbie (age 12): "It affects how people think about you."

DEVELOP CHILDREN'S SELF-ADVOCACY

It is crucial for children to have an active role to make therapy meaningful and effective. This requires a level of self-awareness regarding what they want and need in their lives. To enhance their knowledge about themselves, you can guide them by using self-reflective questions to further develop self-initiative, self-assurance, and resourcefulness.

Assist Children in Getting to Know Themselves and Recognize Their Needs

Self-knowledge and expectations of success are critical for developing self-advocacy. Also necessary is for children to view themselves in a positive light as well as be aware of both their strengths and their difficulties. Recognizing helpful strategies promotes their continuation of success. The monitoring and evaluation of their efforts provides feedback regarding the need for change.

Build Self-Confidence

> **Children might be thinking:**
> *I thought of that idea myself.*
> *I did it all by myself.*
> *I knew I could do it.*

When children develop self-confidence, they are better able to speak up for themselves and handle a variety of situations. They also are more likely to think of solutions when they encounter difficulties and believe that taking action will result in changes. To assist children in building self-confidence, you can recognize times when they speak positively about themselves. Also, give recognition

Curtin, C.
*Strategies for Collaborating With Children: Creating Partnerships
in Occupational Therapy and Research* (pp. 167-186).
© 2017 SLACK Incorporated.

when you observe or hear about a situation in which they identified a solution independently. In addition, highlight their expectations of success and the positive outcomes of their actions.

Fabulous Five: Develop Self-Confidence

- **Recognize positive self-talk.**

As 5-year-old Allie drew a horse, she said, "I'm going to try all nice coloring on this. I'm a good artist drawing turtles and horses. I'm just going to take my time."

"That's a good thing to tell yourself," I replied.

- **Attribute children's identification of a solution to their own problem solving.**

"I'm drawing a crocodile. It's a girl crocodile," Grace said as she drew in her first-grade class. "Eyes are usually black. I got a little green on the eye. So I'll color it black."

"You thought of a good solution, a good idea of how to fix it."

- **Emphasize that children thought of a solution all by themselves.**

While 4-year-old Jeremy ate breakfast at school, a classmate made noises, which became loud. Jeremy crossed his arms and grunted. Then he jumped up, went to the cozy corner, and put on headphones.

When he returned to the table, I said, "You did a good thing by taking a break when it became too noisy. It's great you thought of doing that all by yourself."

- **Recognize children's expectations of success.**

"I'm making a picture," 6-year-old Abby said. "It's going to be really good."

"I bet it will be a good picture," I replied.

As she drew, she said, "I'm picking flowers for my mom and dad. I am really happy because it's spring. We always picked dandelions, and I am in a purple dress. That's me. I'm a good drawer."

- **Acknowledge what children were able to achieve.**

As 4-year-old Ryan connected plastic circles containing slits, he said, "Look, I made a plane. I'm good at making them. See." He turned to Hunter, a classmate who was struggling, and said, "Keep doing it and you'll learn it. Watch me." Ryan demonstrated putting two pieces together.

When Hunter figured out what to do, I said to Ryan, "You are good at building planes, and you're being a good friend to help Hunter."

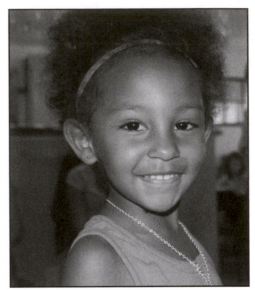

Figure 9-1. Promote the development of self-knowledge.

Identify Ways Children Can Know Their Learning Style, Struggles, and Needs

---

Children might be thinking:
I learn the best when I do….
I know what is best for me.
I know how to help myself.
I know I struggle when….
I know what is hard for me to do.

To advocate for themselves, children need to know what their strengths are, how they learn, what they struggle with, and what they need (Figure 9-1). You can help them increase their self-awareness by encouraging them to think about their lives. Ask reflective-type questions such as, "What helps you learn the best?" or "What gets you in trouble?" For some, you may want to offer books written for children that explain their challenges.

Fabulous Five: Help Children Identify Their Struggles, Needs, and Learning Style

- **Ask, "What helps you learn best?"**

"What helps you learn best?" I asked the second grader.

"In gym, I learned a seal walk. I watched a big kid do it."

"So it helps you to watch someone do it first. Watching helps you learn."

- **Inquire, "What makes learning easier for you in school?"**

"What makes learning easier for you in school?" I asked.

"I ask questions if I need to," 12-year-old Kara replied. "If I still don't understand, I can go to a study session with my teacher."

- **Ask, "What is not so good about…?"**

"What's not so good about school?" I asked 7-year-old Jeffery.

"These kids named Cody and Ryan are mean to me."

"How does that make you feel?"

"Sad."

"What do you do that helps when you see them?"

"I just walk away."

"If it keeps happening, talk to your teacher too."

- **Ask, "What gets you in trouble?"**

"What gets you in trouble?" I asked the second grader.

"I don't pay attention to my body very much," James replied. "When I wiggle, I lose my focusing. When I wiggle, my teacher and kids in my class get frustrated because I shake the table. My teachers get frustrated because I talk when I'm not supposed to, and I don't hear what they are saying."

"What can you do?'

"I can do chair push-ups. I can push my hands together. If I'm in the hall, I can do wall push-ups. I have to write things down to remember. When I get unfocused, I forget what to do. Maybe we could make a card for my desk with these ideas."

- **Inquire, "What have you found you need to do to…?"**

"What have you found you need to do to be successful and do well in your class?" I asked 12-year-old Nicole.

"Sometimes when I am sitting in class, my teacher doesn't like me to sit by my friends because I get distracted. So I found that I just tell my friends that I don't want to talk so I can stay on track. Then I get to stay with my friends."

Ask Questions to Identify Exceptions and/or Possible Solutions

Children might be thinking:
Oh, I can actually do that somewhere else.
I tried doing… and it didn't work, but then I tried doing… and it did work.

To address children's concerns, use a strengths-based approach to assist children in recognizing and identifying their successful strategies. Change your mindset. Move away from looking for what is wrong with children. Instead, look for what they are doing well and build on what they have found to help themselves. Assist children in finding exceptions and solutions that have worked in the past.

To elicit their exceptions, ask them to tell you about a time they did not have difficulty or inquire how they managed despite facing a difficult challenge. You also can ask about a time they surprised themselves and were successful. Explore with them what they have tried or thought about in the past. Ask what has helped them the most in addressing their concerns. These types of questions help children reflect on the successful strategies that are currently in their repertoire.

Fabulous Five: Ask Questions to Identify Exceptions and Solutions.

- **Ask children about times when they did not have the problem or difficulty.**

"What do you want to get better at?" I asked 12-year-old Mia.

"Get better at swimming."

"I know you are on the swim team. What about swimming do you want to get better at?"

"My endurance."

"Anything else you want to get better at?"

"Talking nicer to my brother because I'm mean to him."

"When do you find it is the easiest to talk nice to him?"

"When we're both having fun together and neither one of us is making each other upset."

"So those are times you are able to get along with him. What could you tell yourself so you have more nice times?"

"Be nice to my brother because when we get older I might not see him."

"You said you get along best when you are having fun. Do you think finding more time to do fun things together might help too?"

"Yeah, I could do that."

- **Ask, "How did you manage to… when [mention a difficulty or challenge]?"**

"At first Austin did well in middle school. He even made honor roll. But now he is struggling with his assignments and with math," his mother told me privately before I met with him.

"I heard that you made honor roll your first semester in middle school. That's quite an achievement," I said to the 12 year old. Austin smiled and nodded. "How did you manage to do that when it was your first semester in a brand new school?"

"A lot of studying helped me out. My mom helped me too."

"What did you tell yourself?"

"I can do this. Then sometimes I would sit down and just read the book. I tried to make sure I didn't get off task."

"So it really helped when you focused on what you needed to do and told yourself that you could do it. You believed in yourself. The support of your mom also helped."

"That's right."

- **Inquire, "Has there been a time where you surprised yourself and were able to…?"**

"Has there been a time when you surprised yourself and did something you didn't think you could?" I asked 12-year-old Noah.

"This past week we graded our tests, and I got 89%."

"What did you do to get that good score?"

"Study."

"How did you study?"

"I read the online text and used flash cards."

- **Inquire, "What have you thought might help?" or "What have you tried that helped?"**

"Brandy has a lot of trouble getting ready for school in the morning," her mother said. "It takes her forever."

I turned to the third grader and asked, "What do you think?"

"It's hard for me," she replied.

"Do you want the morning to be easier?" I asked, and she nodded. "What have you tried that helped?"

"It helps if I put my homework in my backpack when I'm done."

"That's a great idea. So getting ready the night before may make it easier," I said.

The three of us talked and decided that at night Brandy would pick out the clothes she wanted to wear for school the next day. She would continue to put her homework and supplies into her pink backpack and leave the pack by the front door.

"What would help you remember?" I asked her.

"Make a list," Brandy replied.

"Okay. Tell me what you need to do every morning," I said. "I'll write it down. Then you can copy and make your own chart." I wrote the number 1 on the page.

"Eat breakfast," she said.

"Number 2. What do you do next?"

"Brush my teeth, wash my face, and comb my hair."

"Then what?"

"Put my lunch in my backpack." Brandy copied the numbered steps for her chart and drew pink hearts around the words.

"See how this works," I said. "Let me know if you need to change or add anything."

- **Ask, "What has helped you the most to…?"**

"You said math is your hardest subject and you want to get better at finishing your work," I said to 12-year-old James. "What has helped you the most to get your math done?"

"I tell myself, 'Just do it. I want to get this done and over, and then I don't have to do it anymore.' And when I'm done, I think about how I did a good job."

"Sounds like you tell yourself to just get it done so you don't have to worry about it. So those words you tell yourself help you face a hard challenge?"

"Exactly."

Help Children Discover and Expand Their Strategies

Children might be thinking:
I have an idea.
Maybe this will help.
My friends give me lots of ideas.
I can help myself. Now I know that works.
Let me decide.
This works best for me.
I know what works best for me.
I like these strategies the best.

To help children help themselves, increase their awareness of the strategies that are already in their repertoire. Next, assist them in expanding the number of helpful actions or applying them in other areas of their lives. Talk with them about their preferences and how and when they want to use the ideas. You also can have children add a personal touch to their strategies.

Increase Awareness of Personal Strategies

As therapy progresses, continue to assist children in recognizing their strategies. Ask the group to share their helpful approaches with each other. To promote awareness, encourage children to think about and identify what they did to get through a difficult situation. You also can mention a specific successful situation and inquire what they did that made a difference. Encourage children to apply strategies that they have used in the past. Ideally, make it a habit to ask for children's ideas before offering your suggestions.

Fabulous Five: Facilitate the Recognition of Personal Strategies

- **Mention children's strengths when trying to identify a strategy.**

Ten-year-old Jake sat in his wheelchair sobbing. The paraprofessional said, "I don't know what's wrong and I can't get him to stop crying."

I walked over to him and said as I gently stretched his shoulders back, "I can see you are not feeling good. I don't know if your teeth are bothering you or if you have leg cramps. First, take deep breaths. I know you're not feeling good, but you have to use your mind to get yourself calm. The more you cry, the tighter your muscles get. It's not helping. Use your mind to think calm thoughts. I know you've done that in the past. You can do it."

After a few seconds, he stopped.

"Good, you calmed yourself," I said, and then asked him to use his communication device to tell us what was wrong.

- **Tell children you have noticed a change and ask what helped.**

"Andy, I remember that in the fall it was hard for you to pay attention to your teacher. But today I noticed you really kept your eyes on your teacher when she was giving directions. What did you discover that helps you with your attention?" I asked the third grader.

"I clear my mind of distractions in the room and I tell myself, 'Focus.'"

- **Have children identify their favorite strategies.**

In January, the teacher and the social worker in the self-contained third- and fourth-grade class gave each student a plastic basket. "This is your own strategy basket. Let's make a list of all the things you can do to keep yourself calm," the teacher said and pointed to the board.

"You can take a walk," Umberto shouted.

"Use headphones if it's too noisy," another child added. The list grew.

The social worker then handed each child five cards. "On each card, draw the picture of the strategy that helps you, and write the words on the back. Make as many cards as you want. When you're done, we'll laminate them and you can keep them in your basket. When you want to use a strategy, just hand us the card."

Umberto drew himself as a stick figure of a boy sleeping at his desk, turned over the card, and wrote, *Ask for a break*. For his other cards, he added *talk to an adult, draw, find a quiet place,* and *use a heavy pillow.*

"Umberto, here's paper to put in your basket for drawing," his teacher said. "Also put your lapbag in your strategy basket."

- **Have the group share their strategies with each other.**

"When you are mad, what do you do to get yourself calm?" I asked the group of third graders as they colored.

"When I'm mad, I take a self-timeout."

"When I'm mad, I go outside and play with my friends."

"I go to my room and tell myself, 'Don't punch anything.'"

- **Ask the group about their strategies and then offer your ideas.**

"When Haley hears loud noises, she stops doing her class work and stares at the wall for 5 to 10 minutes," her fourth-grade teacher said. I explained how the 10 year old's difficulty with sensory processing might be a factor, and we agreed that it would be useful to teach her some sensory strategies.

The next day in the therapy group, I said, "In all the groups, we have been teaching ways to keep calm. First of all, what kinds of things upset you?"

"I don't like when kids say mean things," Sabrina said.

"I don't like it when it gets too loud," Haley added.

"What do you do to stay calm and focused?" I asked.

"I take a big breath," Haley replied.

"I count to 10," Sabrina said.

"Those are good ways. Let me show you a few more ideas you can use when you feel upset or overwhelmed," I said and demonstrated chair push-ups and pushing palms together with force.

Have Children Decide on Their Strategies and Implementation

A critical aspect of collaboration is to ensure that those involved have a voice. For this to occur, children must have a say in decision making. They also must be invited to participate in the process of negotiating and compromising. When determining strategies, listening to what children say is important to them. Acknowledge their feelings and perspectives. As much as possible, honor their choices or try to find ways to compromise.

You can involve children by asking about their favorite strategies and encouraging them to implement them more often or in a different area. Together, you may want to create a photo book illustrating the ideas. You can then read the book to the child. You also could read the book to a class and make the child the expert by demonstrating the strategies. To create a sense of ownership, have them personalize their strategies, such as drawing corresponding pictures. This often appeals to them as they get to use their imagination and be creative. Making them part of the process conveys respect and may lead to meaningful and more effective interventions.

Fabulous Five: Involve Children in Decision Making When Developing and Implementing Strategies

- **Honor children's choices.**

Watching 3-year-old Hank during his first week of preschool, the teachers and I noticed he was W-sitting due to tightness in his leg muscles. The physical therapist brought different chairs to try to see what would put him in the best position. "We just want to find a seat that is comfy for you. Try these," I said to Hank.

We tried a triangle-shaped cushion. It made him slump more. Then we tried a wooden chair with no legs that provided back support and allowed him to sit on the floor with his classmates. Next, we tried a chair with padding that was a perfect fit. His feet touched the ground. His hips and knees were at 90 degrees, but he was sitting higher than his peers. "What do you think, Hank? Do you like this chair?" we asked.

He put his palms on his cheeks, leaned forward, and became teary-eyed. "It's okay," I said. "We are just trying these. Which one do you like?" He pointed to the wooden chair. Recognizing his desire to be like the other children, we honored his choice.

- **Have children figure out a way to consistently implement the strategy.**

Ten-year-old Tory had a history of rocking his body back and forth, jumping out of his seat, and at times rolling on the floor. When I saw him, I asked, "Are you using the strategies you picked to use in class?"

"I can't seem to remember."

"I hear you are good at pushing your hands together when your teacher reminds you. At times, we all need reminders when we learn something new. But now that you're getting older, the next step is for you to do the strategies by yourself. What might help you remember without your teacher's reminders?"

"Hmm. I could draw a picture of me doing pushes and put it on my desk."

"Great idea. Here's some paper."

- **Work together to create a photo book of strategies.**

Four-year-old Dean knocked over a bookcase and threw a wooden toy at his teacher. A few hours later, when he was calm, I met with him. "What happened today?"

"I got mad."

"The pushing and throwing is getting you in trouble and can hurt people. What else could you do?"

"I don't know."

"I have an idea. Let me know what you think. We could make your very own special book on what to do when you get mad. I can even take pictures of you doing the ideas."

"Okay."

"I have a list here. Tell me which ones we should put in the book." After he made his choices, we created the following book with one sentence and a corresponding picture of Dean on each page:

My Strategy Book
When I get mad, my body feels hot and tight.
I tell myself stop.
I blow out a candle with big breaths.
I think of what else I can do.
I can take a break and go to the blue couch and be quiet.
I can use my calming pillow.
I can lift my body off the chair.
I can push my hands together.
I can make myself feel better.
I keep myself safe. I keep my friends and teacher safe.

- **Have the children create a booklet describing their own strategies.**

"Let's make a book of ideas of what you can do if you are upset," I said to the group of 11 year olds. They drew pictures and wrote:

I go to my bedroom and write or listen to music.
I walk away.
I take a deep breath and tell myself, "Do something to keep your mind off of it."
I play with my basketball if I'm outside.
I write a story.

"Thanks for sharing these. You have creative ideas for calming yourself."

- **Encourage children to personalize their strategy.**

"Today you get to make your own mad box. Everyone gets mad at times," I said to the group of 9 year olds in the day treatment. "When you get mad, you can choose what to do. For example, when I get mad, I choose to go for a walk to calm down, and I choose not to hit people because it hurts them and does not make things better.

"You can use this mad box as one way to get calm. Everyone gets a box. You can use these markers to color it and make it your own. When you're done, fill your box with these Styrofoam peanuts. When you start to get mad, you can throw these peanuts as hard as you can."

Dallas drew a black dragon shooting red spikes. Then he grabbed a peanut, threw his arm back like a baseball pitcher, and tried to slam it to the ground.

The group chuckled as the peanut slowly fluttered to the floor.

Promote Self-Monitoring and Evaluation

> **Children might be thinking:**
> *I did pretty good.*
> *I accomplished a lot.*
> *I did a good job.*
> *Keep doing….*

When children are involved in the process of self-monitoring and evaluation, they become more aware of their bodies, feelings, and actions. Doing so promotes self-reflection and gets them more attuned to themselves. Identifying their current state is also an important step for developing self-regulation. Another benefit is that children learn to rely on themselves instead of waiting for feedback from others. They come to realize that they know their own bodies, feelings, and typical ways of doing things and can figure out what to do.

Self-monitoring and evaluation also can provide children with a sense of satisfaction and achievement as they see what they have accomplished that day. They tend to find it rewarding to have a visual representation of their efforts and feel good being able to tell themselves, "Wow, look at what I was able to do today."

Fabulous Five: Involve Children in Self-Monitoring and Evaluation

- **Have children identify a goal at beginning of the session and judge it at the end.**

I showed 6-year-old Robert a paper with the words, *I will…* and said, "Before we start, tell me your goal that you want to try to do during our time together today."

"Be good and try something hard," he responded.

At the end of the session, I said, "Show me thumbs-up if you were good or thumbs-down if you need to get better. Did you write all the letters of your name on the board and practice doing the letter 'b' in a different way?" He put his thumbs up. "Did you finish cutting?" Another thumbs-up. "Did you stay with the game even when it was hard?" Again, he indicated yes. "So did you meet your goal to be good and try something hard?"

"Yeah!"

"I agree."

- **Use a checklist and let children check when each item is done.**

"We've come up with a plan for Connor," his preschool teacher told me. "There is a checklist of the major activities of the day. For each activity, he draws a smiling face if he follows the rules of listening and keeping himself, his friends, and property safe. If he does not, he draws a frowning face. If he has five smiling faces at the end of the day, he gets to pick a small prize out of the treasure chest. That way if he has trouble with one activity, he can recover and try to do better with the other activities. He can always turn his day around."

In the class, I watched Connor carry around his clipboard with the checklist. During opening group, he sat quietly and did not poke his friends as he had done in the past. Afterward, with a serious expression, he took the clipboard and drew a smiling face.

- **Say, "You tell me what you think and then I'll tell you what I think."**

Six-year-old Sadie rubbed her finger over the letters of her name made out of putty. "Now trace the letters with your eyes closed," I said.

She squinted and, without looking, moved her finger over each letter. Then I showed her a paper with her name written using a yellow highlighter. "Next, make the letters inside the yellow lines."

When she was done, I placed her name card in front of her. "Now print your name." When she had copied all the letters, I said, "Check it and tell me what you think. Then I will tell you what I think."

Sadie looked and said, "I did it right!"

"I agree. You did the letters just right."

- **Have children use stamps to reflect their effort.**

When I met 4-year-old Bradley, I said, "We are working on helping you get better at cutting and printing your name. I brought this cool chart." I pointed to the picture symbols for cutting and printing, each with a corresponding row. "If you do try cutting and printing, at the end you can pick out a stamp and the color of ink you want to use. I have really fun stamps. When this is all full, we can show your mom and dad how hard you have worked."

At the end of the session, Bradley picked a sun stamp and purple ink. He smiled as he made a purple sun next to each picture.

- **Have children use a prop to evaluate themselves.**

In the day treatment, I taught the class the Alert Program for Self-Regulation (Williams & Shellenberger, 1996) using the metaphor of a car engine. "Your body is like a car engine. Sometimes your engine may be too slow, too fast, or just right. You want to get your body just right. If your engine is too slow or too fast, use the sensory strategies we have been practicing."

The next week I brought a laminated half-circle. On it were three sections with the words *too slow, just right,* and *too fast* with corresponding car pictures. It also had an attached and movable arrow. As I showed the group, I said, "To help you get to know your body, you can move the arrow to how you are feeling. If you are feeling your body is going too fast or too slow, remember to use our sensory strategies like chair push-ups, pushing your hands together, or taking deep breaths."

As the group started a fine motor activity, Joel began bouncing in his seat and almost fell off his chair. I brought the prop over and said, "Joel, how is your engine right now?"

He stopped, thought for a minute, and moved the arrow to the words *too fast*.

"I see that too," I said. "What do you want to do to get your body just right?"

He responded by putting his hands on the side of his chair and lifting his body.

"Good idea!"

Encourage Children to Seek Information, Find Support, and Think of Alternatives

To become advocates for themselves, children need to gather information that is vital for making decisions. In addition, they need to seek support and use various resources to assist them in the process. Having gained the necessary information and knowing what help is available, they are in a better position of being able to think of alternatives.

Promote Seeking Information and Using Resources

Children might be thinking:
I know who is good at helping me.
I know where to go for help.

Encourage children to discover where information is available and who can help. Ask them, "What can you do to find out about...?" If they do not know, assist them to find the answers. Similarly ask who they can talk to, who has helped them in the past, and/or who they know who is available for support. Let them know they are not alone and that there are people, including you, who will be there for them.

Fabulous Five: Help Children Seek Information and Use Resources

- **Ask children who they can go to for help.**

"When you are at school, who can you go to for help?" I asked 12-year-old Bart.

"My teacher or my friends. I can go to Mr. B. if I need help with my assignments. He's my geography teacher."

"Is he good at helping kids?"

"Yes. He has helped me in the past. He gave me an idea for a game that was my homework."

- **Describe a situation and ask the group who can help them.**

"If someone is being mean to you or your friends, who can you get to help?" I asked the preschool class during our social group.

"My mom, my dad, a teacher," the children yelled out. "My grandma, an adult."

- **Ask, "Who can you talk to if you are having a hard time/day?"**

"Who can you talk to if you are having a hard day?" I asked 11-year-old Doug.

"My mom. She works in a middle school. She knows a lot about the situations. She knows what kids are like."

- **Inquire, "What can you do to find out about...?"**

"What can you do to find out about your assignments if you left your notebook at school?"

"I can just go online and check the school website," 11-year-old Brandon replied.

- **Ask, "Who has helped you when...?"**

"Who has helped you when kids are bullying you?"

"I went to our counselor," 12-year-old Derrick replied. "He's nice. He understands me."

"How did he help you in the past?"

"He talked to the people who were being mean to me."

"It's nice to have an adult like that."

Encourage Children to Think About Possible Strategies and Solutions

Children might be thinking:
I figured out what to do.
I thought of a good solution.
Yea, I did it. I came up with an idea that worked.

As you work with children, continue to teach them to reflect on how to help themselves. Ask questions about the situation and specific circumstances. Select questions that will assist them in clarifying the issue. Then encourage self-reliance by having them determine helpful and effective solutions. You can assist children to create this mentality by telling them to ask, "What can I do to help myself?" Continue to promote self-reflection by soliciting ideas. If their actions are problematic, you can say, "What could you do differently?" or "What else could you say?" Suggest they try their ideas and see what happens. You will find that when children identify their own solutions, they are more likely to use them.

Fabulous Five: Expand Children's Strategies

- **Ask questions requiring children to reflect.**

"I'm not going to write," 10-year-old Ben told his teacher.

"How come? You did the writing last week."

"Because I felt like it."

"What is different this week?"

"I'm tired."

- **Teach children to ask, "What can I do to help myself?"**

Eight-year-old Walker wrote three words and then stared at a crayon box on the table. Because his wandering attention often kept him from completing his work, I said, "Here's the problem. You are trying to write, but you keep looking at that box. I have noticed that sometimes it's hard for you to keep your mind on what you are doing. When that happens, a good thing to do is to ask, 'What can I do to help myself?' So what can you do now?"

"I can move the box," he said, flashing a proud smile.

- **Assist children to identify better solutions.**

"I use 'heck' a lot," 5-year-old Troy said. "My teacher doesn't like it."

"What else could you say?" I asked.

"'Oh my goodness' or 'oh my gosh.'"

"Those are better words to use in school."

- **Ask, "What could you do differently?"**

"I screamed in my sister's ear," 8-year-old Devon said.

"Did that make things better?"

"No."

"What could you do differently next time when you get mad?"

"Tell my mom."

- **Mention what you see children doing and ask for ideas on what would help them.**

"I noticed that when your teacher gave directions, you were looking out the window and you missed what she said. What could you do to help yourself pay better attention to the teacher?"

"Hmm," 6-year-old Belinda said, fidgeting with her yellow pencil. "Could I have a squeeze ball? Sometimes that helps when I use that with you."

I nodded.

Collaborate With Children in Decision Making

To be true partners, children must have a say in decision making. You need to get their input, acknowledge their right to dissent, and recognize choices made both verbally and nonverbally. You want them to have a say regarding their environment as well as the strategies they will be using.

Get Children's Input When Making Decisions

> **Children might be thinking:**
> *This is what I think.*
> *Please listen to me.*
> *Thanks for letting me have a say.*
> *This is what is important to me.*

Only giving children choices for decisions is not the same as giving them a voice. Choice is not voice. Children may not like or want to do any of your choices. Elicit children's perspectives and ask them to tell you more about what they are thinking. If needed, get them the critical information required to make decisions. Inquire about their ideas for handling difficult situations and use guiding questions to think about possibilities.

Fabulous Five: Obtain Children's Input When Making Decisions

- **Encourage children to share their perspective with those making decisions.**

"I don't want to stay there 2 years," 5-year-old Beau said.

"Are you talking about something at school or at home?"

"School. If I don't go to another grade, if I have to stay, I wouldn't like it because it would be boring and I would already know it. I would do the same thing."

"Be sure to tell your parents and teacher what you are thinking."

- **Ask children what they are thinking.**

After spending months in the small, self-contained special program, 11-year-old Jed started going to the regular classroom. To check what he thought about the change, the certified occupational therapy assistant said to him, "Touch my hand if you miss the class with Miss G." After 30 seconds, he touched her hand.

"Touch my hand if you like the sixth-grade class." After a minute of waiting and no touch, she said, "Touch my hand if you would like to do both."

Thirty seconds later, he touched her.

"Thank you for telling me."

- **Give the information needed to make decisions.**

Eleven-year-old Dante was admitted to the children's hospital to control his diabetes. The next day, he met with the dietitian and me in the occupational therapy clinic. After the dietitian explained how to balance what was in his diet using exchanges, I showed him a cookbook of adapted recipes for children with diabetes.

"Pick something you want to make for lunch and you can cook it here," I said. "It's really important to know what you can eat. Although your mom can help you, she is not with you all the time. It is your body. You need to know how to keep yourself from getting too high or too low. We want you to feel good throughout the day."

He thumbed through the book and stopped at the page with macaroni and cheese. After I obtained the ingredients the next day, he cooked his lunch. As he put it on the table, he smiled, looking pleased with himself.

- **Ask for children's ideas on how to handle a situation.**

"We're playing volleyball in P.E.," 10-year-old Amelia told me. "I'm not good at all. I'm the shortest one, and it's really hard for me."

"What do you think you could do to make it better?" I asked.

"I'm thinking about asking my mom if I can take lessons."

"Talk with your mom and see what she says," I replied.

The next week, Amelia stopped by and said, "My mom said okay. I'm taking lessons at the recreation center. I'm getting better."

"Sounds like you had a good idea."

- **Say, "What do you think about doing/using…?"**

When I went into 7-year-old Bobby Joe's classroom, I saw him hunched over his paper. Being left-handed, his wrist was bent and he was printing under his hand. The next day I brought a slant board to his class. "I know you are left-handed, and this slant board has helped other children. It makes it easier to see what you are writing, helps you sit up more, and puts your hand in a more comfortable position. If you don't like this slant board, we can also just turn a binder sideways. It does the same thing. What do you think about trying this?"

"Okay." He placed his paper on it and his wrist straightened as he printed his name. "Yeah, I like it."

Recognize Children's Right to Dissent

Children might be thinking:
I am trying to tell you no.
Listen to me.
I want to do it myself.
I don't want to do that.
Let me try it first, and if I don't get it, you can help.

For children to have a voice, they need to be able to say no and have their wishes respected. Often when children say no, it is viewed negatively as an act of defiance. Instead, when you hear their dissent, explore what children are thinking and want. See if you can explore other options to respect their decisions. Additionally, listen to children when they indicate their decisions through nonverbal means.

Respond When Children Use Their Faces, Bodies, or Sounds to Say No

When safety is not a concern, collaborating with children in therapy means they have a right to say no and have their decision respected. For children who are nonverbal, you have to watch for the various ways this message is expressed. Some may cry, yell, or scream as their way of communicating no. Others may look away, turn their back to you, or drop their head to convey the same message.

Closely observe facial expressions. Look for signs on what they are trying to tell you. If they were able to talk, they would probably be saying, "No, don't do that," "No, I don't want to," or "No, don't. I want to do it myself." When you are able to recognize their message, you will be better at responding in a respectful way.

Fabulous Five: Recognize When Children Use Their Faces, Bodies, or Sounds to Express No

- **Be aware that crying may mean no.**

When the children in the specialized classroom sat down for a snack, I went over to 3-year-old Parker. I removed his straw and poked it into his juice box.

Parker collapsed to the floor and continued to cry for 5 minutes. Seeing the puzzled look on my face, his teacher said, "We have discovered that he wants to try doing things himself first. Then sometimes he will ask for help."

The next week at snack time, I saw that he had a sealed fruit cup. I watched as he struggled with it. Then I put my palm up and waited. He put the cup on my palm, and I opened it.

- **Recognize that yelling or screaming may be a way of saying no.**

Three-year-old Destiny ran into the occupational therapy clinic and sat on a platform swing. I quickly handed her three beanbags to throw at a target. She flung all three and missed. Then she jumped up and ran up and down a small ramp. I brought over a scooter board and said, "Try this."

She pushed it away and screamed, "Aaah."

"You're telling me you don't want this." Then I grabbed a teddy bear, string, and beads. "Mrs. Bear needs a necklace. Come to the table and make her one." Destiny followed me, and when I started to help her with the beads, she said, "Me do." Once she was finished, we tied the necklace around the bear's neck.

- **Recognize when looking away means no.**

"I see we have a new girl in the class. Can you tell me something about her?" I said to the teacher in the specialized class. We both glanced across the room at an 8-year-old girl in a wheelchair.

"That's Carla. She tends to keep her head down and to the side because she can see the best that way. You have to wait 20 to 30 seconds for her to respond. It helps to count while waiting. If she agrees with you, is happy, or is saying yes, she'll make a clicking sound. To say no or if she's upset, she will scrunch her face or look away."

- **Be aware that turning their back to you indicates no.**

When I came in to the preschool classroom, 3-year-old Roland saw me. I sat down in his left side. He immediately turned his back to me.

I thought that his actions indicated that he did not want me to work with him. So I turned to his classmate on the other side and talked with her. Periodically I looked over at Roland's coloring and smiled. When he shifted his body toward me and looked more relaxed, I said, "You're really good at staying in the lines when you color." He smiled. When he started cutting out his picture, he let me help him.

- **Be vigilant for when a child drops his or her head to means stop or no.**

"Levi's nice," 7-year-old Tina said to me.

"Tell him that," I replied.

"Levi, you're nice," she said and began lightly stroking his arm.

He dropped his head to his chest as he cringed.

"When he puts his head down, he's telling you to stop. When you touch his arm like that, it's like an uncomfortable tickle."

Respond to Children's "No" Gestures or Actions

Some children, especially nonverbal ones, also tell you no by their actions. Some may push the object or your hand away or drop to the floor. Others may simply walk away or go back to what they were doing. If they are frustrated, they may even hit you as a message. Again, label what you see, identify the possible underlying message, and make changes.

Fabulous Five: Respond to Children's Gestures or Actions Indicating No

- **Be aware that pushing objects off the table may mean no.**

When I put a jack-in-the-box toy in front of 3-year-old Valerie, she put her arm down and moved it across the table, knocking the toy off.

"You don't want this toy," I said.

Then I placed a vibrating ball on the table.

She reached for it as it bounced around. She held it against her chest and smiled when she felt the vibration.

- **Be sensitive that children's dropping to the floor may mean no.**

In February, the specialized class began making valentines by painting glue on the paper and sprinkling glitter. When 7-year-old Duncan felt the glue on his index finger, he looked at it, shook it, and yelled, "Uuu." He ran to the sink.

When I returned the next day to help the teacher finish the project, the children headed for the table. Duncan saw the valentines and dropped to the floor.

"I know it doesn't feel good when you get glue on your fingers," I said in response to his actions. "Look what I brought." I showed him a tube of glitter glue and a wet paper towel. "You just squeeze the tube, and the glitter and glue come out. If anything gets on your fingers, we can wipe it off with this wet paper towel. Finish your valentine. Your mom will love it."

He hesitated but then stood and joined the group.

- **Recognize that pushing your hand away means no.**

After 3-year-old Tanner completed three puzzles, he pointed to my container. I pulled out a squishy bear. "Would you like the bear?" I asked as I demonstrated squeezing him.

He pushed my hand away.

"No, you don't want that," I replied. "Okay. Let's find something else you would like."

- **Recognize that walking away may mean no.**

I placed a plastic mallet in 4-year-old Cody's hand and helped him to pound a golf tee into the pumpkin. When I removed my hand from his, he walked away. "You don't want to do this, okay." He grabbed two blocks and began banging them together. After a few minutes, I showed him other activities he could do.

- **Recognize that hitting may indicate no.**

In the specialized preschool classroom, Krista struggled to remove the puzzle pieces. She picked at the edges of the pieces with no success. I lifted the puzzle and tipped it over. All the pieces tumbled out. Krista turned to me and started hitting my arm. I moved away as I said, "You are mad. You wanted to take them out yourself."

Respond to Nonverbal Indications of a Choice

When children are nonverbal, you have to constantly observe for any subtle indications of their choices. To let them make decisions, you can use an inviting gesture and wait for them to respond. For instance, you can put your hand out with your palm facing up and wait. If children place their hand in yours, you know they have decided to use your help. Unfortunately, it is not uncommon for adults to forget to ask and wait. Often they will just take the children's hand and lead them to where they want them to go. Or they may provide help without checking to see if the child wants it.

When asking children to decide, let them respond in a way that is comfortable. Some may use sign language to convey their decision. Show them you heard their request or decisions by putting words to their actions. Doing so verifies you understood, respects their autonomy, and reaffirms your belief in their competence.

Fabulous Five: Be Responsive to Choices Made Nonverbally

- **Make an inviting gesture and wait for them to respond.**

On 3-year-old Nancy's first day in the specialized program, she looked around the room. "She's not talking yet," her mother said. "She's also sensitive to touch. She doesn't like to touch or hold things."

I joined Nancy as she walked to the sensory table. She felt the smooth sand for about 10 seconds, but then rubbed her hands. Then she went to another center and sat in a beanbag chair.

After a few minutes, I put my hand out with my palm up and waited. "Can I show you more?" I asked in a soft voice. A minute later, she put her hand in mine. We went over to a child-sized horse, and she allowed me to lift her on the saddle. I gently rubbed her hand on the fluffy mane for a few seconds. As soon as she started to lean over to the side, I quickly responded, "Oh, you want to get off. Let me help you."

- **Allow children to respond in a way that is comfortable.**

Although 4-year-old Ashley talked at home, she did not speak at school. At the beginning of our social group, the special education teacher told the group, "Tell us your name and how you are feeling today."

When it came to Ashley's turn, the teacher waited for her to speak. When Ashley remained silent, the teacher said, "This is our friend, Ashley." Then she held up a page showing children's faces with different emotions. "You can tell us how you feel or just point." Ashley touched the picture of a child with a smile. "Oh, you're happy. Thanks for telling us."

- **Respond to nonverbal requests for help.**

Five-year-old Lindsey slipped her pink jacket on. Next, she walked over to me and put my hand on the zipper. I responded by saying the words indicated by her action: "You want me to zip this for you. I would be happy to help you."

- **Respond to children's nonverbal communication regarding a decision.**

Three-year-old Jillian, who was nonverbal, liked wearing her pink knitted hat. As she played in the sensory table full of beans, the hat fell on the floor. She continued playing and did not retrieve it. Thinking she was done wearing it, I picked it up and started walking to her backpack.

She saw me and started crying. "You're telling me you still want your hat," I responded. "I thought you didn't want it anymore. Here, you can put it back on."

- **Watch for continuation cues.**

Four-year-old Justin bounced on the therapy ball with his feet on the floor. Supporting his body with my hands, I moved him to the left and the right, challenging him to keep his balance. When he was back in the middle, he bounced up and down. After a few minutes, I took my hands off him and he slid to the floor. He rested for a minute. Then he sat back on the ball, looked at me to resume, and signed "more."

I responded, "Okay, we'll do more."

Teach Children to Communicate With Others to Meet Their Needs

One cultural value in the Western world is the importance of teaching children to speak up for themselves and be assertive. This value is not shared by all cultures, and you need to be sensitive to what children are taught by their caregivers.

In the Western world, there are a number of advantages for being assertive. Speaking up provides a chance for children to express their wants and needs, informs others of their desires, and creates an opportunity to negotiate and find solutions. Being assertive facilitates children setting limits with peers, asking for assistance only when they want it, and getting the necessary help from friends and/or adults. After learning this skill and practicing, children tend to feel empowered versus helpless. They also learn that talking, not aggression, leads to better solutions.

Teach Assertiveness

Children might be thinking:
I'm not sure if I should say something.
I don't have the nerve to do it.

Children want to get their needs met but may not know what words to say. Young ones sometimes use hitting as a way to get what they want. For example, if another child tries to take a toy away from them, they may respond by hitting instead of saying, "Stop."

It can be helpful to proactively teach a group or class how to be assertive. Let them know that others will not know what they want if they do not speak up. Encourage them to use "I" statements, such as telling a classmate, "I don't like it when you hit me." You also can coach them in the moment when they are in conflict with a peer. Tell them to avoid name-calling or blaming the other person, such as saying, "You are a...." Emphasize how speaking up with words will increase their chances of getting what they want, whereas aggression will only make things worse and get them in trouble. For some it will be easier to learn if you create a Social Story with pictures and the exact words to use to make requests. In addition, talk about how good it feels when their friends have stood up for them. Encourage them to do the same in return.

Fabulous Five: Teach the Skill of Assertiveness

- **Give children the words to use to express needs that include "I" statements.**

When standing in line, 5-year-old Justin had been hitting anyone who bumped into him. One day as the class gathered in line to go to recess, a classmate put his hands on Justin's back and pushed. He turned around and snarled. Immediately I told him, "Tell your friend, 'I don't like it when you push me. Keep your hands to yourself.'" Justin followed my directions.

- **Teach children to be assertive versus aggressive.**

"My cousin spit on me," 6-year-old Cedric said. "He was mad because I slapped his face."

"What were you mad about before you slapped him?"

"He called me names."

"So then you hit him and he spit on you. Did hitting him make things better?"

"No," he replied reluctantly.

"What words could you use instead of hitting?"

"I could tell him, 'Stop, I don't like that. That's not nice.'"

"Those are good words. And if he doesn't stop, get an adult."

- **Use a Social Story (Gray, 2010) to teach how to make requests.**

After seeing 3-year-old Brandy only playing by herself but often looking at her classmate, the teacher and I talked with her father.

"She's extremely shy," he said.

Together we talked about using a Social Story to help join her peers. We wrote the following:

Sometimes I see my friends playing.
I like to play too.
I can go to my friends and say, "Can I play with you?"
My friends will like that I use my words to ask them.

Later, the teacher read her the story and had her draw pictures of herself and her friends. I helped her practice with different classmates.

- **Encourage children to look at the person and use "I" statements.**

When 4-year-old Derrick tried to grab the shovel, Regina did not let go. He dropped his hold on it but then scooped a handful of sand and threw it at her.

Regina cried as she continually blinked to get the sand out. When she stopped, I said, "Look at him and tell him, 'I don't like it when you throw sand.'"

She marched over to him, put her hands on her hips, and said, "Derrick, I don't like it when you throw sand. That hurt my eyes."

"Sorry," he replied.

- **Teach children to use a strong voice when asserting themselves.**

Three-year-old Rodney started mid-year in the preschool class. His small stature made him look like a 2 year old. "He looks like a baby," one classmate said loudly.

I turned to Rodney and said, "Tell him you're not a baby, you're 3 years old."

Rodney whispered the words.

"Use a strong voice so he can hear you."

Rodney looked at the classmate and repeated the words in a louder voice.

Promote Asking for Help

Children might be thinking:
I want to do it myself.
I need help.
I have to remember to use words.
I know how to stand up for myself. I just don't do it.

Another aspect of self-advocacy is being assertive in asking for assistance when needed. You can teach children this skill by encouraging them to use sign language or words, such as saying, "Help, please" (Figure 9-2). Let them know it is okay to ask for assistance from adults or peers and that using words is necessary because people around them may not notice that help is desired.

Tell children you would like for them to ask when they need or want assistance. Make it a habit to wait and allow them to decide whether and when they want help. If they feel embarrassed because they require more assistance than

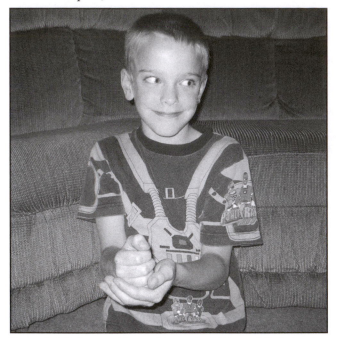

Figure 9-2. Before providing assistance, let children ask for help using words or sign language.

others, suggest that they create an inconspicuous signal to indicate their wish for support. When you let them decide, you show that you recognize their abilities and potential, and do not view them as helpless. You are giving them a chance to show what they know or to try something new without your interference.

Fabulous Five: Encourage Children to Ask for Help When Desired

- **Teach children to use words to ask for help when they want it.**

Three-year-old Jessica stood in front of me and handed me her pink jacket.

"Say, 'Help, please,'" I said.

"Help, please."

"I would be happy to. Thanks for using words to ask me."

- **Teach children to use sign language to ask for help when they want it.**

Five-year-old Cici stood at the coat rack and lifted her coat to put on the hook. When she could not reach it, she dropped her purple coat on the floor and looked at me.

"If you would like help, just ask," I said, and demonstrated the sign language for help by placing my right fisted hand on my left palm and lifting both hands.

- **Teach children to ask an adult or friend for help when they want or need it.**

"This will make a pretty butterfly if you follow the directions," the speech-language pathologist told the group of kindergartners. "Color all the triangles blue and all the squares yellow."

"Look, I traced inside the triangle. Now I'm going to fill it in," Gina said.

Erin kept coloring, and 30 seconds later she turned to her friend Gina. "What color for the squares?"

"Yellow."

"You used a strategy. You couldn't remember the directions so you asked a friend for help. What is another strategy? What if nobody heard the direction? Who could you ask?" Erin pointed her finger in my direction. "Yes. You can always ask an adult, like your teacher, and ask, 'Could you please say that again?' And if you do not understand the words, just ask the person to use different words."

- **Encourage the children to tell themselves, "I just need to ask for help."**

"I'm stupid," Dan said when he did not understand the teacher's direction.

"Instead of telling yourself that, tell yourself that you just need to ask for help," I replied to the second grader. "It's okay. Everyone needs help with something,"

- **Develop an inconspicuous way for children to signal if they need assistance.**

When I observed the third-grade class, I saw Alyse respond with a blank look and inaction for five of the teacher's directions. I saw her that afternoon and said, "When I was in your class, I noticed that it was hard for you to follow your teacher's directions."

"Yeah, sometimes I don't get it and I wonder what I'm supposed to do."

"I know that sometimes it's embarrassing to always be the one asking the teacher to repeat the directions. What some kids have done that you might want to do is ask your teacher if the two of you can create a signal for when you need help. Would you like to try something like that or do you have any other ideas?"

"I like that idea," she said. We then met with her teacher, and everyone decided the signal would be for her to raise her index finger.

Practice Assertiveness

Children might be thinking:
I'm nervous.
This is hard.
Will you come with me?
I found out it is easier to do with a friend or adult I trust.

Becoming assertive requires practice in different situations. For example, children may feel comfortable asking their parents for what they want but may hesitate to speak up with their peers. If you see situations where children are hesitating, find out what they want and if they know what to say. Practice with them the words they can use. Encourage them to speak up and get support from friends or adults if they need it. You can also provide moral support by offering to go with them while they do the talking. Convey your belief in their ability to be assertive and the benefits of doing so.

Fabulous Five: Have Children Practice Being Assertive

- **Explore why children are hesitating to speak up.**

"Are you a customer or a worker?" I asked 4-year-old Alexis in the center designed as a grocery store.

"Nothing."

"What's the matter?"

"I want to play with Janet and Brianna," she replied, pointing to two girls stacking cereal boxes.

"How come you are not telling them you want to play with them?"

"I'm too scared to ask."

Janet overheard the conversation. She took Alexis's hand and said, "You can ask me whenever you want to play. You don't have to be shy."

- **Teach children to ask for and get support.**

While 7-year-old Ryan and I were playing a writing game, he said, "I don't like Jacob."

"Did something happen this morning?"

"No. He just bothers me."

"What does he do?"

"He makes noises with Dylan and Jay."

"What do you do when he does that?"

"Nothing. I just don't like him."

"Have you talked to your teacher?"

"No. I don't want anyone to know."

"How about talking to Mary?" I suggested, referring to the social worker. "She's pretty good about helping kids. Your class is small so you see Jacob every day. You don't want to be grumpy every day because he bothers you."

"Okay."

"There are always going to be kids who bother you. So it's good to figure out what you can do."

"Yeah, so we can be friends."

- **Teach children how they can get their needs met and practice the strategy.**

Ian's mother approached me in the school hallway the week before the holiday break. "Ian has been having problems this past week. He's more whiny and clingy. His kindergarten teacher said he hit a kid who didn't want to read with him. Yesterday when two girls were crying, she said he went in the hall and said, 'I need a break.' He has gone to five birthday parties and just joined a new church group of 25 children."

I also heard from his teacher that the class was preparing for a holiday pageant and everyone was excited. Because Ian had a history of being sensitive to noise and easily experienced sensory overload, his mother, teacher, and I talked about where there could be a quiet space in the class. "He can sit at my desk at the far end of the second room. It's quiet there," his teacher proposed.

Then I spoke with Ian. "I know that sometimes the class can be really noisy. Is that true?" Ian's blond hair swayed as he nodded. "Well, I heard that you had a good idea. One time in class when it was too noisy, you said, 'I need a break.' I talked with your teacher, and she said if you want to take a break, you could sit at her desk where it is quiet. Does that sound okay to you?" He smiled and nodded. "So what can you say to your teacher if it's too noisy?"

"I need a break," he replied. Then, in his presence, I repeated the plan to his teacher, and Ian practiced saying the phrase to her.

- **Offer to go with children but have them do the talking.**

Four-year-old Skyler stood on the playground with her chin down. "Are you sad about something?" I asked, and she shook her head. "Tell me what's bothering you."

"I want a turn on the ball," she replied and pointed to the two girls on the Hoppy-Hop.

"Would you like me to go with you when you ask for a turn?" She nodded. "Let's go over. Say, 'Can I have a turn when you're done?'"

She did, and a few minutes later, a friend gave her a turn.

- **Leave it up to children to speak up or stand up for themselves.**

When observing Heath's class, I saw how he became upset when there were loud noises or commotion. I talked with his third-grade teacher and explored what were realistic options for dealing with sensory overload.

Next, I met with Heath about what ideas he had to keep himself calm. "I talked with your teacher, and she said if the noise is too much, you can ask to go to the quiet space at the back of the class or use headphones with the computer."

"That would be good," he replied.

"It's up to you to ask. So make sure you speak up for yourself."

Promote Standing Up for Others

> **Children might be thinking:**
> *I feel happy that my friend stood up for me.*
> *I feel like my friends care about me and they're really good friends.*

Recognize the times children come to the aid of others. If they are at the receiving end of a friend's assistance, ask them how it feels to have people who care about them. You also can talk about how nice it is to have friends who will get involved and intervene.

As children gain experience being assertive or seeing their friends come to their assistance, they learn about their own strengths and the value of friendship. They discover that having a circle of friends who look out for each other decreases their risk of being bullied. Let them know that the power of one person standing up for the rights of another can make a difference and inspire others.

Fabulous Five: Promote Standing Up for Others

- **Talk about how one person standing up can make a difference.**

"The name of this book is *One*, and the author is Kathryn Otoshi," the special education teacher said to the preschoolers during our social group. "In this story, Red is not a good friend, especially to Blue, and the others are afraid to tell him to stop. But when One stands up to the bully, everyone else does too. Red stops and becomes their friend." When she finished reading the story, she asked, "Now, do the colors want to stand up to the bully at first?"

"No-oo."

"If someone is picking on your friends or you saw a bully picking on someone, what could you do?"

"I would say, 'Stop!'"

"Tell a grown-up," another child added.

"Now what should you do if a bully is hitting you?"

"Protect yourself."

"Run away."

"Tell them, 'Stop!'"

"Get a teacher."

"Those are all good ideas."

- **Ask how it feels to have someone stand up for them.**

"My friend heard Callie was blackmailing me," 11-year-old Summer told me. "She was telling me, 'If you talk to Gavin or his sister, you won't be my friend or come to my birthday party.' My friend Gavin stays late at school since his mom works at the school. Gavin talked to the dean of students. The dean helped me with Callie. He asked her to stop. Three teachers helped. I had a lot of help."

"How did you feel after that?"

"I felt like I was important. My friend cares about me. I feel safe now. Nothing to worry about anymore."

- **Talk about how nice it is to have friends who will stick up for them.**

"My friend, Justin, helped me today," 7-year-old Griffin said.

"What happened?" I asked.

"Ian was being mean. He kept asking me what kind of underwear I was wearing. Justin told him, 'Leave my friend alone. That's none of your business.'"

"It must feel good to have a friend stick up for you."

"Yeah, he's a good friend."

- **Recognize when the children speak up for friends or others.**

"Yesterday my friend, Alyssa, hit her head. She was on the spinning thing on the playground. Anyway, Alyssa hit her head on Kira's head. There was blood everywhere. We found out it was Alyssa's blood. I told them I would take her to the nurse. Ella came over and said, 'I knew this would happen. It's all Kira's fault.' I told her, 'She didn't do it on purpose.'"

"I bet Kira appreciates having a friend like you," I said.

- **Acknowledge when children take action to aid or protect friends.**

When 3-year-old Robin reached for the magnetic blocks on the table, 4-year-old Brent shouted, "No, mine," and shoved her off the chair.

Four-year-old Marco marched over to Brent and said, "Don't push." He helped Robin back up, put his arm around her, and asked, "Are you all right?"

She nodded.

"That's nice you are such a good friend to Robin," I told Marco.

Recognize Assertiveness

> **Children might be thinking:**
> *Talking helped.*
> *I feel good speaking up.*

When you see children speaking up for themselves or others, acknowledge their efforts. Being assertive is not always easy (Figure 9-3). Let them know that you appreciate hearing what they want or need, which allows you to better help them. Also recognize when they handled situations independently and point out the successful results of being assertive.

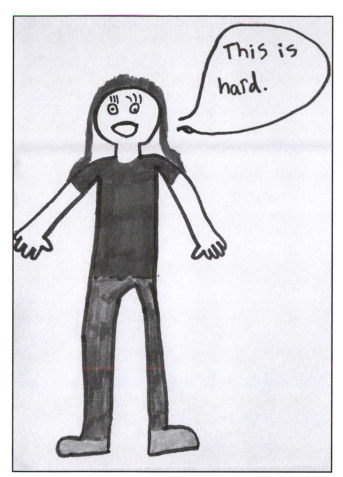

Figure 9-3. For many children, being assertive takes courage.

Fabulous Five: Recognize When Children Are Being Assertive

- **Acknowledge when children speak up for themselves.**

In the preschool classroom, Chase perseverated on keeping all the toys in the same place. He cried and yelled, "No, no, no," if anyone touched the toy fruit. Then he went to 4-year-old Amanda and tried to grab the plastic banana out of her hand to put it back in the container.

Amanda held on to it. "Stop, Chase. I want to play with this."

I intervened and distracted Chase. Then I turned to Amanda and said, "I'm glad you told him what you wanted."

- **Acknowledge the success of their effort when children stand up for themselves.**

While doing a science experiment, 11-year-old Brooke told me, "In this class, Cameron was punching and poking me in the arm. It's been going on for a week. On Friday, after school, my friend Bethany and I went to Mr. D. We told him I needed a new seating arrangement so Cameron wouldn't poke me anymore. Mr. D did that

immediately. Now I'm sitting next to my best friend, Katelyn."

"It's great you said something. That worked out really well. Cameron is no longer poking you, and you are with your best friend. Good for you."

- **Tell children that they took care of the situation all by themselves.**

"Stop pulling my hair," 3-year-old Amanda said to Carson. "Teacher."

"You did good," her teacher replied. "You used your words and told him to stop. You took care of it all by yourself."

- **Thank children for telling you what they need.**

While sitting in his wheelchair, 6-year-old George grimaced. His right hand slowly inched toward his new communication device. Three minutes later, he touched the screen he wanted. The voice from the device said, "My muscles are really tight. I need to stretch."

"Thank you for telling me," I replied, and moved him out of the wheelchair onto the therapy mat.

- **Give feedback when children tell others what they need.**

During the first week of school, Kyle's new third-grade teacher told me, "I was impressed. Kyle approached me and asked for a three-ring binder he could use for a slant board. He said it helped him write better."

"That's great he asked on his own!" I replied. "When he turns the binder sideways, it puts his paper more upright and moves his hand into a better position."

When I saw him later that day, I said, "Mrs. B told me you asked for the binder. You are so smart. You remembered what helped you, and you asked for it."

Have Children Teach Each Other

You show children you believe in them by recognizing their competencies. Acknowledge their life experience and what they have learned. View them as resources for others. Encourage them to share their suggestions, strategies, and words of wisdom.

Have Peers Identify Strategies to Help One Child

Children might be thinking:
My friend is trying to help me.
My friend suggested this—maybe I can try it.
My friend knows what it is like.
My friend knows what to help me with.

As children become older, they place more value on what their peers have to say. They may believe that peers understand them or their situation better than adults. Because peers, unlike adults, do not have power over them, children may be more open to their ideas and more apt to listen. Children will often have a history of confiding in each other, whereas they may wonder if they can trust you. In contrast, at times when adults suggest ideas, children may think they are being told what to do. Also, suggestions from friends may be viewed as a mutual exchange. To promote the sharing of strategies and helpful solutions, encourage children to talk with each other.

Fabulous Five: Use Peers as Resources

- **Ask peers or classmates how they would feel in that situation and what they do to make themselves feel better.**

In the outpatient oncology clinic, 7-year-old Carol heard that she had to be hospitalized for chemotherapy and came into my room crying. When I tried to talk with her, she just stared at the floor. I turned to another child named Tina and asked her, "Is it upsetting for you when you find out you have to go to the hospital?" She nodded. Carol subtly glanced at me and was clearly listening.

"Tina, what do you do to make yourself feel better?"

"I draw."

I picked up markers, paper, and a puzzle. I placed them on the table in front of Carol.

Tina grabbed a puzzle and began emptying the pieces out onto the table.

A few seconds later, Carol started a puzzle and stopped crying.

- **Have a group provide ideas for alternatives.**

At the day treatment, 9-year-old Jack announced to the group, "I was in jail over the weekend for hitting my mom. I wasn't handcuffed. I'm going to court. My dad is getting me."

"Sounds like hitting got you in trouble and you hurt your mom." I turned to the rest of the group. "What else can you do when you're mad that will not hurt anyone?"

"When I'm mad, I go to my room and play music," Robert replied.

"I take a break," another responded.

- **Acknowledge a peer's ideas to help.**

While playing on the playground, 8-year-old Brent saw the look of anger on his friend's face. He went over and said, "If you're mad, breathe in five times, breathe out five times, and then walk away."

"You're being a good friend," I told him a few minutes later. "You gave him ideas on how to get himself calm and stay out of trouble."

- **Encourage children to listen to peers for ideas to help them.**

"Some kid knocked me down, stepped on my hair, and said I was garbage," 9-year-old Alice said in our small group.

"No one wants to sit by her in music and art," Elizabeth, her classmate, added.

"They're jealous because they don't have my red hair."

"When that happens, tell an adult," Elizabeth said. "If an adult does not listen, tell another adult, and if that person does not listen, tell the principal."

- **Ask the group to generate ideas to help a child.**

Nine-year-old Jacob slowly sat down in the chair and slid until his chin was on his chest. He sighed and lowered his eyelids as if he was going to sleep. "Jacob, what is the matter?" I asked.

"I feel low," he said, referring to a metaphor of a car engine. His group previously had learned about how they processed sensory information and had practiced strategies for when their bodies, like car engines, were revved up too high or too low.

I looked around the table and asked, "Does anyone have ideas of what he could do to help himself?"

"He could do chair push-ups fast."

"He could get a drink of water."

"He could put cold water on his face."

Jacob stood up, moseyed over to the sink, and splashed water on his face.

Encourage Children to Pass on Their Words of Wisdom

Children might be thinking:
I'm really happy and excited to tell what I know.
I'm happy you think I am wise and smart.

Children find it refreshing when adults recognize their wisdom. Seniors, more often than children, are thought to be wise. Yet if you ask children, you will find they have a unique perspective of the world and life. You, as well as other adults and peers, can learn from them. Be open to hearing what they have to say and give credence to their knowledge. In addition, provide opportunities and various avenues for sharing their words of wisdom.

Fabulous Five: Encourage Children to Share Their Words of Wisdom

- **Have children write an advice column as a way of helping each other.**

Six-year-old Buddy, sporting a blond buzz cut, shuffled his feet down the hallway and swaggered side-to-side, trailing three girls. When he entered the therapy room, he slid onto the preschool-sized chair, stretched his right arm on the table, and rested his cheek on his makeshift pillow. "I'm so tired," he said.

"How come you're tired?" I asked.

"It's so hard to go from kindergarten to first grade. You have to stay all day. You have to do homework, and you have to go to bed early." He sighed and released a deep breath. "It's sooo hard, and it's not fun."

"You're right. It is a big change," I said. He raised his head and reached for the scissors and red paper.

Later that afternoon, I worked with 11-year-old Chris on his writing and asked him, "Have you ever seen an advice column in the newspaper?"

"Yeah," he said.

"You are very wise, so I'm wondering if you could help a first grader by writing an advice column. You could be Dr. Chris."

"Sure," he said with a smile.

"I know it would be easier for him to listen to another kid rather than an adult." Then I relayed what Buddy had said. Chris chewed on the end of his pencil as he pondered what to write. Then he started his response.

Dear I'm So Tired,

Sometimes schoolwork can be fun, like writing. You can tell what you are thinking. Sometimes you can feel better when you tell someone what you are feeling at that moment or you can just feel good on your own. But mostly when you share a thought you have, if it is sad, happy, or just a daydream you see in your mind, you will feel better about it.

When you start to read, you will find that schoolwork will not be as tiring or boring as it is now. You will feel more comfortable with it.

Dr. Chris

In the next session with Buddy, I read him the letter and added, "I know it's hard now, but like Chris said, school will get easier and can even be fun." Although Buddy remained silent, his eyes softened and he looked relieved.

- **Create an advice book for children to sign when they leave.**

At the day treatment program, the social worker started a Book of Advice. As the children departed the program, they left a contribution. Children wrote:

Try to make friends by playing games.
Be nice to people, especially your teacher.
Don't pout. Talk.
Work hard to learn the rules.
If you get mad, count to 10 and think of a solution.

- **Ask for ideas on handling different situations.**

"Take a minute and write down your words of wisdom for how to get along," I told the two third graders. When they finished, I said, "Please read what you wrote."

"Use nice words," Savannah said.

"When someone is talking, don't shout out," Sarah read aloud. "Wait until they are done before you start talking."

- **Ask the group to share their strategies with each other.**

"What are good ideas that have helped you?" I asked the fourth graders. Their ideas were the following:

1. Tell yourself to focus.

2. If you are playing with something, put it back in your desk.

3. Clear your mind of all distractions in the room.

4. Do your work right away.

5. Don't make noises when you are reading.

6. Breathe in five times and walk away.

- **Create a Kids Helping Kids notebook.**

I held up a notebook and pointed to the title. "This is a Kids Helping Kids notebook. It is a place for you to write down any ideas you think would help others. Later we can share the ideas."

Ten-year-old Mitchell reached for it and wrote:

Tipse for board kids

In school:

1. You can solve a cuple of math problems in your head.

2. You can do some homework.

3. Aske for more work.

4. You can also write about what you are doing over the weekend in your jurnal.

At the movies:

1. You can crunch on some popcorn even slush it around.

2. You can use the bathroom.

3. Solve some questions in your head or make some.

4. Go out and buy an extra large soda and 3 boxes of candy and enjoye.

KEY POINTS TO REMEMBER

- Use therapy to promote children's self-knowledge and expectations of success.
- Help children discover and identify their successful strategies.
- Involve children in identifying and personalizing new strategies.
- Promote self-monitoring and evaluation.
- Encourage children to seek the needed information and use resources.
- Engage children in thinking of alternatives and solutions.
- Collaborate in decision making and be responsive to children's choices.
- Recognize and accept children's right to dissent.
- Teach children to let people know when they want help.
- Teach children how to communicate with others to meet their needs, including how to be assertive.
- Have children use their peers as resources and share their wisdom with each other.

REVIEW QUESTIONS

1. For children to advocate for themselves, they have to learn what helps and hinders them. True or false.

2. Involving children in deciding on and implementing strategies creates a sense of ownership. True or false.

3. Children tend to be unaware of how they are doing in school. True or false.

4. When children figure out their own strategies and solutions, they are more apt to use them. True or false.

5. Children who are nonverbal are unable to tell you no. True or false.

6. Children always want adult help. True or false.

7. It helps to reach for a young child's hand and walk with her or him to where she or he needs to go. True or false.

8. Being assertive is highly valued in Western culture. True or false.

9. It is helpful to give children the words to use if they continually have problems with peers. True or false.

10. It is easy for children to be assertive. True or false.

REFERENCES

Gray, C. (2010). *The new Social Stories book*. Arlington, TX: Future Horizons.

Williams, M. S., & Shellenberger, S. (1996). *How does your engine run? A leader's guide to the alert program for self regulation*. Albuquerque, NM: TherapyWorks.

Become Partners With You as a Guide

Chapter Overview

As you develop a partnership, your role is to guide the therapy process. In this chapter, ways to show that you have integrity and are trustworthy and genuine are discussed. Also included are methods to establish emotionally healthy personal boundaries—an essential skill for therapists. Another topic is about being a fun person and letting your personality shine forth.

Children's Descriptions of What They Think You Should Know

Dr. Clare: "What makes a good therapist?"

Kendall (age 10): "That they're cheerful and also nice. If they let us do fun stuff, that's cool."

Mick (age 11): "Kids have special needs. They need confidence."

Dr. Clare: "What can therapists do to help you get confidence?"

Mick: "They can help you."

Dr. Clare: "How should therapists act?"

Kris (age 8): "Really calm."

Buddy (age 6): "Be happy that you're here. Be nice."

Noah (age 11): "Be kind. Try to stay in a good mood even if you're getting grumpy."

Tina (age 9): "Be helpful."

Hector (age 10): "Be honest and trusting."

Brad (age 9): "They should be nice, caring, and fair."

Guide the Way

As a therapist, you guide children to and through change. Similar to a guide on a nature trail, you encourage them to take the first steps. Together, you choose the destination and the way to get there. You proceed at the children's pace and gradually shift to having them lead. For children to join you, they need to trust you.

Be Yourself

As a guide, you are unique as a person. You are like a diamond—no two are exactly alike. You bring your knowledge of (a) yourself, (b) children and caregivers, (c) occupational therapy philosophy, and (d) your repertoire of skills, strategies, and approaches. Knowledge of yourself entails being aware of your normal ways of being, your physical and emotional states, and the influence of your community and culture. Knowledge of children and caregivers is gained from your education and experience. Your occupational therapy philosophy includes occupational therapy theories, your knowledge about occupations, and various professional trainings and experiences as a therapist. Over the years, you also accumulate a variety of strategies and

Curtin, C.
*Strategies for Collaborating With Children: Creating Partnerships
in Occupational Therapy and Research* (pp. 187-202).
© 2017 SLACK Incorporated.

approaches as well as different skills for handling situations with children. During your time with children, be yourself—be genuine and be fun.

Be Genuine

> **Children might be thinking:**
> *I don't know about you.*
> *You tell the truth.*
> *You don't lie to me.*
> *You're okay.*
> *I can trust you.*

You want to interact with children in such a way that you continually present yourself as a safe person whom they can trust. When you are real, attune to feelings, and assume a positive attitude toward children, you cultivate the bond needed for therapy. Children will watch and quickly sense if you are being fake, which is important because they need honesty for trust. They also will be aware if you accept them for who they are and do not judge them.

Be Real

When you interact with others, it is important to be yourself, with all your strengths and imperfections. Children can sense if you are superficial or insincere. Because children rely more on nonverbal communication, they are very perceptive as to what kind of person you are. If you seem suspicious, the children may wonder, *What are you really like? Will you be mean to me?* If you are not genuine, they also will be leery of you. When children sense this falseness, they will not trust you. Just be yourself. Be honest. Be sincere. You will find that the more natural you are, the more you can relax.

In addition to being real, you also have to accept that you are human, with as many weaknesses as strengths. There are benefits to showing your human side. Children can relate to someone who is not perfect. For example, it is all right to admit that you make mistakes. This allows you to model how to handle problems and still feel good about yourself. Children learn that it is okay for them to fail and that there are ways to deal with imperfection.

Another way children can get to know you is through personal stories. Telling about your life can help children relate to you, especially if they discover you have something in common. Sharing funny life stories can be enjoyable for both of you.

> **Fabulous Five: Be Real**
> - **Be natural.**
>
>   Six-year-old George had a difficult time moving his body and, consequently, hesitated to write. So every time

he attempted to print letters on the board, I bounced an orange plastic figure with a pumpkin head and yelled, "Yahoo."

He smiled. "You're funny, Dr. Clare."

- **Be honest.**

In my first session with 8-year-old Matt, all the children used bamboo tongs to pull pennies out of putty. Matt played with the tongs by stretching the two ends apart and kept pulling until they snapped. I locked my eyes with his and said in a firm but nonthreatening voice, "Listen, I bought these with my own money. These are mine, and I'm upset that you broke them. Do you like it when someone breaks one of your toys?"

"No."

"Well, I don't like my stuff broken either. You have to play with my things right and not break them. Okay, just glue these two parts back together."

Matt fixed them and never broke another item.

- **Show sincerity and tactfulness.**

Craig was a fourth grader who had a gentle personality and limited social awareness. He frequently did not understand appropriate physical interactions. One day as we walked back to class, he smiled and swung his arm around my shoulder.

"Craig, I really like you. You know that?" I said. He nodded. "It's better if you don't put your arm on a teacher's shoulder like that. It's okay to do that with your family and with your friends if they give permission."

"Oh, okay," he replied, moving his arm back to his side.

- **Admit mistakes.**

Seven-year-old Steven stared at the paper with the name *Stephen* on it. "You spelled my name wrong."

"You're right. I'm sorry," I said. "Thank you for telling me."

- **Share personal stories that allow children to get to know you.**

"I have new kittens, and you will not believe what they did," I said.

"What?"

"They jumped in the bathtub with me. I had to shoo them out."

Eight-year-old Corey smiled at that story, and every week after that, we talked about our pets. When Corey's class created a newspaper, he wrote about the story I had told him:

The kittens, Sophie and Sara, jumped in the bathtub. What a sight to see. Sophie also jumped on the lamp shade and swung. The kittens are funny. Dr. Clare's roommate's pupy dug up the rebber tree plant. He also dug up the kittens' litter box. The pupy then fell asleep on Dr. Clare's pillow.

Know Yourself

Working with children can be a journey of learning for both you and them. Maintain an open mind and reflect on the ways you can personally grow as a therapist. Realize that you always have your own issues that you bring to an interaction. One way to become more aware is to ask yourself, "What kind of problems or conflicts do I have?" If, for example, you end up in multiple power struggles with children, you might want to examine whether you have a need for control. Another way is to explore what annoys you. After discovering your issues, you have to find ways to deal with them. Of course, this is a lifelong process.

It is also important to recognize your own needs and limitations. It is not a weakness to acknowledge your limits. All therapists need assistance at some time. Seeking help allows you to get another perspective and to explore other ways to handle the situation. At the same time, be genuine about emphasizing your strengths and talents. Be playful and laugh at yourself.

Fabulous Five: Know Yourself

- **Be open to learning from children.**

In the oncology clinic, the children came for check-ups once a month for 2 years. After a year passed, I knew Mary had to come to the clinic on her 11th birthday. I decided to get her a small present and bought brightly colored pencils and a notepad with musical notes sprinkled around the pages.

"Happy Birthday, Mary," I said. "I have something for you."

She beamed as she unwrapped the package. She fingered the pencils and said, "This is the only present I got."

I was surprised and wished I had bought her something bigger. However, I learned from her that even a small gift or gesture can make a difference.

- **Ask yourself, "What did I learn?" after a difficult situation or interaction.**

In the first session, I watched 12-year-old Roy print with all his fingers clenched around the pencil. Then I said, "Roy, just try to hold the pencil this way for a minute." I gently moved his fingers into a normal writing position using his thumb, index, and middle fingers.

"Noooo. Don't," he yelled and flung the pencil across the table. I quickly changed to a construction activity and thought about what I did wrong. I realized that he might not like being touched. I tried again the next session. This time we talked about it, and I prepared him for trying a different way to hold his pencil. I also had him imitate my fingers holding the pencil correctly so I would not have to touch him. He mimicked my actions and held the pencil in a functional grasp while he printed one word.

- **Laugh at yourself.**

I stood on my toes and stretched my arms as I reached for the wood kits on the top shelf. My fingertips barely brushed against the shelf, so I laughed and said, "I'm too short. I need to be taller. Could you help me?"

"Yeah, you're a shortie," 12-year-old Kurt chuckled as he whisked the kit out of the cupboard.

- **Recognize your feelings.**

In the day treatment, I worked at a table next to the calming area. The first week I had braces on my teeth, I was finishing paperwork. An agitated 9-year-old yelled out in anger from across the room. I ignored his taunts until he said, "Hey, brace-face, look over here."

I did not look but felt myself get annoyed. *Wow, I'm more sensitive about these braces than I thought.* Later, I told my friends about the name-calling and was able to laugh about it.

- **Acknowledge your limits and get help when needed.**

In the specialized program, 4-year-old Jack stood next to the wall and began banging his head on the window.

"Stop!" I said. "That's not safe. You could hurt yourself."

He turned and began thrashing me with both his hands even as I backed away. Hitting was his first response to being told to stop, and this was the fourth time he hit me that day. Although he was not actually hurting me, I found myself feeling frustrated with him. As we often did for each other, I called out to another staff member and said, "I need a break. Could you trade places with me?"

She nodded and came over. I moved to the other end of the classroom, took deep breaths, and began playing with another child.

Establish Healthy Emotional Boundaries

Another essential element for staying genuine in your interactions is to establish emotional boundaries. Setting this boundary is like creating a fence around your home and deciding what to let in and out (Figure 10-1). You can choose what feelings will affect you, as well as what you decide to say and do. Children and caregivers are not there to meet your overall emotional needs. For example, you would not sit down with a group of children and tell them about the argument you had with your family and ask them to help you figure out what to do. Part of having healthy boundaries is recognizing what your issues are, what the children's and caregivers' issues are, and whether there is a problem with your interactions with them.

To set boundaries, you have to be aware of your thoughts and feelings and deal with them in a constructive way. When you find certain children push your buttons and you feel angry, it is important to stop and reflect on what

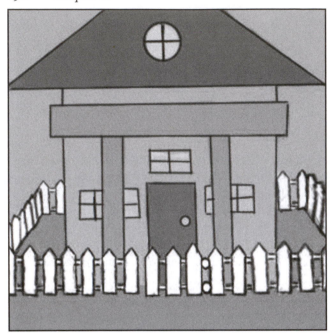

Figure 10-1. Create healthy emotional boundaries by deciding what to let in and out.

happened. Often hot buttons are the result of issues that developed from experience. Therefore, identify and explore your issues that interfere with your work with children.

If you find yourself in a situation with children or caregivers in which you feel angry, you have a responsibility as a professional to handle your feelings and not lash out at others. You may find you do not like being with a child or caregiver. You will like working with some people more than others. Use strategies that will help you act professionally, such as looking for something you like about the person. Reframe the situation and think about all you are learning from interacting with them. This change in your thinking will also change your body language, which children are masters at deciphering. Instinctively, children are perceptive and will sense whether or not you want to be with them.

Setting boundaries also involves recognizing the children's and caregivers' issues. If you are with someone who is out of control and swearing at you, you may have to tell yourself, *This is not really about me.* You also have to realize that there are limits to how much you can help. You may guide and be an influence in people's lives, but ultimately they make their own decisions.

Fabulous Five: Set Boundaries
- **Identify children's issues.**

Four-year-old Riley walked around the playground on her tiptoes and flapping her hands. "Five more minutes," her teacher yelled out.

A few minutes later, the paraprofessional showed Riley a picture of the snack and said, "Time for a snack."

Riley cried from the playground to the class. Once in the room, she threw herself on the floor and tried to open the door. I quickly moved between her and the door to the hallway. She alternated between hitting my leg and sitting on the floor screaming. It was clear she wanted to go back outside. Being nonverbal, I knew she was hitting me because she was frustrated and I was not letting her do what she wanted. When after a few minutes she did not calm herself, I asked one of the staff to bring over her favorite book. She stopped crying as she turned the pages of the book, and 5 minutes later she joined her classmates at the table for her snack.

- **Become aware of what especially upsets you.**

"Try writing a 'J' here," I said to Joy, a second grader.

She stuck out her tongue and blew. Her spit covered my cheek. I felt so disgusted that I stopped the session and left to wash my face. Then I talked with my friend, who was a speech-language pathologist. She suggested different ways of working with Joy. We decided on cotreatment and planned activities to develop her language and fine motor skills at the same time. With two of us in the room, it would be easier to deal with her. This turned out to be a good solution for all of us.

- **Look for what you do like about the children.**

"I burped. Ha-ha. Excuse me," 8-year-old Roy said. A minute later, he laughed again. "I farted. Excuse me." Then he belched for the next 3 minutes.

"Roy, try these tops," I said, hoping to divert his attention. The burping and other bodily sounds diminished as he focused on the activity.

Going home from work, I thought about Roy and realized that I did not really enjoy working with him. Our time together was not very pleasant. I started thinking about what I did like about him and realized I enjoyed the way he beamed whenever he experienced success, even with simple activities. The next session I watched him express delight every time he hit a target, and I found myself enjoying his happy grin.

- **Avoid taking other's actions personally.**

When 4-year-old Andrew kept kicking a classmate, I helped his teacher move him away from the group. "You b****!" he yelled at me. "You're ugly."

I remained quiet and calm. Knowing his dad was in prison and there had been domestic violence at home, I wondered if he had heard such an exchange between his parents. I did not take his insults personally. After he settled, the teacher and I drew a cartoon character showing Andrew what to do when he was mad. Later that morning, I made a point to play with him.

- **Reflect and use self-talk to separate the children's issues from yours.**

On the children's psychiatric unit, the two 10 year olds stood facing each other. "Hey, silly," Justin yelled.

"Yeah, silly is my middle name," Luke replied.

"I know what gets you mad—your momma."

"Don't talk about my mom."

"See, it gets you mad."

"You stinking…." Luke began punching Justin.

When the nurse and I separated the two boys, Luke turned to me and yelled, "Get away from me, you b****!" *Stay calm and ignore his rants*, I told myself.

More staff came, and the two boys went to a calming area to cool off.

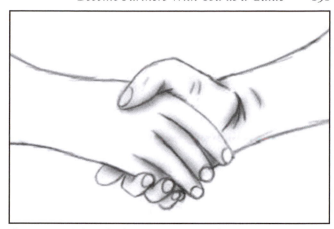

Figure 10-2. Only make the promises you can keep.

Only Make Promises You Can Keep and Show Integrity

How you honor promises is a reflection of your integrity. First and foremost, make sure you only make promises you can keep (Figure 10-2). Avoid making a commitment if you are uncertain or question the feasibility of completing your promise. Second, do not promise to keep secrets. You may tell children that it is all right not to tell about surprises, such as a birthday party or gift. Let them know it is okay to keep surprises but not secrets. This is important because if children tell you they want to hurt themselves or others, or that they are being abused, you must report it. In the beginning, it is better to be honest and upfront than to break your promise later. Third, be specific regarding your plans. Avoid making vague comments such as, "Someday you will get to…." Fourth, be conscientious about following through whatever commitment you made. Finally, for some children you may want to give an outward sign of your promise using a handshake or a note. Your actions show you are trustworthy.

Fabulous Five: Honor Promises

- **Make only promises you can keep.**

"I don't want anyone to break it up," John said as he looked at the boat he created out of blue and yellow plastic strips.

"I cannot promise that because other kids will use these. You know you made your boat pretty quickly. You could just make it again next time."

"Yeah, I'll make a bigger boat next time."

- **Do not promise to keep secrets.**

In the oncology clinic, 12-year-old Debbie talked with a child psychiatry intern. In their session, the intern promised that their conversations were confidential, so Debbie revealed that her stepfather touched her inappropriately. She hospitalized Debbie on a psychiatric ward over a weekend and tried to intervene with her family. The family refused to come to the hospital for a meeting. I saw Debbie on Monday in the oncology clinic, and the first thing she asked was, "Do you think I'm crazy?"

"No," I said. "I think you are just in a bad situation."

"If I had known she was going to tell everyone, I wouldn't have told her."

- **Be specific instead of vague when making promises.**

"I want a turn," 6-year-old Zach said as soon as he saw the musical top.

"Everyone will get a turn today, I promise. Let's go around the circle. Spin three times, then pass it to the next person."

- **Do what you promise.**

"In three minutes it will be time to stop."

"But I don't want to stop," 6-year-old Eddy said. "I want to keep playing with the putty."

"Would you like me to bring it back?" I replied, and he nodded.

Over the weeks, I kept my promises and brought the desired toys back to the group. A month later when I said it was time to end, Eddy said, "But I want to play with these tops."

"She's going to bring it back, so you don't have to worry. Right, Dr. Clare?" 6-year-old Dottie said.

"Yes, I will. I keep my promises."

- **Give an outward sign of your promise.**

Abraham colored half of his car picture, raised his head, and said, "I want to do that maze game."

"Okay, when you're done coloring, I'll get the game for you." A couple of minutes later, he was paged to the school office but balked at going. "I know you wanted a chance to play the game. I promise you that you will play it next time. Let's shake on it. A shake is a promise that you will get to do it the next time we meet."

He clutched my outstretched hand, shook it, and walked to the door.

Be Supportive

> **Children might be thinking:**
> *Thanks for listening.*
> *I feel safer.*
> *That was a nice thing to do.*

For children to trust you, they have to know that you are a safe person. Your words and actions will show that you can provide emotional support. This may be done by showing acceptance, staying open, and being a good listener.

Show Acceptance and Openness

For children to feel comfortable expressing themselves, they need to know you are open to hearing whatever they may say. They will watch to see if you are accepting of who they are and if you view them in a positive way. When they are given the message that they are valued instead of being judged, they tend to relax and be themselves. To give this message, you can listen when they ask to talk to you and avoid discounting their perspectives or feelings. You must be aware of your own preconceived notions or expectations and be willing to change. Also, help children view themselves in a positive way by reframing and converting their perceived weaknesses into strengths.

> ### *Fabulous Five: Be Open*
>
> - **Avoid discounting children's perceptions or feelings.**
>
>   Ken looked at the paper on the table. "I hate writing."
>
>   "Is it hard for you?" I asked the kindergartner. He nodded. "I understand. If writing is hard, then it is probably not fun to do. What I want to do is make writing easier for you because I know your teachers still expect you to write. But I want to do something different to make writing more fun." I poured some salt in a tray and began printing his name.
>
>   Ken pulled the tray closer and swirled his finger in the salt.
>
>   "Try doing your name," I said.
>   He hesitated, but then made a "K."
>
> - **Be cautious of preconceived notions or expectations.**
>
>   When I received the occupational therapy referral, I stopped at the nursing station to read 12-year-old Gerry's chart. In addition to describing the status of his leukemia, the intern reported that he was a gang member who resided in a detention home after committing a burglary. I passed a uniformed guard in the hallway as I entered his room. Expecting to see a tough character, I was surprised to view a skinny, mild-mannered boy with scrawny shoulders.

> I introduced myself, and we began talking. After we discussed his family, interests, and routines at the detention home, I told him, "I really don't know very much about gangs. What is it like to be in a gang?"
>
> "I'd like to get out, but the only way you can leave is if you are dead."
>
> Two years later, I was happy to hear that Gerry's cancer was in remission, he had been released from the detention home, and his family moved to another city to give him a new start.
>
> - **Convert perceived weaknesses into strengths.**
>
>   Ten-year-old Al argued anytime he could, and he often landed in the principal's office. One day I told him, "I've noticed that you're really good at arguing, but the teachers do not appreciate it. There is a way to argue constructively in a positive way. It's called debating. Here's my idea. Every time we meet, you will get 1 minute to present an argument. Let's start with something about sports teams. Then it's Jose's turn. If you talk for a full minute and do not interrupt each other, you will get a point. We'll see how many points you can get. What do you think?"
>
>   "Okay!" In the next session, the two boys came prepared, and Al grinned as he presented his case.
>
> - **Reframe perceived weakness.**
>
>   When 9-year-old Adam accidentally colored outside the line, he said with disgust, "My stupid brain. I'm so stupid."
>
>   "Your brain may work a little differently, and I'm sure some things are harder for you. But Albert Einstein's brain worked differently too, and he was very smart," I said, pointing to Einstein's picture hanging in the class. "Just because coloring is hard for you does not mean you are stupid."
>
> - **Be open to what children tell you, including possible personal matters.**
>
>   "Can I talk to you?"
>   "Sure."
>   "I'm a little embarrassed about something that I'm wearing," 11-year-old Elena said. "My mom says you don't have to tell others what you are wearing."
>
>   "She's right. Some things you do keep private," I replied. "Sounds like you are growing up."

Be a Good Listener

For children, having a trusted adult to confide in is like having a security blanket. That person becomes a source of comfort. Like their soothing favorite blanket, it is reassuring for them to know that the adult, usually a parent or teacher, can help them. As you build a relationship, they will tend to trust you as well. Support them by giving them your full attention, being a good listener, and guiding them in addressing their feelings.

Fabulous Five: Be a Good Listener

- **Give children the opportunity to talk about difficult experiences or situations.**

I heard that 7-year-old Aaron's teenaged brother had committed suicide. So when he returned to school, I met with him individually. We went to a quiet place, and I sat in silence while he played with putty.

"You haven't seen me in a long time," he said.

"I know. I've missed you," I replied.

"My mom is in the hospital. She got real sad because my brother died."

"How are you doing?"

"I saw his coffin. I cried a couple of times. My dad said not to tell kids but I can tell teachers."

"How is your dad doing?"

"He's not crying that much anymore."

- **Walk and talk.**

"I had to go to the emergency room last night. My throat started swelling," 10-year old Sarah said as we walked down the school hallway. "I watched a movie and got a Popsicle in the middle of the night. I got to push a button and someone came right away. It was like room service. It was scary. I thought I was going to get a shot."

"That would be scary. Are you feeling better now?" I asked, and she nodded. "Oh good, I'm glad you're okay."

- **Answer questions.**

"I came first," 3-year-old Olivia said because she was the oldest in a set of triplets. "I'm going to have a boy baby and a girl baby."

"Can I have a baby if I'm in the middle?" her sister asked.

"Oh yes. When you grow up, you can have a baby."

- **Explore concerns.**

"I'm a little nervous about next year," 10-year-old Tanya said.

"What are you nervous about?"

"Going to the mountains with my class for Outdoor Lab. The only time I've been away from home is to stay with my grandma."

"Is there something you can bring that would make you feel more comfortable?"

"My dolphin."

"The other thing you could do is to be with a friend who makes you feel safe. Who could you be with?"

"Taylor is my friend."

- **Clarify concerns or worries.**

"We're moving to a new house, and I don't get to take my toys. I have to leave them all behind," 4-year-old Hunter said.

"Let's check on that," I replied. "We'll talk with your mom when she comes to pick you up." At end of the school day, I approached his mother with him by my side and said, "Hunter says he has to leave all his toys at the old house. He's worried about that."

"Oh no, Hunter," his mother said. "We're cleaning out some of the old toys you don't play with anymore. But you will definitely take all your favorite toys with you."

Offer Support

Let children know you are there for them. You can give this message by making a comforting or nurturing gesture. You can invite children to talk with you if they wish. Whether or not they choose to talk, convey that you are always there to listen. You also can be helpful by empathizing with them and telling them their feelings are typical.

Fabulous Five: Be Compassionate

- **Provide silent support.**

As the teacher read a story to the preschoolers, 4-year-old Sam jumped up, ran over, and pushed 3-year-old Danielle. The staff quickly moved Sam away.

Danielle started to cry, so I put my arm around her and pulled her next to me. She snuggled against my side, and her body started to relax.

- **Make a nurturing gesture.**

On the day the children demonstrated their homemade Australian didgeridoos to their parents, 9-year-old Ethan scanned the room with a frown on his face. "What's the matter?" I asked.

"My mom is not here."

"So you're disappointed your mom didn't come?"

"Yeah, she said she was going to try."

"Something must have come up. I see they have punch and cookies. Would you like me to get some for you?" He nodded.

- **Tell children, "If you tell me what happened, maybe I can see if there is something we can do."**

I saw a tear roll down 8-year-old Cherelle's cheek. "If you tell me what happened, maybe I can see if there is something we can do," I said.

Cherelle words tumbled out. "He knocked me straight into the wall and a tree. I hurt my shoulder."

"I can see why you're upset. Do you want to go to the clinic?"

"No, I'll be okay," she said bravely.

- **Tell children they may feel better if they talk about what is bothering them.**

When 10-year-old Tory walked into my room, tears trickled down his cheeks and his lips trembled. "You look upset. What happened?" He shook his head. "Sometimes you feel better if you talk about it. Did someone say something to upset you?" He shook his head again. "Did someone do something to upset you?" He nodded. "Was it a teacher or a kid?"

"A kid," he said, his voice quivering.

"What happened?"

"I don't want to talk about it."

"That's okay. I'm always here to listen if you want to talk."

- **Tell children you had a similar experience and felt the same way.**

"I was scared last night," 5-year-old Jamie said. "I had a scary dream nightmare. I was on my grandma's boat and it turned into a monster. I sprayed paint on the monster and it turned back into a boat."

"I've had bad dreams too. I wake up and my heart is racing. It can be really scary to have a nightmare."

Be Fun

> **Children might be thinking:**
> *You're funny.*
> *I like being with you.*
> *That's funny.*
> *I like playing around you.*

When you work with children, continually show the fun side of your personality. Be funny and playful (Figure 10-3). Joke and laugh. Do comical imitations. Children will enjoy being with you.

Be a Fun Person

You can show that you are a fun person in simple ways. Just making funny faces with exaggerated expressions can make children smile. Also showing excitement in a child-like fashion is captivating. Wearing unusual clothes, such as crazy-looking socks, shows that you can be whimsical and light-hearted. Chuckling indicates a playful perspective, and using a silly tone of voice can make you appear goofy, which they love.

> ### *Fabulous Five: Be Funny*
> - **Make funny faces.**
>
>   In the kindergarten, I sat next to Sheila as she drew. When she looked up at me, I smirked, scrunched my eyes, and lifted my shoulders. Seeing my enjoyment of being with her, she broke out into a smile.
> - **Show excitement.**
>
>   The occupational therapy student waved her hands in the air and said, "Check this out! It's brand new. There are three tops. You have to attach the top to this control

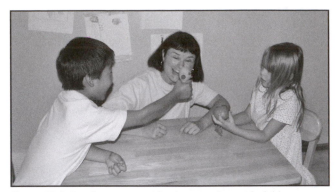

Figure 10-3. Be a fun person and enjoy your time with children.

piece, twist it, and push the button to release it. First, get the large top to spin. Then do the same thing with the smaller tops, and try to drop them on top of the spinning top. It's hard but fun."

- **Wear fun clothes.**

"Wow, I like those," 7-year-old Sharee said, pointing to my white socks with black spots.

I grinned and said, "Thanks. These are my cow socks. My brother gave them to me."

- **Remember to laugh.**

The two first graders and I stacked the blocks into a swaying tall tower. "Don't sneeze," I said with a smile.

"Achoo," the boys teased, pretending to blow. We laughed as they knocked it down.

- **Use a silly tone of voice.**

When 10-year-old Ken aimed for a target, he missed and hit me with a small bean bag. Using a high-pitched voice, I laughed and said, "Oh no, don't hit me. Hit the target."

Be Playful

Another way to show you are a fun person is to play with words or tell funny stories. Exchanging corny jokes can be hilarious. Applying everyday expressions in an unusual way and using old-fashioned phrases can be attention getting.

> ### *Fabulous Five: Use Playful Words or Stories*
> - **Play with words.**
>
>   "I'm pleased you're doing so well," I said.
>   "I'm pleased you're pleased," the fifth grader replied
>   "I'm pleased you're pleased I'm pleased," I said.
>   "I'm pleased you're pleased I'm pleased you're pleased."
>   We both giggled as we walked back to her class.
> - **Tell funny stories.**
>
>   When I went to get Chris, his first-grade class was learning about dolphins and other sea life. So as we did our

activity, we talked about sea creatures. Chris started cutting, but when he kept making mistakes he started to cry.

"Hey, Chris, you know what? I have a friend who worked with dolphins. And guess what happened? A dolphin fell in love with him. Every time he went in the water, the dolphin followed him around and gave him kisses." I lightly tapped Chris' shoulder with my arm, demonstrating dolphin kisses, and he started to smile.

- **Tell goofy jokes.**

The week of Halloween, 8-year-old Peter started picking up ghost-shaped erasers with tongs. "What did the baby ghost say to the bully?" I asked.

"What?"

"Leave me alone or I'll tell my mummy," I said, and we both chuckled.

- **Use everyday expressions in an unusual way.**

The preschool teacher started an exercise group by saying, "Everyone sit on the floor and put your legs out. Now lift your toes up and say, 'Hi, toes.'"

"Hi, toes," echoed throughout the room.

"Now, point your toes down and say, 'Bye, toes.'"

"Bye, toes," the children repeated and laughed.

"Next, put one leg over the other and give it a hug. Now do the other one."

"So he won't be sad," 3-year-old Heather yelled out with a smile.

- **Use old-fashioned phrases.**

Four-year-old Rita raced to the table and started grabbing all the objects. "Hold your horses," I bellowed like a cowboy. "Give me a chance to show you what to do." Rita stopped in her tracks and smiled.

The next week, when she wanted the group to wait for her, she yelled, "Stop the ponies."

Joke and Laugh

When you joke about yourself, you model self-acceptance and convey that you do not always have to take life too seriously. Showing enjoyment when children tease you gives this same message. It also can be fun to tease another adult if you know he or she will not mind. Some children like to be teased in a playful manner. However, be careful to avoid any kidding that could be interpreted as being hurtful. Often it is better to joke about the situation rather than about an aspect of their personality. Consider that younger children tend to be more literal. So if you say, "I am pulling your leg," they will think you are going to tug on them. They will not understand that you are joking. Using objects in a comical way is another means of eliciting laughter. When teasing is done in a kind-hearted manner, it can be a delightful experience for both you and the children.

Fabulous Five: Joke and Laugh

- **Joke about yourself.**

When I went to get a child from his second-grade class in the day treatment, he was learning about bats. "When I was in Australia," I said, "I hiked in the woods and saw hundreds of bats hanging in the trees."

"I saw a bat," a classmate said.

"Yeah, you've seen me in the morning," the teacher said, and everyone chuckled.

- **Tease another adult if you know the person will not mind.**

My friend, Mrs. S., was a speech-language pathologist. We shared a room that was divided by a folding wall. Although we could not see each other, we could hear what the other person was saying. Rose, a fifth grader, received both speech and occupational therapy. In my room, Rose started making a book about wizards, and as she wrote, she said loudly, "Mrs. S. was a witch with a big nose."

"Hey," we heard a voice yell through the wall. Rose and I started laughing.

- **Use playful teasing.**

In the morning it was warm, but by noon the temperature dropped. Five-year-old Darren borrowed his teacher's black fleece jacket, and the sleeves hung a foot over his hands.

"Darren, you shrunk. That jacket doesn't fit you anymore," I said, and we both laughed.

- **Use objects in a comical way.**

I held a hairbrush next to my ear like a telephone. "Hello, Kyla."

The 3-year-old with long blonde curls laughed. "That's not a phone."

Grinning, I picked up a shoe and held it to my ear.

Smiling, she squealed, "That's not a phone." I laughed.

- **Enjoy when children tease you.**

On Monday morning, 6-year-old Joel was barely awake when we started batting a Koosh ball back and forth with rackets. I swatted the ball, and it bopped Joel on the middle of his nose. "Well, that woke me up," he laughed.

I started laughing too. "I can't believe I did that."

When he saw me the next week, he smiled as he pointed to where I had hit him on the nose. We both chuckled.

Use Imitation

You can create a fun experience by asking children to imitate your silly actions. Some may react with disbelief but enjoyment that you are acting like an out-of-the-ordinary adult. It also is pleasurable for them if you imitate their actions or their ideas for an activity. Incorporating the imitation of superheroes or cartoon characters into therapy is playful. At times, it is also good to ask children to imitate you. You may be surprised at how accurate they are in depicting your mannerisms and sayings. It also is a wonderful opportunity to learn how they perceive you.

Fabulous Five: Incorporate Imitation

- **Have children imitate you.**

In the day treatment, the two first-grade boys had to walk with me to another building. "Let's pretend we are a marching band. Get behind me and march." We moved in single file, and I waved a ruler like a bandleader. The boys grinned as we marched in time.

- **Imitate the children's actions.**

Walking to the next school building, 6-year-old Loni yelled to Jordan and me, "Look at me." He stomped his feet and raised his arms to his side with his hands hanging down. Like a bouncing scarecrow, he continued the walk he invented and was quite pleased when Jordan and I imitated him.

- **Incorporate imitations of superheroes or cartoon characters.**

Six-year-old Harry walked in the room wearing a T-shirt with a picture of the Incredible Hulk showing his bulging muscles. I handed him a stress ball in the shape of a lion and said, "Be like the Hulk; squeeze this hard."

"My muscles are getting strong like the Hulk. I've been working out at home."

- **Follow along with children's imitations of movie or television characters.**

Four-year-old Polly held a golden-haired doll and said, "This is Tinkerbell." As she flitted around the room, she added, "I'm Peter Pan."

"Hey, Peter Pan," I replied, "fly over here and check this out."

Her wispy bangs swayed as she sauntered over to the table and reached for the scissors and paper.

- **Ask children to do imitations of you.**

"You're weird," Bob said to Lucas, another first grader.

Turning to the third member of the group, I said, "What do I usually say?"

"Be nice to each other," Juan said as the other two listened.

"What else do I usually say?" I asked with a smile.

The boys took turns imitating my voice and phrases. "You say, 'Today we're going to play a fun game.'"

"'Today we are going to finish our cards.'"

"'Try your best.'"

"'Don't say you can't do it.'"

"'Don't shake the table while he's writing.'"

"'Say nice things.'"

"'Do nice work.'"

"'I like your work.'"

They grinned as they imitated my facial expressions. Juan pulled his chin down, made his mouth into an oval shape, opened his eyes wide, and looked up in the right corner. Bob crinkled his brow the same way I do, and I laughed.

Know About the Ways of Children

Naturally, the more you learn about the way children think, the easier it will be to work with them. Consider what the world is like from their perspective. Taking their viewpoint will help you better understand their feelings and actions. In addition, be sensitive to their needs, especially their need to be liked.

Be Sensitive to What Children May Be Thinking

Children might be thinking:
Oh, you're nice.
You understand.
You like me.
I like being with you.
We have similarities.

It is to your benefit to gain knowledge on how children see their world. This helps you approach them in a respectful way. At the same time, be conscientious about how your presence and actions affects them and can influence their thinking.

Learn the Ways Children Think

You will quickly learn that children are open and honest. They often will tell you what they think regardless of whether it is good or bad. They may say what they like about you. Children also may tell you if you appear too skinny or fat. They may say what they like or do not like about your clothes. In addition, be prepared that they will ask questions about your life and give their opinions about that too.

Keep in mind that younger ones tend to be literal. For instance, one child said he was going to draw his face. He proceeded to put his head down on the paper and traced around it. Younger children also have a different sense of time and tend to be more present oriented. Always be sensitive about doing anything that appears babyish or is perceived to be for the other sex. They find it insulting if they think you are treating them like a baby or go against their cultural norms.

Fabulous Five: Learn the Ways Children Tend to Think

- **Be ready for honesty.**

"You're really old," 6-year-old Sara said.

"How old do you think I am?"

"Seventeen."

"You're right," I replied, laughing to myself.

- **Be prepared for children to be curious about your life.**

"Are you married?" 6-year-old Brad asked the special education teacher during a group.

"No, I'm single."

"Well, you need to get yourself a man and get married."

"When I'm older, I'll marry you," soft-spoken Jose said.

The teacher smiled, and everyone resumed writing.

Five minutes later, Ray wrinkled his eyebrows and said, "Now why is Jose marrying you?"

"Oh, we're not getting married. It was a nice offer, but I'm too old to marry Jose."

- **Be sensitive about doing anything children might perceive as babyish or only for the other sex.**

I handed 6-year-old Anthony a pole with four gold pinwheels attached to a string. "Try swinging this in a large circle."

Anthony swung once and placed it on the table. "You're making me do a girlie thing," he said with disdain.

"You think it's girlie?" I asked, surprised.

"Sorta."

"Oh, let's do something else then."

- **Remember that younger children tend to be literal.**

After a local shooting at a high school, the staff at the day treatment program talked with the children about their feelings and worries. The staff were surprised when 6-year-old Mark raised his hand and said, "I got shot. I got shot right here." Then he pointed to his upper right arm, paused for a moment, and added, "But at least I won't get the measles."

- **Be aware that younger children have a different sense of time.**

In June, 3-year-old Cora went for a ride on a train named Thomas. For the next 2 months, she said, "Last week I saw Thomas."

When I left her house after my weekly appointment, she said, "See you tomorrow."

"See you next week. In 7 days I will see you again," I replied. "Have a nice week."

Be Aware That Children Are Affected by Your Presence and Actions

Realize that you may influence children more than you know. This becomes evident when you see them imitating you or other adults. It also is good to assume that children are always listening. They may repeat your exact words or tell others the strategies you have discussed. This means you have to be careful that whatever you say is okay for them to repeat. In addition, they may notice subtle things you do. Children are often barometers to the emotional climate of their surroundings. They will react if there is major stress at home or at school. They are sensitive to how you are feeling and your mood. For instance, if you are in a bad mood, they may respond by being restless or easily frustrated or mad. It is a good practice to think about how you are coming across.

Fabulous Five: Recognize Your Influence on Children

- **Be aware that children often imitate the adults in their lives.**

"We get to wear pajamas to school," 4-year-old Corrine said.

"I'm going to wear…." the three preschoolers said in unison, but all their answers mingled together and were indistinguishable.

Corrine imitated her teacher by waving her upright index finger and yelling, "One at a time. One at a time."

- **Realize that children often repeat your words.**

"How old are you?" Brandon asked.

"One hundred," I said.

"No you're not."

"My grandmother says you never ask a lady her age," I said with a smile.

Later that week we went on a field trip to the beach. On the bus, Amy asked a nurse her age. Brandon looked at them and said, "You never ask a lady her age."

- **Recognize that children can be affected by your mood or feelings.**

One time I had an allergic reaction, and when a staff member saw me a week later, she asked, "Are you feeling better?"

"Yeah, but I was really sick. I'm still not over it," I replied with a tired voice.

Seven-year-old Darryl sat at the table with me and continued playing while we talked. At the end of the session, he went into the next room and I overheard him tell the teacher, "Dr. Clare is sick." The worry in his voice was evident.

I went to him and said, "Oh, Darryl, I'm okay. I have an allergy like when you sneeze around dust. I just have to stay away from what I'm allergic to and then I'm okay. I'm getting better."

"Oh good," he said, relief crossing his face.

- **Be prepared that children listen and pass on your strategies.**

"Make four brown triangles and color them inside the butterfly wings," the certified occupational therapy assistant said to the kindergartner.

"Guess what? My teacher taught us a really cool strategy. Trace down and around. Then color." He continued his commentary as he drew. "This is a triangle. Look, I traced it inside, now I'm going to fill it in."

- **Be aware that your actions may make an impression on children.**

In class, 6-year-old Leonard created letters in a tray filled with salt. To clean up, I made a funnel out of paper. "Help me put the salt back into the bottle," I said to him.

A month later, the school administrator came to observe me, and I introduced the children at the table. As we sat down, Leonard told my boss, "Dr. Clare recycles salt."

Be Cognizant About the Needs of Children

Children might be thinking:
Do you like me?
Thanks for talking to me.
Thanks for listening.
Thanks for caring about me.

As you work with children, learn their general and individual needs, then do what you can to meet those needs. At the same time, base your expectations on their developmental level versus their chronological age. Also, be careful if a child is taller or bigger than others of the same age that you do not expect them to act older.

Recognize Children's Needs

A primary need of children is that they want to be heard. They want you to listen and respect what they have to say. Another crucial need is to know about and to have a general understanding of what is happening around them. Often adults underestimate how aware they are. Of course, the amount of information shared is dependent on their level of understanding. You also will find that they react to stress in their environment. Be prepared that some children need to keep their hands busy while they talk. Finally, they will appreciate knowing that you will miss them if they are gone.

Fabulous Five: Be Conscientious About Children's Needs

- **Recognize that children want to be heard.**

As I walked down the school hallway, I passed a girl I did not know. She waved at me and said, "I have to tell you some news. My grandma went to the clinic and someone screamed in her ears and she didn't get her pills. She's old. She needs her pills."

"Well, I hope she's okay," I replied.

- **Be aware that younger children may need to keep their hands busy while thinking or talking.**

Seven-year-old Mary finished cutting the pieces for her pop-up book. While she was trying to think of a story to put in her book, she opened and closed the scissors on the edge of the table. I handed her scraps of paper. "Here, cut these while you're thinking." As she snipped the scraps, she created her story of the wizard and his magic stew.

- **Be sensitive to what is happening in the environment that may upset children.**

Dewey, who was very sensitive to loud noises, sat at a table next to Tessa and Tara. The two girls started squealing, "Yee! Yee! Yee!" Every few seconds, the sounds became louder and higher pitched.

One minute later, Dewey became overwhelmed by the noise and started rocking in his chair. In a low, deep voice, he yelled, "Pull hair! Pull hair!"

Everyone quickly moved away from Dewey to give him the space needed to calm himself, and at the same time we tried to quiet the girls. Afterward, I recommended to the teacher that the staff offer Dewey a choice of headphones or going to a quieter place as soon as the class got too noisy.

- **Realize that children want to know what is happening.**

"Today we are going to make letters out of Play-Doh," I said.

BJ used a rolling pin to flatten the dough, and the other children around the circular table repeated sounds to themselves. "Da, da, da. Ee, ee, ee," echoed in the room.

Mick kept singing a radio slogan.

"Our teacher is really sick," the paraprofessional said to me.

I moved away from the table and said, "Tell me about her over here."

All the children at the table stopped making sounds, and the room went quiet as she whispered to me. After talking, I went back to the table and reassured the children, "Your teacher is sick. She is getting better and will be coming back soon."

- **Talk about missing children who are unable to attend a session or have left.**

As we headed for the therapy room, I said, "Howie moved to another city, so he will not be in our group. I'm going to miss him. I always miss kids when they leave."

"Why did he move?" 8-year-old Martin asked.

"I don't know."

"I've known him since first grade. Maybe the house got too small or they lost it in a bet."

"Families move for all kinds of reasons," I said.

"I'll miss him too," Martin said.

Recognize the Need to Be Liked

Children can usually sense whether or not you like them and want to be with them. At times, some may be doubtful or uncertain about your feelings toward them. Others may interpret your actions with the meaning that you do not like them. Address their concerns. It can be helpful to say, "I like you," "I like being with you," or "I like playing with you." Others may wonder if you have favorites. In addition, some may believe they have to give you a gift to be liked. Convey to children that you care about them for who they are.

Fabulous Five: Be Aware of the Importance of Being Liked

- **Recognize that children need to know that you like them.**

Four 9-year-old boys sprawled on the floor while they colored pictures of desert scenes. As I walked by, one child said, "I like you, Dr. Clare."

"I like you too." Then I looked at the other boys and realized they might wonder how I felt about them. So I added, "I like all of you."

- **Be cognizant that children need to know that you like them as much as others.**

"We need to put this blue sand back in the bag because I will be using it with other kids."

"Do you like them better than me?" 5-year-old Brian asked.

"No one more than you," I replied with a grin.

- **Be aware that children may question whether you like them.**

"Why don't you ever see me?" 7-year-old Drew said, looking dejected.

"It's not because I don't like you. I do like you. It's because you don't need extra help. Do you want me to stop by and see how you are doing?" He nodded with a grin.

- **Separate your feelings about the children from their behavior.**

In the preschool classroom, 4-year-old Jeremy left the group on the rug, ran to a bookcase, and pulled two bins off the shelf. "You have a choice," I said. "You can go to the cozy corner to get yourself calm, or you can take big breaths now and go back to the group."

In response, he darted over to the cozy corner filled with large pillows, a blanket, and stuffed animals. He threw himself on the floor, kicked his feet in the air, and cried.

I stood quietly watching him in my peripheral vision and looking like I was attending to his teacher. After a few minutes, he calmed. Realizing he was not getting any attention from me, he jumped up and raced back to the group.

Later in the day, when the group went back to the rug, I sat next to him and said, "I like you, Jeremy."

"I wish you could come every day," he replied.

- **Consider the motivation of the children's gift giving and respect the gesture.**

"I have a surprise for you," Rena said as she handed me an unwrapped piece of candy.

"Thank you for thinking of me," I said to the 5 year old with a runny nose. "That's a nice thought. I'm going to save it for later." Because I was unsure of where the candy had been, I wrapped it in paper, waited until lunchtime, and threw the candy in the wastebasket in the staff lounge, where I was sure Rena would not see it.

The next day, I went to her class. After working with her for a half hour, I said, "I'm so glad I get to spend time with you."

Be Responsible for Your Role

Children might be thinking:
You say nice things.
You care about me.

When there is a problem, it is easy to think that it is the other person's fault without considering your role. This may lead to a prevailing view that the children need to be "fixed." Yet you must consider your role in every interaction. Recognize and take responsibility for your assumptions, attitudes, and approaches. Reflect on how you handle tough situations, including the nonverbal language you use during those times. Learn to choose your words and reactions carefully. Respond to children in a way that gives the following messages:

- You are a safe person who will treat them with respect no matter how they act.

- You are modeling caring ways to respond to difficult situations.

- You will help them learn successful approaches for getting what they want.

Recognize Your Assumptions, Attitudes, and Approaches

Children might be thinking:
Are you going to yell at me?
Are you going to be mean to me?

Taking responsibility for your reactions requires a process of self-reflection. You need to know what your assumptions are about children. You can start by examining your history. What were your parents' assumptions and expectations regarding how you should act? For instance, in some families, whining is viewed as an annoyance and is not tolerated. Explore whether you hold the same beliefs and views as your parents. Ask yourself the following questions: Do you expect them to do exactly what you say every time regardless of what they think? Do you assume their actions are communication, or do you tend to think they are just being naughty? Do your expectations match their developmental level? Do you believe that because you are an adult, you must be in total control?

As you interact with children, create a habit of analyzing the situation whenever there is a problem and examining how you contributed to it. For example, children might have reacted to the tone of your voice or the way you worded your request. Look for what is your issue and not theirs. Think about how you typically react. Be open to learning from your mistakes and try to discover ways you can prevent conflict. Be flexible and try different approaches.

At the same time, continually reflect on your strengths, especially which approaches are successful. Strive to use a positive approach in your interactions. In addition, be aware that your reactions to children's actions are learning experiences for them.

Fabulous Five: Recognize Your Assumptions, Attitudes, and Approaches

- **Recognize that annoyances or irritations may be related to your family history.**

"I waaant that," 6-year-old Derek whined at me in a squeaky, high voice.

Ugh, his whining drives me crazy, I thought. I wanted to repeat my mother's words: "I'll talk to you when you stop whining." I took a deep breath and said, "Please ask me using different words." I modeled for him a regular tone of voice as I said, "Say, 'Could I please have that?'"

He followed my request with a normal tone of voice, and I immediately reached for the toy he wanted.

- **Recognize if your first thought is to blame the children.**

During our social group in the preschool classroom, I said, "We're going to practice ways to calm yourself when you are mad." I demonstrated and the class copied taking

deep breaths. Next, I pushed my palms together. As they pressed their palms together, counted to 10, and released them, I thought, *I see Martin just standing there. He's not cooperating.*

When the practice ended, Martin said, "I couldn't do those because I hurt my hand this morning."

Oh, I thought, *that's why he wasn't participating.*

- **Ask yourself if you have a high need for control.**

On the first day back in January after a 2-week break, I sat with the preschoolers on the rug. I was just starting to feel better after being sick for 4 days. When the teacher started to read a book, 3-year-old Aston jumped up, ran to a center, and began playing with blocks.

"Aston, it's not time to play with blocks," I said in a firm voice with a frown on my face. "You need to go back with your friends on the rug."

I waited, but he did not move. Feeling frustrated, I was ready to tell him there would be consequences if he did not return to the group. I thought for a minute about how when I'm tired or sick I often revert to using a controlling versus empathetic approach. With that realization, I shifted my approach and said, "What's wrong? You usually stay with the group."

"I miss my mommy. She went on the trip."

"Oh, you're sad your mom is gone. You have her picture in your backpack. Would getting it help you?"

He nodded and retrieved the photograph. Holding his mom's picture in his hand, he rejoined the group.

- **Reflect on whether you expect children to do exactly what you say before hearing their perspectives.**

As I guided a group of preschoolers to a table, 4-year-old Colton crawled under it.

"You need to come out now and sit down," I said in a firm tone of voice. He backed farther away from me.

After taking a deep breath to regain my cool, I sat down on the floor so I was not peering over him. I changed my demeanor and asked, "Are you okay? Are you upset about something?"

He said, "I'm supposed to go to my friend's house after school. I don't want to be at school. I want to go now."

"So you're telling me it's really hard to wait." He nodded, and I continued, "Let's find something fun for you to do now to help."

He crawled out, and I put the putty he liked on the table.

- **Realize what you focus on affects your actions.**

In the day treatment, I found myself focusing on Cordell's unwanted actions. When I realized that, I decided I needed to change. I told myself to watch closely and tell him any time I saw him do something right or positive.

In the next session, the 7-year-old passed a box of pencils to Pedro, who was sitting at the other end of the table. Immediately I said, "Cordell, that was a nice thought. Thanks for passing those pencils."

Use a Positive Approach

> **Children might be thinking:**
> *You say nice things.*
> *It's okay to be with you.*

Make a conscious effort to only use a positive approach and focus on children's strengths. This means that when you direct children on what to do, you use positive statements. You may want to start with a compliment, if culturally appropriate. Be sure to state what you want them to do versus focusing on what not to do. Continually watch closely for anything good the children are doing and decide to focus your attention on positive actions, such as helping another person. Some children just want adult attention and may use negative actions, such as hitting or fighting to get noticed. In those situations, find ways to give attention to ANY positive actions. Another approach is to make requests or ask questions in such a way that it is hard for them to refuse.

Fabulous Five: Use a Positive Approach

- **Use positive statements.**

"Today we will be tracing the letters of your names with colored glue and sprinkling salt over them. What color do you want?" Six-year-old Steve picked blue, and Bill chose yellow.

As I helped Steve, Bill sat quietly. A few seconds later, I turned to Bill and said, "Thank you for waiting so nicely. Do you want me to help you with yours?" He nodded.

After a couple of minutes, I switched to helping Bill. I turned and asked Steve, "Do you remember how Bill waited nicely for you?" Steve nodded his curly-topped head. "Could you please wait patiently just like Bill did?" Steve stayed in his chair while Bill worked.

At the end of the session, I said, "Thank you for being patient and for being so nice to each other."

- **Give more attention to positive actions than negative actions.**

"We are going to make a book, and the four of you need to draw pictures." Eight-year-old Justin started right away, whereas the other three wiggled and fussed in their chairs. "Justin, it's great how you started right away. I really like the car you're drawing," I said. The other three children twisted their heads toward Justin. I turned to them and said, "I bet your drawings will be good too. It's time to get started." The three children began drawing.

- **Shift children to positive actions.**

Three-year-old Russell ran away from the table where his classmates were playing with putty. He grabbed a toy lawn mower and walked in circles. Knowing that he enjoyed helping the teacher and that it was time to stop, I brought a clear plastic bin over to him. "Russell, you are a super good helper. Take this bin and tell your friends to put the putty in here."

He dropped the lawn mower and walked over to the table. "Friends!" he announced. "Put the putty in here."

- **Use a positive approach.**

As I went to give directions, two girls started chatting with each other. "Everybody listen," I said. "I want you to have enough time to do our fun activity. If you're talking and I'm talking, you will miss the directions. I want to make sure you know what to do."

- **Approach in a way that is hard to refuse.**

Lonnie's previous occupational therapist told me about his emotional problems and how he often tried to avoid doing any work. Sometimes when she would go to see him, he would hide under a table. So the first time approached him, I said, "I believe in using toys for therapy. Is that okay with you?" He nodded. "Good, I'll see you next week." Then I left, which did not give him a chance to refuse. Because he was curious, the next week he came willingly to the first session.

Realize Your Reactions Are a Learning Experience for Children

> **Children might be thinking:**
> *Do you like me?*
> *I feel safe with you.*

How you interpret children's actions affects your reactions. It is always best to honor their spirit and view it in a positive light. This includes recognizing their good intentions and considering their actions as communication. Also, be flexible and open to their ideas.

You want children to think for themselves and learn from their experiences. When children's actions appear defiant, be grateful that they have spirit that may be used on their life journey. Rather than perceiving children as bad, think about how you can facilitate their growth by helping them channel their strong will in a positive direction.

Fabulous Five: Recognize That Your Reactions Are Learning Experiences for Children

- **Enjoy children's spirit.**

"How does this puzzle work?"

"Figure it out," I replied, knowing he could do it.

Seven-year-old Dan rotated the wooden piece one twist and tried to ram it in place. "I can't. What do you expect me to do—ask King Kong for help?"

I laughed. "Not a bad idea. Do you think he's available?" We grinned at each other.

He fiddled with the piece until it fit. "Hey, I got it." He then manipulated the next six puzzle parts with ease.

"Time to go," I said, and began walking down the school hallway. Dan followed for five steps and then plopped on the ground. I kept walking, subtly peeking behind me and swallowing my chuckles. Surprised that I did not stop, Dan stood and ran down the hall to catch me. *I'm going to have fun working with him*, I thought.

- **Appreciate children's strong will.**

When 4-year-old Allison joined her three classmates at the table, she stared at the paper. Then she crumpled it, threw it, and kicked it as a floated to the ground. She folded her arms and turned her body away from the table.

Although I maintain a neutral face, I laughed to myself and thought, *Wow, now that's really dramatic! Allison is good at making a statement.*

- **Acknowledge children's good intentions and point out what to do differently.**

Ten-year-old Dave insisted on showing 7-year-old Sarah how to connect her device to the printer. He snatched it out of her hands and pushed her aside. He took the cable and tried to connect it. When Sarah reached toward him, he snapped, "I'll do it." Sarah became quiet and backed away from him.

Afterward, Dave and I went into another room. "Dave, I think you were trying to help, but the way you helped is not a way to make friends. You were too pushy and didn't give Sarah a chance to try. I really believe you have a good heart and wanted to help her do it right. But when you push people and yell at them, it makes them mad. They won't appreciate your help. You could have helped her more by just telling her what to do, then she could learn how to do it by herself."

"Okay," he said.

- **Assume that the action is communication.**

Nine-year-old Albert printed his name and grunted, "Hee-hee." Then he slapped and pulled Collin's arm.

"Oh, you want him to do your name," the teacher said, and she helped Collin trace over Albert's name. Albert clapped with delight.

- **Go along with children's ideas.**

The three children played the game Operation, removing plastic body parts with tweezers. "I don't want to play anymore," Mariah said.

"How come?" I asked.

"I don't know."

"Okay. Just watch." We went around the table and passed her twice. The third time, she said, "I changed my mind. I want a turn."

"No problem. You're next."

KEY POINTS TO REMEMBER

- Be yourself—be genuine and be fun.
- Show acceptance and openness and truly listen to what children say.
- Establish emotionally healthy personal boundaries.
- Be reflective about your role in all interactions.
- Show integrity and only make promises you can keep.
- Be a really fun person.
- Learn as much as you can about how children think.
- Be aware that one of children's basic needs is to be liked.

REVIEW QUESTIONS

1. It is not okay to tell children if you have made a mistake. True or false.

2. You should berate yourself for what you did wrong in a difficult situation. True or false.

3. A child is screaming swear words at you and calls you a nasty name. What can you tell yourself regarding how to react?

4. Why must you follow through on any promises you make?

5. You read in the 9 year old's Individualized Education Program that he has hit others, refused to do schoolwork, and tried to run out of the building. You should tell yourself to start looking for his strengths and interests when you first meet him. True or false.

6. Name at least six ways you can show children you are a fun person.

7. A child critiques the clothes you were wearing. How can you respond?

8. Children look for signs that you like them. True or false.

9. When children are playing, they are oblivious to what is going on around them. True or false.

10. The 7 year old refuses every time you ask her to do something. You become more irritated with each request and start wishing you do not have to work with her. What can you tell yourself at this point?

11

Set Respectful Limits

CHAPTER OVERVIEW

Keeping children safe is top priority. This requires you to be vigilant and set limits on children's actions that could harm themselves or others. In this chapter, there are details on how to establish rules of respect, set safety limits, use a caring and respectful approach, and prevent problems. Additionally, there are ideas for helping a group settle and allowing children to save face.

CHILDREN'S DESCRIPTIONS OF WHAT THEY THINK YOU SHOULD KNOW

Dr. Clare: "What is important for therapists to know when they work with kids in a group?"

Rachel (age 8): "Talk to everyone. Make sure kids share."

Justyn (age 9): "Make sure they're not wild because if they're really wild they may bounce all over the place."

Isiah (age 6): "If they're hyper, you can tell them to calm."

Ken (age 10): "Have things that everyone likes."

Kris (age 8): "Be calm because then they might do the same."

Dr. Clare: "Why is that important?"

Kris: "They have to be calm to work with you."

ESTABLISH A POSITIVE RELATIONSHIP

When you are with children, you have a responsibility to keep them both physically and emotionally safe. Children want and expect respectful limit setting. They need to feel secure. They need to know that, first, you will not hurt them nor let others hurt them. Second, you will not allow them to hurt themselves, hurt others, or destroy property. If children see that you do not have control, they often will become scared. Consistently show by your words and actions that you will set respectful limits and thereby create a framework of safety.

Show Children You Will Set Respectful Limits

In the beginning, when you set limits children may perceive you as being mean or not liking them. But once they realize you are keeping them safe and protecting them, they appreciate it. It is important to keep in mind that the

Curtin, C.
Strategies for Collaborating With Children: Creating Partnerships in Occupational Therapy and Research (pp. 203-224).
© 2017 SLACK Incorporated.

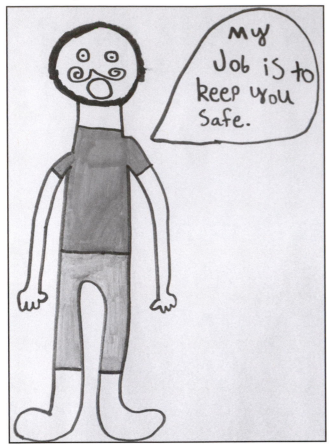

Figure 11-1. Show by your words and actions that you will keep children safe.

purpose of limit setting is to keep children protected and help them grow (Figure 11-1). It is not about overpowering or intimidating them. Let children know what is or is not okay to do. At the same time, it is crucial to convey that you care about them.

Establish and Implement the Rules

> **Children might be thinking:**
> *I'm glad you're setting the ground rules. They help me follow what to do.*
> *This is what I have to go by. If I don't do this, I'll get in trouble.*
> *If other people aren't being nice to me, I'll tell.*
> *You're nice, and you like other people to be nice too.*

Rules define how everyone should act when they are together. They may vary depending on children's ages and the situation and setting. Three basic rules that apply to all are that no one is allowed to hurt themselves, others, or things.

Establish and State the Rules

When possible, have children establish the rules, write down their wording, and display them as a visual reminder. In other situations, state what rules you have in that setting. Keep the list simple so children can remember them. Describe the rules by telling them what to do versus saying, "Don't...."

For younger children, it is best to use picture cues with the corresponding words. To ensure their understanding, give details about each rule and have them demonstrate the correct actions. Review them often. When children understand the rules, they are better able to follow them.

Fabulous Five: Teach the Rules

- **Have group members establish basic rules or guidelines.**

"We have to set group rules," I said to the group of fifth graders, pointing to a blank sheet of paper hanging on the board. "Of course the school rules are that you treat yourself, your friends, and all things with respect. What other rules should we have that will help us get along? I'll write them down for us."

"Take turns and share."

"No bad words. Only one person talks at a time."

"Be nice."

"No laughing at mistakes."

"Keep your hands to yourself."

- **State your rules.**

In the first session, I told the group of second graders, "I have two rules. First, you have to be kind—only say kind things and not mean things. Second, if you want something that is in my cart, you have to ask me. I will get it out for you."

The group nodded, showing they were listening.

- **Tell children what to do versus saying, "Don't..." when stating rules.**

"We get to go to the aquarium," the preschool teacher told the class. "We get to ride the bus there. Here are the rules for the bus. Number one is to talk quietly and use your inside voice. Number two is to stay sitting down."

"You might bang your face if you stand up," 3-year-old Darius added.

The teacher nodded and continued, "Number three is to wear your seatbelt. Buckle yourself in so you don't get hurt."

"You can't run in the school bus," 3-year-old Tracey said.

"Number four is to keep your hands inside."

"Yeah, something could hit your hand," Tracy added.

"Number five is to step off the bus," the teacher said, "and stay with an adult."

"If you jump out of the bus," Darius said, "you'll get hit."

"We want everyone to stay safe so we can have a fun time."

- **Use picture cues with words to show the main rules.**

On the first day of class, the preschool teacher pointed to a chart with pictures of the rules. She touched each picture as she read it. "Here are our rules. Number one: I keep myself safe." She slid her finger to the right, pointing to two pictures that were more detailed examples of that rule. "To keep myself safe: I listen to the teacher and I walk. Rule number two: I keep my friends safe." She moved her finger to the right for more examples. "To keep my friends safe, I use nice hands and nice words. Our last rule is I keep my things safe. To do that, I put away my toys. I use gentle touch with my toys."

- **Be consistent in implementing the group rules.**

The third graders met to start their newspaper. "What do you want to call it?" I asked them.

Ruby began, "I have an idea. I think we should call the paper…."

"*The Knight News*," Tom blurted.

"Hold on, Tom. Ruby is talking. Remember our group rule of just one person at time. We want to hear what you have to say after Ruby is done."

When Ruby finished, I turned to Tom and asked, "Now, what are your ideas?"

Establish Rules of Respect for Each Other

Create a climate of caring that enables children to work together. Start by establishing the basic rules of respect that specify how to act each other. Talk about the importance of using nice words and actions not only in therapy, but also in their lives.

A second way to promote caring is to ask children to be helpers to each other. Putting them in the helper role highlights their competencies and gives them an opportunity to discover the rewards of giving. Often what follows is that group members start volunteering to help one another. Also, notice and comment on any other compassionate gestures. For instance, you may say, "What a good friend you are," or "I'm sure your friend really appreciates that."

Depending on the group, you may need to further clarify the rules of respect. This often occurs during a time of conflict. You want to promote sharing, taking turns, and waiting patiently. Instead of tattling, encourage them to talk to each other and figure out possible solutions. Let them know that their friends will appreciate being asked before they touch, grab, or knock down their friends' projects. Also, teach the lesson that people will do more if they are asked politely including the use of "please" and "thank you," whereas demanding or barking an order creates resistance.

At the end of the session, take a minute to state the caring actions seen. Emphasize how they are a wonderful group. Children will learn that caring for others can be a gratifying experience.

Fabulous Five: State the Rules of Respect

- **Present rules in a way that conveys that you respect the children and believe in their maturity.**

"Welcome to our wonderful group," I said to 5-year-old Bradley, who came in the middle of the school year. "This group is so good about helping each other, sharing, and being nice to each other." The group members beamed as they listened. "Taylor, can you show Bradley how to start the pattern for the scarecrow?" I asked, and he nodded with a smile.

- **Tell children to only use kind words.**

"When we are together, how should we talk with each other?" I asked the group of second graders. "What are some good ways?"

The children responded:

"No yelling."

"Use a quiet voice. Talk it over if you're mad. Don't hit."

"Don't be rude."

"If someone took my eraser, I would say, 'This is my eraser and I want it back.'"

"Be kind and say nice things."

- **Let children know they need to ask before touching others' things or projects.**

"What do we need to remember about touching others' things?" I asked the group of kindergarteners.

"Ask and don't grab," Terry replied.

"What words can you use if you want to help someone build?"

"Can I help you?" Matt added.

- **Tell older children to ask before hugging others.**

When 7-year-old Clark headed for his teacher with outstretched arms, she said, "Clark, it's so nice you want to give me a hug. What could you ask me before hugging?"

"Can I give you a hug?"

"Yes," she replied with a smile. "At school it's good to ask before hugging someone."

- **Present the expectation that children will have to wait and take turns.**

"This is our baking group," I told the three girls on the children's psychiatric unit. "We get to make chocolate chip cookies, bake them, and eat them for snack today."

Seven-year-old Salinas smiled. "I love cookies!"

"In this group we have to work together to make them. That means everyone has to help, wait, and take turns."

Establish Essential Safety Limits

> **Children might be thinking:**
> *Am I going to get in trouble?*
> *You're mean.*
> *You don't like me.*
> *Are you going to hurt me?*
> *Oh, I am safe with you.*
> *No one is going to hurt me.*

Safety always comes first. You do not want children to hurt themselves, hurt others, or damage property. You have to show that you will consistently ensure their well-being. Stopping them implies that you will stop others from doing the same to them. It is critical that you do not give mixed messages in which you say one thing and do something else. If you state a consequence, you have to follow through with it. It also is crucial that if you disagree with other adults, talk with them in private and not in front of the children.

Demonstrate That You Will Keep Children Safe

It is normal for children to test limits to see what you will do. It is a discovery process for them. With some, there is a honeymoon period. They may follow all directions at first so they can check out what you are like. Then some will test you. They are deciding whether you mean what you say and are dependable. It is important for you to be consistent about what are considered acceptable or unacceptable actions. Although you may vary in what you allow, it is easier to start off stricter and then lighten up. After the children see that you mean what you say and will keep them safe, they tend to relax.

> ### *Fabulous Five: Show Children You Will Keep Them Safe*
>
> - **Tell children to keep themselves safe.**
>
>   Two second graders were playing tug of war on top of a large boulder.
>
>   "That's not safe," I said.
>
>   "We have to stop because that teacher said so," the young girl snipped.
>
>   A teacher behind me said to them, "No, you need to stop because it is not safe."
>
> - **Stop children from hurting themselves.**
>
>   Ten-year-old Harry made a mistake. As he erased it, he said, "I'm stupid," and started hitting his head on his desk.
>
>   "Harry, stop!" I said. "You are hurting yourself. And stop telling yourself that."
>
>   "That's what my dad says when he does something wrong."

"Well, that's not a good message to tell yourself. It's okay to make mistakes. Everyone does." Later, when he made another mistake, I reminded him, "It's okay to make mistakes. Don't be too hard on yourself. That's how you learn."

- **Stop children from being mean, being rude, or hurting others.**

Eight-year-old Tony mumbled in a goofy tone of voice, and Mike whispered to him, "You're retarded."

Tony continued making sounds.

"You're stupid. I hate you," Mike yelled.

"Stop," I replied. "If Tony is bothering you, use nice words to tell him to stop."

- **Be consistent so your actions match your words.**

Seven-year-old Audrey threw yellow beanbags at bowling pins as she swung high on a platform swing. She stopped and arched her back as if she were going to do a back flip off the swinging board. "Audrey, stop. That's not safe," I said, looking at the 2-foot drop to the mat. She hesitated for a minute and resumed the back flip. I caught her in midair. "Audrey, that was not safe. You could have gotten hurt."

"I didn't get hurt," she said with a huff.

"Well, I care about you and do not want you to get hurt. I need your promise that you will not do that again."

"I won't get hurt," she insisted.

I took the swing down and said, "When I hear a promise from you, I'll put the swing up again." In the next session, we started with a drawing activity. After she agreed to be careful, I hung up the swing.

- **Be consistent with other adults.**

"It's time to clean up," the preschool teacher said to the class.

"No. I don't want to clean up," Jessie yelled, stomping his feet. Then he kicked the wooden blocks surrounding him.

Because it was his first week at school, the teacher said, "I know you are still learning what we do at school. Everyone helps clean up. Just put three blocks in the bin and you'll be done."

"No," he said, folding his arms across his chest.

"Everyone line up to go outside. Dr. Clare, will you wait with Jessie until he puts those blocks away?" the teacher asked.

I agreed, and the rest of the class left. In a soft but firm voice, I said, "First put three blocks in. Then you can go outside." I waited quietly.

After a few minutes, he threw the blocks in the container and said, "Next time don't let them go outside without me."

"Just clean up and then you can go with the group," I replied.

Be Cognizant of Your Role When Setting Limits

When giving a directive or telling children to stop an action, you want to do it in a way that increases the likelihood that they will respond. First of all, you need to gain their attention before saying anything. Often, calling their names makes them turn and look. Then you want to convey your message with the least number of words. If you rant or ramble on and on, children get lost in your words. They may not be sure what you want them to do. It is also more effective if you get closer to them versus yelling across the room.

An important aspect is to be patient and give children time to respond. Some need extra time to process what you are saying, to calm themselves, and/or to decide whether to do what you are asking of them. If you bombard children with constant talking and expect an immediate response, you may find that they will either shut down or act out. If you find yourself frequently telling children to *stop*, try instead to find ways to get them started in the right direction.

Fabulous Five: Be Cognizant of Your Role When Setting Limits

- **Gain children's attention before setting limits.**

While sitting on the rug with his classmates, 3-year-old Dylan swiveled and turned his back to his teacher. When his eyes met mine, I pointed to my eye and then pointed to his teacher, giving him the message that he needed to look at her. He responded by shifting back to face his teacher.

- **Use the least number of words when setting limits.**

Five-year-old Allen came into the classroom with a scowl on his face. He grunted when classmates talked to him. After playing with manipulative toys, the group went to the rug. Allen ignored his teacher's request for him to join the others. He began racing around the room and then started to climb up on a two-tier bookcase.

"Stop! Put your feet on the floor," I said as I ran over and helped him climb down. "It is my job to keep you safe."

- **Be close by the children when giving directives or setting limits.**

Four-year-old Bailey started to pull a stuffed animal out of her classmate's hands.

Seeing the distressed look on the classmate's face, her teacher yelled from across the room.

Bailey continued tugging on it until the teacher was within 2 feet of her.

"Stop. Your friend had that first," she said. "If you want a turn, you need to say, 'Can I have a turn?'"

Bailey listened and repeated the words.

- **Give children time to respond to your directives.**

At the end of the day, 4-year-old Brandon's class walked over to the rug. He threw himself on the floor and did not budge. I showed him a picture symbol of a child sitting and said, "Go sit on the rug so we can sing our goodbye song." Knowing that he depended on the routine, I placed the card on the floor in front of him and waited. About 30 seconds later, he picked himself up and ran over to the group.

- **Give more start versus stop directives.**

The first week of preschool, 3-year-old Connor crawled around the rug. He rubbed one girl's shoe, touched the next child's T-shirt, and lifted up a girl's dress. Thinking that he was trying to make friends, his teacher said as she demonstrated, "Here in preschool, if you like someone you can touch your thumbs together. We call them thumb kisses." The class then practiced.

Ten minutes later, when Connor headed toward the classmate, I said, "Use thumb kisses."

He smiled and put his thumb up, and the classmate touched it.

State Limits in a Caring Manner

Children are more apt to follow what you request if you use a caring versus demanding tone of voice. They tend to be more willing to stop an action if you say you care about them and do not want them to get hurt. Your request implies that it is in their best interest to stop before something bad happens. For instance, instead of yelling, you can tell them, "Watch your step. I don't want you to bump your head when you go under the slide. That would hurt."

You also can set respectful limits by choosing words that do not convey blame or put them in a position of having to admit wrongdoing. Cue children to follow their peers who are acting appropriately. Another helpful way is to model the action you desire or ask a peer to show the children what to do. Children appreciate a caring versus controlling attitude as you keep them safe.

Fabulous Five: State Limits in a Caring Manner

- **Let children know that you are asking them to stop an action because you care about them.**

Seven-year-old Dean jumped on the mini-trampoline, stopped, and started to step onto a scooter board.

"Stop! I don't want you to get hurt," I shouted with concern, but not in time. Both of his feet were on the scooter board for a few seconds before Dean lost his balance and I caught him. "Please listen to me. I want to keep you safe. I care about you and don't want you to get hurt."

- Use wording that does not convey blame or require children to admit wrong-doing.

Six-year-old Donovan played with marbles and magnets on the table. One marble rolled off the table. "Please pick up that marble by your chair," I said.

"I didn't drop it," he insisted.

"It must have just rolled off. Please get it so we do not lose it."

He leaned over and scooped it in his palm.

- Model the action you desire of children.

At the bottom of the staircase, I put my index finger to my lips and whispered to 8-year-old Sasha, "We need to go back to class quietly."

She whispered back, "Okay."

- Have peers model what to do.

"One of my goals is to get Seth to stop sucking his thumb," his grandmother said.

"In class, he only does that when the class is on the floor and the teacher is talking," I replied. "We can definitely work on that."

The next day I taught the 4-year-old to hold his hands with his fingers laced together. Whenever he started to suck his thumb, I smiled and demonstrated what to do. His classmates quickly learned too.

The next week when he started to suck his thumb, I said, "Marco, show Seth what to do."

Marco tapped Seth's arm and said, "Here, look at me. Put your hands together." They smiled at each other, and Seth moved his thumb out of his mouth.

- Cue children to follow what other children are doing.

Four-year-old Felicia stood at the door and demanded, "I want to go outside."

The teacher pointed to the table full of toys and said, "Look at what your friends are doing. They're cleaning up. The way to go outside is to help your friends clean up."

Felicia curled her lip but moved in slow motion toward the table to help.

Use Reasonable Consequences

If safety is not a concern, you have to decide whether pursuing an issue is worth it. Some situations you can just let go and not make a big deal out of it. However, if children are not being safe, you may need to set consequences. The purpose of doing so is to make it a teachable moment versus punishment. You want them to learn to do something more appropriate. Consequences have to be reasonable and fair. When possible, avoid using the word *never*. In addition, if the consequence is delayed too long, younger children will not understand the connection. You also can point out natural consequences that are a result of their actions.

Fabulous Five: Use Reasonable Consequences

- **Decide which issues are worth a possible struggle.**

Damon walked in the room looking irritated. He looked at pictures and decided to color.

After 5 minutes of silence, I commented, "You're good at coloring within the lines."

The third grader crumpled the paper and threw it in the wastebasket. I sensed that he was looking for a reaction from me, so instead of having him redo the page, I sat quietly and waited.

Then he grabbed another paper and began coloring again.

- **State consequences in a matter-of-fact way.**

Five-year-old Freida flicked her paintbrush in the watercolors and sprayed blue paint over the sink and her shirt. "It would be better if you paint over here," I said, pointing to the paper-covered table.

"I don't want to."

"All right. I would hate to see you get paint on your pretty pink shoes, but it's up to you."

She crinkled her eyes as she thought about it, and a few seconds later she moved to the table.

- **Have consequences within an age-appropriate time frame.**

Three-year-old Lenny and his mother walked to the parking lot. Suddenly, Lenny ran ahead and started climbing on a concrete structure. "Get down and come back here," his mother yelled. He ignored her and climbed higher. "If you don't get down, you won't get to watch TV tonight," she threatened, but to no avail. She walked over and pulled him down.

Later, in a tactful way, I suggested to her that consequences for a 3-year-old should be more immediate, and we discussed different ideas of what she could do, such as saying, "It's unsafe for you to climb up there. If you don't come down now, we will not have time to get ice cream."

- **Set fair and realistic consequences.**

Three-year-old Mitch walked past Jake's block structure. Mitch swung his fist and knocked it down.

Jake began to cry.

"Look at your friend," I said to Mitch. "How does he feel?"

"He feels happy."

"I see tears, which tells me he feels sad. Jake, what can Mitch do to make things better?" I asked.

"He can help me rebuild it," Jake replied.

"That sounds like a good idea. That's fair."

Mitch started to wander away with a toy car in his hand, showing no interest in rebuilding. I guided him back and said in a neutral but firm voice, "First you help Jake make his house, and then you can play."

- **Point out naturally occurring consequences.**

"Everyone stand up. We are going to dance," the pre-school teacher said.

Three-year-old Eric rolled on the floor.

"Stand up," I repeated to him. "You could get stepped on."

Eric ignored me and remained on the carpet. The teacher turned on the music, and the other children danced around him. Then one child stepped on Eric's hand. "Ouch," he yelled.

"Stand up," I said. "Then you will not get hurt."

Help Children Learn the Connection Between Unsafe/Unwanted Actions and Consequences

The purpose of consequences is to help children learn to stop doing unsafe or unwanted actions. For them to learn, they need to understand the direct connection between the two. They need to know that when they do a specific action, a specific consequence will follow. Having consistency and predictability assists in this learning process.

Another way to solidify the connection is to show a picture symbol of the unsafe/unwanted action with an arrow leading to the resulting consequence. You also can have children reenact the scene but end with an appropriate action. This allows them to experience what they should do. If children are using unwanted actions to gain adult attention, ignoring them often works. They learn that doing an unwanted action does not get them the attention they desire. You may also make the connection by saying, "If you choose [state action], then you choose [state consequence]." Encourage them to make good choices. Make direct connections to facilitate children's learning.

Fabulous Five: Help Children Learn the Connection Between Unsafe/Unwanted Actions and Consequences

- **Use the same consequence with a specific action.**

In the specialized classroom, 3-year-old Melissa flung a wooden block, just missing a classmate's head. As we consistently did, I calmly took her hand, and together we walked over to the block. With my hand over hers, I had her pick up the block and drop it in the bin so she would understand how to handle blocks properly.

- **Show picture cues of an unsafe/unwanted action and corresponding consequence.**

Four-year-old Wes whacked a staff member with his fist. In response, she showed him a page with two picture symbols showing a child hitting and an arrow leading to the second picture of a child sitting. "You hit, you sit," she said as she walked him over to a chair.

She then showed him a file folder with the picture symbol of a child sitting. After a minute of sitting, she added a happy face without saying a word. When he started to get off the chair, she removed it. Wes sat back down. After sitting for 3 minutes, he earned three happy faces. Then the staff member said, "We keep each other safe. We use gentle touches. Go join your friends."

- **Have children reenact the scene ending with the appropriate action(s).**

Three-year-old Athena walked over, pushed a classmate off a chair, and sat down.

I calmly moved her off the chair and asked the classmate, who was not hurt, "Would you please sit back in the chair so we can show Athena how to use words."

She agreed. Then I told Athena to say, "Could I please sit there?" She repeated the words, and the classmate stood. "Now say, 'Thank you.'" She did, and I thanked the classmate.

- **Ignore children when they are using undesirable actions to get adults' attention.**

The preschool teacher handed everyone a picture cue of children sitting in a group. They all headed over to the rug, except 4-year-old Bryan. He ran in the opposite direction and crawled under a table. He then looked to see if staff would follow. In the past, giving him attention only prolonged these situations. So I stood and faced the group but kept him in my peripheral vision. After a minute of being ignored, he stood and ran over to the rug.

- **Tell children that if they choose [state action], then they choose [state consequence].**

"Everyone gets a beanbag to use with our song. Hang on to it. Keep it in your hand. If you choose to throw it, then you are choosing not to use it. Make a good choice," the preschool teacher told the class.

When the singer in the song directed the children to place the beanbag on different body parts, 4-year-old Jordan threw his beanbag in the air multiple times. The teacher caught it and said, "So sad. You chose to throw it, so now you don't have a beanbag for a minute." After the minute passed, she asked, "Are you ready to hold on to it now?"

He nodded, and she gave it back to him.

Make Sure Children Are Capable of Following Your Request

Children might be thinking:
I'm not sure what to do.
I can't do that.
That's too hard.

Consider whether children are capable of doing what you ask before you give directions or make requests. If you find they are refusing or not following through, remember that the first thing you should ask yourself is, "Do they have the skills and do they understand?" Think about why they are acting that way. It is often a lack of communication skills. They may not know the necessary words to express their needs or feelings. Make sure your expectations match what they are able to do.

Fabulous Five: Make Sure Children Are Able to Do What You Want Them to Do

- **Explore and address underlying reasons for children's actions that end up getting them in trouble.**

As 9-year-old Bryant followed his classmates back from recess, he bumped into the wall and ricocheted back, knocking two boys. "Hey, quit it," one yelled. When the class reached the doorway to their room, the line came to a halt. Sid bumped into Bryant's back. Bryant turned around and pushed Sid's shoulder.

After observing this incident, I talked with Bryant's teacher and explained how Bryant seemed to have limited body awareness. I told her that he also had a history of being sensitive to touch. We talked about possible strategies, like having him be the first or last in line but not in the middle, where he was more likely to be bumped. I also talked with Bryant, and together we identified the strategy of saying, "Stop. Give me some space," if someone was standing too close.

- **Check if children understand your request.**

"It's time to line up," the kindergarten teacher announced on the first day of school. Twenty students formed a line, but Shane stood to the side. "Get in line," the teacher repeated.

"Shane, stand behind Nikki. She's wearing the purple shirt," I said. Shane looked from left to right and wrinkled his eyebrows. "Look at what the other kids are doing. Do you know what 'behind' means?" He shook his head. I placed my hands on his shoulders and gently guided him to the line. "Here is Nikki; now you are behind or in back of your friend."

- **Make sure children are capable of following the directions.**

I observed 9-year-old Rudy writing in class and noticed that he wrapped his feet around the chair legs, which kept his body from moving.

"Put and keep your feet in front in you," his teacher ordered. He shifted his legs, and his feet dangled 4 inches from the ground. I left the class and returned with a footrest. I explained to his teacher that the footrest would allow him to keep his feet in front and hold his body still, which would also make writing easier for him.

- **Consider whether children have the needed communication or play skills.**

Four-year-old Tony began tickling Whitney. She grimaced, stood, and moved to a chair farther away. The next day, Tony ran up to his friend Clint, stuck out his stomach, and did a belly bump. Clint felt down and cried.

At our planning meeting that week, his teacher said Tony was frequently in trouble. The other children were complaining, and no one wanted to play with him.

"From what I observed, it looks like Tony wants to play with friends," I said. "But he doesn't know how and ends up hurting them. I think he has good intentions."

The group agreed. We created a Social Story on how to ask friends to play and read it to him.

- **Match difficulty level to children's skills.**

At the day treatment, 10-year-old Carl constantly had trouble in physical education (P.E.). One day he threw a scooter board at his teacher. The next day, I went to observe him and watched his teacher tell the group to stand on one foot and bounce a ball underneath the raised foot. Carl lifted his right foot up and started to bounce the ball, but after 3 seconds he lost his balance. Then he started throwing the ball against a wall and catching it. When his teacher saw him, she was upset that he was not following her directions.

Later that day, I tested Carl's motor skills and discovered that his balance was at a 4-year-old level. I shared the results with his P.E. teacher, and we talked about how his difficulty in P.E. was more a problem of delayed skill development rather than a lack of compliance. She adjusted the expectations. I also talked with Carl, and we started intervention. By the end of the school year, he could complete the same P.E. activities as his classmates.

Examine and Change the Environment to Prevent Problems

Children might be thinking:
It's boring here.
What's that over there?

Instead of assuming that all problems are the children's fault, think about what is happening in the environment and consider what *you* can change. Are the surroundings boring or distracting? Is there anything you can add, simplify, or eliminate that will make the situation better? Can you set up the environment with appropriate choices and let them choose? Figure out what can be done to prevent problems.

Fabulous Five: Make Changes in the Environment to Prevent Problems

- **Add to what is missing in the environment to eliminate difficulties.**

Five-year-old Gary threw pebbles on the slide and grabbed children's shirts as they slid down. Throughout recess, the school staff continually yelled at him to stop. Because there were no toys in the sand box, I thought about how there was nothing else for him to do. The next day, I brought two buckets and four shovels to the playground and handed them to him. "Here is something fun," I told Gary. "See what you can build."

A group of children gathered around him and asked, "Hey, can I play with you?" He smiled and nodded, and they joined him in the sand.

- **Have enticing and therapeutic toys or activities ready before children arrive.**

In the last two sessions, every time I suggested an idea, Logan automatically said no. So before the kindergartner entered the room in the third session, I placed two toy figurines on the table that were good for hand strengthening.

"Hey, it's a monkey," he said when he walked in the room. He lifted the toy and squeezed the buttons that made the monkey flip.

- **Change one aspect of the environment to prevent problems.**

"What's the weather like today?" the preschool teacher asked, pointing to a weather chart.

"Cloudy," the class yelled in unison. As the teacher continued with the opening group, Evan turned his back to her and flapped his T-shirt. Then he put his left arm around another child's shoulder for a few seconds until the child pulled away. Next, he rolled on the floor, bumping those around him.

I left the classroom and returned a few minutes later with a beanbag chair. I whispered to Evan, "Here, I brought something special for you. This is your own chair to sit on during group time. Stay on this chair. It's really comfortable."

He snuggled in the chair and sat still. The next week, his teacher reported that he continued to like his chair and stayed in his own space.

- **Simplify the environment.**

"We are trying to get Norm to stay in one center," the preschool teacher told me just before school started. That day, Norm chose to play with the blocks. He built one structure and knocked it down. Then he wandered out of the area to his right and ran to the sand table. The teacher directed him back. He fiddled with a truck and then wandered off to his left. Again he was guided back.

He's getting too distracted, and there are too many openings to this center, I thought. I moved a table next to the shelves to block one exit. I sat down, blocking the other exit. Then I gave him another bin of manipulative toys to use with the blocks, and he stayed put.

- **Prevent distractions.**

In the first session of the school year, the three 9-year-old boys chose a stress ball in the shape of an earth, star, or moon. As they squeezed the balls for hand strengthening, each child told what he did over the summer.

"This summer I went to a lake," Adrian said. The other two squirmed in their seats and grabbed the pencils on the table. They began poking the pencil tips into the stress balls.

"Please just squeeze the stress balls," I said, and the boys reluctantly dropped the pencils. In the next group, I only put the balls out and kept the pencils on my desk until we needed to write.

Prevent Problems

It is wiser and easier to prevent problematic situations than to have to deal with them (Figure 11-2). Continually observe and analyze what is helping the children. Try to understand the situation from the children's perspectives. What do the children want? What are the children trying to tell you? Do the children understand the direction or request? Create your own theory on why the children are acting the way they are. Then problem solve how to prevent confrontations.

Always consider if the children's language comprehension or delayed skill development is a factor. Also, preparing children ahead of time is important because it prevents a clash of expectations. If children know what to expect, they are less likely to start thinking, "I want…," causing you to have to say no. Recognize what have been problems in the past. Use this information to anticipate and prevent the same occurrence.

Let Children Know What to Expect

Children might be thinking:
Now I know what you expect of me.
Now I know what is happening.

One of the best preventative approaches is to let children know what to expect. Be proactive by preparing them for what will happen and when. Also, talking about the benefits of following expectations improves the likelihood of children responding.

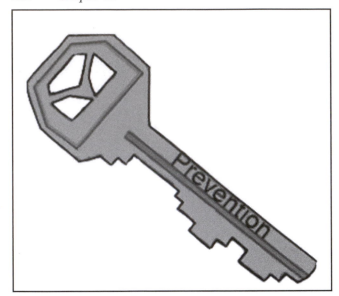

Figure 11-2. Prevention is key.

Be Clear About What to Expect

When you are clear about what will happen, there are no surprises or disappointments. A visual schedule and a routine make events predictable. Also, a group routine means a child will be following what the peers are doing. This eliminates you having to tell the child what to do. Clearly stating the rules before starting an activity helps prevent unwanted actions. Another option for alerting children to what will happen and preventing upset feelings is to create a number strip with a picture of the next activity at the end. This is especially useful for those who understand pictures more than words.

Fabulous Five: Let Children Know What to Expect

- **Prepare children for what to expect.**

At Halloween, 7-year-old Sid sorted skull and spider rings using tongs. He became entranced with a skull ring and slipped it on his middle finger. "You can wear and play with that ring here, but you will have to give it back before you leave the room," I said. At the end of the session, as we talked about his Halloween costume, I held out my palm to cue him to give me the ring. He dropped the ring in my hand and left without a fuss.

- **Use a visual schedule to show expectations,**

"Liam has been having multiple meltdowns," his kindergarten teacher told me. We discussed how the meltdowns often occurred near the end of the day, when he appeared to be on sensory overload.

"The routine use of a weighted vest and doing activities involving deep pressure sensation may help him," I said. "If he sees his twin brother wearing a weighted vest, he

does too, but he always declines if it's offered by a teacher. Liam likes to follow his visual schedule. Let's just add a picture symbol of the weighted vest."

His teacher and mother agreed.

The next day, Liam looked at the picture cue and put the weighted vest on by himself.

- **Create routines so children know what to expect.**

After testing 9-year-old Ashton's fine motor skills, I asked him to copy a sentence so I could have a sample of his writing. "No, I hate writing," he replied, folding his arms to emphasize his point.

"That's okay," I responded. "We can do things to make writing easier."

The next day, I said to Ashton's classmate, "Russell, please tell Ashton what we do in our group."

"First we squeeze stress balls to make our hands stronger. Then we practice some cursive letters in salt or putty. Then we do writing. A lot of times we make a book, and then we play a fun game." Ashton listened and then followed his peers in all the activities.

- **Clarify the rules before beginning an activity so the children know what to do.**

"What are the rules before we start the game?" the certified occupational therapy assistant asked the four fidgety 6 year olds.

"Keep your fingers out of your mouth," Sharlene said, her hand cupped beneath her chin.

"Yeah, no licking fingers," said Lewis, shifting his eyes to Todd because he tended to tap his buck teeth.

"Keep the dice on the board," Allison added.

"Uh-huh. The first time the dice go off, you get a warning. The second time you lose your turn. The third rule is to make sure you do not knock anyone off. No bowling, please. Let's have fun."

The group nodded in agreement.

- **Have a number strip with a picture of the next activity at the end.**

"Drew refuses to stop," his preschool teacher told me. "He has been throwing himself on the floor and yelling when I ask him to stop playing on the computer."

To help him adjust, I made him a strip with a row of numbers 1 through 5, each one attached by Velcro. At the end of the strip was a picture of the next activity, also attached by Velcro.

The next day, 5 minutes before Drew was to get off the computer, I showed him the strip and said, "You have 5 more minutes." One minute later, I removed the number 5. "You have 4 more minutes." I continued the countdown. After removing the number 2, I said, "You have 1 more minute." I pointed to a picture of blocks that was at the end of the strip and added, "Play in blocks." When I removed the number 1, he stopped with no tantrum.

Mention the Benefits if Expectations Are Followed

You can assist children in responding to your expectations by talking about the benefits that come afterward. Purposely choose wording that (1) states the expectation and (2) describes something good that will follow. One helpful strategy is to say, "First [state expectations], then [state benefit]." This is a way to simplify what is expected into only two thoughts: the expectation and the benefit. Use as few words as possible. For instance, say, "First clean up, then playground." Also helpful is using similar phrasing that describes the benefits being contingent on completing the expectations. This type of wording shifts children's thinking from, "I want…" to "After I do… I get…."

Fabulous Five: State the Benefits if Expectations Are Followed

- **Tell children, "First… then…."**

"During group time, Justin has been holding a stuffed dinosaur," his preschool teacher told me. "He likes to squeeze it, and the dinosaur helps him sit still."

The children entered the room and began playing with the toys and puzzles on the floor. After they played for a while, the teacher announced, "You have 5 more minutes." When it came time, she told the class to clean up.

"I want the dinosaur," 3-year-old Justin demanded, leaving his blocks on the floor.

"First clean up, then dinosaur," the teacher responded, repeating it until he started to pick up the blocks.

- **Say, "I will… when you…."**

In the specialized program, 3-year-old Caleb liked to keep a toy car in his hand throughout the day. Before going to the playground, however, all the children had to put their toys or favorite objects in a basket located next to the door. They could retrieve them when they came back inside. During Caleb's first week, he cried when he heard he would have to part with his car. When he refused, the rest of the class went out.

His teacher closed the door and said, "I will open the door when you put the car in the basket. There's a big truck on the playground you can play with."

After his teacher waited quietly for 5 minutes, Caleb dropped the car in the container.

- **Say, "Yes, you can… when/after you…."**

Four-year-old Asher sat on the tricycle, ready to start riding.

"Wait," I said as I placed my hand on the handlebars. "You need a helmet."

"I want to ride the bike," he demanded.

"Yes, you can ride the bike after you put on the helmet. The helmet protects your head if you fall."

Begrudgingly he allowed me to assist him in putting it on his head.

- **Say, "When you… then you can…."**

When it was time to go to the playground, the preschool teacher handed each child a picture symbol of a coat and said, "Get your coat. It's time to go outside."

As everyone donned coats, Mike stood at the door. I looked at him and pointed to the coat rack.

He started crying and tried to push the door open. I stepped between him and the door. "It's snowing out," I said. "It's cold. You need your coat."

When he did not budge, his teacher brought over his coat. Mike shook his head. "When you put your coat on, then you can go outside," she said. A few minutes after the other children left, Mike reluctantly put his coat on.

- **Say, "When I see you… I will know you are…."**

"Everyone come to the rug," the preschool teacher said. "I have a special message."

Three-year-old Casey came to the rug but kept rolling back and forth.

"Casey, when I see you sitting, I will know you are listening. Please sit and listen."

He stopped and sat with his legs crossed.

"Today we get to go to the park and have a scavenger hunt. That means we are going to look for different things. Everyone has a list with pictures of what to look for. We are going to have a fun day!"

Anticipate and Prevent Problems

> **Children might be thinking:**
> *You help me with my problems.*
> *It's better this time.*

Anticipate challenging situations and be creative in finding ways to prevent difficulties. Observe for children's tendencies and be one step ahead of what they might do. For example, if a child has a tendency to bolt out the door when going to the water fountain, position yourself in front of the door. Also, try to discover what tends to upset the child and, if possible, remove the object or change the situation.

Fabulous Five: Anticipate and Make Changes

- **Anticipate and address problems with children's perceptions.**

I brought two magnet sets into the kindergarten and knew both children would want the larger set. "I want this one," Monika said, pulling the larger box toward her.

"I want that one," Judson demanded.

I handed him the smaller box and said, "The magnets in this box are stronger. You get to play with the strong ones." He opened the box and started building a house.

- **Think of possible problems before children come to the session and plan ways to prevent the problems.**

"You can really tell that Debbie does not have good body awareness," I told the school psychologist. "She comes in the room with food smeared on her cheeks, bumps into kids in the hall, and often kicks me under the table."

That afternoon, I hung a 4-foot sheet of yellow paper for the group. I could foresee 6-year-old Debbie drawing off the paper onto the wall, so I drew a thick black 3-inch border around the paper to cue her where to stop. "Here's the frame for your picture. Color inside the frame," I instructed everyone.

"I'm drawing a big flower," 6-year-old Debbie said as she made sweeping motions for the leaves and touched the border. "Whoopsie."

"Stay inside the frame," I cued her again.

She sketched an outline of a daisy. "Look, Dr. Clare, I'm almost done. I'm doing good." I smiled in response.

- **Point out and discuss potential problems.**

Lying on his stomach, 9-year-old Cliff pushed the scooter board 5 feet and threw the turtle beanbag at the clown target. "I've got a good arm," he said as the turtle sailed into the clown's mouth.

"You do," I replied. Then he missed the next three throws and only had one beanbag left. "Marley, I need you to retrieve the beanbags for Cliff, and when it is your turn, he'll get them for you." Marley ran and stood directly behind the target. "Are you going to get upset if you get hit in the head?" I said with concern.

"No, I'll catch it."

"Why don't you get your hands up and ready just in case it comes close to your head."

Cliff threw and missed.

"Too high. Got to go lower," Marley yelled.

- **Discover what upsets the children, and change or prevent the situation.**

After his family moved in the middle of October, 4-year-old Logan transferred into the specialized preschool class. The teacher told me about his last school and added, "Mom said that he easily gets on sensory overload, and when he melts down it is hard for him to calm himself. He also hits and pushes."

The first day, Logan appeared fearful and kept going to the cozy corner, a quiet place with a beanbag chair, pillow, and blanket. He watched the group from a distance. The next day, the teacher showed him a blue cube chair, which he liked. A few days later, he came in and another child was sitting in his chair. "That's my chair," he yelled, starting to cry. He tried to push the classmate out of the chair.

Having seen that Logan viewed the chair as being comforting and safe, the teacher and I decided to designate the blue chair as his. We put another cube chair out for others to use.

- **Head children off at the pass.**

When the group from the specialized class went to the library, Yelena ran ahead and sat in the rocking chair that her second-grade teacher used while reading books. "Please move to your chair over here," her teacher said.

Yelena stayed put in the rocker and began wailing. Everyone in the library turned their heads and stared. The next time the class went to the library, her teacher walked ahead of her and sat in the rocking chair. Yelena looked for a chair and settled into her seat without a ruckus.

Use a Respectful Tone of Voice and Nonverbal Signs to Indicate "Stop"

Children are more likely to stop their actions if you ask them to cease in a respectful and supportive tone of voice. This lets them know you care about them even as you are setting limits. You also can use nonverbal signs to let them know you want them to stop. Using nonverbal signs, such as shaking your head, conveys your message in a simple way. Taking this type of approach can help them stop without embarrassing them or creating a scene.

Use a Supportive Tone of Voice

> **Children might be thinking:**
> *Oh, I better stop.*
> *You're not mad at me.*
> *You don't want me to feel unhappy, bad, or scared.*
> *I like how you used the tone you used rather than yelling at me.*

Your tone of voice is a critical element when setting limits, and it affects children's reactions. Staying calm with an easygoing approach is good for defusing a situation. If you sound harsh, demanding, or controlling, they will often think you are mean. Some may become angry and be more determined not to listen to you. Some may feel belittled. Others may feel hurt. Purposely choose a tone of voice that conveys that you care and want the best for them.

Fabulous Five: Use Supportive Tone of Voice

- **Use noncritical statements in a neutral voice.**

Seven-year-old Shawna screeched in the seat next to me. "Whoa. Inside voice, please," I said. Then I pointed to my ears, grinned, and added, "My ears work just fine." Shawna smiled back.

- **Use a nondemanding tone of voice and ask children to repeat what you said.**

Six-year-old June looked at her classmate flipping through a book of pictures that looked like a movie. "I want a turn with that flipbook too."

"You will get a turn when Susan is done," I replied, then gave her the choice of three other activities. She chose the magnets but said two more times, "I want a turn."

"What did you hear me say about that?" I asked in a gentle voice.

"Wait your turn."

"I promise you will get a chance to play with the book too."

- **Maintain an easygoing versus controlling tone of voice.**

At the beginning of the baking group, two second graders giggled for about 3 minutes. "I think you like to laugh a lot," I said to the girls with a smile.

"Dr. Clare. Auntie Clare," Lily teased and laughed.

"I'm not your aunt," I said with a chuckle. Lily and Linda laughed again. "Okay, let's think about making these chocolate chip cookies. Lily, we need you to add the flour." Giggling, she reached for the measuring cup.

- **Speak respectfully by talking to children in a way that is not belittling.**

Dee squeezed a hole puncher and made a star. "Dr. Clare," a staff member called. I turned away from Dee for 5 seconds, and when I glanced back, the 9-year-old was pressing the hole puncher on her hand.

"Is that a good idea?" I asked in a calm voice.

"No."

"What could happen?"

"Maybe it could hurt my hand."

"Yes, I don't want you to get hurt. Please don't do that."

- **Use the speed, volume, and tone of your voice to guide.**

Each week, the occupational therapy student taught the third-grade class at the day treatment different sensory strategies they could use to keep calm in class. During the second week, she instructed, "Let's try a chair push-up. Put your hands on the side of your chair and push your body up."

The five children groaned as they lifted their bodies in the air and then dropped back to the chairs with a loud thud.

She whispered slowly, "Let's try again and see how quietly you can do it." This time they moved slowly and silently.

Give a Nonverbal Message for Stopping

Children might be thinking:
Am I going to get in trouble if I don't stop?
I see you want us to stop.
You don't want me to get embarrassed.

When setting limits, you can choose to use nonverbal signs as a subtle way to stop an action. By not using words, you can convey your message in a quiet manner. This can limit distractions to a group and prevent embarrassment to the child. One way is to use culturally appropriate signals for stopping. This may include shaking your head, hand gestures, or even sign language. Another option is to create together a unique signal that all involved can understand.

Fabulous Five: Show a Nonverbal Sign to Indicate Stop

- **Shake your head.**

Two 6-year-old boys started poking each other in the ribs. I looked in their direction. When our eyes met, I shook my head and they stopped.

- **Use a subtle hand gesture to convey a message.**

Dan continually tapped his pencil on the side of the table. His fourth-grade teacher nonchalantly walked up to him and gently put her palm on his hand to let him know he needed to stop. He glanced at her, stopping tapping, and resumed writing.

- **Gesture without saying a word.**

"I'm not doing this anymore. I need to rest," 6-year-old Simone said. She moved off the chair, plopped on the carpet, and kicked her legs in the air. I held up my palm to indicate stop. She dropped her legs to the floor. I waited without saying a word. After about 3 minutes, she peeked at me to see if I was watching her. With my palm up, I curled my fingers and beckoned for her to come back to the table. She strolled back and sat on the chair.

- **Use sign language to define limits.**

While the teacher was reading a book, 3-year-old Paul wandered amongst the sitting children. He smiled and patted each head as he passed. Because Paul knew basic sign language, I made the sign for "stop." I pointed to his beanbag chair and signed the word "sit." He watched me, then walked to his spot and nestled in the chair.

- **Create a nonverbal signal to cue children to stop an action.**

Although Scott was a fifth grader, he had a habit of talking in an infantile manner. At times, his speech would become more nasal with a slight stutter. The other children often made fun of him. To help him stop this habit, a staff member talked with Scott, and together they created a signal of touching the index finger to the chin. From then on, whenever he talked like a baby, staff would give him the signal. Without the other children knowing it, he received the message and resumed talking normally.

Help the Group Get Settled

When a group of children become unruly or too loud, let them know you want them to be quiet. This can be done nonverbally or with words. You also can address a ruckus by making changes to what you are doing or adding something new. Often this captures their attention. Another way to regain control of the group is to ask them to take action.

Show Your Desire for Quiet

> **Children might be thinking:**
> *But I want to tell my friend….*
> *It's too loud.*
> *That hurts my ears.*

You can help a group settle down by giving a clear message that you want them to be quiet. One way to indicate this message is the use of gestures and a soft tone of voice. Ironically, talking in a whisper tends to be more successful than trying to shout. Children will often stop talking to listen to what you have to say. Giving a countdown signal or waiting patiently for all group members to become quiet also works. Having the child who is quiet go first in the activity can be a motivating factor in decreasing the noise level.

> ### *Fabulous Five: Indicate Your Wish for Quiet*
> - **Use hand gestures and a soft, soothing voice.**
>
> "What should we do today?" I asked the group of fourth graders.
>
> Five children shouted their ideas at the same time. I raised my hand and then lowered it slowly to indicate the need for them to lower their voices. Then, in a soft and caring tone, I said, "You have lots of ideas. When you all talk at once, it is hard to hear you. Let's take turns and use an inside voice to say what you are thinking."

- **Use whispering to calm.**

The three preschoolers screeched as they snatched the Play-Doh off the table. "Whoa," I said as I pulled the Play-Doh toward me. Then I said softly, "It's too crazy and noisy when everyone is grabbing and yelling. Whisper, 'I'm ready,' when you want to start."

"I'm ready," each child whispered back.

- **Give a hand signal indicating a countdown.**

The group of third graders grew increasingly loud. "Everyone look," the teacher said. She held up three fingers and, as she lowered each one, said, "Three, two, one." Then she touched her index finger to her thumb, making a circle. "Zero noise."

- **Say, "When everyone is quiet, then we can start."**

"Please sit down," the occupational therapy student said. "I have something really cool. I can't wait to show you." The third graders made a beeline for the table but started shouting at each other. "When everyone is quiet, then we can start." The group stopped and turned their heads toward her.

"What are we going to do?" Kari asked.

"I'm going to show you," she replied as she pulled out a tumbling tower game. "This is going to be fun." Then she demonstrated how to take out the bottom block without tipping the tower.

"I can't wait to do this," Quinn said with a grin.

- **Tell the children that whoever is the quietest will go first.**

During the last week of school, the kindergartners bounced as they sat on the floor, and their voices became increasingly loud. I put the game board between them and said, "Whoever is the quietest will go first."

"I'm going to zip my mouth," Jackie said, pressing her lips together without uttering a peep while the other two giggled. "Jackie gets to go first," I announced.

At the beginning of the next session, Jackie said, "Whoever is the quietest gets to go first."

Make Changes or Add Something New to Help a Group Settle

> **Children might be thinking:**
> *Somebody might get hurt.*
> *What's that?*
> *Good, we get to move.*

Another approach for helping a group settle down is to change the current situation. If you find children are running wildly around the room or are in constant motion, have them sit on the floor. Children will tend to shift quickly to a quieter state. An additional strategy is to change to a different type of activity. If they are not interested in the current activity, switch to a contrasting one. For example, if they are sitting, have them stand. If they are manipulating small objects, have them do large movements. Adding something new tends to capture children's attention, which in turn helps them to stop what they are doing. Props, including toys, are eye-catching, especially with younger ones. A mystery or a surprise can also quiet a group in seconds.

Fabulous Five: Make Changes or Add Something New

- **Have the group sit on the floor if they are restless.**

Travis and Tate ran around the room and threw toys in the air. "Come over here and sit with me," the occupational therapy student said to the first graders, patting the carpet in front of him. They stopped and plopped on the floor. In a soft voice, he said slowly, "You are winding yourselves up. It's time to calm down." They sat quietly. "Now I can show you our game," he said, and then gave the directions.

- **Introduce a new or novel object, toy, or activity.**

The three 5 year olds started laughing as they wiggled in their seats.

"Hey, check this out," I said in animated voice.

Curious, the children turned toward me.

"I want to show you my special markers. First you color with one marker. Then use this special maker to trace, and it changes the color." There was silence as they began to color.

- **Change to a different type of activity if the group is restless.**

"Watch me, and then make the letter 'P' on your board," I instructed.

"Poop, poopsie, poopie head," 3-year-old Jill giggled while rolling on the floor.

"That's not nice talking," said Tristan, and I nodded in agreement.

Lance took the chalk and marked his foot.

"Lance wrote on his foot," Jill giggled, and they both laughed.

"Finish the letter," I said. "It's time to go to the table and cut out your penguin."

Once they sat down and started cutting, they became quiet.

- **Use props to help a group settle.**

The two preschoolers were jumping in place and yelling, "I want to start." Another 3 year old ran into the room and tripped over Tamara.

I held a clown marionette and raised the puppet's hand to his mouth. "Mr. Clown says, 'Shh. Shh. You need to sit in a circle. We are going to build a monster and we'll take turns. I'm going to sleep, so use your quiet voice.'" I laid the clown against a bin, looking like he was asleep.

A minute later, Tucker yelled, and Tamara put her index finger to her lips and said, "Shh. The clown is sleeping."

When I raised my voice, Tamara whispered, "Shh!"

"You're right." I turned to the clown and said, "Sorry, Mr. Clown. Go back to sleep." The group spoke softly for the next half-hour.

- **Use mystery or a surprise.**

The three children ran in circles laughing. When I placed a box on the table, the group of second graders stopped and gathered around the table. "What is it?" Andrew asked, intrigued.

"It's a surprise. Sit down and I'll show you."

Ask the Group to Take Action

Children might be thinking:
I can do that.
I know the answer.

The third major approach for getting control of a group is to ask them to take action. You may want to tell them to close their eyes and give them a suggestion regarding what to think about. This strategy quickly eliminates any visual distractions. Another tactic is to request an answer to a question. Children will have to shift their attention to you in order to respond. You also can clap and ask the group to clap back, which can easily turn into a game if you vary the tempo of the clapping. Another way is to have them copy a movement or sing a song with a variety of motions. The use of calming strategies such as deep breathing also can lower the level of activity.

Fabulous Five: Have Children Take Action

- **Have children close their eyes for calming.**

Five-year-old Evan pulled his bottom eyelids down and laughed. Roxana rolled on the floor. "He's making us laugh. I have the giggles today."

"Close your eyes and think about your favorite toy."

They quieted as they wrinkled their faces with their eyes shut.

- **Ask the group to respond to a question.**

Four-year-old Jolie ran ahead of me and yelled, "Come on, Dr. Clare. Let's have some fun. Hurry. Hurry." We joined the other two preschoolers sitting on the floor and started a bear hunt game with corresponding hand motions.

"Let's climb a tree," I said, and we all pretended to scramble up the tree with our hands. "Do you see a bear?" I asked, and we looked right to left.

"No," everyone replied. Jay jumped up and circled the room like a zooming bee.

I brought him back to the group by asking him a question. "Jay," I said, "where do you think we should go next to look for the bear?"

"In the water," Jay said as he ran back to the group.

"Okay, everyone swim." The children did the crawl stroke. "Now where do we go?"

"In the house."

The group pretended to open the door, and I said, "Oh no. It's a bear. Run with your hands." We all slapped our thighs, sounding like a drumroll. I whisked my right hand across my forehead and said, "Whew. We are safe."

- **Clap your hands and have children clap back.**

When four boys yelled, 6-year-old Jordan shouted to me, "My teacher claps her hands and we clap back. You should do that."

"Okay. Thanks for the idea," I said, and clapped three times.

The boys responded with perfect rhythm.

- **Tell group members to follow your movements.**

Three preschoolers pulled out Legos and began building. Lorna and Luis looked at me and started talking at the same time about what they wanted to build. Their voices became louder to the point of almost screaming. Connie covered her ears, raised her shoulders, and opened her mouth, ready to yell. I quickly said, "Connie, is it too noisy for you?"

She nodded.

"Lorna and Luis, it's getting too noisy. Everyone put your hands together and wiggle your fingers. It's a butterfly. Put your butterfly on your tummy." The group quieted and moved their hands to their stomachs.

- **Have the group use strategies involving deep pressure sensation or deep breathing.**

When the group of third graders at the day treatment became unruly, I said, "Stop! I need everyone to be quiet." I waited a minute. "It looks like a lot of people need to calm down. So everyone put your hand on your stomach and take 10 slow, deep breaths. You should feel your stomach moving." Afterward, in a slow and calm tone of voice, I said, "Okay, now we can talk about what happened."

Choose Your Words and Reactions When Setting Limits

Another way to be responsible for your role in the interactions with children is to consciously choose the wording you use and your reactions to what they do. At the same time, make explicit that your intention is to help versus boss them around.

Select Your Words Carefully

> **Children might be thinking:**
> *No, I don't want to.*
> *I can't.*
> *Can I trust you?*
> *You really care so much about me. You're trying to help me.*

The careful choice of words can prevent a power struggle. When you ask children to do something that they have to do, avoid asking, "Will you…?" or "Do you want…?" or ending your sentence with "Okay?" These questions imply that you are giving them a choice and it is fine to say no. Then, if they decline, you are in the awkward position of insisting they go against their wishes. Similarly, starting a request with "Can you…?" can be interpreted by children to mean, "Do you want to?" or "Do you have the ability to do it?" They can easily say no to this type of phrasing.

Be aware that saying the word *don't* often makes people want to do that action. For instance, when you are at a museum and are told, "Don't touch the painting," you start wishing you could touch. Some children think being told "don't" is a dare to do it. Try to find other words to get your message across. You can emphasize an expectation before there is a problem by using words such as, "Like always…." In addition, it is helpful to describe what you see and want stopped. Use neutral words that do not convey blame.

> **Fabulous Five: Choose Your Wording**
> - **Avoid saying, "Do you want to…?" or "Will you…?" or ending your request with, "Okay?" when it is not a choice.**
>
> I went to get Ryan in his first-grade class in the day treatment. He was coloring with his head close to the desk and pressing the crayon hard on the paper. "He's A-N-G-R-Y," the paraprofessional spelled out. Then she turned and asked him, "Do you want to go with Dr. Clare?" He shook his head.
>
> "Do you want to finish coloring before we go?" I said. He nodded. I whispered to her in a gentle tone, "Next time, please don't ask, 'Do you want to?' when it is not a choice." She nodded in agreement, realizing what she had said.

- **Say, "Try" versus "Can you...?"**

"What's that?" 6-year-old Olivia asked.

"It's blue sand for making letters."

As Olivia ran her fingers through the sand, the occupational therapy student said, "Can you use your finger to write your name?" Olivia ignored the student and drew a face.

"Try using your finger to write your name," the occupational therapy student said, and Olivia started the "O."

- **Be aware that saying, "Don't" often becomes a dare or may create a desire to do the action.**

As we made letters in salt, I said, "Don't eat the salt because all the kids have touched it."

Immediately 5-year-old George stuck his index finger into the salt and tasted it. He scrunched his face and said, "Yuck."

- **Start with, "Like always..." and state the expectation to convey a message of consistency.**

As we headed to another school building, Winston, who was holding a red pencil in his hand, raced Will. "Walk," I shouted to the first graders, and they slowed down.

"I won," both boys yelled in unison.

"I know you are both fast runners. Just make sure you walk when you have pencils in your hands. You don't want to get hurt," I said.

The next week as we went to the other building, I repeated, "Like always, be sure to walk while carrying your pencils. I don't want you to get hurt."

- **Say, "I see [describe action], and that tells me...."**

"Debbie, I see your pencil flying all over the table. It almost hit Hannah," her third-grade teacher said. "That tells me you are not being safe. Hold on to your pencil."

Decide How to Respond

> **Children might be thinking:**
> *You're funny.*
> *You care about me.*
> *You're kinda nice.*
> *You want me to get it right, and you want to help me.*

How you respond to children is a choice. It can be detrimental if your first response is always that of a serious authoritarian. This approach sets up the dynamic of you against the children. Instead, you can convey that you want to work and be together. One way to do that is to agree with them. Another way is to laugh, joke, or make light of the situation. Reacting with a puzzled or surprised look suggests that you are trying to understand them. You also may want to give a compliment regarding what they are doing or saying, and then state your concern.

Fabulous Five: Respond Intentionally

- **Respond with, "I wish we could too."**

"I don't want to stop," 6-year-old Walt insisted. "I want to keep playing with you."

"I wish we could keep playing too. I like being with you, but I have to go see another boy. Would you like me to bring this toy back the next time?" He nodded.

- **Laugh and joke as a response.**

"Do we have to do ALL of these?" 7-year-old Glenda said, looking at four puzzles.

I laughed and said, "Yes, we're going to be here all night. Did you bring your pajamas?"

"Noooo," Glenda giggled.

- **Make light of the situation.**

The day after a blizzard, I told the group of first graders, "I didn't get much sleep because of the snow storm. I had to shovel a lot of snow. I'm really tired, so I need you to try your best today."

The group started the butterfly cutting activity. Kenau cut one wing and then yelled, "This is too hard."

I grinned and said, "Listen. I'm already tired and a little crabby. We both can't be crabby on the same day. This is hard on purpose. It's to help you learn."

He smiled in response.

- **Act puzzled or surprised.**

Six-year-old Justin made an "n" instead of an "h."

"Oh, just add a line to the 'n.' Don't erase," I said.

He waved his hands in the air and stomped his feet. "I want to erase. I don't want to add a line."

I crinkled my eyebrows and said, "I don't understand. The way I suggested is easier. When you erased before, you ripped the paper. Make it easy on yourself." He reluctantly added the line.

- **Compliment, then express concern.**

Corey talked constantly while the other first graders colored their dinosaur book covers. "Corey, you know a lot of interesting things. One thing I am concerned about is that you're not going to finish your book if you keep talking and do not start to color."

State Your Good Intentions

> **Children might be thinking:**
> *Oh, you're going to help me.*
> *You want to help.*
> *Maybe I shouldn't get mad at you.*
> *Maybe you are trying to help me feel better and get things done.*

At times, children may view you as someone who is trying to control them by telling them what to do. They may think you are being mean. This perception can lead to a desire to rebel. You may need to clearly state that your intention is to help and not to control. In addition, tell them you are trying to make it easier or better for them. You may also want to ask them how you can be of assistance or suggest how you can help them achieve what they want.

Fabulous Five: Give the Message That You Are a Helper

- **Let children know you are trying to help.**

Seven-year-old Saul tried a number of pencil grips, which did not seem to help. When I started to show him how to hold the pencil between his index and middle finger, his eyes became teary and he said harshly, "That hurt when I tried it before."

"Stop a minute. The way you are talking, you sound mad."

"I always talk like that," he snipped back.

"I'm trying to help you. The way you write now is going to make your hand tired when you have to write a lot. So I am just trying to figure out how we can make this easier for you."

"Oh," he whispered.

- **State that you are not trying to be mean.**

Holly held the scissors with her thumb down and in the larger loop, which made cutting awkward. Pointing to the scissors, I said to the 4 year old, "Try moving your thumb into the smaller loop and cut with your thumb up."

Holly yanked the scissors and paper toward her body and gave me a look of disgust.

"I'm not trying to be mean. I'm trying to show you a way to make the scissors work better."

- **Assist children in understanding your intentions.**

"Your 'B' is going the wrong way."

I want to do it my way," 6-year-old Lisa-Marie said.

"Am I trying to help you or make it harder for you?"

"Help me," she whispered.

"Yes. Give yourself a chance to learn."

- **Tell children you will help them obtain their wishes or desires.**

Seven-year-old Clark scrambled up the curly slide in the park, colliding with a descending little girl. "Clark, use the ladder so no one will get hurt," I said.

"But I like going up the slide this way."

"Then you need to wait. I will be your lookout and tell you when there are no kids. Wait for the okay sign to go. I just want to make sure you and the other kids do not get hurt."

Three children swished down the slide, and Clark waited. I checked the top of the slide, raised my thumb up, and said, "It's okay now." He grabbed the sides and wiggled up the slide like a caterpillar.

- **State the expectation and then say, "What can I do to help you?"**

"Your teacher said you have to answer the questions on this paper. I see you looking around and not getting anything written. What can I do to help you?" I asked the first grader.

Myrna shrugged. Then she said, "You can get me headphones. Sometimes that helps."

Help Children Save Face When Setting Limits

It is important to always consider how you can assist children in saving face. This means you help in a way that does not require them to admit that they are wrong, they have no control, or they are different. Thus, you provide a way for children to avoid embarrassment and maintain a sense of control.

Avoid Embarrassing Children When Setting Limits

Children might be thinking:
I don't want to look stupid.
Someone might laugh at me.
Don't make me look bad.
Can we talk later, not now?

Humiliating children is not a good way to teach them a lesson. It just teaches them that adults can be mean. The best approach is to avoid being demeaning and embarrassing them as you help them learn better ways to act. You can still be firm and keep them safe without belittling them.

Help Children Look Good in Front of Their Peers

In all your interactions with children, you do not want to embarrass them. Continually ask yourself, "Will my actions make them look bad to their peers or cause them to be laughed at by others?" If they perceive themselves as being berated or belittled, they may feel humiliated or angry. To save face, some may act like clowns or worse to show others that your words or actions do not affect them.

If you need to point out what they are doing wrong, try to talk to them in private. Be subtle and avoid calling attention to what you are doing. You may want to talk or interact with everyone in the group so one child is not singled out. You also may help them save face by telling them you have done the same thing too.

Fabulous Five: Avoid Embarrassing Children When Setting Limits

- **Talk to children in private.**

"Hey," Jessie shouted. "I want that top."

"Jessie!" 5-year-old Carlos screamed, covering his ears with his hands. "She was saying that too loud and making my ears hurt."

I involved the group in an activity and said, "Carlos, I can see that upset you. Let's go over here and talk." We walked a few feet away, but I kept the group in my sight. "Carlos, what can you do to let someone know they are talking too loud and that bothers you?"

"Tell them stop."

"Yes, and be sure to say it in an inside voice." Then I spoke with Jessie privately.

- **Use a normal tone of voice when setting a limit to avoid embarrassing children.**

The preschoolers sat on the rug while their teacher read them a story. Kayla listened for a few minutes but then leaned back until she was lying on the floor.

"Sit up so you can see the good book," I said in a normal tone of voice. "A good part is coming."

She popped up and turned toward the teacher.

- **Tell the group what is expected instead of just telling the child.**

As I started to give the directions to the activity, 4-year-old Seth started talking to the child next to him. Rather than calling Seth's name, I told the group, "I need everyone's eyes and ears. I'm trying to tell you what to do so we can get on to our fun game." When all eyes were on me, I gave the directions.

- **Present the limit as a concern.**

When I looked over, I saw that 4-year-old Rashon had built a 3-foot tower with large wooden blocks. As he started to add another one, I said, "Please stop. I am concerned that the tower could fall on your head and hurt you. If you want a tall tower, use the cardboard blocks."

- **Tell children you have done the same thing when asking them to stop an action.**

In the second-grade class, Becca leaned out of her chair 2 inches toward Candace. "Becca, you are too close to Candace. Sit back in your chair. Sometimes I get excited too and do not realize how close I am to someone."

Offer a Different Explanation

Another way to help children save face is to attribute the difficulty to being a problem with the situation. By offering a different explanation or perspective than the view that something is wrong with them, you allow them to look good to others and feel better about themselves. In addition, if you find that they are refusing to do something, you can quickly move out of a potential power struggle by saying, "Oh, you just want to watch." Instead of giving them the message that they are being defiant or are not trustworthy, use an approach that allows them to maintain their self-respect.

Fabulous Five: Offer a Different Explanation

- **Reframe by providing a different perspective.**

As we started walking to Seth's first-grade class, he asked, "Can I walk myself back?"

"No, I always walk kids back to class," I responded.

"You're mean," he said.

"I like you, and this way I get to spend a few more minutes with you."

He stopped, grinned, and gave me a hug. The smile stayed on his face as he walked all the way back to class.

- **Identify the difficulty being with the situation instead of the children.**

On a nippy day, 5-year-old Jacob ran around the room in circles. Instead of chiding him for being too active, I said, "I know you didn't get to go outside for recess. I have a challenge for you. Let's see how many chair push-ups you can do."

- **Give a reason for your request that does not imply the children are bad or in trouble.**

The two talkative boys sat on the floor in the back of the group. They bumped shoulders and laughed. "Patrick and Paxton, come up to the front so you can hear better," the teacher said in an even tone voice. The 6 year olds moseyed to the front and stopped talking.

- **Say, "Oh, you just want to watch," if children are refusing.**

"Today I want to show you some ideas of what you can do to help yourself. You can do these if you feel wiggly," I said to the preschool class, shaking my shoulders, "or if you want to get calm." I held up a picture of a boy pushing his palms together. "Everyone push and take a big breath. Now relax." Then I showed a picture of a girl blowing on her finger. "Pretend you are blowing out all the candles on your birthday cake. Take a super big breath and blow."

Everyone tried except Luke. I walked over to him and held out my finger, "Try blowing." He sat still and tight-lipped with a smirk on his face. "Oh, you just want to watch," I said, and continued with the next picture.

- **Find a way that prevents a problem without making children look bad.**

"We've discovered that Erik has been taking supplies from the classroom," his third-grade teacher told me.

In my first group in the class, I gave each child putty and tongs and then counted the mini-erasers. "Everyone gets 10." At the end of the session, I recounted them.

"Why do you count?" Erik asked.

"So I can make sure I have them all and none have fallen on the floor."

Avoid Backing Children Into a Corner

> **Children might be thinking:**
> *I'm doing this because I want to.*
> *I'll think about it.*
> *Maybe I can do it later.*

If you make a demand and do not give choices, children may feel like they are backed into a corner with no escape. In this situation, they may submit but feel angry or humiliated. They may fold their arms and not move. Or they may feel the need to fight back. Unless they are in immediate danger (e.g., running into a street), always try to give choices and help them save face.

Give Choices and Have Children Choose Between Options

One way to guide children is to establish what needs to be done and then provide two choices in that realm. For example, you may say, "Do you want to clean up the blocks or the toy cars?" Cleaning up is not a choice. This approach helps them switch from thinking, "I'm not doing it," to "Which one should I do?" Other options are to let them decide which one to complete first and to pick when, where, or how they will do the action or activity. Even with children who are starting to become agitated, you can state the expectation and then ask if they can do it by themselves or if they need your help. This choice gives them time to think and hopefully regroup. Giving choices is a way to help children feel more in control.

> ### *Fabulous Five: Provide Specific Choices*
>
> - **Give two choices for what has to be done.**
>
> "He's sitting in the teacher's chair," the children yelled, pointing to 3-year-old Joey.
>
> "You can sit in that chair or this one," I replied, gesturing to empty seats. He took the plate and shoved it across the table. Then he picked up the fork and spoon and threw them. I moved the place setting out of his reach. He moved out of the teacher's chair and took one boot off and threw it. I caught it midair. "Not safe. We keep our friends safe. You're mad you can't sit in the teacher's chair."
>
> Joey sat down on the floor and did not move. I waited for about a minute and then said, "You can sit here or there." When he saw some orange slices on the table, he picked one of the chairs I had pointed out closest to them.

> - **Give children the choice of which action to complete first.**
>
> "Tucker, pass the glue. Barbie needs it too."
>
> "No, I won't," he yelled, overturning the glue bottle and throwing the scissors on the floor.
>
> "Now you need to clean that up," his kindergarten teacher said.
>
> "I'm not doing it," he shouted, sliding down until his head rested against the back of the chair.
>
> I turned the glue bottle upright to minimize the required cleanup and obtained wet paper towels. I sat next to Tucker without saying a word for about 2 minutes, giving him a chance to settle. Then I slid the paper towels toward him. "Here, I brought these for you. What do you want to do first? Pick up the scissors or wipe up the glue?"
>
> He stomped, stooped, and snatched the scissors off the floor. Then he stuffed the paper in his palm and began swishing it over the glue-covered table.
>
> - **Mention the time frame and allow them to decide when to complete the action or activity.**
>
> "I don't want to do my card," 7-year-old Elise said.
>
> "Everyone is finishing the cards today. Do you want to do it now or in a few minutes?"
>
> "In a few minutes." She completed a drawing of her dog, then waved her purple pencil with a pink heart eraser and said, "This is my magic pencil. It brings me good luck."
>
> "Use your magic pencil to finish your card so you can take it with you."
>
> - **Provide children with choices regarding where or how but not whether the activity will be done.**
>
> The 5 year old started running around his classroom. I grabbed the activity sheet and said, "Chris, where would you like to sit to color? Your desk? The floor? The table?"
>
> "The floor."
>
> "Okay," I said, grabbing a red beanbag chair to help him get comfortable and handing him a clipboard for his paper.
>
> - **Ask children if they can do it themselves or if they need help.**
>
> As the preschool class lined up at the fence, 3-year-old Trent ran in the opposite direction back to the playground. I went after him. He climbed the ladder and slipped inside the tunnel. "That's not safe," I said. "Look where all your friends are. It's time to go and play inside." Trent stared at me and did not budge. "Can you do it yourself or do you need help?" Reluctantly and in slow motion, he came out of the tunnel.

Give the Option to Say No or to Not Use Your Idea

When you present your ideas as options, children are more open to hearing what you have to say. By making suggestions or allowing them to say no, they tend to mull it over and consider if it is something they want to do. If they agree, they are more likely to follow through. State their choices in a neutral way and be clear that they can accept or decline. This lets them save face if they want to say no.

Fabulous Five: Give Children Options

- **Present your idea as information.**

Seven-year-old Paul pulled out a glob of putty and plopped it on the table. "Let me punch it flat," he said, and pounded the putty with his knuckles.

"It flattens better if you use your palms," I said in a helpful tone of voice.

He pressed his right palm and left an imprint on the putty. "Nobody has my same fingerprints," he said.

- **Present the direction as a suggestion.**

I handed 4-year-old Craig the two construction pieces and said, "You can make a monster. Hold the pieces close to each other and then snap together. You don't have to do it this way. It just makes it easier."

He followed my directions and said, "Look, it's a three-eyed monster."

- **Suggest an idea of what you want the children to do and add, "If you want."**

I walked the two boys back to their classrooms. First, we stopped at the kindergarten doorway. Because Ryan, the first grader, constantly moved, I said, "I need you to wait here for just a minute before we go to your class. While you are waiting, you could try standing on one foot if you want."

He began counting as he lifted his leg and balanced on one foot.

- **State what the options are.**

Tom picked the black scissors, which left the purple pair on the table.

"I want the black scissors," 7-year-old Sam said.

"The purple ones are good too," I replied. Sam folded his arms and frowned. "After you're done cutting, you can pick whatever building toy you want."

Sam stared at the scissors. "I'll start cutting when he's done."

"That's okay. That's your choice. But you are using the time you have for building. It would be better to start cutting now and not wait."

He scrunched his lips, picked up the scissors, and started cutting.

- **Say, "Here's an idea. Tell me what you think."**

As Hal waited in the lunch line with his first-grade class, he turned sideways and threw himself into the wall, hitting the children around him.

I happened to walk by and said, "You could hurt yourself and your friends doing that. Here's an idea. Let me show you something else you could do." I placed my palms on the wall and began doing wall push-ups. "Try this."

He tried it, then smiled when I said, "Oh, look how strong your arms are. What do you think?"

"I like it," he replied.

KEY POINTS TO REMEMBER

- Establish the rules of respect and create a climate of caring.
- Show children you will set limits and keep them safe.
- Use reasonable consequences to help children learn.
- Let children know that you care about them and are concerned for their well-being.
- Be proactive in preventing problems.
- Incorporate strategies to gain control in a group situation and help the group settle and get focused.
- Use your nonverbal language and tone of voice as a subtle way to stop unwanted actions.
- Choose your wording and reactions carefully.
- Always allow children to save face by providing options when setting limits.

REVIEW QUESTIONS

1. Three-year-old Logan finds a stick buried under the rocks on the playground. He picks it up and starts swinging it, just missing a classmate. What can you say?

2. You need to tell children the rules before you expect them to comply. True or false.

3. Tell children what not to do when stating rules. True or false.

4. What tone of voice should you use when setting limits so that children know you mean what you are saying?

5. You get the group's attention and begin giving directions for the activity. Five-year-old Carly turns her back to you, takes a magic marker, and draws on the table. You should have her wipe off the marks with a wet

paper towel, then you should check if she understands the words you used in your directions. True or false.

6. It is best to prevent children's unwanted actions than to deal with them later. True or false.

7. Children do not respond to nonverbal gestures indicating stop. True or false.

8. Talking louder works better than whispering to get a small group quiet. True or false.

9. To avoid having children say, "No," what words can you say instead of, "Do you want to…"?

10. If children are refusing to participate, what can you say to help them save face?

Teach Children to Regulate Their Emotions, Thoughts, and Bodies

CHAPTER OVERVIEW

In addition to setting limits, an equally important responsibility is to teach children specific methods for regulating their emotions, thoughts, and bodies. In this chapter, I will present strategies that are mainly based on Western cultural values. Included are ways to assist children in recognizing their feelings and acceptable actions. Also discussed are techniques you can teach children for self-regulation and conflict resolution. In addition, there are approaches for dealing with emotions in a crisis.

CHILDREN'S DESCRIPTIONS OF WHAT THEY THINK YOU SHOULD KNOW

Dr. Clare: "How can therapists help you with your feelings?"

Syndey (age 12): "You should ask what is troubling me."

Dr. Clare: "If you are feeling sad, what can therapists or teachers do to help you feel better?"

Marco (age 12): "They could try to cheer you up, like telling you about the good things in life."

Emily (age 11): "They can pull me aside from class to get myself together, like if my dog died. Pull me aside to tell me it's okay and to help me feel better."

Kaylee (age 12): "If I feel sad because someone hurt me or bullied me, they could tell me to get the kid's name and the next time I see them tell the kid's name so they could tell the kid to stop bullying me. It's not nice."

Dr. Clare: "If you are feeling mad, what can therapists or teachers do to help you feel better?"

Olivia (age 12): "If I am mad, they can help me calm down so I don't hurt anyone."

Brian (age 11): "Take me in the hallway and talk to me."

Dr. Clare: "If another kid is very angry, what can therapists or teachers do to help you?"

Leah (age 11): "I would probably want to talk to someone so I don't feel scared and would feel comfortable coming to school every day and know it's a safe environment for me."

Marco (age 12): "If a kid was going to beat me up, talk to me and tell the principal."

Dr. Clare: "Why is it important to learn what to do with someone acting like a bully?"

Mallory (age 11): "You should know because if you don't, it could become worse and worse. And if the bully doesn't stop, he could become a criminal."

Curtin, C.
Strategies for Collaborating With Children: Creating Partnerships in Occupational Therapy and Research (pp. 225-252).
© 2017 SLACK Incorporated.

GUIDE CHILDREN TO A CALM AND POSITIVE STATE

It is important for you to know how to help children with self-regulation. Children coming to therapy have often had multiple experiences of failure. As they face challenges, they may have feelings ranging from being thrilled with their success to being angry about failing. Furthermore, it is common to work with children in groups. With a mix of personalities and interests, conflict is inevitable. Another common scenario is for children to talk about their feelings and concerns while they are involved in an activity. In these situations, it is vital for you to know to help children in the moment. Also important is to know resources for more serious concerns. In addition, your knowledge about sensory modulation and associated strategies is a valuable contribution for helping children learn how to become calm and stay in a positive state.

Teach Children to Recognize and Describe Their and Others' Feelings

Everyone has feelings that affect what they think and do. Young children often act out their emotions without recognizing the specific feeling they are experiencing. To help them talk instead of impulsively acting out, they need to know a variety of feeling words. Next, they have to learn how to recognize their and others' feelings. They learn that all their feelings are valid but they have to handle them in a way that is not harmful. What is considered an acceptable expression of emotions largely depends on their family's, community's, and culture's views, which may vary depending on the children's gender.

Teach Feeling Words

> **Children might be thinking:**
> *I'm learning new words.*
> *I like playing games.*
> *That was a good story.*

When children do not have the words to describe their feelings, you have to interpret their sounds, facial expressions, and body language. You have to guess what emotion their grunting, grimacing, or grandstanding represents. By teaching feeling words, you enable them to verbally communicate with you and others about their internal state. This is helpful in creating a common language because they are then using words you both understand.

Teach Vocabulary of Feeling Words

The first step is to teach children a variety of feeling words. Some children may only know the words "happy" and "mad." They may say they are mad when they are feeling sad, frustrated, hurt, or bored. Expanding their vocabulary allows them to better label their emotions. Having more detailed information means you can guide them in how to deal with their feelings.

Fabulous Five: Teach Vocabulary of Feeling Words

- **Teach feeling words.**

Six-year-old Craig printed the first two letters of a word but then started scribbling. "Craig, are you frustrated or bored?"

Craig kept scribbling.

"Do you know what 'frustrated' means?"

He shook his head.

"It is when things do not go right and you feel like you can't do it and go 'Ugh.'" I folded my arms, raised my shoulders, and let out an exasperated gasp. "So are you frustrated or bored?"

"I'm bored."

- **Model the use of feeling words.**

The children heard that a staff member's horse had died. "I could make a card for Nina," 9-year-old Nicholas said.

"That would be so nice," I replied. "It's very sad when you lose an animal."

"I lost an animal."

"Cat or dog?"

"Dog. I cried a lot. I still miss my dog. It's sad too."

- **Give children the feeling words to use.**

Six-year-old Sharon pulled on her pink socks, but when she tried to stuff her right foot into the white tennis shoe, a bent tongue stopped her. "Aah," she wailed.

Her teacher walked to her and said in a gentle tone, "Say, 'I'm mad at the shoe.'"

"I'm mad at the shoe," she half-said, half-wailed.

"Say it again softer."

"I'm mad at the shoe," Sharon said in a normal voice.

"If your shoe is bent, you can fix it by pulling it. Pull here."

Sharon yanked, straightened the inside of the shoe, and slipped it on her foot.

- **Say the feeling to match the children's words or actions.**

Byron tossed a ball at a target and missed. "Stupid thing," he said.

"Frustrating, huh?" I commented.

- **State your feelings and ask children if they felt the same.**

There was a loud crash, and I jumped. "Wow, that scared me. Did it scare you too?" I asked.

"Yeah," the kindergartner said.

Use Activities to Teach Feelings

Children enjoy learning through activities. You can teach them about various feelings and matching facial expressions. One way is to read books with vivid pictures of the emotions and match your tone of voice. Another way is to use a game requiring them to identify a specific feeling or indicator. You can also help them learn by telling them an emotion and asking them to draw what their faces would look like. Using props containing feeling words or stamps of different expressions are additional options. While doing these activities, ask children to tell you about a time they felt a specific emotion. This helps them connect the feeling words to their own personal experiences.

Fabulous Five: Involve Children in Activities to Teach Feelings

- **Read a book about feeling words.**

"The title of this book is *Glad Monster, Sad Monster*, and the authors' names are Ed Emberley and Anne Miranda," the special education teachers said to the preschool class. She read about the first monster's feeling happy and then asked the group, "What makes you glad or happy?"

"Know what makes me happy? That I'm going to be riding on a two-wheel cycle soon."

The teacher read the next page about a sad monster. "What makes you sad?"

"I get sad when someone breaks up my blocks and I have to build again."

"When my brother kicks me."

"What worries you?" the teacher asked after reading about a scared monster.

"When I see spiders."

"I'm scared of thunder."

The teacher continued reading about an angry monster and asked, "What makes you angry?"

"When my brother doesn't help me clean up."

"When my mom tells me to do something I don't want to do."

"When someone takes my dollies away."

- **Incorporate games involving recognizing emotions.**

"We have a fun game," I told the preschoolers in our social group. "It's a concentration game. Turn two cards over and if their faces are the same, you get to keep the two cards. If they are different feelings, put them back."

When the children made a match, I asked what feeling was shown by the face on the cards.

- **Make a prop using feeling words.**

In the small group of second graders, we made dice out of a paper pattern. We then wrote different feelings on each side of the dice. When the group was done, I asked, "The question is 'How do you feel at school?' Roll the die to find out."

Debbie rolled her die, and it landed on the word *Upset*.

"Tell us about a time you felt upset at school."

"Sometimes I get upset when no one plays with me."

- **Use stamps of faces with different emotions.**

"These are stamps of faces showing various feelings," I said to the preschoolers. "Pick one and stamp it on your paper next to the words, 'I feel….' Then tell me about a time you had that feeling."

Four-year-old Ella reached for the sad face, put it on the inkpad, and pressed it on her paper. "We just moved. I feel sad because I miss my friends."

"It is sad to say goodbye to friends and not get to play with them."

- **Draw faces associated with feelings.**

I handed 5-year-old Jason a dry erase maker and a laminated picture of a head. "Draw a face showing he is scared."

He drew eyes, nose, and a circle for the mouth. "I was scared this morning. I looked under my bed and I shivered. It was dark. I thought there was a monster there. But it was only my clothes."

Teach Children to Identify Their and Others' Feelings

> **Children might be thinking:**
> *I'm not sure what I'm feeling.*
> *I'm feeling….*

When children can label and articulate their feelings, they tend to have more control over their actions. Being able to identify a specific feeling influences their self-talk and resulting actions. They become more aware of their internal state and often less impulsive in their actions. By learning to recognize others' emotions, they can develop empathy and understanding. They also learn to make decisions on how to act by reading the feelings conveyed by another's nonverbal language.

Assist Children in Recognizing Their Own Feelings

After children have learned a variety of feeling words, the next step is to assist them in recognizing their emotions. Checking in with children or starting a group by asking how they feel is one way. You can have them practice making faces associated with each emotion, such as saying, "Show me a surprised face." When children are in difficult situations, you can mention two possible feelings they may have and encourage them to talk.

Children are better able to figure out what to do when they can recognize and articulate their feelings. For instance, if they realize they are mad, they may decide to talk with the offending person. If they realize they are sad, they may seek comfort. Sharing their feelings with peers promotes a mutual exchange and a deeper level of friendship. Being able to identify their emotions also is a vital step in developing empathy. It helps them relate and understand what others are feeling.

Fabulous Five: Support Children in Recognizing Their Feelings

- **Ask children how they are feeling.**

"How are you feeling today?" I asked 4-year-old Adler.

"I feel proud."

"What did you do?"

"I put my shirt on all by myself," he said with a smile.

"Good for you." I grinned both for his accomplishment and because his shirt was on backward.

- **Have a group make faces connected with different feelings.**

In our preschool social group, the special education teacher said, "This book is called *The Way I Feel* and is written by Janan Cain." On each page was a child with a different feeling. After reading a description of one feeling, she said, "Everybody make a mad face."

The children folded their arms, squinted their eyes, and tightened their lips.

The teacher continued reading, and with each new feeling she asked the class to make a matching face.

- **Start group by asking each person how they are feeling.**

The speech-language pathologist, special education teacher, and I started the small social group by saying to the preschoolers, "Tell us your name and how you're feeling today."

"My name is Erin, and I'm feeling happy. My friend is coming over for a play date."

"My name is Jasmine, and I'm happy too."

"My name is Mason, and I was nervous this morning. The garbage truck made a lot of noise and woke me up. I told my mom."

- **Provide two possible feelings children might be experiencing.**

The specialized class went into the school library, and 6-year-old Emily dragged her feet with her chin down and her eyes half-closed. When a classmate grabbed a book she wanted, she began wailing.

Her teacher whispered to her. Emily stopped crying to listen. "Are you mad about not getting the book or are you tired?"

"Tired."

"Well, you have two choices. Be tired and have a good day or be tired and have a bad day. I hope you make it a good day. We can tell your dad you need more sleep."

- **Help children sort out their feelings.**

In the day treatment, a younger child was so angry he started to lose control. He threw chairs in the classroom and was quickly escorted by two adults to a calming area. On the way, he spewed curse words.

Two boys and I were working at a table by the calming area. At the beginning of this disturbance, I quickly positioned myself between the two boys and the path of the angry child. "It's noisy here. Let's move to the other room," I told the boys. As we walked, I asked Neal, "Did that make you feel mad or scared?"

"It makes me mad because of the noise. It makes me feel like punching someone."

"But then you would get in trouble. What else could you do when you feel mad?"

"Just walk away."

The other boy chimed in, "Then he would come up to you."

"No," I said, "because staff would keep you safe."

"He might push me," Neal added.

"I know it's scary when someone is that mad, but staff will keep you safe."

"Yeah, staff will keep us safe," Neal and the other child said at the same time.

Assist Children in Learning the Signs and Triggers of Their Emotions

To assist children in dealing with difficult situations, ask them what they find upsets them. Inquiring gives you the opportunity to learn what they have recognized as problematic. If they do not know, your questions may get them to think about it. Similarly, look for the antecedents to their actions. Watch for what happened before outbursts, meltdowns, or withdrawal. Was the environment chaotic and noisy? Did children start crying following interactions with specific people? Once upsetting situations are identified, discuss with them what you have noticed. Ask for their ideas on what to do. Together you can figure out more ways to prevent or handle the situation.

To help children deal with their feelings, it is also important that they recognize their physical signs related to emotions. They can then use those signs as cues to think about how they are feeling in the moment. For instance, if they feel their muscles tightening, they can tell themselves, "Oh, I'm starting to feel mad." When children can recognize the triggers and signs of their emotions, they are better able to understand and respond to stressful situations in a constructive way.

Fabulous Five: Help Children Learn the Signs and Triggers of Their Emotions

- **Help children learn their physical signs of emotions.**

"How do you know when you are mad?" I asked 12-year-old Kiera. "How does your body tell you?"

"Sometimes if I get really, really mad, I start to choke up and cry."

- **Ask what situations tend to make them mad or upset.**

"What situations do you find tend to make you mad or upset?" I asked 11-year-old Jan.

"I get mad if someone is constantly picking on me and they don't stop when I ask them to."

- **Describe what you observe to be triggers for their outbursts.**

"I can't write," 6-year-old Tabitha yelled after she made a mistake. She threw herself on the floor and kept screaming, "I'm stupid. I hate myself."

"I can see you're upset. This would be a good time to take a break."

She stomped over to the beanbag chair and let it engulf her. When she was calm, I joined her on the floor. "I notice you get really upset every time you make a mistake." She nodded. "Everyone makes mistakes. I do too. Give yourself a chance to learn. Next time you make a mistake, tell yourself, 'It's okay. I can fix it.'"

"It's okay. I can fix it," she mumbled to herself.

- **Ask children how they can handle situations that continually upset them.**

"What do you tell yourself when you keep getting mad at the same people or situation?" I asked 12-year-old Troy.

"Leave them alone and maybe they won't bother me anymore."

- **Describe for children the physical signs you see indicating their emotions.**

"I am so mad," 12-year-old Carson said as he scrunched his lips and raised his shoulders. "I'm having a horrible day. A new kid took my seat at my lunch table. Another kid called me names when he pointed to my new cap. I had to go to the principal, and I put my new sunglasses down in class and someone took them."

"That is a lot. I'm sorry. It's been a really bad day for you. I can see in your face and body how mad you are. Your face is red, and your mouth and body are really tight. You look like you are trying to hold it together."

"Yeah," he snarled back.

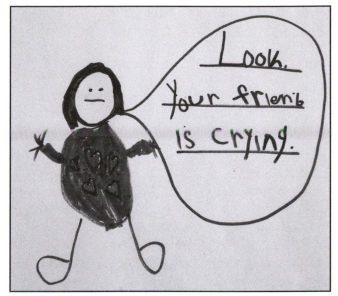

Figure 12-1. Assist children in learning how to recognize other's feelings.

"You've had such a bad day. What do you think would make you feel better?"

He thought for a minute and said, "I think I will ask my mom to take me to the gym so I can lift weights. That makes me feel better."

"That sounds like a good idea. I hope tomorrow is better for you."

Teach Children How to Recognize Others' Feelings

Another important life skill is to be able to recognize and read others' emotions. If this ability does not come naturally, it can be enhanced by giving explicit clues for what to observe (Figure 12-1). Point out visible signs of feelings, such as saying that crying is often seen with sadness. Create a game requiring children to recognize various facial expressions. Have them create a collage showing differences in body language. You can have one child demonstrate a feeling and the others guess. When there is conflict, have children look at the other person's face to encourage them to consider the other's feelings.

When children can recognize others' emotions, they are better able to be empathetic and resolve conflict. They also learn that others may feel differently from them and that feelings can change over time. In addition, they discover that reading others' emotions gives them crucial information on how to interact with others.

Fabulous Five: Teach Children How to Recognize Others' Feelings

- **Point out visible signs of feelings.**

"Look at this picture," the teacher said to the preschoolers. "How is the boy feeling?"

"Sad."

"How do you know that?"

"He's crying."

"Yes, and his head and eyes are down. You can see it in his mouth too." On the next page of the book, she asked the same question.

"He's happy."

"How do you know?"

"He's smiling."

- **Create a game about recognizing facial expressions.**

"We get to play bingo. It's really fun," I told the preschoolers in the social group. I handed each one a card I had made containing rows of faces showing different emotions. "When I pick a word, you put a chip on the matching face." I reached into a bag and pulled out the word happy. "Everyone look for a happy face."

"I got one," Beatriz said. "I hope I win."

A few minutes later, Dominique put her last chip on and shouted out, "Bingo!"

- **Create a collage of different facial expressions and body language.**

I passed out paper, scissors, glue, and a variety of magazines to the third-grade class in the day treatment. "Today, you get to make a collage. On one half of your paper, cut out and glue pictures of people who are happy. On the other half, put pictures of people who are angry or upset. Look at their faces and the way their bodies are to determine how they are feeling."

- **Have one child show different feelings while the group guesses.**

"Today we are going to play a guessing game," I told the preschoolers during a social group. "I am going to tell Jake a feeling. Watch his face and guess what he is feeling. Now cover your ears." I whispered to Jake, "You are happy you got a present. Show them a happy face."

He smiled, and the class yelled, "He's happy."

"You are surprised you got a puppy."

He made his mouth into an oval shape.

"Happy, surprised," they yelled.

"He's surprised," I said. Then he showed the following feelings: mad someone took his toy, sad his fish died, and frustrated that he could not tie his shoe.

With the frustrated face, the class yelled, "Mad, mean, frustrated."

"Sometimes," I said, "it's hard to tell if a person is mad or frustrated, so you just have to ask. You guessed all the answers. You won the game."

- Say, "Look at your friend, does he/she look… or…?"

Just as I said, "We have 2 more minutes," 5-year-old RJ dumped over a bin of blocks.

Billy ran over and started putting the blocks away. RJ crossed his arms and grimaced.

"Billy, thanks for helping," I said. "But look at RJ's face. Does he look happy for the help or mad?"

"Mad."

"Yes, I think he's trying to tell you that he'll put the blocks away himself."

"Yeah," RJ replied, placing the blocks back in the bin.

Teach Children Desired Actions

Children might be thinking:
I'm in trouble.
I wonder what will happen.
Maybe I could try these ideas.
That might help me feel better.
Oh, I see what to do.
Now I know.

To prevent unwanted behavior, teach children what to do. Assume that their current actions may be the only way they know how to handle their feelings. Be mindful that children who act like bullies may not know other options for getting what they want. See if children have the skills and strategies for dealing with difficult situations. You would be surprised at how often the answer is no. For instance, adults will often tell a child to stop kicking, pinching, or hitting. They expect the child to stop and not do it again. If children do not know, teach alternative actions using objects, words, pictures, photographs, or stories that match the children's learning style.

Teach Alternatives by Telling or Showing What to Do

To start, make it a habit to tell children what to do when redirecting them. This gives them an idea of other options and cues them on what is expected. It also shifts their thinking about their current actions to thinking about other possibilities. Telling them what to do can become a teachable moment. See Table 12-1 for how to change from telling children what NOT to do to describing what TO do.

When setting limits, it is common for many people to tell children, "No," or "Don't…." They may say, "Don't hit," or "Don't push." They assume that the child knows the right thing to do. If you grew up in a family that used this approach, you may think this is the only way. You may use these words as your first response. Yet there is another way. If children are about to hurt themselves or others, use

TABLE 12-1	
TELL CHILDREN WHAT TO DO WHEN REDIRECTING THEIR ACTIONS	
INSTEAD OF SAYING	**SAY**
No.	Stop.
Don't touch.	Look with your eyes.
Don't throw rocks.	Keep the rocks on the ground.
No running.	Use walking feet.
No pushing. No touching others.	Keep your hands to your side. Hug yourself. Keep your hands in your lap.
No shouting. No yelling.	Use your inside voice.
No fighting.	Tell your friend, "I would like a turn, please." Or ask, "When can I have a turn?"
No running away. No hiding.	Stay with your friends.
You are not paying attention.	Look… or Look what your friends are doing.
No hitting.	Stop. Use your words (give the exact words or phrase to say).
No bad words.	Use nice words.

the word, "Stop," and intervene. In other situations, try to eliminate saying, "No," or "Don't." Guide them by telling or showing alternatives. You can tell them to do an action that is the opposite of the unwanted one. It also helps to use the same keywords or phrases and/or pairing verbal cues with sign language.

Remember to ask yourself, "Do they know what else to do?" Have your first thought be that children are lacking the skills instead of willfully trying to be naughty or irritate you. Make a landmark decision to change your assumptions and automatic way of reacting.

Fabulous Five: Teach Alternative Actions

- **Tell children what to do versus what not to do when setting limits.**

Three-year-old Dana decided to play the Native American drum. I handed her a drumstick with a leather covering and said, "Just hit the drum with this drumstick."

"Not our eyes," Dana said as she shook her head to make the point. "If we hit our eyes, our eyes will pop out and we have to get them fixed at the doctor."

"Just hit the drum."

- **Tell children to do an action that is the opposite of their unwanted one.**

At the school's outdoor field days, two third graders, Erik and Martin, started to shove each other. One flicked the red visor off the other's head.

I stepped in between them. "Today is a day for fun, not fighting."

I sat down, and Martin started flicking my ankle. To get him to stop, I reached down and extended my hand. "Shake my hand."

He raised his foot instead.

I held the heel of his shoe, shook it like a hand, and said, "Hi, Mister Foot."

He grinned back.

- **Give a verbal cue using a key word or phrase.**

"Although Roman has wonderful things to say, he talks nonstop," the preschool teacher said during a planning meeting.

"It would help if we all use the same words to let him know when it is time to listen," I said.

"Let's say, 'Turn on your listening ears,'" his teacher suggested, and the group agreed.

- **Pair a verbal cue with sign language.**

While the preschool teacher read a book in the specialized classroom, three staff members repeatedly told children to sit down. The noise level increased, and few children paid attention to the book.

Later, when the staff met, we talked about how to change the situation. The next day we taught the class sign language for "stop," "sit," "more," and "all done." The children practiced, and the staff began using the signs throughout the day.

A week later, I saw Randy rolling on the floor. Without saying a word, I signed, "Stop. Sit." I pointed to his chair. He moved to his seat but looked at me instead of the teacher. I pointed to my eyes and then to the teacher reading the book, and he shifted his attention to the book.

- **Show children other ideas of what to do.**

Three-year-old Trent threw a red rubber ball that bounced off the wall and just missed hitting another child. As he ran to retrieve the ball, I quickly grabbed a green bucket and turned it on its side. "It's okay to throw the ball outside, but when you are inside, just roll it. See if you can roll it into this bucket five times."

Use Photographs, Picture Symbols, or Objects to Cue Children

Some children learn better when you use photographs, pictures, or objects instead of just words. This can especially help younger ones or those who are visual learners to understand what they are supposed to do. One approach is to show them a photograph of themselves or others doing the desired action.

The use of picture symbols that are printed or on a mobile device is another teaching tool that promotes comprehension. Additionally, you can incorporate objects such as a visual timer to cue them regarding what to do. These strategies not only increase understanding, but may also eliminate a power struggle. Children may be more likely to follow pictures or objects cues than verbal directions. They may balk if they feel like adults are ordering them around but respond differently to nonverbal signs.

Fabulous Five: Teach Using Objects or Body Cues

- **Show a photograph of children doing the desired action.**

"During opening group, Deana has been pinching the children around her," the preschool teacher said.

"It might help to define a space for her to sit so her peers are out of reach," I replied.

"I can get her a cube chair."

"I'll bring a weighted pillow for calming. Then if we tell her to keep her hands clasped together, she can't pinch."

The next day I took a photograph of Deana smiling as she sat in the chair with the weighted pillow on her lap and her hands folded. I laminated the photograph. When she reached for others, we showed her the picture, and she responded by putting her hands together.

- **Use a picture symbol to show what to do.**

When the preschool class made a line to go to the library, 3-year-old Mickey ran to a center and started playing.

"It's time to line up," I said, showing him a picture symbol of children in a line. "Let's go. We're going to get books. Maybe we can find a book about trucks. I know you love trucks." I tapped the picture symbol and then pointed to his classmates.

Mickey dropped the toy and went to the line.

- **Show a series of pictures of what to do.**

"When I call Dayton's name, he doesn't look at me or stop what he is doing," his preschool teacher said. "He's been getting in others' spaces and putting his hands on their faces. He is getting so close that he ends up spitting on them when he talks."

After we discussed the situation, we decided to make a cue card to get his attention and a Social Story for maintaining personal space and playing with friends. On the cue card were three pictures symbols: a boy, eyes, and ears. When the teacher wanted his attention, she placed the strip in front of him and said, "Dayton. Look. And listen." This captured his attention, and he began listening to his teacher.

- **Use a visual timer to cue children about how much time they have.**

"Every day, Bruce's first choice is to be on the computer. He doesn't want to go to any other centers," his preschool teacher told the special education team. "If other children come near him, he yells, calls them names, and pushes them away."

The teacher and our team discussed different strategies and decided on using a visual timer. He could start on the computer, but after 15 minutes he would need to choose another center and give other children a turn.

The next day, a visual timer was placed next to the computer. His teacher moved the knob to 15 minutes, showing a large area of red that decreased as time passed. "When the red is gone," she said, "you have to stop and go to another center." When his time was up, his teacher pointed to the visual timer and helped him change. The following day, he watched the timer and stopped on his own accord.

- **Use an object to represent desired action.**

Three-year-old Travis rolled on the rug, bumping into the children around him. Then he started rolling away from the group. I grabbed a green carpet square and handed it to him. "Look what I have for you. It's your favorite color. Sit on this."

He marched to the front of the group, knocking children in his path, and sat down on the carpet square. The next day he brought the same square to group and plopped down on it.

Create Stories, Comic Strips, or Images to Teach Children

Other avenues for teaching desired actions are the use of Social Stories (Gray, 2010), comic strips (Gray, 1994), or images. You can write a story that explicitly describes the situation and outlines what children can say or do. Adding pictures to the story can increase the clarity of the message. Similarly, you can draw a comic strip showing the situation and a different strategy than the current undesirable one. Having children draw the pictures for the story or comic strip can increase engagement and ownership.

Children with delayed communication and/or play skills may need to learn a script that teaches them the words to use. For instance, you would teach them what to say if they want to join a group who are already playing. Another option is to use a Power Card (Gagnon, 2001), in which their favorite superhero or character defines the actions to take. Also helpful is the Incredible 5-Point Scale (Buron & Curtis, 2012), in which numbers are attached to variations of behavior, such as the volume of their voices.

Fabulous Five: Use Stories, Comic Strips, or Images to Teach Children

- **Write a story explaining what children are to do in a certain situation.**

On Gary's first day at kindergarten, the teacher rang a soft bell and said, "Time to go to the next center."

Gary stood but did not move. A classmate came over and sat down. "That's my chair," Gary screamed, pushing the child out of the chair.

Assuming that he did not understand, the special education team wrote the following story and read it to him before he started to play:

In my classroom, I get to go to centers. When I hear the timer, it is time to clean up. Then my teacher tells us to go to the next center. I will go to the next table. I will sit in a different chair. This is okay. I like centers!

Gary was then able to make the transition.

- **Draw a comic strip showing what to do.**

"This is the third time today you have had to leave the group because you hit someone," I said to 4-year-old Justin after he sat quietly for a few minutes. "Do you like to get hit?"

"No. But I wanted the truck and Kris would not give it to me."

"Did hitting help you get the truck?"

"No."

"What else could you do to get the truck?"

"I don't know."

"I believe you. Let me show you what else you could do." I drew a number of boxes. In the first box, I added two stick figures, with one holding a truck. "Here, this is you, and here is Kris." Then I drew a bubble for the dialogue. "You could say, 'Kris, could I please have a turn?'"

In the next box, I drew Kris again and had him say, "No, I want to play with the truck."

Then I drew Justin. "You could say, 'When you are done, could I have it next?' Kris says, 'Okay.'"

In the next scene, I had Justin say, "I will just get another toy."

In the last box, I had Kris say, "Here," as he handed the truck to Justin. "Justin, then you say, 'Thank you.'"

I walked with Justin back to the play area and had him practice the scenario with Kris.

- **Teach a script.**

Three-year-old Ginny saw her classmate, Maria, holding a new baby doll. She walked over and tried to grab the doll out of Maria's arms. A tug-of-war ensued. "I had the baby first," Maria yelled as she pulled the doll closer to her. Ginny responded by hitting her.

Knowing that Ginny's language skills were delayed, I created a small book with four pictures and a script of what to do and say. On the first page were the words *I say, "Can I have a turn?"* On the second page was *"I wait."* On the third page was *"My friend gives me the toy."* On the last page was *I say, "Thank you."*

We practiced looking at each picture and saying the script during regular activities and when conflict occurred. Using pictures, we also practiced ideas of what to do if classmates did not want to share, such as offering a trade or finding another toy.

- **Use a Power Card (Gagnon, 2001).**

"Gerry is stuck in his play. He only acts like Spider-Man and does not play with the others," his preschool teacher said about the 5 year old. "Sometimes he gets wound up and keeps running around the classroom."

"We could try using a Power Card," I suggested. "That's when you make a cue card that has his superhero telling him what to do. So Spider-Man would be telling him instead of you."

"Let's try it," his teacher said.

On the card, we put a picture of Spider-Man and wrote: *Spider-Man says, (1) walk in class, (2) stay in your center, (3) let me sleep when you are in centers and play with friends.*

- **Use the Incredible 5-Point Scale (Buron & Curtis, 2012) and attach numbers to actions.**

"The two new boys in my class have really changed the dynamics," the preschool teacher told me. "They are always talking, even when I'm reading a book. The other kids are distracted by this, and it's hard to keep everyone's attention."

The next day I brought in a chart showing the Incredible 5-Point Scale, with 5 being the loudest volume and 1 being quiet. Next to each number was a picture of children with words inside a thought bubble, ranging from multiple words to none. The teacher hung the chart up and attached a clothespin to the desired number and corresponding volume. At the beginning of different activities, she pointed to the charts, moved the clothespin, and announced the level of volume. She held up the same number of the fingers to emphasize. The entire class responded. The teacher used this strategy throughout the rest of the school year.

Clarify What to Do

Another aspect of teaching children appropriate actions is to give detailed information on what to do. Clarify when, where, or in which circumstance their current actions are acceptable. State the purpose of an object being misused. Clarify exactly what other actions they could do. It is also helpful to state what they have to do differently to get their desires met. Be clear in defining the particulars. When given details instead of vague statements about their actions, they are better able to learn and make changes.

Fabulous Five: Clarify What to Do

- **Clarify when the action is appropriate.**

Six-year-old Brent ran down the school hallway. A preschooler stepped in front of him, and the two nearly collided.

"Use walking feet in school," I said. "When you're outside for recess, you can run and run and run."

- **Clarify where or in which circumstances the action is acceptable.**

Seven-year-old Valerie ran into the school hallway, wrapped her arms around her friend's neck, and squeezed tightly.

Seeing the distressed look on her friend's face, the certified occupational therapy assistant said, "Valerie, it's okay to hug people at home, like your mom and dad. Here at school when you see your friends, give them a big smile, wave hello, or say, 'Hi.' If you want to hug a friend, ask first."

- **Say the purpose of an object being misused.**

Six-year-old Kylie took the plastic knife and rocked it on her hand. "The knife is for the putty, not for hurting yourself." I moved the blue putty closer to her. "See if you can cut this in six pieces."

A few weeks later, I placed the knife, a rolling pin, putty, and small figurines on the table.

"I want the roller," Rita said.

Kylie snatched the knife and the lion figures.

"What do you need to remember about the knife?"

"Use it for cutting putty, not our hands."

I nodded in agreement.

- **Clarify what else children can do.**

Three-year-old Nat sat with his classmates at the table. "Today we get to play with Play-Doh," his teacher said as she handed Nat a clump.

"I don't like Play-Doh," he said, throwing it on the floor.

"Play-Doh stays on the table," I said. "If you don't like touching it, you can use cookie cutters. Or, if you are done, you can just put it back in the bag."

- **State what the children have to do differently to get their desires met.**

"What letter is this?" the kindergarten teacher asked.

"I know, I know," Stewart shouted, stepping forward.

"Ouch," his classmate said when Stewart bumped his shoulder.

"Stewart, your teacher will only call on you when you are sitting and raising your hand," I cued him.

He swiveled his body and returned to his place on the floor.

Help Children Deal With Their Feelings

It is common in therapy to work with children who have difficulty dealing with their emotions, especially intense ones. These children often have a history of failure leading to frustration, nervousness, and/or anger. Some are sensitive and quickly become upset. It is helpful for you to know a variety of strategies for calming.

Teach Children Ways to Regulate Their Feelings, Thoughts, and Bodies

---

Children might be thinking:
How can I help myself? I need to think.
You're making me think.
I'm learning what to do when I feel….
That helps me get calm.

It is beneficial for children to have a repertoire of self-regulation strategies. To regulate their feelings, thoughts, and bodies, they have to learn how to calm themselves, change negative or aggressive thoughts, modulate sensory stimulation, adjust their arousal level, and control any impulses to hit or harm another. Often, the children who frequently get in trouble do not know any helpful strategies. They have to be taught.

For all children, it is best to teach and practice the strategies when they are not angry. However, there may be times when you need to teach them in the moment. For instance, when a child is screaming and hitting, show him or her a card with pictures of four different calming strategies and have him or her point to the one he or she chooses to use. Eventually you want children to use the coping strategies without any assistance from adults.

Promote Self-Calming and Changing Negative or Aggressive Thoughts

For children to develop self-reliance and regulation, they have to know how to calm themselves. They need to learn that they have control and can deal with intense emotions.

To help children learn this, you and other adults have to give them time to soothe themselves and regroup. When you see children who are upset, it is natural to want to comfort them. For those who have not learned self-calming, however, it is better to give children time to comfort themselves. You can show your support and respect for them by quietly waiting a few minutes before intervening.

To help children change negative or aggressive thoughts, give them alternative statements they can tell themselves. For the times when they are too upset to talk to you, stand within their hearing and discuss with another person what other children have done to help themselves. Creating a personal calm-down book or having a box with their favorite objects can also be used for calming.

Fabulous Five: Promote Self-Calming and Changing Negative or Aggressive Thoughts

- **Give children time to calm themselves.**

At the beginning of the session, Claudia's mother put her on the therapy mat in the occupational therapy clinic. Looking like a 1 year old, the 3 year old was finally sitting without support.

As I took her shoes off, she leaned to the right. Reacting to the slight movement, she started wailing. "That scared you," I said in a gentle voice. I calmly waited a couple of minutes until the wailing turned into a whimper. Then I brought over her favorite musical toy.

- **Give children a saying to repeat for calming.**

When a classmate took his toy, 4-year-old Davis wrapped his arms around her neck and bit her.

The teacher intervened. Later, when he was calm, his teacher taught him to say, "My eyes are looking. My ears are listening. My voice is quiet. My body is calm." He repeated the saying twice. Then whenever his teacher saw him starting to get upset, she went to him. Together they would repeat the words, and then he would say them on his own.

- **Have children create and use a box containing objects for calming.**

Four-year-old Ian jumped in front of the first child in line to go to the playground. His teacher told him, "Go to the end of the line."

He marched back, scowled, and squinted. A few minutes later, he pushed the child in front of him. A second teacher moved between the children. Ian then pushed the teacher, who immediately had him move away from the group. "You are hurting people. I think you are still mad you are not the line leader today. It's time to take a break. Let's get your castle box."

Ian followed the teacher, sat down, and opened the box containing crayons, a notebook, a fidget toy, a stress ball, and interlocking cubes. He became calmer as he started to draw. A few minutes later, he joined the group outside.

- **Discuss with another person, within the children's hearing, strategies they could use to calm themselves.**

Before the occupational therapy student walked into the class, Chase's fourth-grade teacher had chastised him. When Chase came to his group, his face was red, his lips were pursed together, and he refused to talk.

"Chase, I need you to look at me and talk. I'm not going to know what's wrong if you don't tell me," the occupational therapy student said in a kind voice.

Chase turned the chair so his back was to her.

"Chase, please look at me."

With his back still to the occupational therapy student, he moved off the chair and sat on the floor.

Speaking in Chase's direction, I said, "I think you're trying to tell us you're too upset to talk. Sometimes when kids are upset they need quiet time to get calm." I turned to the occupational therapy student and said loud enough for Chase to hear, "Sometimes it helps to count to 10 and then take deep breaths. Then, after cooling down, it helps to talk with someone about it. It doesn't have to be us."

After waiting quietly for about 5 minutes, Chase still looked upset, but when shown two activities, he chose one. The next time we met, the occupational therapy student talked with him about what had happened.

- **Create a calm-down book.**

In a joint session with the school psychologist, she told our group, "You get to make your own special book and draw pictures of yourself on the pages." She handed a copy to each third grader and read:

"Sometimes I get angry! I can make my body feel better by relaxing. I can use the calm-down steps: One, ask myself, 'How do I feel?' Two, take three deep breaths. Three, say, 'Calm down' to myself. Four, if I need to, talk to a grown-up about it. Then, whenever you get upset, get your book to help you calm down."

Have Children Identify and Adjust Their Arousal Level

Children need to be able to modulate sensory stimulation and adjust their arousal level to be alert and calm. To do so, they have to learn to recognize when they are over- or understimulated, as well as the demands of the current situation. For instance, in class they have to be able to recognize when they are too sleepy or, in the other extreme, moving excessively. It also is important to learn to recognize patterns, especially when they are responding to sensory stimulation with undesirable actions. Once they have gained that self-knowledge, the next step is to learn a variety of sensory strategies and determine which one works best for them.

Fabulous Five: Have Children Identify and Adjust Their Arousal Level

- **Have children identify their arousal state.**

Using the *How Does Your Engine Run?* program by Williams and Shellenberger (1996), I told the group of third-grade boys in the self-contained class, "Our bodies are like engines. Sometimes our engines run too fast and sometimes too slow. You want to get your engine just right. Show me what it looks like if your engine is too fast."

The boys bounced in their chairs and waved their arms from side to side.

"That's right. Now show me what it looks like if your engine is too slow."

They slouched down with their heads on their chests.

"You're right again. It's like being sleepy, or you just don't feel like moving. Now show me just right."

They sat up straight and looked wide awake.

"Now you look like you are ready to learn."

- **Present sensory strategy that have helped other children.**

Red-faced and grimacing, the angry fifth grader followed the special education teacher into our room. "George is wound up. He needs to calm down. Can he join you?"

"Sure. I have an idea that might help." As I pulled out two stress balls and a weighted pillow, George sat down, crossed his arms, and stared at the floor.

"Here, put this pillow on your lap. Some kids like it." Then I handed him the earth and moon stress balls. "Slowly squeeze these 10 times as hard as you can and see which ball is harder."

"Ten, nine, eight…." he counted down as he clenched his fists. "The earth is harder," he said calmly.

- **Assist children in recognizing patterns of being over- or understimulated.**

The kindergarten teacher approached me and said, "I keep noticing that Kerry is going to the clinic nurse right after he has P.E. The nurse said he complains of headaches."

"It's really loud in the gym during that time," I replied. "I wonder if he gets on sensory overload and goes to the clinic because it is quiet. I've seen him be sensitive to loud noises in class too."

Later I observed him in the gym, and afterward we talked. "Do loud noises bother you?" I asked, and he nodded. "I hear you have been going to the clinic after P.E. I know the clinic is really quiet. I've talked with your teachers and your mom about how to help you feel more comfortable. When it gets too loud or it just feels like too much, you have some choices. You can use earplugs, you can ask your P.E. teacher for a break, or you can use headphones in your class."

"I want to try the earplugs."

His mother obtained a special earplug that he began wearing in his left ear to filter out the noise during the school day, and his visits to the clinic decreased.

- **Teach strategies to obtain the just-right arousal level for the situation.**

In kindergarten, Tanner spent more time walking around the room than sitting at his desk. One day I carried in a cushion filled with air and said to him, "I heard that sometimes it's hard for you to stay seated at your desk. So I brought this to help you stay in your chair. It is real comfy. Kids usually like it, and it moves a little. Try it and tell me what you think."

"Why does it have these bumps on it?"

"To help you stay on it and not slip off."

He plopped on the pillow and said, "I think it's really comfy."

Then I taught Tanner that when he felt restless, he could also put his palms together with his elbows up and push.

The next year, I observed him in his first-grade class during the first week of school. As several children moved around the class, Tanner stood up nonchalantly, pushed his palms together with force, and then calmly walked to the computer.

- **Have children identify the best sensory strategies for staying alert and calm.**

Knowing that 12-year-old Brian needed extra movement in class, I asked him, "When it's hard to sit still in class, what do you do that helps?"

"I say, 'I need to go to the bathroom.' When I come back, it's easier for me to concentrate."

Teach Self-Control Strategies

In order for children to have self-control, they need to be able to stop their train of thought and actions in addition to controlling their bodies. For instance, if a classmate takes a toy from them, children have to learn to inhibit an impulse to hit and stop thinking of retaliation. They have to learn to change their thoughts so they can let go of their anger, forgive, and forget.

A vital lesson for self-control is to learn to tell themselves, "Stop!" This verbal cue helps them to freeze and think before acting. Doing so can prevent them from reacting impulsively. Some children do better when taught to pair the word *stop* with the corresponding sign language or hand gesture. If their hands are making the sign, they are not as likely to be using their hands to hit. Also teach them to tell others to stop using a firm voice.

Two fun ways for younger children to learn how to control their bodies are the use of stop-and-start movement songs and games. You can play songs that cue children when to move and dance and when to stop. Similarly, games such as Red Light, Green Light can be used. In this game, children run when told "green light" but have to stop immediately when they hear the words "red light." By teaching strategies for self-control, children learn how to help themselves.

Fabulous Five: Teach Self-Control Strategies

- **Teach children to tell themselves, "Stop!"**

When 6-year-old Jill tried to print her name, she wrote the wrong letter. She recognized her mistake and, as was her usual response, automatically hit her head with her fist.

"Stop! You are hurting yourself," I said. "Say, 'Stop! I keep my head safe.'"

She repeated my words.

"Now say, 'I'm frustrated.'"

Again, she repeated the words.

- **Teach children to tell others to stop unwanted actions.**

"Does calling someone names hurt on the outside or the inside?" the special education teacher asked.

"Inside," the preschool class yelled back.

"That's right. It hurts your heart. It makes you feel sad. If someone calls you names, tell them to stop."

- **Pair the word *stop* with corresponding sign language or hand gesture.**

To help Keith learn self-control strategies, I helped him make a picture book of what to do if he became angry. Then the teacher and I had him show the pictures to the class and demonstrate each strategy. On one page were two picture symbols: a stop sign and hands making the sign language for the word *stop*.

"If your friends say or do something mean, tell them to stop," I said, pointing to the symbols.

"Do this," Keith said as he made the sign with his hands.

The rest of the class imitated him.

Later that day, Keith saw a classmate flicking another. He ran, retrieved his book, and pointed to the page. "Stop! You don't flick friends." Because they were surprised to have Keith tell them to stop, the two children moved away from each other.

- **Use stop-and-start games.**

During the monthly meeting between special education staff and preschool teachers, one teacher said, "The afternoon class is really rowdy. Two or three are very impulsive."

"Try using stop-and-start games," the social worker suggested, and the teachers agreed.

The next day, the teachers brought a green and red card out to the playground. They gathered a group of children and said, "We're playing a game called Red Light, Green Light. Go over to the sidewalk. When you see the green card, run. As soon as you see the red card, stop. If you keep running, you will be out of the game."

"This is fun," one child yelled out as they ran across the grass.

- **Use songs requiring stop-and-start movements.**

"The Freeze Dance activity teaches self-regulation," the director told the parents of a new preschooler during a tour. "The teacher plays the music, and the children dance. When she stops the music and holds up a card, the children have to stop and imitate what they see on the card."

Teach Relaxation Techniques

Children can feel changes in their bodies when they are angry or upset. Their muscles tend to tighten in their mouths or fists or throughout their body. To counteract the physical response to their emotions, teach children relaxation techniques. Teach children to use deep rather than shallow breathing (Figure 12-2). With younger children, have them feel their chest move as they take big breaths. Then tell them to blow on their index finger so they can feel the amount of air passing. Let them know that this is a technique that adults frequently use.

Another method to relax their bodies is to count to 10. Saying the numbers helps their mind shifts away from their anger and gives them time to regroup. Purposely tightening their muscles and then relaxing can remove the tension in their bodies. Sensory strategies such as pushing their hands together or trying to pull them apart can provide a calming sensation. Knowing how to relax their bodies is vital for maintaining self-control.

Fabulous Five: Teach Relaxation Techniques

- **Demonstrate deep breathing for calming.**

"When you are mad, here is something you can do to calm down," I told the preschoolers. "Put your hand on your tummy. One, take a breath. Move your hand up. Two, take more breaths. Move your hand up again. Three, more breaths." Then I held up my index finger. "Now blow out your birthday candle."

The class practiced this every week. One day when a 3 year old saw his mother looking upset, he said, "Mom, you should try blowing out a candle."

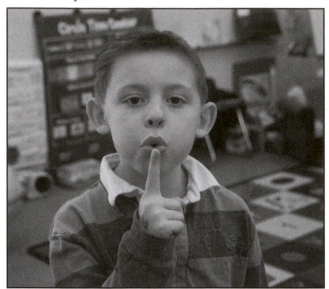

Figure 12-2. Teach children deep breathing techniques.

- **Show the tightening and then relaxing of one's body to get calm.**

"Make your body like a robot," the social worker said to the preschoolers as she demonstrated tightening all her muscles. The class followed her example. "Okay. Now relax. Be like a spaghetti noodle." The class responded by swinging their arms around.

- **Demonstrate pushing hands together with a deep breath for calming.**

"If your body is moving too fast and too wild, this is something you can do to get yourself calm," I told the group of kindergartners. "First rub your hands, then push your palms together and take a big breath."

"Sometimes I get too wild at home," Scott said. "It hurts my heart when my mom yells at me."

"It is upsetting to have someone yell at you. Try the pushes and see if it helps you get calm.

- **Show how to pull hands apart and take a deep breath to get calm.**

"Put one hand up toward the ceiling. Now put one hand down and try to pull your fingers apart. As you pull, take a deep breath," I said, demonstrating.

The next week when the class practiced this strategy, 4-year-old Raul said, "I taught my brother that one."

- **Demonstrate counting to 10 for calming.**

"Pretend you are squeezing a ball," I told the preschool class as I made a tight fist. "Now count to 10." After the class said the numbers, I said, "Now shake your hands out." Adam's mother, who was volunteering in the class, smiled as the children wiggled their hands.

Two months later, she told me with tears in her eyes, "I told Adam to put his game away. He got really angry, but he stopped and counted to 10. Then he calmly handed it to me. Thanks!"

Use Visuals for Calming

Visual materials such as pictures can be helpful for calming. When children are very angry, they often yell. Younger children often cry. The noise level tends to escalate and adds to the commotion around them. If they are having a meltdown due to being on sensory overload, talking only adds more. When upset, some children also may repeatedly tell themselves you are mean, it's not fair, and they are not going to listen to anything you say.

To help them shift thinking about their anger, show them visuals that help them identify their feelings and calming strategies. You can ask them to point to a related face on a poster of children with different feelings. They also can point to the intensity level of their anger on a feelings thermometer (see www.csefel.vanderbilt.edu). In addition, giving children an "I need a break" card allows them to calm themselves. When they are getting upset, they can hand it to the teacher without words and remove themselves from the maddening situation. Another option is to show them pictures of their choices for relaxation or sensory strategies. You can ask them to point to their choice and remain quiet and calm until they do.

Using a visual does not add to the noise level. Helping children identify their feelings and showing them choices for calming shifts their focus away from their anger. They can start thinking about how to get calm. Asking children to point makes it easier for them to respond versus asking them to say their choice.

Fabulous Five: Use Visuals for Calming
- **Show pictures of calming strategies.**

Four-year-old Danny marched around the classroom. Then he walked over to the shelves and began pulling and throwing the bins of manipulative toys to the floor. Plastic pieces flew in all directions. I quickly grabbed a paper with three pictures of calming strategies and went to him. "Stop! That is not safe. You are mad." Showing him the page, I said, "Point to what you are going to do to get yourself calm."

He looked at the pictures of taking a deep breath, going for a walk, or going to the calming area. He pointed to the calming area.

"Okay. Go there and take a break." He did, and 5 minutes later he returned to the group.

- **Tell children to use an "I need a break" card.**

Five-year-old Trevor was seen repeatedly hitting children when he was on sensory overload. To change this common reaction, I showed him a card with the words *I need a break*.

"When there's too much going on around you," I said, "give this card to your teacher. It says 'I need a break.' Then you can go get a drink of water in the hall. Take a break instead of hitting. Hitting only gets you in trouble. Would you like to draw yourself on the card so it is yours?"

He nodded and began drawing.

- **Have children look at a feeling thermometer.**

One day when a classmate would not give him the toy car he wanted, 4-year-old Donald took a block and whacked him on the head.

"Donald hit me," the child cried, and the teacher intervened.

When I was in his class the next day, I saw him grimace when a classmate reached for one of his favorite trucks. I gave the classmate another truck and, holding his favorite red one, I said, "Donald, come with me." We walked over to the chart showing a thermometer going from white at the bottom to different degrees of red at the top. At the bottom was a child with a calm face, and at the top was a child looking livid. "Point to how you feeling. Are you a little mad, mad, or really, really mad?"

He touched the middle of the thermometer.

"When you are feeling mad, take a deep breath and then use your words. Tell your friend you want to play with the red truck first and then he can had a turn."

- **Use a poster of feeling words and facial expressions and have the children point.**

When 4-year-old Ian stomped into the classroom, we went to a poster of various faces portraying different feelings. "How do you feel right now?" I asked, gesturing to the poster.

"I feel like all of them."

"You look upset," I replied, pointing to the corresponding face.

"That's right. I'm mad. My brother's mean. He broke my truck."

- **Show pictures of sensory strategies.**

When the noise in the classroom escalated, 5-year-old Marcos started yelling, "Aaaa!"

I brought over a strip with pictures of wearing headphones, taking a walk, or putting on a weighted vest. "I know it is loud in here, and you are upset. What do you want to do to feel better?"

He pointed to the headphone picture, walked over to the shelf, and put them on.

Help Children Manage Their Feelings

> **Children might be thinking:**
> *You're paying attention.*
> *I feel better when I talk it out.*
> *You're helping me cope.*
> *Talking it out helps.*
> *You care about me.*

During children's time with you, they will often talk about their experiences and emotions. In a group or classroom situation, you may also be with them when they become angry, scared, or frustrated. At these times, help them clarify what they are feeling, what happened, and what they can do.

Promote Constructive Handling of Anger

When you see children are angry, acknowledge that. Encourage them to use their successful strategies for self-calming or offer additional ideas. Afterward, if they have hurt someone's feelings, have them figure out what they can do to make the situation better. Also discuss constructive ways to deal with anger in the future.

> ### Fabulous Five: Assist Children in Addressing Their Anger
>
> - **Let children know it is okay to feel angry but what is important is what they do.**
>
> The school psychologist and I had helped the third grader learn ways to manage his anger. During the year, Brandon became less explosive. In the spring, he started working with an occupational therapy student to learn a special typing program on a computer. He practiced the row of home keys twice.
>
> "Try it again," the occupational therapy student said in a gentle voice.
>
> He folded his arms, slumped in the chair, and put his chin on his chest.
>
> The occupational therapy student moved to the computer and said, "Okay. Tell me what to type."
>
> "I don't like you," he shouted.
>
> In a firm voice, I said, "That is not okay. You may be angry, but it is not okay to hurt people's feelings like that."
>
> "Well," he whimpered, "why do I have to keep practicing? I'm not stupid."
>
> "It takes everyone a lot of practice to learn typing. It is okay to feel angry and frustrated. Next time say, 'I'm mad. I need a break.'"
>
> - **Ask children if they feel mad.**
>
> While making a picture, 10-year-old Doug stuck his tongue between his lips and blew a raspberry.

"Please stop making those noises," I said.

He stopped drawing and said, "You can't tell me to stop." He sat still, stared at his picture, and pushed his lips out. "You can't tell me to stop. I'm going to spit on you."

"Doug, I like you. You don't need to do that. Are you mad at me?"

"Yeah, you can't tell me to stop."

"Asking you to stop making those noises is just like when everyone asks you to stop burping loudly. I can see that upset you. Let's do something fun." I pulled out a construction toy that Doug liked, and he started to build.

When I passed him in the school hall later that afternoon, he said, "I like you too, Dr. Clare."

- **Encourage children to use their successful strategies when mad.**

"When I'm mad, I scream and kick," 4-year-old Justin said. "And when I go to my bedroom, I kick the door."

"What could you do instead?" I asked. He shrugged. "I remember last week you told us that when you have scary dreams, you tell yourself, 'I can be brave.' You had a great idea. When you are mad, use your idea and tell yourself, 'I can be calm and take deep breaths.' You can also tell yourself, 'I'm the boss of my body and I can calm down.'"

- **Acknowledge feelings and offer an alternate strategy to aggressive actions.**

Seven-year-old Oliver growled behind Ed's back. Ed swung around and put his nose an inch away from Oliver's nose. I quickly stepped between them before a punch could be thrown.

"He growled at me," Ed yelled.

I looked at Ed and said, "It's okay to be upset. Use words to tell him to stop."

- **Help children figure out what to do if they make someone mad.**

"You're a baby," 4-year-old Rachel snipped at her classmate.

"I am not," Chandler replied, and stomped away.

"Rachel, look at your friend's face. Does he look happy or mad?" I said.

"Mad."

"Chandler, come back. Are you mad?"

"Yeah," he said.

"Tell her why."

"Don't call me a baby. I don't like it."

"What could you do to help him feel better?'

"I can draw him a picture." As she drew, she said, "Here's me and here's Chandler. How do you spell sorry?"

I printed the word, and she copied it. Then she ran over and gave him the picture.

Address Children's Scared Feelings

Let children know that being scared is a normal reaction to a frightening experience. When they tell you their fears, explore what scares them and why. Validate their feelings and offer reassurance or comfort. Prepare the children if you know an activity has scary elements. Then if they are hesitating, support them in facing and overcoming their fears.

Fabulous Five: Reassure Children Who Are Scared and Help Them Face Their Fears

- **Acknowledge that everyone gets scared.**

At Halloween, 6-year-old Jack said, "If I saw a vampire, I would kick him. I never get scared."

"It's okay to get scared. Everyone gets scared at some time."

- **Soothe or comfort scared children.**

When the specialized class went on a field trip to a farm, 8-year-old Andrew followed his classmates to see the horses. But when the large stallion came to the fence, Andrew started crying and saying, "Go home. Go home."

"That horse is big. I will keep you safe. Let's move away from the horses," the speech-language pathologist said, taking out picture symbols to show him what fun activities were next. "Look, next we are having lunch, then a fire and marshmallows, and then we ride a fire truck." They walked over to the antique fire engine parked in the driveway.

He stopped crying, pointed, and said, "Fire truck."

- **Offer reassurance when children feel scared.**

"We are having a fire drill today. It is practice for what to do if there is a fire," the preschool teacher told the class.

When the alarm sounded, I helped the teacher usher the children outside. After we came back in, 4-year-old Emily said to me, "I'm glad we're alive."

"Were you scared?" I asked, and she nodded. "Did you see how we helped everyone and kept you safe?" She nodded again. "We will always help you."

"My mom's grandma died. She is up in the sky. If we die, we have to go to heaven."

- **Acknowledge that an activity or experience may be scary.**

During the week of Halloween, I placed a plastic stress ball on the table and said to the first grader, "This is scary looking. The eyeballs and blood inside it are pretend. If you want to try it, you can squeeze as hard as you can because it's unbreakable."

Shelby snatched it and molded her fingers around the ball. She squeezed, and the bloodshot eyes popped out the side of her hand. "Are they real?"

"No, they're fake. They are pretend. They're plastic."

"What's this red stuff? Is it plastic or real?"

"It's not blood. That's plastic too," I reassured her.

She started squeezing, and the eyeballs squished back and forth. She smiled and said, "They're so slippery." When it was time to go, Shelby rolled the ball to me and said, "Bye, Mr. Eyeballs."

- **Help children face their fears.**

"Try it. We'll all be with you," 4-year-old Katie told her classmate, Tania. Katie turned to me and said, "She's afraid to go up the stairs to the slide because she fell one time."

"These are high steps. I'll help you," I replied, looking at Tania. "When you go up, put your hand on the rail. For each step, find a place to hold on." I followed as Tania went up. Once she was sitting on the slide, I asked, "Do you want me to stand at the bottom?" She nodded.

I quickly backed down the steps. She moved an inch forward but held tightly to the sides of the slide. When she did not move again, I asked, "Do you want me to hold your hand as you go down?"

"Yes."

I held on and slowed her rate of descent. After assisting her two more times, I said, "Do you want to try it on your own now?"

"Yeah."

When she reached the bottom, I told her, "Say, 'I did it!'"

Tania raised her arms and said with a smile, "I did it!" She continued without my help, following her friends as they went down the slide.

Help Children Deal With Frustration

It is common for children to experience frustration when facing a challenge. Some expect perfection the first few times they try something new. Children often become upset if the activity is difficult, if they are unsuccessful, or if people do not do what the children want. Some believe that if they try again, they will just fail. They may question their competencies. Others may give up or destroy whatever they are doing or making.

Help children learn how to tolerate the uncomfortable feeling of frustration. Start by identifying whether they feel anger, boredom, or frustration. When they say they are bored, check to see if it is really frustration. Then tell them to use the words, "I am frustrated."

Encourage them to view challenges as something to be conquered. Have them tell themselves that with each try, they will learn more or will get better. Explore other strategies they can use, such as taking a break, getting help, or trying a different method. If they are frustrated with another person, assist them in talking together. You can also lighten a tense situation by using humor. In addition, you can model or role-play how to persevere.

Fabulous Five: Increase Children's Frustration Tolerance

- **Offer a strategy for dealing with frustration.**

Nine-year-old Bud cut a piece of paper to fit his home-made book on knights and started copying a sentence. As he printed, he said, "I don't know how to make a 'T,'" but then he proceeded to make the letter.

"The next letter is 'h,'" I said.

"I'm doin' it," he snarled, but he wrote an "n" instead of an "h." He clenched the paper, crumpled it, and cried out, "I hate this paper."

"I understand. You feel frustrated when things don't go right."

"Yeah, and I'm not going to do this."

"Everyone makes mistakes. You look like you need some time to get calm." I handed him a stress ball and said, "Try squeezing this ball. That helps kids feel better."

Bud curled his palm around the ball and squeezed hard.

"Squeeze five or 10 times."

"Ten times," he said, smiling.

After counting down to zero, I handed him a new sheet of paper and said, "Okay, cut this again and just write two words."

- **Be aware that when children say, "This is boring," they may think the activity is too hard.**

Seven-year-old Zach made a pop-up book in the shape of a wolf. He added wiggle eyes and was pleased with the results. When it came to writing the story for the book, he erased his printing every few minutes and started grunting. "This is boring," he said.

"It looks like you are getting frustrated with the writing. Maybe it would be better if you stopped and finished the writing next week."

- **Use humor to alleviate frustration.**

When 8-year-old Billy could not remember what he had previously learned, he grimaced and clenched his hands.

In response, I started to sing, "Memory, memory, where are you? Come back."

He smiled.

- **Model how to deal with frustration.**

I brought a new spinning top that, when given the right force, flips over and spins, looking like a mushroom. As the second graders watched, I tried spinning it 10 times with no luck. "Boy, this is frustrating," I said. "It's really hard, but I'm not going to give up. I'm going to keep trying." After 10 more tries, I finally was able to get it to flip, and the group clapped.

- **Role play how to handle a frustrating situation.**

Seven-year-old Max kept making the same mistake and let out a loud sigh. I asked, "Max, when you sighed like that, were you thinking, 'I keep making mistakes. I can't get this. I'm frustrated'?"

"I was thinking, 'This is hard!'"

"Max, instead of just sighing, use words and tell me what you are feeling. Let's pretend I'm you and you are me, Dr. Clare." I imitated making the same mistake four times. I took a deep breath, dropped my shoulders, and let out a sigh. "Okay, you are Dr. Clare. What do you say?"

"Use words. Say you are frustrated."

Using Max's voice, I said, "I'm frustrated. I want to quit and give up."

"No, don't give up. You can do it."

"Okay, I won't give up, but I need a break."

Address Children's Worries

As children talk, listen for their worries or concerns. For instance, when one foster child was upset, he would often yell at a classmate, "You're bad. You're going to get taken away," indicating his fear. It is common for them to be worried about being safe. They may wonder if they, their families, homes, and pets are safe. They may get anxious thinking something bad might happen, be leery of the unknown, or be concerned about their comfort level. Think about what their experiences, especially traumatic ones, are like from their perspective. Be aware that at times, children will blame themselves for an event, such as a divorce or parents fighting. Provide reassurance and explanations of the situation. You also can help them by watching for subtle signs of anxiety, guessing at the underlying worry, and checking to see if you are right. In addition, you can assist children in dealing with their worries by teaching ways to relax and to communicate their fears to others.

Fabulous Five: Ease Children's Worries

- **Encourage children to talk about their worries.**

"I'm afraid of fire," 5-year-old Bridget told me.

"How come?"

"I saw the burnt trees on TV when there was a fire on the mountain."

"Were you scared that your house might burn down too?"

"Yeah, but my mom said we're safe."

- **Explore underlying worry.**

At the beginning of our session, 7-year-old Vanessa sat down and blurted out, "Kayla said if I didn't invite her to my birthday party, she would kick my butt."

"Are you worried she might hurt you?" She nodded with a distressed look. "Should we go and talk to your teacher and tell her about that?"

"Okay."

- **State possible worry.**

"Time to line up for recess," the preschool teacher announced.

"It's dark outside," 4-year-old Josh said as he looked at the gray, overcast sky. "We shouldn't go outside."

"I see you didn't bring a jacket," I said. "Are you worried that you might be cold?"

He nodded.

"Do you want to borrow one of our extra coats?" I asked, and he reached for the one I offered him.

- **Consider what worries children might have after seeing or experiencing a traumatic event.**

When I walked into the specialized classroom, I saw three 11 year olds, who were nonverbal and immobile, sitting in wheelchairs in front of the TV. They were watching continual coverage of wildfires engulfing numerous homes and were not able to move away. I asked the inexperienced teacher to turn it off and said to the boys, "Those houses are far away. They are not here. It's sad that happened, but you are safe. Your family is safe. Your home is safe."

- **Explain what will happen to eliminate children's worries.**

"Everyone line up. We are going to get our pictures taken," the preschool teacher told the class.

Three-year-old Austin burst into tears.

"It is not like a shot," his teacher reassured him. "It does not hurt. Remember when I took your picture in class? It didn't hurt."

His crying changed to sniffling.

Decrease Nervousness

Some children are shy and afraid of being with or talking to others, especially if they do not know them. They need reassurance and to feel safe before they will talk. Even if they are too uncomfortable to speak, they do appreciate being acknowledged. Gently and gradually give them the opportunity to participate without any pressure to talk.

Children also may feel nervous if they are trying something new, are concerned about losing, or are fearful about looking bad in front of their peers. They may focus more on their nervousness, which can generate more anxiety. They may tell themselves they cannot do the activity, so it is not worth trying. Some may seek soothing from others or from whatever calms them. For instance, a 3-year-old boy practiced singing a familiar song with his class. With delight, he sang the loudest and the most off key. However, the next day when his class performed in front of parents, he stood quietly with his fist in his mouth. He was just too nervous. To help break the cycle of perpetuating more anxiety, encourage them to use relaxation techniques, such as deep breathing. Promote self-talk that is reassuring and builds confidence. Provide encouragement and recognize when they think about trying again. Talk about how helpful it is to get the support of others and to be open to assistance.

Fabulous Five: Reduce Nervousness

- **Bring shy children into the conversation.**

As 4-year-old Gavin gathered toys, he said, "I love Superman."

"I love horses," Anne added.

I turned to Felicia, who was fiddling with a toy with her head down. "What do you love?"

She raised her head slightly and whispered, "I love Tinkerbell."

- **Ask about a time they overcame nervousness.**

"Tell me about a time you overcame your nervousness," I said to a group of sixth graders.

"During fifth-grade field day with a different school in the same district," Crystal responded, "we were competing for ribbons. I was doing the 50-meter dash. I was the smallest and the rest of the girls were really tall. I thought they were going to win. I was really nervous I was going to lose because everyone was so tall. We went in the five lanes, and five go at a time. They pick random so you don't know who you are up against.

"My friends in the bleachers were watching and cheering for me. I was very happy about that. I knew I would do better because they were with me. Then I was called up to race. There was a fake gun, which scared me. The gun was shot. I ran for my life! I almost fell over the finish line I was running so fast. I was so close in the second lane. I couldn't see if I was first. I looked back, and they were all behind me. I got first place!"

"Congratulations," I said. "Sounds like having the support of your friends really helped you."

- **Acknowledge positive self-talk.**

"The first time I rode my bike, I crashed into the mailbox two times," 7-year-old Kaylee said. "The first time I pedaled, I kept thinking I was going to fall, and I didn't focus on what I was supposed to do. I was so nervous. Then I told myself, "If I am nervous, I'll fall. If I'm not nervous, I won't.""

"Did that help?"

"Yeah."

"What you tell yourself can make a difference."

- **Talk about getting support.**

"I have to give a whole speech in front of my class," 11-year-old Laura said. "My teacher said that if it helped, she would stand next to me. She knows I have stage fright. I told her that would be great. I've never had a teacher help me get over my stage fright."

"Getting support is a good strategy when you're nervous."

- **Acknowledge when children tell themselves they can try again.**

"Yesterday in band class there was a chair test," 12-year-old Brittney said. "There are five chairs in the flute section. The first chair is for those who are the most advanced. Second and third chair are advanced, and fourth and fifth chair are more beginners. I was in the third chair and was challenged by someone in the fourth chair. I knew the music really well and practiced it the night before and in class.

"When it came to the test, the competitor played first. She's only played the flute for 1 year. I've played for 3 years. She played with only little mistakes and then I played and messed up a lot. I was nervous and my flute was messed up. So I had a disadvantage. She won third chair and I was moved to fourth. The worst part was that in front of others, he switched my music to beginner's music, and I have to play that at the concert. It's music that's not challenging for me. And my friends are in first and second chair. I am going to ask my teacher if I can challenge her again this month with different music."

"So you're telling yourself to try again and give yourself another chance. Is that giving you hope?"

She nodded.

Respond to Feelings of Sadness

No matter where they are, children more often than adults tend to cry aloud when they are sad. Their tears are an obvious sign of their sadness. Others may show their feelings nonverbally. They may stop and stand still with their heads down while their peers are playing. Their eyes may be downcast and their mouths droopy. When you see children in this state, explore reasons for their glum looks and acknowledge their feelings.

Some children will talk about their experiences, like the 3-year-old child who said, "It's a sad day. My frog died. We had to bury him." Empathize by acknowledging their pain and expressing your hope that they will feel better. Comfort them and, if possible, help them find a solution to the situation that is making them sad.

Fabulous Five: Provide Empathy and Comfort When Children Feel Sad

- **Explore the reason for sad looks.**

"Carrie, you look sad," I said.

"I'm sick," the 8 year old replied. "My heart's not feeling good."

"What's the matter?"

"I'm still upset about my friend leaving. She moved to Chicago for life."

- **Acknowledge their sadness.**

When I went into the second-grade class, Martin jumped up, wrapped his arms around my leg, and started crying. "My dog Eddie ran away," he said through his tears.

"Oh, that is so sad. I'm sorry that happened to you," I said softly.

His teacher overheard our conversation and said, "I have a book about losing a pet. I can read it to the class this afternoon."

- **Show empathy when children are sad.**

"You can take your drawings home and give them to your parents," the preschool teacher told the class.

"I can't give mine to my mom," 3-year-old Valerie said in a sad tone of voice. "I live with my aunt now. We took my mom to the hospital and left her there."

"You miss your mom?" I asked gently. She nodded.

- **Comfort children who are sad.**

"Goodbye. Have a good day at school," Sue's mother said to the 3 year old.

Sue started crying and hugged her stuffed puppy.

I took the puppy and, pretending to be it, said, "I'm sorry you're sad. It's hard to say goodbye. Let me give you kisses." I raised the puppy to her cheek. "Kiss, kiss, kiss."

She stopped crying and smiled at me.

- **Help children find a solution to the situation that is making them unhappy.**

On the playground, 4-year-old Jared stood by himself with tears streaming down his cheeks. "You look so unhappy," I said. "Tell me what's wrong."

"Jessica and Alyssa won't play with me."

"Sometimes friends take turns with who they play with. Can you find another friend?"

"No."

"Let's go over and try talking to the girls."

"Why is he crying?" Jessica asked when she saw him.

"He's sad because he hasn't had a chance to play with you. Could he join you?"

"Sure. Here, everyone hold on to the outside of the hula hoop and spin." The three laughed as they twirled around.

Assist Children in Learning How to Handle Conflict

In addition to learning how to keep themselves calm, children also have to learn ways to negotiate and resolve conflict. This can be challenging for them because negotiating means they may not get exactly what they want or they may have to wait. If there is a power imbalance, children also need to know how to protect themselves from those acting like bullies.

Teach Ways to Negotiate and Resolve Conflict

Children might be thinking:

I'll try to find something we have in common and see if that helps.

It's good to know what to do if we're not getting along.

Teach children a process and variety of strategies for handling disagreements. First let them know that they can say, "No, thank you," if they do not want to negotiate. Convey to them that by saying those words in a polite and respectful way, they are more likely to be heard by others.

When there is quarrel, teach them the following process of negotiation: (1) decide to talk with each other and think about that person's feelings or perspectives, (2) listen to what each one says, (3) see if there is any common ground and shared needs/desires, (4) explore alternatives, and (5) decide on a solution and plan.

It is also helpful for them to know different negotiation techniques. For instance, they can consider taking turns, trading, or sharing. Help them think of ideas around shared needs and common ground or meeting each other part of the way. Encourage them to shift from thinking about winning to compromising. Emphasize how this is an important skill for making and keeping friends.

Fabulous Five: Teach to Negotiate and Resolve Conflict

- **Teach to say, "No, thank you."**

Four-year-old Edwin built a house out of magnetic tiles. He was adding a roof when Mark came over and took one tile off. "No, stop," Edwin yelled, swinging his arm toward Mark.

I turned to Mark and said, "You have to ask Edwin if you can help him."

"Can I help you?" he asked, but Edwin shook his head.

"Just tell Mark, 'No, thank you,'" I said.

"No, thank you."

- **Describe a difficult situation and ask children how to handle it.**

The preschool teacher held up a picture of two girls grabbing the same doll. "Look at this picture. They are fighting. How could they solve their problem? What can they say?"

"Please," one yelled out.

"Could I have the doll, pretty please?" another said.

"Yes. They could use nice words like 'please.' One could get another doll and see if her friend would trade. Or they could take turns."

- **Teach children to use cards with pictures of different solutions.**

"Dr. Clare and I brought presents for your class," the special education teacher said. "We have a very special box called a solution kit. Solution means an idea on how to make things better. Inside the kit, there is a ball to squeeze. If you are mad or having trouble with a friend, you can calm your body down by squeezing the ball and counting to 10.

"When you are calm, you can look at these pictures to solve your problems. There are ideas like sharing, trading, saying please, and asking a teacher for help. You can look at these picture cards to figure out what to do."

Later in the day, when 4-year-old Carrie became upset with a friend for not sharing, she said, "I need that box."

The teacher pointed to the kit on shelf. She then showed them the cards and helped the two girls decide on a solution.

- **Ask, "How can you solve this problem when you both want…?"**

Two first graders grabbed the one pair of red scissors. "I want red," they both demanded at the same time.

"I have a pretty blue pair," I said, and they both shook their heads. "How can you solve this problem?"

"Hey, do you have any more red scissors?" Elizabeth suggested.

I looked in my cupboard. "No, but I found a purple pair."

"Purple is my favorite color," Elizabeth said, handing the red pair to Bella.

- **Ask the group, "What can you do so that everyone can…?"**

"They're not being nice," 4-year-old Collette said to me, pointing to two girls holding hands and dancing to music.

"She's not being nice," the girls replied.

"They won't dance with me."

"What can you do so that you are nice to each other?"

The three thought for a minute. "We could do a different dance and all dance together."

"That works," I replied.

All three smiled and, holding each other's hands, they danced in circle.

Support Standing Up to Those Who Act Like Bullies

> **Children might be thinking:**
> *I'm scared to ask.*
> *I don't know what to say.*
> *Will I make the situation worse?*
> *I think my friend would help me, so I should help them.*
> *Maybe I should get help.*

Bullying can entail belittling, threats, intimidation, and/or bodily harm. It can be taunts, rumors, drawings, and/or exclusion from peers. It may occur face-to-face, behind children's backs, or online (i.e., *cyberbullying*). At greater risk for being targets are children who are different from their peers in any way. Those who act like bullies want to have power over their victims. It takes courage to stand up to them, and doing so can be scary.

Children may hesitate to do anything because they fear that their actions may be ineffective or make the situation worse, or that the person might lash out more. They do not want to be perceived as a tattletale and worry about being shunned by their peers. They may hesitate to tell caregivers because they believe adults cannot help, and they fear retaliation if they intervene. Children may feel helpless and powerless.

It is vital, of course, to have bullying prevention programs and policies in all schools, organizations, and settings. It is also important for children to know that they have options and their actions can be effective. One option they have is to tell the person to stop. If necessary, teach them words they can use and practice using a firm voice. They can ignore or walk away from the person. Let children know, however, that if these options are ineffective, they should seek peer and/or adult support. They will find that having the support of friends decreases the feeling of vulnerability and makes it easier to stand up for themselves. If they want your assistance, talk with them and together decide on a plan.

> ## Fabulous Five: Support Standing Up to Those Acting Like Bullies
>
> - **Encourage children to use their words to confront those acting like bullies.**
>
> Unprovoked, 3-year-old Alex jumped up and ran across the room. He extended his arm, made a fist, and began whacking 4-year-old Denise. She began crying.
>
> I moved Alex away from the group, and the teacher comforted Denise. After I talked with him and she stopped crying, I asked her to come over to Alex. "Use your words and tell him you don't like to be hit."

"Don't hit me. I don't like it," Denise said. "You're not keeping my body safe."

Alex hugged her in response.

- **Promote ignoring when being bullied and then getting support.**

A third grader walked by and taunted Matt, "I saw your boxers."

"Is he playing or being mean?" I asked Matt.

"He's being mean. He's in the pack, and he does that a lot."

"What do you do?"

"Ignore him. He gets in trouble a lot."

"Does he ever get you in trouble?"

"No."

"Ignoring is a good thing to do. He's the one having problems, not you. If he continues, your teacher can help you too."

- **Encourage children to walk away and get support.**

"I had a bully at my dad's baseball game. He said, 'Get away or I'm going to beat you up.' Then he threw my bike in the mud. So I ran away. My parents believed me. My neighbors stood up for me and saved my life. He's mean, and I'm only going to the park if my neighbors are with me."

"Sounds like you have a good plan," I told the 8 year old. "It helped when you walked away and had others help you."

- **Recognize the courage it takes to confront those acting mean.**

"This one girl was spreading rumors about me," 12-year-old Noel told me. "She told one of my friends that I didn't like to hang out with her. So I went up to that girl and said, 'Have you been saying these things?' She said, 'I don't know what you're talking about.' I told her, 'Well, if you are saying these things, you need to stop because they are rude and not true.'"

"What did she say?" I asked.

"She turned and went to her locker. She didn't look at me or talk to me for a week, but she stopped."

"That takes courage to do. Your confronting her made a difference."

- **Affirm that talking to an adult can help.**

"I made Cori all pissed off for talking to Garrett," 11-year-old Aimee told me while she drew. "I was outside. She threw the ball and hit me in the head. I told the playground assistant and she told the dean of students. Then he talked to Cori and called me down during seventh period to talk to me. My friends said, 'Oh, you're in trouble.' I told them I wasn't. Cori said she was sorry."

"Sounds like talking to an adult really helped," I said, and she nodded.

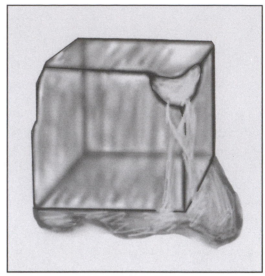

Figure 12-3. Prevent meltdowns by defusing tense situations.

Handle Emotions in Crisis Situations

If you work in settings where children are more likely to lose control (e.g., day treatment programs, psychiatric hospitals), it is important to get formal training in crisis intervention. There are specific techniques for stopping aggressive actions and preventing harm to children, other people, and yourself. The following are general guidelines because children may lose control in any setting, including school.

These ideas are to help neutralize a situation until assistance can be obtained. You must intervene if the safety of the children or others is in jeopardy. Of course, as mentioned previously, it is better if you can prevent problematic situations. If prevention is not possible, the next best step is to intervene quickly before a situation becomes explosive (Figure 12-3). It is similar to putting out a fire. It is easier to extinguish a spark than contain an out-of-control and spreading fire.

Shift Focus to Regaining Control

Children might be thinking:
I'm so mad.
I feel enraged.
I feel scared.
I feel unsafe.
You keep me safe.
You don't yell at me.

At all times, watch for signs of any situation that might become volatile. Try to learn children's body language, especially those who have a history of losing control and hurting themselves or others. Observe to see if they have a certain look or movements that show their anger. Become a master at reading the warning signs, and intervene quickly. You can defuse a possible crisis situation by addressing their feelings, helping them get their needs met, or giving ideas on how to resolve the situation. If necessary, you may need to ask the child to move away from the group.

When intervening, acknowledge any attempt children make to regain control. You also may want to provide two options that will both allow the children to save face and stop the crisis that is brewing. Another approach is to eliminate an audience. If they know their classmates are watching, some may become excited by doing something they know is not allowed. A crowd mentality may develop in which the peers may encourage them to continue. Although the classmates may laugh, they also may feel scared because they do not know what will happen. By eliminating the audience, you may eliminate some of the fun associated with showing off to peers.

Fabulous Five: Defuse a Brewing Crisis Situation

- **Watch the children's faces and body language and intervene at the first sign of angry or tense looks before the situation escalates.**

"I want that truck," 4-year-old Alex said as he tried to pull it away from Dylan.

Dylan held the toy tightly, not letting go. Alex grimaced and tightened all his muscles. He raised his shoulders and made his hands into fists.

Because he had hit another child earlier that week, I immediately intervened. I pulled out a ring of picture cards showing different solutions to conflict. Picking out two pictures, I gave Alex two choices. "You can ask Dylan for a turn when he is done or you can find another toy and see if he wants to trade."

"Can I have a turn when you're done?" Dylan asked, repeating my words.

Alex nodded.

- **Eliminate the audience in a crisis situation.**

In the last few minutes of our newspaper group, PJ jumped on top of a chair and raised his arms up as if he were king. The other children grinned at his antics. Rather than give him attention, his teacher said, "It's time for recess. Line up." The class hustled to the door with their backs to PJ. "Who wants a ball?" the teacher asked.

"I do," one boy said.

"I do too," PJ said.

"Come join us in line," his teacher replied, and he lowered himself to the ground.

- **Intervene quickly if children say or do something that could be mean or hurtful to another child.**

We were playing the game, Don't Spill the Beans, by picking up beans with tweezers and placing them on a hanging cup that spilled when there was too much weight. Savannah snapped the tweezers like lobster claws and reached toward Frankie's ear.

"Savannah, stop," I said, and she turned toward me. "I know you are playing, but you could hurt Frankie with those tweezers."

- **Present two options that allow children to take action without admitting they are wrong.**

"I got in a fight yesterday. I really hurt him too," Victor bragged with a smile. He became more excited as he continued telling the details of the fight even after I asked him to stop.

Finally I said, "Victor, you have two choices. You can either stop talking about the fight or you can leave the group. What is your choice?"

Although he was not happy that I interrupted him, he did stop. Later, the two of us talked about the consequences of fighting and other ways of handling anger besides violence.

- **Acknowledge the children's attempts to maintain control.**

On my first day in a class in the day treatment, I asked the children about their strengths, interests, and goals. Ten-year-old Terry had just returned to his desk after taking a timeout break. I waited 5 minutes and then approached him. "What do you like to do for fun?" I asked.

"I don't want to talk to you." He popped out of his chair and ran to a table.

I waited a few more minutes and then said, "That's okay. I know you are trying to get calm. I understand that talking to me would not help you right now." I waited another 5 minutes, then moved closer to him. "You do not have to talk. I just want you to know that next week, we'll be starting a group in here. When you feel more relaxed, I would like to talk with you and get to know you better."

He participated in the group the following week.

Be Cognizant of Your Role in a Crisis

Children might be thinking:
You're not going to hurt me.
You're trying to help me.
You're staying calm.
You're not scared.

How you handle yourself in a crisis is a major factor in determining whether the situation improves or becomes worse. You have to balance being calm and firm without appearing threatening. You need to take action that conveys that you want the children to regain control. Although there are no guarantees, there are approaches that are more likely to defuse a situation.

When children lose control and hurt others, it often scares them and their peers. The situation may also scare you, although you have to remain calm. Your actions will show if you, as the adult, have control and answer the children's ever-present question, "Will you keep me safe?" At this time, shift from making demands to helping them regain control. Step out of any arguments or power struggles. Your agenda now is to help them become safe and calm. To do this, you must use firm but nonthreatening body language. You also must give a short but clear message on what action they need to take. If children have lost control, do not expect them to act rationally. In addition, do not take it personally if they swear at you or call you names.

Use Firm But Nonthreatening Nonverbal Language

Your body language is a key element in defusing a tense moment. Nonverbally, you have to give the message that you are a caring, calm, and respectful person and you will not hurt them. Some children go into a fight mode and look to see if you will be aggressive back. Nonthreatening moves include the following: keeping more personal space than usual, approaching from the side, using minimal and slow movements, and maintaining a neutral tone of voice.

Children may perceive the following actions as aggressive: invading their personal space, yelling, peering down on them, using harsh tone of voice, making fast or unexpected movements, or getting in their face—nose to nose. If they perceive you to be aggressive, they are more likely to hurt you. If children start to run, one of the best ways to get them to stop is to stop chasing. Of course, if they are running into a street or an unsafe area, you have to run faster!

Fabulous Five: Recognize Your Role in a Crisis Situation

- **Use a neutral and firm tone of voice in a deliberate and slow manner.**

Frazier began swinging a wooden stool in circles and said, "You could use this as a weapon."

Using a calm but firm tone of voice, I said, "Please stop. You could hurt someone."

"It could be a weapon."

"This stool is for sitting, not hurting someone."

- **Approach children from the side.**

Although 12-year-old Derrick had only been on the psychiatric unit for a few days, he had already hurt three staff members. The first day I met with Derrick, we were in the occupational therapy room, which was connected to the unit. When we started talking about his family, a scowl crossed his face. Derrick dashed out of his chair and

---

darted to the doorway. He leaned against the thick wooden door and spread his arms. I was trapped in the room.

I moved to his side, steadied my breathing, and held my body still. Determined not to show the fear I felt, I said in a firm tone of voice, "You need to open that door." After 2 minutes, which felt more like an hour, he moved aside and opened the door.

- **Stay calm and collected.**

Everett walked over to the locked occupational therapy room on the psychiatric unit. He kicked the door and yelled, "Let me in so I can tear the place apart." Other staff quietly gathered to keep both of us safe, although we all stood at least 8 feet away to allow Everett space.

In a neutral and firm voice, I said, "Get yourself calm. When you show me you are calm and in control, we can go in." I waited, but he was unable to regroup. Seeing all the staff, he followed their suggestion that he walk to his room to help himself cool down.

- **Use minimal and slow body movement.**

Griffin stomped down the stairs, and when he reached the basement, he turned and yelled at Brady, "Leave me alone." Brady moved to the other side of the room.

"What's wrong? Did something happen?" I asked in a concerned tone of voice. I moved slowly until I was 3 feet away to show my support.

"Yeah. Brady took my backpack on the bus, and the driver didn't do anything."

"That would be upsetting. Did you get your pack back?"

"Yeah."

"Did you tell Brady that you didn't like him doing that?"

"No."

"It might help if you do."

- **Stop children who are running by not chasing unless they are in harm's way.**

Corbyn bolted out of the kindergarten class and raced down the school hallway. When he saw me following him, he laughed. He stuck his thumbs in his ears and wiggled his fingers. "Chase me."

I stopped, stood still, and waited without saying a word. Then I waved my hand in a come-back gesture. He hesitated for 2 minutes, then dragged his feet as he returned.

Give a Clear Message

When children are getting upset and their behavior starts to escalate, first let them know you want to talk and help them. Next, say that you will wait for them to get calm. You can give cues, such as, "We can talk when you stop yelling," or suggest that they take deep breaths. Another option is to have children tell you when they are ready to talk. It is best for you to maintain a calm presence and be quiet while waiting. This gives children an opportunity to regain self-control.

If you find children are starting to hurt themselves or others, tell them to stop and give a clear message regarding what you want them to do. Be vigilant in using a neutral tone of voice, and recognize that children's life experiences may affect their interpretation of your voice. Use the fewest words possible with a firm and nonthreatening tone. For example, if a child is about to throw a chair, you would say, "Stop! Put the chair down." When you give a directive with just two to four words, the child is more likely to hear what you are saying. If you yell, children will often become frightened, and some will respond in an aggressive way. When children are angry, also avoid asking questions and demanding a response because this will only lead to a struggle.

Fabulous Five: Provide a Clear Message About What to Do

- **Tell children you will talk to them when they stop yelling and then say, "I can wait."**

While his classmates sat on the floor, John rolled back and forth with his head on the ground. "My brain is heavy."

"What month is it?" the kindergarten teacher asked.

John sat upright and raised his hand. "I know. I know. I know."

His teacher called on another child, and John put his hand in his lap.

The teacher wrote *Dear superstars* on the board. John stood and yelled, "Look, would you erase 'superstars.' I don't like 'superstars.' You have to write 'Dear boys and girls. It's Wednesday.' That's what you write on Wednesday. I don't like 'superstars.'"

"Sometimes we use different words," his teacher replied.

"No. No. NO," he screamed, thrashing his arms and just missing a classmate's head.

"You are not being safe. It's time to take a break," I said.

He ran into the hallway, collapsed on the floor, and started screaming.

I partially closed the classroom door and said, "We can talk when you stop yelling. I can wait." I stood for a few minutes without saying a word.

He calmed and said, "I have something to tell you. I lost an eyelash."

"So that upset you?" I replied.

"Yeah."

"Are you ready to go back to class?"

He nodded.

- **Ask children to let you know when they are ready to talk.**

"I want to be on the computer," 7-year-old Carrissa demanded.

"When it is your turn, I will let you know," I replied.

She flopped on the floor, hid her face with her fingers, and started crying.

"When you stop crying, we'll talk. Perhaps we can find something else for you to do while you are waiting. Raise your hand when you are ready to talk."

After a few minutes, she gradually lifted her hand.

- **Tell the children, "Stop. Take big breaths and get yourself calm so we can talk."**

On the psychiatric unit, 11-year-old Clayton had been in trouble all morning. When he came into the occupational therapy room, he took one look at his wood project and started yelling and repeating, "I'm not doing this."

"Stop. Take big breaths and get yourself calm, then we can talk about it," I said, and waited quietly until he settled.

- **Be aware that children's responses to a crisis situation are affected by life experience.**

On the psychiatric unit, 5-year-old Bart's right hand covered the closed scissors with only the sharp point showing. He started swinging the scissors. "Bart. Stop! Put the scissors down," I said with a slightly raised voice.

He leaped toward me, wrapped his arms and legs around my left leg, and tried to bite my knee. I placed my palm on his forehead to hold his head back and limped into the unit hallway with Bart still attached to my leg. The staff then helped him to a calming area.

Afterward, I reflected on the situation. I knew Bart had been abused, and whenever he perceived a situation to be threatening, he would attack before being attacked. I was surprised, however, that he reacted to the subtle variation in my voice.

- **Use a short phrase with the fewest words possible and give a clear message on what you want the children to do.**

"It's Victor's turn. You have to wait," the preschool teacher told 5-year-old Russ as the children passed around a toy.

He stood, started kicking the children sitting next to him, and then ran to the other side of the room. "I hate you. I hate this place," he yelled as he knocked over a bookcase full of toys. He then started throwing the wooden blocks, just missing one child's head.

I approached him on his side and, with a calm and firm voice, said, "Stop! Put the block down."

Everyone was silent as I waited quietly. He raised his arm as if he was going to throw it, but then dropped the block on the floor.

"Good choice," I said, then walked with him to a quiet space so he could get calm. Later, the teacher and I created a Social Story on what he could do and what words he could say if he has to wait for a turn.

Have Children Use Calming Strategies to Regain Control

Children might be thinking:
I'm starting to feel better.
I'm letting out my anger.
I'm letting out my worries.
I'm calming down.

When children are about to lose control or already have, it is your responsibility to try different strategies to assist them. You want to find ways for them to self-calm and use appropriate approaches for getting their needs met. You have to do this in a manner that allows them to feel respected and save face. One way to help them regain control is to acknowledge that you heard what they desire. Other useful approaches are taking a break, getting a drink, using deep pressure sensation, leaving a contentious situation, or moving to a quiet space. For some children, counting and taking deep breaths helps in regaining control.

Fabulous Five: Use Calming Strategies
- **Acknowledge what you think the children want.**

   Three-year-old Vera climbed on top of Jackson, trying to grab a flashlight out of his hand. When he did not let go, she started hitting him.

   "Stop, you are hurting your friend," I said as I pulled her off and moved her to a chair.

   She cried and tried to kick me. I moved behind her and waited a few seconds. Then I said, "You want a turn with the flashlight." She kept crying and I repeated, "You want a turn with the flashlight." She nodded. "Okay, let's go back. Say to your friend, 'Can I have a turn?'"

- **Have children take a break and move out of a problematic situation.**

   When 11-year-old Chase took his classmate's book on superheroes, the teacher said, "Chase, give the book back."

Using a low voice, Chase started preaching, imitating his pastor. Staff on the specialized unit recognized this as his sign that he was about to lose control and likely hurt someone.

"Chase, let's go for a walk and get a drink," the teacher said, knowing that a quiet walk usually helped him. Two staff members accompanied him and remained silent as they walked. When he returned, he gave back the book.

- **Decrease stimulation.**

   After the first-grade class returned from a field trip to the fire station, they made fire chief hats. "I want a hat. I want a hat. I want a hat," Heath said, each repetition getting louder.

   I could hear him in the school hallway, so I stepped into his class. The teacher knew me well because I worked with Heath. "He ripped his first hat. Could you help him make another one?" his exasperated teacher asked, handing me another nearly completed hat.

   I squatted down to Heath's eye level and said, "You will get a hat. Let's go where it is quiet and relax for a few minutes. Then I will help you finish your hat."

   We walked across the hall to an office and he continued to rant, "I want a hat."

   "Here, sit in the beanbag chair," I said, and I gave him a weighted pillow, which he placed on his lap. After a few minutes of silence, I said, "There was a lot going on this afternoon, like going to the fire station and riding a loud and bumpy bus. I know it was a change from what you usually do. I know you want a hat. As soon as you are calm, we will work on the hat."

   After five minutes of deep pressure and taking 10 long breaths, we went to the table. To ensure success, I held the paper hat and Heath manipulated the glue bottle. He put on the finished hat and nodded his satisfaction.

- **Use counting to give children time to regroup.**

   Eight-year-old Jeff stomped into the classroom, grabbed his desk, and slammed it to the floor. Then he lifted the chair to shoulder level.

   "I'm going to count to five, and you need to put the chair down. One. Two. Three. Four," I said slowly, hoping this would give Jeff time to regroup. Jeff lowered the chair an inch at a time. "Good choice," I said.

- **Provide a quiet space for calming and do not talk to children during this time.**

   In the day treatment, 7-year-old Seth started screaming and was told to go and sit in a chair away from the group to get himself calm. He stormed over and threw himself on the chair. After his inexperienced teacher talked to him nonstop for a few minutes, he screamed, "Shut up," and started kicking the wall.

Process What Happened During a Crisis Event and End on a Good Note

Children might be thinking:
That scared me.
That got me in trouble.
Do you still like me?
You're not leaving mad.

After a crisis is over, remove yourself and allow time to calm down. It is not unusual for you to feel scared or upset. You may want to get support by talking to colleagues and getting feedback. Once calm, ask yourself what you learned from the experience. Process the situation by reflecting on the following questions:

- What could have prevented the situation?
- Did I miss any cues?
- What approach did I use, and was that a contributing factor?
- How could I handle it differently?
- Do I need to change the environment or my approach?
- What will help children? Do I need to teach children coping skills?

In any event, help the children reflect on their actions and figure out what to do differently in the future. End your time with the children on a positive note.

Fabulous Five: Process What Happened Before, During, and After the Crisis

- **Reflect on how your role in the interaction contributed to the crisis situation.**

One day on the psychiatric unit, four boys were making wooden cars. Seven-year-old Cassidy raced to snatch a mallet just as Trevor reached for it. Trevor tightened his jaw, reached over to Cassidy's car, and raised the mallet, ready to smash it. I made a quick turn, frantically waved my hands, and rushed over to intercede. When Trevor saw me moving toward him, he lunged and grabbed a fistful of my hair. As I was trained, I pulled his hand in a way that resulted in a release.

I thought about the scenario later and realized I had moved too fast. Trevor seemed to interpret this as intimidating. I learned from that incident to be conscious of how I move during a crisis.

- **Talk to other adults about the incident.**

Four-year-old Russell started the day with a scowl on his face. "He's had a rough morning," his mother said to the teacher. "He did not get much sleep."

Russell sat in a cube chair for opening group. When the others leaned against his chair, he pushed their shoulders and yelled, "No."

"Move over and give him some space," I told them.

Russell then played quietly for the next half-hour in his center. He assembled a marble game and smiled when he dropped the marble and it rolled through the plastic tubes.

After two more class activities, the teacher said, "It's time to line up to go outside."

Russell moved behind Sam, and a few seconds later he shoved Sam to the ground. Sam started crying as he rubbed a red bump on his head.

When I asked Russell to move away from the group, he kicked me. Then he picked up a chair and threw it. "You are not being safe," I said, motioning for him to go to a quiet area. He did. A few minutes passed, he calmed down, and we talked. Russell joined his class on the playground.

When the children left for the day, I talked with the rest of the staff. "That surprised me when he threw that chair," I said. "I'm glad it didn't hurt anyone."

"I thought he was okay after being in centers," one teacher said.

"Me too," I replied.

"Next time he seems agitated in the morning, we may want to watch him more closely and give him extra breaks."

"And make him a helper," I said. "He likes that. He could be the one to carry the basket of toys to the playground."

- **Ask children how they would feel if someone hurt them.**

The day after 7-year-old Donny tried to choke a classmate, the social worker met with him and asked, "What happened that got you in trouble?"

"I squeezed Ashley's neck."

"Do you like to get hurt?"

"No."

"How would you feel if someone squeezed your neck?"

"Mad."

"If it makes you angry, don't you think it upsets them?" Donny nodded. "Do you like people to be mean to you?" Donny shook his head. "People don't want you to be mean to them. If you get mad and feel like hitting, stop and think for a second. Ask yourself, 'Is this what I would want somebody to do to me?'"

- **Help children reflect on their actions.**

On a snowy day, I went into the first-grade class at the day treatment and told Charlize, "Put on your coat before we go next door."

"I don't want to wear a coat."

"It's cold out, and the coat will keep you warm," I said.

She began stomping her feet and, with a burst of fury, slammed the desk and chair to the floor. The teacher took her to a quiet place to calm down.

Later, she put the coat on and we talked about what happened. "So did pushing the desk and chair get you what you wanted?"

"No. I got in trouble."

"What could you do differently next time?"

"Follow directions."

I nodded and said, "I wanted you to wear your coat because it was really cold out. I care about you and don't want you to get sick."

- **End the interaction on a positive note after setting a limit.**

Four-year-old Haley tackled Jake and hit him with a block.

"Stop!" I said firmly as I pulled her off him. "You are hurting your friend." I took her to a place away from the group and showed her a picture of blowing on a finger to cue her to take deep breaths.

"Go away," she screamed at me. "I don't like you."

I moved away to give her space to calm down but kept her in my peripheral vision to ensure that she was staying safe.

When she settled down, I read her a short book on what to do when feeling mad and had her apologize to Jake. Then I walked with her to the play kitchen. I drew circles and cut out pretend cookies.

She smiled when I offered her a paper cookie.

KEY POINTS TO REMEMBER

- In Western culture, it is important for children to be able to recognize and identify their feelings.
- Children need to learn a variety of feeling words in addition to "happy" and "mad."
- Teach children how to recognize the signs and triggers of different emotions.
- Assume children lack the skills or strategies when you see unwanted behavior and teach them what to do.
- Match the method of teaching (e.g., words, pictures, stories) to children's learning style.
- Assist children in dealing with different feelings.
- Teach children strategies for regulating their bodies, thoughts, and feelings.
- Diffuse crisis situations by staying calm and helping children regain control.
- Neutralize a crisis situation by approaching children in a calm, nonthreatening way and helping them regain control and learn from the experience.

REVIEW QUESTIONS

1. Why is it important for occupational therapists to have expertise in dealing with children's feelings?
2. When children are able to tell you their feelings, their self-control improves. True or false.
3. Why is it necessary to find out what happened before a meltdown?
4. Some children have to be taught how to recognize what others might be feeling. True or false.
5. Punishment is the best way to stop unwanted behavior or actions. True or false.
6. Social Stories (Gray, 2010) provide children with the details on how to act in a certain situation. True or false.
7. Name at least three visual methods to cue children what to do.
8. Sensory strategies do not help children regulate their bodies. True or false.
9. When children are losing control and screaming, it is best to get in front of them and tell them to stop. True or false.
10. After a crisis, examine whether you made the situation better or worse. True or false.

REFERENCES

Buron, K., & Curtis, M. (2012). *Incredible 5-point scale: Assisting students in understanding social interactions and controlling their emotional responses.* Shawnee Mission, KS: Autism Asperger Publishing.

Gagnon, E. (2001). Power cards: *Using special interests to motivate children and youth with Asperger syndrome and autism.* Shawnee Mission, KS: Autism Asperger Publishing.

Gray, C. (1994). *Comic strip conversations: Colorful, illustrated interactions with students with autism and related disorders.* Arlington, TX: Future Horizons.

Gray, C. (2010). *The new Social Stories book.* Arlington, TX: Future Horizons.

Williams, M. S., & Shellenberger, S. (1996). *How does your engine run? A leader's guide to the alert program for self regulation.* Albuquerque, NM: TherapyWorks.

Avoid Power Struggles

CHAPTER OVERVIEW

Therapy is a more pleasant experience when you know ways to avoid or move out of power struggles. In this chapter, there are empathetic, playful, and creative approaches for guiding children to mutually beneficial outcomes. Also described are tactful ways to help children learn from their actions.

CHILDREN'S DESCRIPTIONS OF WHAT THEY WANT YOU TO KNOW

Dr. Clare: "If you are doing something wrong, what can a therapist or teacher do instead of yelling at you?"

John (age 12): "Talk to me. Ask, 'What's going on?' Check in for my thoughts."

Lauren (age 11): "They could tell me to try again and try to help so that I could do better so they don't make me feel unhappy."

Dr. Clare: "If you are doing something wrong, instead of embarrassing you in front of others, what can therapists or teachers do?"

Monique (age 11): "They could pull me aside and tell me to get better so I can join class again and do the right thing."

Carolyn (age 12): "If we are in a group, they can pull me aside and work with me to fix my problem and do something right the next time."

John: "Let it go once. But if it happens again, talk to them. Go to a separate room."

Dr. Clare: "How can a therapist or teacher help you if another child is very angry and is yelling and throwing things?"

Lauren: "They can help me get out of the way so I don't get hurt. They can make me feel confident to come back to class."

Sam (age 12): "Stop the other kid and calm him down. Move me or let me move myself."

Monique: "They can keep me safe. They can help the kid calm down and come back to class so then I wouldn't be scared."

MAINTAIN A POSITIVE RELATIONSHIP

With an authoritarian approach, an adult makes a demand and children are expected to respond or acquiesce; this often creates a win-lose dynamic. This approach is appropriate if children's safety is at risk (e.g., if a child is running into a street). For other times, however, it is better is to maintain a positive, collaborative approach. You create a win-win dynamic by guiding the interaction to prevent power struggles or, if needed, guiding the interaction to a resolution that is good for you and the children.

Curtin, C.
Strategies for Collaborating With Children: Creating Partnerships in Occupational Therapy and Research (pp. 253-274).
© 2017 SLACK Incorporated.

A power struggle is a situation in which one makes a request or a demand of the other person and the other person refuses to engage or comply. The refusal can be either verbal (e.g., saying, "No, I won't") or shown through behavior (e.g., ignoring the request). A power struggle can also develop when there is a difference in opinion or beliefs, and each side becomes entrenched in their position (e.g., saying, "I am not going to do that because it is not fair"). The more skilled you are at avoiding these struggles, the more enjoyable your time together will be.

Eliminate Power Struggles

When you and children become embroiled in a power struggle, everyone has the desire to win. It is not uncommon to find yourself trying to win by becoming authoritarian and demanding that children obey. You may give this message by raising your voice in a stern manner, hovering over children, and making threats. You may even say the exact words your parents said to try to make you obey. However, it is detrimental if your first and only way of responding to a struggle is an authoritarian approach. This approach can be harmful because people (including children) usually do not like to be told what to do and tend to respond by rebelling. In addition, if you are rigid and controlling, it limits your options because you are more focused on winning than thinking of alternatives. The more ultimatums you use, the more likely you are to get in a power struggle.

Thus, a demand in an authoritarian manner often leads to confrontation, and in my experience adults often do not win in confrontations with children. Ironically, you will have more control of most situations if you use a variety of nonauthoritarian approaches. Thus, when you work with children you need to monitor how you present requests or demands and how you respond to the children. Use more guidance than ordering them around.

Promote Mutual Understanding

Children might be thinking:
I want….
You noticed how I feel.
You're not yelling or screaming at me.
I'm glad you asked.
You listened to me.
You are right; I am worried/upset.
You're trying to help me get what I want.
You're comforting me.
You care about me.

You can help develop an understanding of each other's perspectives in a variety of ways. When you respond to children's actions with empathy, you give the message that you are trying to understand. Second, checking with the children regarding the reason for their actions allows you

to learn about what they are thinking and feeling. It gives them an opportunity to tell you what they want. Third, letting them know you heard the underlying message of their actions is reassuring to them. Finally, giving them information and sharing your point of view gives them a chance to change their thinking. When the focus is on listening to each other's perspectives, it is easier to work together to create change and avoid getting involved in a struggle.

Respond to Children's Actions With Empathy

The quickest way to defuse a power struggle is to respond to children with empathy. Using this approach changes the mentality that you and the children are on different sides and only one person can win. Using empathy gives children the message that you are joining them by considering what they may be feeling or experiencing and by attempting to understand (Figure 13-1).

If there is not a safety issue, try to make this approach your default one—the response you use without even thinking. When you see an unwanted/undesirable action, take the children's perspective and think about why they are acting that way. Are they upset with a peer? Are they frustrated? Keep in mind that they may be tired or feeling sick. When nonverbal children are unusually cranky or having frequent meltdowns, it is often a sign that they are getting sick and do not feel well. If appropriate, make an empathetic statement about the possible cause. Respond to unwanted actions with a soft and caring tone of voice. You also can say, "I'm concerned/worried…." State what the children might be feeling and suggest options for calming or resolving the situation. Let them know you want them to feel better. Also, by considering their feelings there may be times when it is wise to respect their wishes for you to back off.

Fabulous Five: Respond to Actions With Empathy

- **Attribute an action to being tired, feeling sick, or having a bad day.**

One morning when Tracy, who was nonverbal, came into the specialized preschool classroom, she dropped to the floor and started crying.

"That's unusual," one staff member said, and we all agreed. As the day went on, she frequently pulled on her ear and cried with every transition.

"I don't think you feel good. I think you might be sick," I said in a caring tone of voice as she rolled on the floor. "Let me find something you like." I brought over her favorite toy to comfort her. After she played with it for a few minutes, she went to her center.

The teacher called her mother, who picked her up and took her to the doctor. She was diagnosed with an ear infection.

- **Respond to unwanted actions with a soft, caring voice.**

The preschool class danced to the music and froze when it stopped, assuming the body position shown on the card. Children were tightly packed in one area and kept bumping into Robert. He reacted by swinging his arm and knocking over one child.

"Robert hit me," the child cried.

Because I had previously seen that he was sensitive to touch, I said to him in a soft, caring voice, "I see the kids are bumping into you, and I know that upsets you." He nodded. I continued, "But you can't hit; that hurts them. Let's go talk to your teacher and see if everyone can spread out more when they are dancing." He followed me and listened.

Next, I helped him talk to the child he hit. From then on, the teacher made sure the other children gave Robert more space during that activity.

- **Make an empathetic remark about why they may be upset.**

"Five more minutes," the preschool teacher yelled to her class on the playground. When she rang the bell, 3-year-old Michael continued riding the tricycle that he had just mastered that week. When I put my hands on the handlebars to stop the bike, he began crying.

"You're sad you have to stop. You love riding this bike. It's time to go in and have a snack."

He reluctantly got off the bike and went to the teacher.

- **Label feelings and suggest something calming.**

When it was time to change centers, 3-year-old Lane dropped to the floor and started crying.

"It makes you sad to leave the water table," I said. "Let's find something you like in blocks. I know there's a train. You like trains." He took my hand and followed.

- **Respect their wishes.**

During free play, 4-year-old Tyler played with interlocking cubes. I sat down next to him and began making a chain with cubes. He forcefully grabbed the chain from my hands and started taking the cubes off.

Because he was nonverbal, I thought about what he was trying to tell me. "Oh, you want to play with these by yourself," I said. "Okay." I pushed all the cubes on the floor toward him. "I'll just watch you."

He continued connecting the cubes by himself.

Gain an Understanding of Children's Explanations for Their Actions

When you are trying to make sense of the meaning of children's actions, you have to examine the situation for cues and make your best guess. You can say, "I see you

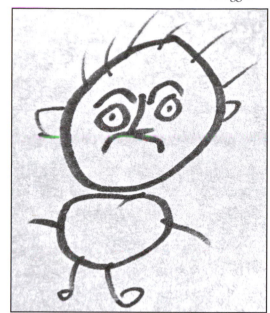

Figure 13-1. Make responding with empathy your first approach.

[state the action seen]" and ask what the children want. An additional way is to state one possible emotion conveyed by the observed action. For instance, you may ask, "Are you [state feeling]?" They can agree or disagree. Another way is to say, "I wonder if you are feeling [state feeling] because [state possible cause]." If children do not want to respond, they will at least know you are trying to understand. If you are wrong, they may say, "No, I am…."

To discover their own explanations for their actions, just ask. Be sure to also explore reasons for not wanting to do something. Also, check if something upsetting happened prior to their current actions. Always try to acknowledge their perspective and feelings and address their concerns.

Fabulous Five: Gain an Understanding of Children's Explanations for Their Actions

- **State the action you observe and ask what the children want.**

Four-year-old Bonnie ran her fingers through the bin of crayons while the other children colored. Then she grunted, shoved the container across the table, and started to leave.

"Bonnie, I see you looking mad that you didn't find what you want," I said. "What you are looking for? Come back and let me know."

She stomped to the table and said, "I want a blue crayon."

"I'll find one for you. I'm glad you told me. When you use words and say what you want, it's easier for me to help you."

- Use the phrase, "I wonder if you are feeling [state feeling] because [state possible cause]."

"What do you want me to bring next week?" I asked 7-year-old Mark.

"Nothing," he muttered, staring at the Silly Putty.

"I wonder if you're disappointed because you didn't get to play with the putty."

He nodded.

"I'm sorry we ran out of time. Do you want me to bring the putty back or the magnet game?"

"The putty." A minute later, Mark said, "I'm not mad anymore."

"How come?"

"Because we talked about it."

- State one possible feeling conveyed by their actions.

Six-year-old Robbie cupped his hands around the lettered dice, shook, and let the dice spill onto the table. "I see the word 'go,'" he said, and just as he reached for them again, Brooke snatched the dice. Robbie grimaced, folded his arms, and started bouncing in his chair. Then he dashed out of the room into the hallway and curled up on the floor in an open closet.

"Robbie, are you upset because Brooke took your dice?"

He nodded. "I'm upset I didn't get to finish."

"So you are telling me you just want a chance to roll the dice once more?" He nodded again. "Okay, let's do that." He returned to the room. After the other children left, I said to Robbie, "It would really help if you would use your words when you're upset. I can't read your mind. If you just run out of the room, I don't know what you are upset about. But if you use words, then I can help you."

- Discover children's explanations for their actions.

Five-year-old Troy snorted 10 times while he fiddled with the brown crayon.

"How come you're making that noise?" I asked in a curious tone of voice.

"It clears my mind."

I smiled and said, "Well, now that your mind is clear, it is time to start coloring."

- Explore why children do not want to do something.

"Have you ever played Hangman?" the occupational therapy student asked.

"No, and I don't like it," 8-year-old Collin said.

"How do you know you don't like it if you have never tried?"

"I tried once."

"Let's just give this game a try. Play one time."

"N. O. No."

"Just play one game. If you don't like it, then you can stop," the occupational therapy student said.

"Okay," Collin said. For a few seconds he sat and stared at the paper.

"Do you want me to give you a word?" I asked.

"Nope."

"I'm wondering why you don't like this game," I said.

"It's boring because you have to tell letters. It's spelling, and I'm not good at spelling."

"So it's frustrating for you when you don't know how to spell the word," I said. Collin nodded. "I have an idea. You and I can be partners. We'll do this together. That way you don't have to worry about spelling." Collin agreed and was pleased when he picked a word that stumped the occupational therapy student.

Clarify Children's Desires

The more specific and clear children are in their messages, the more you will understand them. If they are vague, for instance whining or grunting, ask them to tell you what they want. Another way to clarify is to ask them to use words when their actions indicate a message. You also may directly ask, "What are you trying to tell me?" Encourage them to say their thoughts and provide details. For children who are nonverbal, ask them to show, point, or look with their eyes at what they want. Provide a communication device, if needed, to express their wants and needs.

Fabulous Five: Identify What They Want or Are Trying to Say

- **Say to younger children, "Tell me what you want."**

Three-year-old Peggy pointed to the cupboard, jumped up and down, and grunted.

"Tell me what you want," I said.

"The blocks," she whispered.

"Okay. Here they are. When you tell me what you want, it's easier for me to help you."

- **Ask children to use words when their actions seem to indicate a message.**

Holding a small blue ball over 5-year-old Jason's head, I said, "This ball has magic dust, and it makes you into an animal so you can do an animal walk. What animal do you want to be?"

Jason just stared at the floor with his arms folded.

"Do you want to be a bear?"

He did not move.

"Jason, I can't read your mind. Tell me in words what's bothering you."

"I don't want to write today," he grumbled.

"I am glad you told me what you were worried about. You don't have to do any writing. Are you ready to have some fun?"

"Yeah," Jason said as he looked up at me.

After he roamed the room as a majestic lion and rambled as a crab, I said, "I'm glad you talked to me. When you were just staring, I didn't know what you were thinking. How come you didn't want to write?"

"It's boring. I've been writing all morning."

- **Ask, "What are you trying to tell me?"**

An occupational therapy student brought in a recipe for an apple snack. "I brought this for you to copy so you can start your own cookbook."

"My brother makes waffles," Joe said.

"Maybe you can make this recipe for him," she replied.

"He doesn't need recipes. I don't need recipes." Joe stared at the paper.

I suggested, "Maybe Joe doesn't want to do the cookbook."

"No," Joe said in a way that hinted I was wrong.

"What are you trying to tell us?" I asked.

"We don't like apples."

"Do you like pears?" the occupational therapy student replied. "We can change this to pears."

"Yeah."

"Do you still want to make this recipe?"

"Yeah, I do."

- **Encourage the children to say their thoughts instead of just saying no.**

"It's time to write your sentence."

"No."

"Oh, are you still drawing?"

"Yes."

"Instead of saying 'no,' just tell me that you need more time to draw."

- **Have children show, point, or look with their eyes to what they want.**

When the preschool class went to the pumpkin patch, 3-year-old Tristan, who was nonverbal, needed assistance walking.

First the class went to a maze made out of hay bales. "Point to where you want to go and I'll help you get there," I said. Using his index finger, he directed me. Then the class went to pick pumpkins. We walked around and around. Tristan kept shaking his head. Finally, we came across a large group of pumpkins. He pointed his finger at the largest one and smiled.

I laughed and said, "Of course, you want the biggest one."

Check if There Is a Mismatch

As you spend time with children, continue to observe their nonverbal language. Learn what signs they use to show their feelings. They may be certain looks or sounds.

Watching for these cues helps you sense their feelings and be empathetic. When you see their feelings expressed nonverbally, ask them what they are thinking or feeling. Check if you see a mismatch between any of their words, facial expressions, body language, or actions. This gives them a chance to talk and clarify how they feel. Telling children you are worried or concerned about them also lets them know you care.

Fabulous Five: Watch for Concerns Expressed Nonverbally

- **Say, "You look [state feeling]."**

In his class on Monday morning, 4-year-old Brady pushed all papers, markers, and scissors to the other side of the table. He puckered his lips and lowered his blond eyebrows.

"You look upset," I said.

"I'm not upset. I'm sad. I pinched myself. You know how come?"

"How come?"

"The seat belt did it. And I didn't get to kiss my mom goodbye."

"Oh. It sounds like you've had a rough start to your day."

"Yeah," he replied, slowly reaching for his paper.

- **Inquire, "What's wrong?"**

"You don't look like yourself. What's wrong?"

"Shiloh's not happy with me," the first grader said.

"What happened?"

"I don't know."

"It's upsetting if someone is mad at you and you don't know the reason why. It might help if you go and talk with her."

- **Tell children you are worried or concerned about them, then ask how they are feeling.**

Seven-year-old Jane dragged herself down the stairs and pouted as she walked into the room. She started the activity half-heartedly, but then began forcefully flinging pieces in the air.

"I'm concerned about you," I said. "Have you had a hard morning?"

"No."

"How was your weekend?" She stared at the floor. "Is it just the Monday blues?" She just fiddled and grunted in response. "Jane, you are not yourself today. You seem grumpy. Is something wrong?"

"My stomach hurts. I threw up last night."

- **Observe and explore mismatches between voice, facial expressions, actions, or previous ways of acting.**

As 8-year-old Kevin tried to write his name on his homemade valentine, he wrote his letters above the line.

"Grrr," he said as he erased. He tried again. This time he wrote *Valentinee's*. He sighed abruptly. "That's not right." He erased again.

"Kevin, you seem more frustrated than usual. Are you okay?" He opened his mouth and showed his broken front tooth. "What happened?"

"I hit it on the table at home."

"Are you going to the dentist?"

"No, we don't have enough money."

"I'm sorry that happened to you."

- **Ask, "What are you thinking/feeling?"**

Ken sat quietly at the table with a scowl on his face.

"What are you thinking?" I asked the second grader.

"At recess, Mike was swinging his coat around and hit someone. He was right in front of me. Sometimes he punches people too."

"How did that make you feel?"

"Makes me feel bad."

"Was it scary for you or more upsetting?"

"Both. He's smaller than me," he said, as if trying to convince himself.

"If he upsets you, what can you do?"

"I moved to the end of the line."

"That's a good idea. It's good you are talking about it."

Let Children Know You Heard What They Think and Want

Some children will keep repeating themselves and not listen to you until they know you heard what they think and want. It is important, therefore, to listen carefully and acknowledge what they desire. The act of listening also shows you care about them. Then you may want to take action that shows you will honor their request at a later time. You may want to agree with them or respond with, "You are right," and then provide your explanation or request. Children respond better when you say, "Yes, you can, after…" versus "No, you have to…." You can also make a connection between their conversation and your request.

Fabulous Five: Let Children Know You Heard What They Wanted

- **Identify the children's desires.**

"This is my ball," 6-year-old Skip said.

"Remember when we started I said you could play with my toys but you have to give them back," I replied.

"No, this is mine and I'm keeping it."

"You want to have your own ball. I think you really like my ball a lot, and now that I know that, I can bring it back."

"Skip has one in his backpack," his paraprofessional said.

"Oh, let's get your ball so you can put it in your pocket." He hesitated, then dropped my yellow ball on the table.

- **Take action showing that you will honor the children's requests at a later time.**

At the end of the session, I packed my supplies into my canvas bag. Four-year-old Todd rushed over to me holding his new Scooby-Doo game. "I want to play this," he said, thrusting the box at me.

"Oh dear. It's time for me to go. We don't have time to play this."

"But I wanta play this," he demanded, and started running in circles.

I reached for the box. "Let's look at the directions so we will know how to play it the next time I come." We sat on the couch and examined the board and all the playing pieces. "This will be fun for us to play next time," I said, standing to leave. He walked me to the door and waved goodbye.

When I returned the next week, I told him we could play his new game.

- **Agree with children and restate their concerns or desires, followed by your request.**

At the beginning of the newspaper group, 7-year-old Monty spotted a monkey wind-up toy on my desk. He pointed and said, "I want to play with that."

I nodded and said, "Sure, you can play with that after you do one page for the newspaper. I will make sure we save time to play at the end of group."

He reached for paper and began sketching his favorite sports car.

- **Acknowledge what children are saying, then connect the request to the children's conversations.**

Bud pointed to a water game on my desk and said, "I want to do the crab game."

"Okay, you will get to do that game after we're finished with our group's game," I said. Then I pointed to the tongs the other children were using. "These tongs are like pinchers. Be like a pincher crab and pick up these fish erasers."

- **Respond with, "You are right."**

The group had finished their newspaper, entitled *Occupational Therapy Tribune*.

"Colleen, just sign your first name on the cover of the paper."

She wrote her first name and started to write her last name.

"Only your first name."

"But we are always supposed to write our first and last name."

"Yes. You're right, usually you do, but for this paper we are only using first names."

Explain or Reframe

> **Children might be thinking:**
> *Thanks for telling me.*
> *I'm glad you're not saying no.*

When you give children an explanation or help them view a situation differently, you are showing respect. Instead of just telling them what to do, talk with them. Children appreciate it when you take the time to do so.

Promote Children's Understanding

The more children understand a situation, the less anxious or worried they may feel. It also may prevent them from getting angry if they understand why they are not going to get what they want. In addition, it is easier to follow rules if the reasoning behind them makes sense. Clarifying how their current actions might affect them also can be beneficial. Sometimes telling them the easiest way you have found will help them understand better. When providing an explanation, keep it short and match the children's level of understanding. Do not go overboard with lengthy explanations.

Fabulous Five: Help Children Understand the Situation or Your Reasoning

- **Assist children in understanding the situation.**

In his kindergarten class, George matched the letters to corresponding pictures. Then he looked at the picture of an egg and searched for the letter "e," but it was not in the box. George yelled, "No, no, no," flapped his hands, and jumped up and down.

"It's not there," I said. "I know it's frustrating."

"No, no, no. It should be there."

"It's like when you lose a toy at home; it's just missing."

George sat back in his chair.

- **Explain the reasoning behind the rules.**

"I like guns," 3-year-old Terry said as he pretended to shoot a classmate.

"We don't talk about guns at school because guns hurt people," I replied. "We want people to be safe and not get hurt."

"Yeah, you can die from them."

- **Talk about the necessity of knowing the directions.**

Six-year-old Brady walked over to the blue paper in the shape of a lake dotted with 10 cards, which had attached paperclips. He lifted the fishing pole with a magnet on the end and swung it in circles, missing all the fish.

"Please stop a minute. Let me tell you how to play this game," I said.

He dropped the pole, ran to the table, and whimpered as he covered his head with his arms.

"You have to know the directions to play the game and have fun."

"I don't want to fish."

"But you haven't tried the game yet. It's really fun."

"But it's too hard."

"Just try it one time."

He held the pole, and I directed the string. Two seconds later, he hooked a card. The speech-language pathologist read the card, and Brady looked pleased to give an answer.

"I wonder which card you will get next," I said as he resumed fishing.

- **Explain to children what might happen if they continue what they are doing.**

Three-year-old Tessa tipped the chair back, balancing it precariously on two legs. "Please keep the chair on the ground. You might fall back and hit your head," I said in a caring tone of voice. She looked up at me and then plopped the chair back on the floor.

- **Point out to children that you are demonstrating the easy way.**

"Put the hole puncher on the table, slide the paper in, and push. If you do it this way, it will be easier for you."

Five-year-old Harry lifted the punch in the air and struggled with the paper.

"The hole puncher works better if it is on the table," I hinted. "Try it that way and see if you think it is easier."

He placed the star punch on the table, inserted the paper, and punched with ease.

Change Children's Mindsets

Children often respond when you reframe the situation. You can do so by offering a different perspective than what they might be thinking. If they think they did something wrong, they may worry about getting in trouble. Some may even try to run away to avoid any consequences. Instead of thinking you need to punish them, use a caring approach. You can let them know that you are not mad and they are not in trouble. This can eliminate the worry. Then they are more likely to participate in a conversation on what else they could do to make things better.

Some children will get upset just by thinking that you are going to say no to their request. You can address this by clearly stating, "I'm not saying no." For others you can mention how you enjoy being with them as a way to get them to change what they are doing. Another tactic for children who are having difficulty at the end of the session or day is to point out how well they have been doing. Tell them they have had a good day and encourage them to continue to do so. What you also are implying is that you believe they have the ability to regroup.

Fabulous Five: Respond in a Way That Changes Children's Thinking

- **Tell the children you are not mad.**

Sally Jo sauntered into the room with slumping shoulders and a stiff smile. She snatched a piece of paper, printed four letters, and then scribbled circles, creating a spiral. Her pencil slipped off the paper, and she marked the table.

"Please stop," I said to the second grader. "I know it's Monday, and it looks like you're having a hard day. I'm not mad. I'm concerned. What's wrong?"

"My dad yelled at me this morning."

- **Let children know they are not in trouble.**

Five-year-old Jordan walked into the therapy room, looking agitated. "Let's play dominoes," the group decided, and they started taking turns lining the tiles in an S-shaped pattern.

When Gus took Jordan's turn, Jordan jumped out of his chair and yelled, "That's not fair. It's my turn," and bolted out the door.

I asked another therapist to watch the group and followed him to the next room. "It's all right. You're not in trouble. I'm just concerned that you're feeling so upset. Let's go back and figure out a way to make things better."

Keeping his chin on his chest, he followed me back.

- **Tell children you are not saying no.**

"I want to play with that musical top," 4-year-old Dema demanded.

"Wait a minute," I said, searching through the cupboard.

"But I want to play with the top," she insisted in a louder voice.

"I'm not saying no. I'm saying wait. Give me a chance to find it."

- **Tell children you enjoy being with them.**

"Work makes me fall asleep. I'm way, way too tired here. Can I take a 10-hour nap?" 6-year-old Warren asked.

"I like you, Warren. I enjoy being with you. Let's move around to help you stay awake, and then we will play our game. Be sure to go to bed early tonight."

- **Talk about having a good day.**

In the last 5 minutes of class, 7-year-old Jeffery threw the small board on the floor. "You've had a really good day. You only have a few minutes left before school is over. Just put the board away."

He stooped over and picked up the board.

Make Alternatives or Requests Seem Beneficial or Appealing

> **Children might be thinking:**
> *That looks like fun.*
> *I want to do that.*

You can get younger children to shift from their current actions by dangling an enticing object in front of them or demonstrating a fun activity. Children tend to respond if you make your request sound appealing and beneficial. Avoid a power struggle by capturing their attention, piquing their interest, and creating a desire to change.

Use Appealing Objects or Activities

One way to get children to change what they are doing is to entice them with a novel or favorite object. Often this gains their attention and enables you to guide them to something else. You can also refer to something they like as a way to motivate them to change. Another way to get them to do what you want is to make a request in the form of a compliment. Ask disruptive children to be helpers. Often they feel flattered and will do what you ask.

Fabulous Five: Make Your Requests Appealing

- **Capture interest with a novel or intriguing toy or activity.**

When the room became too noisy, 3-year-old Damian started crying and hitting his head with his palm. I quieted the other children, but he continued. I went and pulled a new toy out of the cupboard. Holding it in front of him, I pushed the button, which activated a spinner inside the toy.

Intrigued, he stopped crying and reached for the toy.

- **Say, "Look…" with animation.**

After the preschool teacher in the specialized class finished reading the book, she handed each child a picture symbol of where to go for centers. I was in the art center and worked with the children as they rotated from one center to another. When the teacher handed 4-year-old Trent's picture symbol for art, he dropped to the floor and did not budge.

I brought over a plastic claw in the shape of an alligator. "Trent, look," I said as I pulled the handle and the alligator's mouth opened.

He jumped up and immediately followed me to the art center. I handed him the alligator. He pulled the handle and scooped up beanbags.

"That alligator is hungry," I said. "Feed him some more."

Trent smiled and continued.

- **Say, "This is something you like."**

Four-year-old Hansen rolled back and forth on the rug. "Hansen, come sit on your chair," I said, pointing to a cube chair. "Your teacher is going to read a book. This is something you like. I know you like the stories." He stopped and moved into the chair.

- **Make requests in the form of compliments.**

After 7-year-old Scott made five animal figurines with clay, the table needed to be washed. I said, "You're so strong, I need your help. Here's a wet paper towel. Use your big muscles and rub the clay off the table."

Smiling, Scott grabbed the towel and began scrubbing the table.

- **Put children who are disruptive into helper roles.**

When everyone was sitting on the floor, 6-year-old Juan tickled the girl in front of him. She moved away. He then started to poke another boy with his index finger.

"Juan, come here. I need your help. Hold this," I said, handing him a poster board. He stood still and held the board up high as I read the directions off the poster.

"Thank you. I appreciate it."

"Sure. I'm a good helper."

Highlight the Benefits of Changing Current Actions

One way to get children to shift what they are doing is to emphasize the benefits of changing. It helps to present your request in a way that suggests they will be doing themselves a favor if they comply. For instance, you can tell children to move their chairs so they will be more comfortable, or say, "Let me show you how to hold the scissors so they will work better for you." Expressing concern about what they might miss can gain their attention. You also can assist them in learning by pointing out the positive results of a change. When they hear compassion in your voice and realize you are considering their best interests, they often listen.

Fabulous Five: Talk About the Benefits of Changing What They Are Doing

- **Emphasize the benefits of doing an activity or action.**

In the kindergarten class, Carla looked at the booklet and said, "I'm too tired to draw." She folded her arms on the table and rested her head on them.

"I know it's hard to be at school on Monday. How come you're so tired?" I asked.

"I didn't sleep much."

"Okay, take a minute break, rest, and then start drawing." I turned and watched a child who was drawing.

After a couple of minutes, I looked over at Carla. Knowing that she liked to please her father, I said, "You did really well on the first page of your book. I'm sure your dad will really like this. Do this second page so you can take it home."

She slowly lifted her head off the table and picked up a pencil.

- **Present a direction in a way that implies the children will be doing themselves a favor if they comply.**

Six-year-old Beverly perched on the edge of her seat a foot away from her desk and stretched to reach her work.

"Bev, move your chair in closer so you will be more comfy," I said. She nodded and scooted the chair next to the desk.

- **Tell children you are concerned they are going to miss the directions.**

Eight-year-old Anna May rolled the pencil between her two index fingers and giggled with her classmate.

"I'm concerned that you two are not going to know what to do. Then you will be lost," the occupational therapy student said. When their eyes shifted to him, he stated the directions for the writing project.

- **Highlight the positive results of a change.**

Seven-year-old Grant talked in a gruff, unintelligible, raspy voice. When he switched to his usual voice, I said, "I like when you talk like that because then I can understand you. What you have to say is important to me."

- **Say, "I just want this to turn out good for you. Try it this way."**

Eight-year-old Paula shoved all the pages of her Halloween joke book into the stapler. "Wait," I said. She grumbled at having to stop. "I just want this to turn out good for you. If you staple all of these pages together, you will not be able to open your book. Try it this way," I said, and demonstrated stapling the corners of the pages.

Use a Different Approach

> **Children might be thinking:**
> *Maybe you're not so bad.*
> *You're funny.*
> *Hey, that's fun.*

When you maintain the attitude that it is better to enjoy being with children more than controlling them, you can be open to using a variety of approaches. Of course, you will always take action to ensure their safety. Many times, you can get children to change what they are doing by using play, surprise, or challenges (Figure 13-2). It also works to make them into teachers or shifting to a joint venture.

Use a Play Frame

Children tend to respond better when you use a playful versus a serious approach. Play is associated with fun, not anger. Using this approach can help children shift from thinking, *I don't want to do this* to *I want to have fun*. This can be effective because if they think you are playing, it is

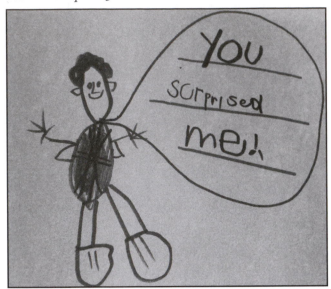

Figure 13-2. Use an unusual approach to avoid a power struggle.

easier to listen to you. They also will not feel like you are giving orders and telling them what to do. Often you can incorporate toy figurines or pretend play as a way to start or stop an action. As they are playing, you also can state your expectation and weave it in as part of the activity. Surprising them with a playful twist or being humorous also works.

Fabulous Five: Use a Play Frame

- **Use toy figurines.**

"I don't want to fish," 5-year-old Felipe said as the other children waited.

The occupational therapy student pulled a tiger-striped cat figurine out of the bag, placed it on the table, and said, "Meow. Get me a fish for lunch. It's fun to fish. I wonder what kind of fish you'll get."

Felipe looked at her and said, "I'm going to get a fish for the cat." His magnetic fishing rod swayed from the left to right and finally snagged a blue fish. "I got one."

"What letter is on it?"

"It's an 'A.'"

"Okay, everyone write the letter 'A.'" At the end of the session, she said, "Did you like this game?"

"Yeah, I like the game," Felipe replied. "I want to play it forever."

- **Use pretend play to stop an action.**

Three-year-old Dylan held a plastic airplane and pretended to fly it. He made zooming noises that became progressively louder. The teacher asked him multiple times to be quieter, but he continued to be loud.

I joined him in the center and began building with blocks. "I'm making an airport," I told him. "Now I am the traffic controller. I tell the planes where to fly and

land. I'm on the radio. Hello, Pilot Dylan, where are you flying to, New York or California?"

"Arizona," he yelled.

"Oh, I have my headphones on. That's too loud. Talk softer please," I said in almost a whisper. I gestured from the top of my head to my ears to indicate my pretend headphones.

In response, he lowered his voice as he flew the plane.

- **Incorporate limits into children's play.**

Five-year-old Jim threw putty on the table to make a pretend pizza. To let him know that I wanted him to keep the putty on the table, I said, "Keep the pizza on the table. We don't want it to drop on the floor and get dirty. Then we couldn't eat it."

- **Start with the children's actions and add a playful twist.**

I heard crying outside my therapy room in the pediatric oncology clinic. Three-year-old Joey was stomping his feet and waving his hands as his distressed mother tried to soothe him. She handed him toys. He took each toy and slammed it to the ground. With each thud, the wailing intensified.

I stepped into the hallway to help, and a toy car whizzed by me. I retrieved it and handed it back to him. When he tried to fling it to the ground again, I caught the toy midair and tossed it back, creating a game of catch. He flashed a look of surprise, captured the car against his chest, and stopped crying. We continued the game. His mother looked at me with gratitude.

- **Use humor to defuse tense situations.**

Paul's aggression and tendency to be oppositional landed him in the children's psychiatric unit. On his first day, the 10 year old strutted into my therapy room as if he were in charge. He immediately began repeating everything I said and looked at me as if challenging me to a fight. The three other boys stopped what they were doing.

I smiled and said, "Dr. Clare is beautiful," hoping that he would repeat it.

"Dr. Clare is…UGLY," Paul responded.

The other children held their breath, waiting for my reaction.

"Paul is nice," I said lightheartedly.

"Thank you!" he replied, and we all laughed.

Incorporate an Out-of-the-Ordinary Approach

An out-of-the-ordinary approach tends to catch children by surprise. Because this is not a typical response by adults, they often will stop what they are doing. Using a toy or a prop to make a point gains and keeps their attention. Incorporating an unexpected reaction or making an intriguing offer captures their interest. With older children, you can demonstrate and exaggerate the children's actions or expressions. When they see how silly you look, they tend to smile or laugh.

Fabulous Five: Incorporate an Out-of-the-Ordinary Approach

- **Use props to make a point regarding limit setting.**

Nine-year-old Shay shuffled through papers on my desk and started reading one page.

"Are you supposed to be at my desk?" I asked.

"No."

"Come sit at the table." She moseyed over and slid into her chair. I rolled a ball painted like an eyeball toward her, smiled, and said, "Just remember I have my eye on you."

- **Use a prop to indicate stop.**

Seven-year-old Dan reached for his game piece when it was not his turn.

"Hey, no fair," Alan said, annoyed.

Two minutes later, Dan rocked in his chair and bumped the board. "Dan, please be careful," I said, and everyone stopped to listen.

The next time the group met, I brought a new game and a 2-inch stop sign glued to a Popsicle stick. Within three minutes, Dan started shaking the table. While the others kept playing, I showed Dan the stop sign, and he settled back in his chair.

- **Use an unexpected action.**

I walked down the hall of the children's psychiatric unit until 9-year-old Ned raised his arms like a scarecrow and scooted sideways to block my passage. I gently clasped his hands and started to dance with him, twirling him around as if we were doing the waltz. When I let him go, he was no longer in my way. I smiled, thanked him for the dance, and continued. He looked dazed when I glanced back at him.

- **Make intriguing requests or offers.**

I wanted to see if 4-year-old Lenny had mastered three prewriting shapes. I brought a clipboard over and said, "Lenny, I just need you to draw a cross, a circle, and a square. It will not take long."

"No," he said emphatically, crossing his arms.

I waited 20 minutes and tried once more. Again he refused. Then I looked over at the center that was a pretend coffee shop and said, "If you draw, I'll buy you a cup of coffee."

"Okay!" he replied with a smile. He quickly copied the shapes.

I went to the center and ordered coffee. "Do you want cream and sugar?" Lenny nodded. I pretended to give the worker money, and she gave me an empty cup. "Here you go, Lenny. Be careful, it might be hot. Enjoy your coffee."

- **Demonstrate and exaggerate the action you want children to stop.**

The group moved different body parts to music. Carrie sat without moving a muscle. "Give it a try, Carrie," I said, but she still did not move. "Come over here to the side so we can talk." She followed me to the edge of the room. "How come you're not doing anything?"

"I don't know how to do it."

"I know it's hard for you, but you can't just sit there."

"But I like to just sit there."

"Carrie, it won't help you to just sit. If it's hard, I will help you, but you have to try too." I crossed my arms, wrinkled my face, and stuck out my lips into an exaggerated pout. "You can't just sit there looking crabby." She giggled at my face. We returned to the group, and she tried the next activity.

Create a Challenge

Offering a challenge is one way to redirect children's behavior. If they are doing something they should not do, say to them, "See if you can [state the challenge]." They will often try because they perceive it as a dare or a test of their abilities. The key factor is picking the right challenge. Make the challenge to be whatever you want them to do. You can ask them to do something that sounds fun, do more positive actions they have already shown, or do the opposite of their current behavior. Another strategy that tends to be appealing to them is to suggest they try to be the best or compete against each other. A challenge will often help children shift to trying something different.

Fabulous Five: Create a Challenge

- **Challenge children to figure out a different way of acting.**

Nine-year-old Tim tapped his ruler like a drumroll, and the two other boys laughed. "Figure out a way to make it stop and be quiet," I challenged him.

He fingered his ruler and said, "I could put it in my desk."

"Sounds like a good idea."

- **Make a challenge that incorporates the opposite action.**

"Three, four, five," 8-year-old Matt counted as he hit the Koosh ball with a racket. Then he whacked the ball and laughed when it hit the ceiling light.

"See how many times you can hit it softly," I said.

He lightly tapped the ball, and it only bounced 6 inches.

- **Point to what children did right and challenge them to do more.**

"Everyone gets a board, a marker, and an eraser," the teacher said as she passed out the materials. Then she told a story and instructed the children to make "gentle rain" on their boards whenever the music played. Four-year-old Gregory started making dots as directed, but then switched to making lines.

I pointed to his raindrops and said, "These are just right. See if you can make more like these."

- **Offer a group challenge.**

The group of first and second graders had a tendency to stomp down the stairs, which disrupted the third-grade class. "Who can go down the stairs the quietest?" I challenged them. Immediately the children start tiptoeing down the stairs. "Wow, you're good," I said.

"I won," a first grader said.

"Everyone was good."

- **Make a fun challenge.**

Seven-year-old Dane stopped at his teacher's desk and spun the chair. "Teacher's chair," the teacher said. "Here's a chair for you." She slid his chair next to his hands. "Be like a truck driver and drive your chair to your desk."

"Zoom, zoom," he said as he maneuvered the chair to his desk.

Have Children Be Teachers or Change to a Joint Effort

When children start to engage in a power struggle, you can often circumvent an argument by making them into a teacher. This role gives them control and allows them to tell you what to do. Ask them to teach you the action or activity that initially you wanted them to do. Sometimes you can make a mistake on purpose and encourage them to correct you. Another way to move out of a struggle is to say that it will be a joint effort to complete the request. Often they will be agreeable if they see that you will help them. You also may want to compromise and meet them halfway. Acknowledge the children's perspective and be open to considering that not everything has to be done your way.

> ### Fabulous Five: Make Children Into Teachers or Change to a Joint Effort
>
> - **Make a mistake on purpose and ask children to teach you the correct way.**
>
> "Do you like clowns or butterflies better?" The 6 year old tapped the clown picture. "This is a following directions activity."

"I know what it is. It's a dot-to-dot page."

After the clown's face appeared, I said, "RJ, put your name on the picture."

He drew a circle. "Oh, you're going to write your name in the circle. He printed the "R" and stopped. I wrote "CC" on another paper and asked, "Is this right?"

"No, it's RJ."

"Could you fix it for me?"

"I'll show you," he said, and he finished his name.

- **Ask the children to instruct you as a way to change their problematic actions.**

When I walked in the first-grade classroom, the teacher pointed to a child sitting on the floor with his arms hugging his chest. "Vinnie is supposed to be listening to an audio book, and then he has to write his answers."

I went over to him and said, "Hi! How does this machine work?"

"I'll show you," a classmate offered.

"No, I'll show her," Vinnie insisted, bounding over to the audio player.

- **Put the children in a teacher's role.**

"It's time to go back to class."

"I don't wanta," 7-year-old Shari shrieked in her high-pitched voice.

"Shari, I need your help. Show me where your class is."

"Okay," she replied, and we left the library.

- **Shift to a joint effort.**

When Marcus dropped a half-inch metal ball on the floor, I said to the 6 year old, "Please pick up that ball so we don't lose it."

Marcus ignored my request. He curled his lips, fiddled with a blue magnet, and then dropped it.

"I know it's frustrating when that happens. Hey, I'll pick up this magnet. You pick up the ball."

He hesitated for 5 seconds, then recovered the ball.

- **Meet halfway.**

Sitting on an office chair, 8-year-old Reba rolled between the teachers' desks and opened five drawers.

"What are you looking for?" I asked.

She did not answer and rolled to another desk.

"Let me give you a ride," I said, pushing her to the table.

She pushed herself 1 foot away.

"What color do you want to use?" I said, holding up the watercolor tray. She pointed to blue, and I put the paint on the table.

She scooted the chair toward the table and started painting.

Weave Children's Actions or Words Into Your Request

When you go along with whatever children are saying or doing, there is less likelihood of resistance. It is similar to following the flow of a river. First you need to recognize what they are doing. Then make your request part of their current actions. Another option is to use their exact words in your request. You also can acknowledge any steps taken or discuss what they want. An additional strategy to avoid a power struggle is to describe their actions and tell them to do the same actions. For example, if they are wandering around the room, you can say, "I see you are looking out the window. Take a few minutes to look and then come join us."

Fabulous Five: Comment on What They Are Doing

- **Interpret the children's actions or behavior.**

Six-year-old LaToya used tongs to separate miniature animal figurines and put them into two buckets. When she finished, I said, "We have another fun activity," and put out my palm for her to give me the tongs. She slid her hand with the tongs under the table. "Are you trying to tell me you want to keep playing with the tongs?" She nodded. "Okay," I said, and reached for putty and small bunny erasers. "Make up a game using the tongs."

- **Describe the children's actions, tell them to do that action, then state what you want them to do.**

In class, the three preschoolers snapped tongue depressors to make dinosaur bones and glued them onto a picture of a T-Rex.

"Dane, please come join us and make some bones," I said. He crossed his arms and sat on the floor.

"Oh, I see you need a break. Sit and relax for a minute, then come over and make your own dinosaur. It's really fun," I said, then turned my focus back to the group. Four minutes later, he rose and meandered over to the table.

- **Acknowledge any action taken by children, then restate the direction.**

The kindergarten teacher told the children to color the flowers on the paper. Then they were to cut and glue them on a poster board. Traver strolled to the bin and picked purple scissors. I watched him as he wandered the room looking lost and then said, "I see you picked your scissors. That is one step. Have you colored your flower?"

"Not yet," he said.

"The paper with the flower on it is on the cupboard. That is your next step," I said, pointing him in the right direction.

- **Integrate the request as part of the children's current action.**

In the specialized program, 8-year-old Jack wandered around the room, pushing a cart loaded with books. As he passed by the group's table, the certified occupational therapy assistant put some used paper towels on the top shelf of his cart. "Please take these to the trash can." As he headed to the trash can, she said, "Thank you."

- **Use the children's words in the directions.**

"I'm going to use my hand claw," 5-year-old Hunter said as he curled his fingers into a bear claw.

"Use your hand claw to work the clothespin." I pointed to a brown container and animal-shaped mini-erasers. "Put the animals in the bear den."

Make Changes

Children might be thinking:
I'm overwhelmed.
You made it easier.

You can often avoid power struggles by being willing to make changes. You may want to adjust your expectations, change the environment, or remove whatever is the source of difficulty. It also can help to weave children's words or actions into your request. Another approach is to convert their actions into something positive.

Adjust What You Expect or Do

Be considerate and adjust what you expect or what you are doing. Keep in mind that everything does not have to go the way you want. Be flexible and shift from thinking about how to get your way to thinking about how to work together. Be sensitive to when children are not feeling well or are just having a bad day. You also can help children adjust by teaching them what is acceptable or giving them something more appropriate to do.

Fabulous Five: Adjust

- **Adjust your expectations if children are having a difficult time.**

The week 6-year-old Bradley heard that his foster family decided not to adopt him, I pulled out a selection of his favorite toys. I thought about how it would be best to use this session for comfort rather than challenging tasks. "I know it's been a hard week for you," I said with compassion. "Pick whatever toy you would enjoy."

He reached for the magnetic blocks and started to build a robot.

- **Simplify or modify the demand.**

"Krista is having a hard day. She has already been to the principal's office," her first-grade teacher said.

Krista joined my group in the class and colored her flower picture. When she was done, she left the table and looked at a bobbing figure. "Krista, come back and put the crayons away. Then we can do something else."

She put two crayons in the box, then popped out of her seat and again wandered around the room. I stuffed in six more, leaving four on the table. "There are just a few crayons left. Get them in the box."

She headed back and wiggled the crayons into the box.

- **Say only one step or action at a time.**

In music therapy, the fifth graders chose their instruments. Larry sat at the piano. He looked at a picture showing a hand with a pointed index finger and repeated, "One finger. One finger."

Harry blew the harmonica. Strumming a guitar, Gus rocked vigorously in the rocking chair. Sam shook a leather strap with bells five times. Then he flung the bells in the air, jumped up, and flapped his hands. "Hee-hee," he squealed.

"Sit down and don't throw the bells. Watch the teacher," a staff member yelled. Sam did not respond.

Knowing he did better following one-step directions, I said, "Sit on the chair, Sam." After he sat down, I handed him the bells and said, "Hold on to them." A few seconds later, I added, "Shake the bells."

"Quiet," announced the music therapist, and everyone stopped. "One, two three, start." Each child played his or her own melody, sounding like an orchestra tuning their instruments.

- **Change to acceptable phrases.**

Two boys taught 9-year-old Judson to say, "Son of a b****," knowing he would not understand the meaning of the curse words. They laughed every time he cursed.

Then Judson tried the phrase in class. His teacher smiled and responded, "Oh no, the phrase is sunny day. Say, 'Sunny day.'"

"Sunny day."

"It sure is. Wonderful day, isn't it?" He nodded.

- **Give children something else to do.**

As the teacher walked around the room getting the children to volunteer for classroom jobs, 8-year-old Rusty flicked his fingers on his cheek. Then he rocked his desk back and forth. With a grunt, he pushed over the desk, just missing Madelynn.

His teacher signed as she said, "Not safe." She lifted the desk and, realizing he was bored, handed him a tissue. He wrapped his hand around the tissue and wiped his desk like windshield wipers until it was his turn to pick a job.

Substitute or Remove Anything Problematic

If an action is a habit, it is unrealistic to think it is easy to change. Instead of telling children to quit doing what is

their usual way, think of what could be done to replace that action. For instance, if children are pushing others when they stand in line, telling them to tap the sides of their legs will keep their hands on themselves. Similarly, you can use an appealing object or activity to trade for or to replace an inappropriate one. If children are misusing an object or distracting others, subtly remove the object. In addition, avoid conversations that you know will lead to perseveration or unwanted topics.

Fabulous Five: Substitute or Remove Anything Problematic

- **Incorporate an action that prevents the action you want the children to stop.**

Seven-year-old Dale squeezed the purple gel ball with two hands. "Squeeze the ball with one hand," I said, but he ignored me. I handed him another stress ball and said, "Squeeze this one in your other hand and see which one is harder." He grasped the two balls and contemplated the difference.

- **Offer a trade.**

Seven-year-old Marisela waved the magnet over the metal clips and smiled as they connected to each other.

"I want a turn," her classmate said.

Marisela responded by attaching the magnet to the table leg to hide it.

Because I knew she liked to play with putty, I said, "I will trade you the putty for the magnet." She reluctantly ended the hiding game.

- **Replace an inappropriate object or action with an appropriate and appealing one.**

Four-year-old Frances stuck a fragile figurine in the purple putty. I quickly scooped up a solid plastic fox and said, "Here, this fox wants to hide in the putty." Frances wrapped his fingers around the fox and handed me the figurine.

- **Remove a problematic object.**

Seven-year-old Jodi pounded on the stapler as I gave the directions. The pounding drowned my voice. I slowly put my palm on the stapler, moved it out of her reach, and repeated the directions.

- **Avoid engaging in problematic conversation.**

"My baby ceiling fan is boring. When I move I'll have two ceiling fans in my home. One is upstairs and one is downstairs. Do you have any ceiling fans?"

I had heard that 6-year-old Cole often perseverated and would talk about fans for hours, so I responded, "No. So what is your favorite class?"

"Math."

Convert Actions or Conversations Into a Positive Frame

In situations in which you want children to change their actions, you can convert what they are doing into something positive. One way to do this is to define a different purpose for their actions. You also can interpret their actions and then say what you believe they may want or need. Even if you think they are purposely not following directions or participating, you can pretend that they have positive intentions. For example, state to the children that you think they are doing you a favor. Similarly, steer conversations about violence to a more neutral topic.

> ### *Fabulous Five: Convert Actions or Conversations Into a Positive Frame*
>
> - **Change the purpose of the children's actions.**
>
> Three-year-old Nadine lifted her cup and began pouring water on her plate. I went over to a potted plant and said, "Nadine, bring your cup here. This plant is thirsty. It needs water." She ran over and emptied the water into the dirt.
>
> - **Translate action into words regarding children's perceived need.**
>
> The three preschoolers sat in a circle drawing pictures with pastel markers. Peggy drew a pickle with two eyes and a smile and said, "That's you, Dr. Clare." Stefanie made one squiggle line, then stood and headed to the other side of the room.
>
> "Come back and join us, Stefanie," I said. "We miss you. I think you are telling me you need some help."
>
> She nodded and said, "I don't know what to draw." Then she returned to the group.
>
> - **Change talk or actions portraying violence into a positive frame.**
>
> Five-year-old Arthur connected the plastic parts into a shape that resembled a gun. "I'm gonna zap you."
>
> "That looks like a magic wand," I said. "Make me a queen or a princess."
>
> "You're a queen."
>
> - **Convert the action into a positive.**
>
> "Robin, feel the pumpkin," the speech-language pathologist said to the group of second graders. Not wanting to participate, Robin slid the pumpkin away from her in my direction.
>
> "Oh, you are showing me the pumpkin," I said. "Thanks for thinking about me." We passed it around the table.
>
> "Tap it," the speech-language therapist said.
>
> Again, Robin pushed the pumpkin to me. "Oh, you want me to tap it for you. Okay. You can just watch," I said, and then tapped it.
>
> - **Pretend the children are doing you a favor.**
>
> One morning, 5-year-old Ivy either balked or did the opposite of my every request. As I sat across from her, she fished for an alphabet letter and snagged the letter "v." She manipulated the two pink rulers, making an upside-down "v," and smirked at me.
>
> "Oh, you made the 'v' for me. Thanks," I said, then reversed the rulers. "And if we make the letter this way, it's for you."

Adjust Your Attention

One consideration in your interactions with children is to recognize the effect of your attention on the situation. There will be times where it is better to limit the amount of attention you give to their actions. Other times it is a better approach to divert their attention or change the focus away from problematic conversations or actions.

Limit Your Attention to Children's Actions

> **Children might be thinking:**
> *You saw me do something good.*
> *You're not watching me.*

Unless there is a concern about safety, make a conscious effort to give your attention to children who are doing well. You can do this by watching them and making comments about their positive actions. Likewise, ignore actions you want children to stop. Then watch to see if you are getting into a pattern of giving extra attention to the children who are getting in trouble. It is very easy to slip into this pattern without realizing it. Then they learn that the more trouble they stir up, the more adult attention they get. Some learn that if they cry or scream, adults will come running and they will get what they want regardless of the impact on others. You have to find a way to break this cycle. You can start to ignore the behavior and teach them another way to express their desires or deal with their feelings. Also, watch and comment when you see them do something positive. Another way to limit your attention to negative actions is to tell children what needs to be done and then look away. At times, this can prevent the start of a power struggle. Also, avoid locking eyes because this can become a nonverbal challenge leading to a struggle to see who will win.

> ### *Fabulous Five: Limit Your Attention*
> - **Give attention to children who are doing well.**
>
> The group started a newspaper, but instead of writing, Dan tipped his chair back and twirled a pencil in his hand.

Then he started mumbling, "I'm not doing this," periodically looking at me to see if I was going to make him write.

For a few minutes, I talked with the children who were working and ignored Dan. Then I went up to him and said, "Dan, you know a lot about cars. It would be great to have an article on cars. Just write down a few ideas for today, or at least find some pictures we can use for the paper." He wrinkled his forehead, but then started looking through books.

- **Avoid giving attention to actions or behavior you want to stop.**

On Brian's first day at his new school, the teacher pointed to the calendar as part of the morning routine.

"F***," the 6 year old yelled.

"Just ignore that," the teacher cued everyone in the room.

"I can spell poop," he said, turning his head and looking for a reaction that did not come.

"Brian, what is the weather today?"

"Windy," he replied.

- **Watch for a pattern of attending only to negative actions.**

As 4-year-old Noah walked by a group of boys playing with blocks, he kicked over their tower. "Hey," they shouted.

A few seconds later, another child yelled, "Noah kicked me in the leg." Staff rushed over to intervene.

Noah ran and kicked a girl sitting on the floor. She started crying, "He kicked me in the chest." Noah continued running, scooped up a plastic block, and threw it, hitting a teacher in the cheek.

Later that day, the teachers and the special education team met to discuss the earlier events. "Noah is getting a lot of attention from adults and peers," I said. "It's hard because you can't ignore him when he is hurting people. We have to find a way to start catching him when he's good."

"We could make sure we spend at least 5 minutes playing with him at centers," one teacher suggested.

"Maybe we could make him a helper too," another said.

"I'll make a book with photos of him doing different sensory and calming strategies. That way we can teach him what to do when he is upset." Then the group discussed what the consistent consequences would be if he hurt another person.

- **Tell children what needs to be done and then shift your attention away.**

As the group of preschoolers watched the teacher reading, 3-year-old Jasmine turned around and started poking my leg.

"Look at the book," I said, pointing to the teacher. "You are missing a good story." Then I shifted my eyes to the book and ignored Jasmine. After a few seconds of trying to get my attention to no avail, she turned back.

- **Avoid locking eyes.**

After going to the restroom, Nick and Nadia wandered the school halls and laughed loudly. "Quiet voices," I said as I stepped out of my office. Nick saw me and walked away from me, which was the opposite direction of the kindergarten. I nonchalantly walked toward him and then passed him without making eye contact. He reversed direction and headed away from me, right into the classroom.

Shift Children's Attention

Children might be thinking:
Oh, what's that?
I want to do that.
That looks like fun.

In situations in which children are doing something they should not be doing, shifting their attention away from their current action or activity can help. This especially works well with younger children. To get them to stop, you can use diversion tactics or guide the conversation or actions to more appropriate ones.

Divert Children's Attention

When young children are crying or engaged in undesirable activities, use distraction to capture their attention, thus shifting their thinking to something else. This approach is more effective for younger ones or those functioning well below their same-aged peers. For these children, instead of using words to divert their attention, it is better to use objects or sensations. You can draw their attention by making interesting sounds, feeling an object, or doing a fun action they would like to try. Showing them a toy or favorite object is also enticing. When they see that there is something more interesting or fun, they tend to stop what they are doing.

Fabulous Five: Divert Children's Attention
- **Distract by making sounds.**

On the first day of preschool, 3-year-old twins Jay and Lance ran to their mother in the doorway. Their baby sister was nestled in a sling against their mother's chest. Holding the twins' hands, they all started to walk out. Halfway there, Lance dropped to the floor and screamed. I ran over to assist and took Jay's hand because I had spent most of the day in his classroom. The mother was then able to calm Lance.

When we made it to the parked car, Jay tried to get in and cried when I stopped him. To give his mother more time to buckle the other two in their car seats, I picked up a dried leaf. While crumbling it in my hand, I said,

"Squish, squash, squish, squash." Jay stopped crying and smiled. I put a leaf in his hand and continued making sounds until it was his turn to get in the car.

- **Divert children's attention with a toy.**

In the occupational therapy department at the hospital, 3-year-old Gabriel headed for the kitchen. I quickly pulled out a musical toy from the cupboard in the children's area and said, "Gabriel, come here. Check this out." He turned around out of curiosity and headed back to me.

- **Distract with touch.**

Three-year-old Cody wandered around the rug where the rest of the class was seated. When his teacher began reading a book, I realized that he did not understand the words in the book. I wanted him to sit with the group and at least look at a simpler book.

I gently guided him to sit between my outstretched legs. I then put a touch-and-feel book in front of him. Using hand-over-hand assistance, I rubbed his hand over the soft fur attached to the picture of a horse. He turned the page and touched the next animal's fur.

- **Entice using a favorite object to divert attention.**

Three-year-old Bruce alternated between flapping his hands and flicking his ear. His teacher showed him the picture symbol for group time and pointed to the other children sitting on the rug. Bruce threw himself on the floor and started crying. The teacher brought over his favorite album containing photos of his family and friends at school. Bruce stopped crying to peek at the book. When he reached for it, the teacher guided him over to the group. As soon as he sat down, she handed him the book.

- **Distract with a fun action.**

As the children in the specialized class played in the gym, 4-year-old Rollin ran to four stacked mats in the corner. I followed. He started doing somersaults on them but then decided to somersault off the mat, which was a 2-foot drop. I caught him before he landed on the gym floor.

"That's not safe," I said. I quickly grabbed a wand with an attached blue streamer and waved it in the air. "Run with this. It's really fun." I placed it in his hand, and he started running.

Change Children's Focus

Another way to avoid a power struggle is to change children's focus. Doing a quick exchange of toys or objects often prevents younger children from getting upset. By substituting one object for another, they are able to focus on the new object and are not left empty handed.

If you find children are balking about doing an activity and refusing to even try, shift to something you know they will attempt. You also may want to move away from a point of contention. If they are refusing or doing the opposite of what you are requesting, change your wording. Use different words that are more to the children's liking. Eliminate the part they are determined not to do. Similarly, steer conversation about violence or inappropriate topics to more neutral and acceptable ones. If necessary, discuss and try to resolve underlying issues at a later time.

Fabulous Five: Change Children's Focus

- **Do a quick exchange to change children's focus.**

When I saw 3-year-old Jeremy's mother, I said, "We see that he loves to hold a car in his hand. It would help us if you could put one of his small toys from home in his backpack. Then at the end of the day we can exchange his home toy for the school toy." His mother agreed.

The next day when it was time to leave, I took his toy from home out of his backpack and said, "Here's your cool blue car." I put that car in his hand and in one quick motion removed the school toy. From then on, before going home he switched cars on his own.

- **Shift the conversation or activity to a neutral one and discuss the issue later.**

As soon as 8-year-old Lauren saw me, she balked at the doorway. "I don't wanta write," she announced. Then, as if she were in a Shakespearean play, she flung her arms in the air with a dramatic flair. "Writing makes me feel like I'm in an ocean of sadness."

I smiled and said, "Have you acted in any plays? It seems like you would be a good actress." She shook her head. "Okay," I said. "We will do something besides writing."

Later we talked about her frustrations with the writing.

- **Change the focus away from children's refusals.**

When I told 6-year-old Trenton to draw through three mazes and take his time, he kept repeating, "I can go fast."

I stopped saying, "Take your time." Instead, I pointed to the maze and said, "Stay on the road. Don't go in the water. You don't want the alligators to bite you."

He slowed down and said when he was finished, "I didn't get bit."

- **Ask questions to guide children to different actions.**

"Everyone get your coats and then come sit down with me," the preschool teacher told the class.

Jasmine headed to the dollhouse instead of the coat rack.

I walked over and said in a curious tone of voice, "Jasmine, what color is your coat?"

"Pink," she said with a smile.

"Oh, show me your pretty pink coat."

She stopped playing, went to the coat rack, and pointed to it.

"It's pretty. Put it on. It's time to go home."

She responded by sliding the coat on and joining the group.

- **Guide the conversation to another topic.**

"Did you see *Friday the 13th*? I loved all the blood," the first grader said.

"No, horror movies scare me too much," I said. "Have you seen the movie about the talking mouse?"

"Yeah, it was good."

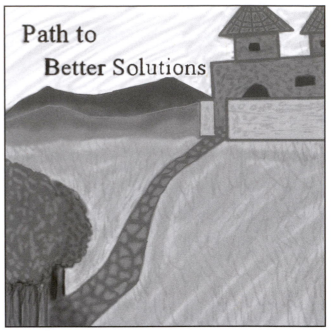

Figure 13-3. Guide children on the path to better solutions.

Promote Children's Self-Awareness of Their Actions

When working with children, you want to help them grow as people. One way to foster this growth is to increase their self-awareness. This can be done by being truthful with tact and pointing out how their actions limit themselves. You also can use guiding questions to promote self-reflection and problem solving (Figure 13-3).

Be Truthful With Tact

> **Children might be thinking:**
> *I'm not sure I like what you are saying.*
> *You're honest.*
> *You're trying to help me.*
> *Maybe I can trust you more.*

Sometimes children are not aware that they have choices in how they act. One life lesson, of course, is to learn that you are responsible for your actions and there can be consequences for the choices you make. Also, some are unaware of their habits and their impact on others. You can help children grow by talking to them with honesty and tact. In a respectful way, convey that you care about them and that your intention is to make things better for them.

Fabulous Five: Confront With Honesty

- **Point out children's responsibility for their own actions.**

Adrian was on a point system in his third-grade class. One day he refused to do an assignment and, consequently, did not earn his points. He walked into my room and began circling the table. "It's not fair. It's not right. My teacher has got to give me those points." He kept repeating, "It's not fair."

"Adrian, you're mad at the wrong person." He stopped and stared at me. "You are the one who chose not to follow directions, and because of that you did not earn your points."

- **Provide tactful feedback to help children look normal to peers.**

Seven-year-old Gil bent his elbows and flapped his arms each time he became excited. "You know when you move your arms like that, some kids might tease you. Do you see your teacher waving her arms like that?" I said softly.

"No."

"Do you see me doing it?"

"No."

"Well, I have an idea of one thing you could do instead. May I show you?" He nodded. "When you feel excited and want to shake your arms, you can put your hands on the side of your chair and push up. Try it."

He did a chair push-up and visibly relaxed.

- **Confront with tact and honesty.**

The kindergartner played with my eight tops and especially liked a small blue one. At the end of the session, I said, "Carol, spin the tops three more times and then it will be time to go. When you're done, put them in this bag."

I turned my head for a few seconds, and when I looked back, I saw all the tops in the clear plastic baggie except for the small one. "Let's look for that blue one so I know it's there for you next time."

Looking sheepish, she reached into her pocket and pulled it out.

"Don't take my toys. If you like it, I will bring it back so you can play with it. But don't take it," I said in a serious tone of voice. "You wouldn't like it if I took your toys, would you?" She shook her head.

- **Point out the effect of their actions on others.**

Four-year-old Jake curled his fingers, growled, and began tickling a classmate's back.

"Stop," Darien yelled, moving away.

Jake turned to another classmate and grabbed his shirt.

"Quit it," Blake yelled, scowling at Jake.

"Jake, look at your friends' faces," I said. "They don't like you touching them that way. If you want their attention, ask them to play with you."

- **Help children see a pattern in what they do and how their actions impact their lives.**

I observed 6-year-old Dan on the playground and saw him interrupt a game, to the other boys' dismay. That afternoon in our session, I set up wooden dominos in a "V" pattern for him to knock over with a beanbag. He watched me, then swiped the blocks with his wrist and rearranged them. "Do you want to play with me or just do this by yourself?" I asked.

"With you," he said with surprise in his voice.

"Do you realize that you knocked down my dominos without even talking to me? When you're playing, people often get upset if you don't ask first. How would you feel if I knocked down your blocks right before you were going to throw?"

"I wouldn't like it."

"To get along with friends, it helps if you check with them first. Ask if it's okay to join in or change the game."

Discuss How Children's Actions Affect Them

> **Children might be thinking:**
> *I'll listen.*
> *Okay, I'll give myself a chance.*

At times, children will hold back and not give themselves a chance to grow. When this happens, be specific on how they are making it harder for themselves. Then describe what they can do differently. Let them know that it is unacceptable to use a diagnosis as an excuse not to do something when you know they can do it. Look at the core issue underlying a refusal. Are they afraid of failure? Do they doubt their abilities? Encourage them to give you and themselves a chance.

Fabulous Five: Talk About How Their Actions Are Limiting Them

- **Point out to children how they are making a task harder.**

"You need to do this again so I can read it," Cole's teacher said.

I leaned over his desk to try to help. "It looks like you need to put more space between each word," I said.

Eight-year-old Cole covered his paper with his arm and rushed to rewrite the sentence.

"Oh dear, this second one is messier than the first," I said. "Now your teacher will ask you to do it a third time. If you think about it, you are making it harder on yourself because you are rushing and not letting anyone help you. I have a few ideas, if you will let me show you."

- **Talk to children about how their current way of acting is getting them in trouble.**

I went to talk to 4-year-old Hunter after he smacked a girl. He had been told to leave the center. "So what happened?" I asked.

"Paige took my toy, so I hit her."

"Did hitting make things better or get you in trouble?"

"Got me in trouble."

"Let's figure out what else you can do so you don't get in trouble. What can you do if she takes your toy again?"

"Umm, I could get a teacher to help me."

"That's a good idea!"

- **Avoid letting children limit themselves by a diagnosis.**

In the first part of the motor test, 9-year-old Tammy cut quickly and carelessly. Then I read the test directions to draw a line through a crooked path. She zipped through the task in 2 seconds and said, "There, I'm done." There were numerous errors.

"Please slow down and do your best," I said.

"Well, I have ADD," she said, referring to attention deficit disorder.

"I work with lots of kids with ADD. I know it may take more effort to concentrate, but please try to do your best. You're in charge of your own body." I had her redraw the line through the maze, and this time there was only one error.

- **Tell children, "Please give me a chance to…."**

"Here's the game. Use the…." I started to say, but before I finished, 7-year-old Gabriel grabbed the frog figurines and pitched them into the purple pot. "Gabriel, you didn't let me finish. I was trying to tell you about the game. Please give me a chance to tell you the directions so you can play the game with us."

"Okay," he murmured.

"Use the tongs to put the frogs in the pot."

- **Point out how the children are not giving themselves a chance.**

"Please sit down."

"I don't wanta sit down," the 8 year old grumbled.

"Please sit down so I can show you some fun things."

"No," Tom said, even as he slowly lowered himself into the chair. When I put four construction toys on the table, he blurted, "No," and folded his arms across his chest.

"No? I haven't even shown you what your choices are. Give yourself a chance to have some fun. You don't have to make yourself miserable."

I left the toys on the table, sat back in the chair next to him, and waited. Ten seconds later, he picked up a toy and started building with it.

Use Guiding Questions to Find Better Solutions

> **Children might be thinking:**
> *You're making me think.*
> *I better think about this.*

You can ask questions that guide children in the right direction. For many, you can promote self-reflection both before and after a situation. For others, your questions may cue them about how to act. Use questions rather than advice to guide their thinking. Children become more engaged and can learn when they have to provide the answers.

> ### *Fabulous Five: Use Guiding Questions*
> - **Ask children, "Are you helping by doing that?" or "Are you making things better?"**
>
>   "I want to be first in line," Alvin said, trying to bulldoze his way in front of two girls. They raised their arms and did not let him pass.
>
>   The kindergarten teacher opened the door, and Alvin raced into the room, shoving three chairs to the floor to show his anger.
>
>   "Are you making things better by pushing over chairs?" I asked.
>
>   "No," he said with a pout.
>
>   "I understand it's frustrating when you don't get what you want. It would be a good idea to pick up the chairs before you get in trouble."
> - **Ask children how they can handle a situation or feelings.**
>
>   "I need my glue. I don't want to share," 5-year-old Quinn said.

"Mara needs some too. What can you do?"

"I don't like sharing my glue. I'll go get one for her."

"That sounds like a good idea."
- **Use questions that cue the children on how to act.**

"When we go back to class, do we run or walk?"

"Walk," the three kindergartners shouted in unison.

"Loud or quiet?" I whispered.

"Quiet," they whispered back.

"You're right."
- **Ask children what they need to remember.**

"Squeeze this gel ball with your fingers," I said to the second grader. "But if you push it down on the table, the ball will pop."

One minute later, Lou tried to flatten the ball against the table.

"What do you have to remember about this ball?"

"It can pop," he said.

"Yes, and if it breaks I'll have to throw it away and you will not get to play with it again."
- **Ask, "What did you learn?"**

Eight-year-old Felicia flattened the blue glittered putty and pinched the edges with a teeth-shaped clip. "Here's something you can do with these teeth," she said. "You can make designs. Pretty cool, huh? I never thought of that. Now I have."

Then she clamped the clip on the putty and pushed a plastic rolling pin over her creation, causing the clip to break into pieces. Felicia raised her head and froze, waiting for my reaction.

"What did you learn?" I asked in a calm voice.

"Not to keep the teeth on the putty while you're rolling," she replied, and I nodded.

Promote Self-Reflection and Problem Solving

> **Children might be thinking:**
> *I figured that out on my own.*
> *I fixed my own problem.*

Teaching children to reflect on their actions and problem solve alternatives fosters the development of self-control. They learn that their thinking and feelings affect what they do. A second lesson is that they can stop and think before acting. A third lesson is that they can problem solve for themselves. When they discover that they can figure out solutions on their own, their confidence increases. In addition, they decrease their reliance on adults to resolve their difficulties.

Fabulous Five: Promote Reflection and Problem Solving

- **Point out how the children's thinking affects them.**

"I hate writing," 8-year-old Joel said.

"If you say you hate it, you're telling your brain not to learn it," I replied. "Instead you can tell yourself it will get easier with practice."

- **Encourage children to think before acting.**

Six-year-old Hannah aimed the open scissors toward her dazzling red hair, which was pinched between her index and middle fingers.

"What will happen if you do that?" I asked.

She stopped, smirked, and said, "My mom will get mad."

"Use the scissors just for cutting paper."

- **Cue children by saying in a nonjudgmental tone of voice, "Think about what you are doing."**

Seven-year-old Travis climbed on top of the therapy table and yelled, "I'm a crazy monkey."

Because I was close enough to catch him if he fell, I said, "Stop and think about what you are doing. Is that safe?"

"All right, I'll get down."

- **Promote children's problem-solving abilities.**

The two preschoolers had their hands on the new ball, and each was trying to take it. "I want it," they both yelled.

I came over and took the ball. "Oh dear," I said. "It looks like we have a problem. You both want to play with the ball. What can we do about that?"

"I can go first," Jay said.

"No, I want to go first," Kenny replied.

"That's one idea. You could each take a turn. Because you both want to go first, what is another idea?"

"We could share and play a game together," Jay proposed.

"What do you think? Would that work?" I asked, and the boys nodded. "You came up with a good idea. I'm glad you figured out what to do."

- **Have children discover ways to prevent recurring problematic actions.**

Twice the 9-year-old boys walked out of my room with my therapy toys in their pockets. When I asked them to search for the toys, they returned them.

In the following session, I said, "I need your help. The last few times, my toys have disappeared, I think kids accidentally walked out with them. I buy these with my own money. I need ideas on what we can do to prevent— do you know what I mean by 'prevent'?" They nodded. "To prevent kids from accidentally taking my stuff. Here's paper you can draw or write ideas."

Sal buried his head in his arms and mumbled, "I don't have any ideas."

Jonathan drew a hand and wrote in it: *Remember—do you have something?* He handed me the paper and said, "Show us this at the end of group."

"This is a way to check so you're not taking anything accidentally," I said. "It's like if a friend comes to your house and takes your things home. That can be upsetting, and you want to prevent it. Thanks for your good idea."

KEY POINTS TO REMEMBER

- Avoid power struggles by using a variety of approaches.

- Make responding with empathy your first approach if safety is not an immediate concern.

- Listen and try to understand each other's perspectives.

- Find constructive ways to meet the children's needs expressed by their actions.

- Highlight appealing and beneficial aspects of following your request or expectations.

- Use playful, out-of-the-ordinary, or unexpected actions to circumvent a struggle and lighten the situation.

- Adjust, make changes, eliminate problematic objects/ situations, or frame children's actions positively to prevent a confrontation.

- Avoid giving your attention to unwanted actions, and use distraction to divert children's attention.

- Help children learn by being truthful with tact, pointing out how their actions affect others, and encouraging them to problem solve and find better solutions.

REVIEW QUESTIONS

1. When you find yourself continually reprimanding a child, you need to find ways to interact more positively with that child. True or false.

2. Recess is the last activity of the day. The class goes in, but a 4-year-old girl hides under a slide. When you move around the slide, she moves farther away and laughs. Parents are watching. What can you say to get her to come inside?

3. You must insist that children immediately respond to all of your directives. True or false.

4. A 5-year-old boy snatches the playground ball from another boy and runs away. Three boys chase him, grab the ball back, and kick it to each other. He goes to the door and sits down with his back to the playground. You see what happens and can see that he is upset. What can you say?

5. You see a preschooler walk to the center full of blocks to play with a new toy as the rest of his class sits at their tables. What can you say to him using the following sentence?: "I wonder if you are [state feeling] because [state possible cause]."

6. You are in the kindergarten classroom sitting at the table with Ashley. The teacher tells the class they need to color, cut, and glue four pictures on a science sheet showing a seed growing into a plant. Ashley looks at the paper and says, "I don't want to do this." Name three approaches you could use as a response.

7. Children respond more positively when you use a serious versus playful approach to avoid power struggles. True or false.

8. Give children more attention when they are demonstrating unwanted actions. True or false.

9. Diverting young children's attention is often effective in stopping unwanted actions. True or false.

10. Name three possible questions that can help guide older children to think about better choices for their actions.

Co-Create Educational Experiences That Are Challenging and Fun

CHAPTER OVERVIEW

Experiences in therapy need to have the elements of fun and challenge. Fun activities are enticing and motivating. The just-right challenge promotes growth. In this chapter, I will discuss the fourth dimension, which is about how to work with children to co-create meaningful educational experiences. Included are ways to assist children in getting started, making decisions, and creating a desire to face a challenge. Also described are child-friendly ways to give directions, make therapy fun, and be fair when setting up activities and deciding who goes first.

CHILDREN'S DESCRIPTIONS OF WHAT THEY THINK YOU SHOULD KNOW

Dr. Clare: "What is important for therapists to know when they work with kids?"

Alex (age 9): "Make it fun."

Rachel (age 9): "Know kids' personalities, what they like, and what they're good at."

Emilio (age 6): "Do fun things."

Dr. Clare: "Why should therapists be fun?"

Vinnie (age 9): "So kids don't think you are boring."

Jane (age 9): "Then you can laugh and have fun. My teacher puts on funny hats. She has a tiger you can sit by."

Chris (age 9): "You can have funny jokes."

Dr. Clare: "Why should therapists use toys for therapy?"

Vaughn (age 10): "Toys make your hands better to pick up things. They're good for you because your hands get more stronger. The games teach you eye-hand coordination."

Harry (age 6): "It's good to have toys for playing and for fun. I like them."

Sherry (age 11): "If kids can't walk or talk, they can still use toys."

Dr. Clare: "What's good about occupational therapy?"

Lynn (age 12): "It's fun. There's a variety of things to do and choose from. It's good to have fun. Without occupational therapy, clinic would just be boring. Get stuck with needles and leave. Who wants to be bored? Who wouldn't want to have fun? I don't have fun at home."

WORK TOGETHER TO CREATE EDUCATIONAL EXPERIENCES

As a therapist, you want children's time with you to be a positive educational experience. Through therapy, you help children build on their strengths, develop new abilities, and see or experience themselves and/or their world differently.

Curtin, C.
Strategies for Collaborating With Children: Creating Partnerships in Occupational Therapy and Research (pp. 275-300).
© 2017 SLACK Incorporated.

One important life lesson for them to learn is that they have to challenge themselves to grow. Children seen in therapy have often experienced multiple failures and, consequently, tend to avoid taking risks. These children often gravitate to activities they know they can do successfully. This limits what they can learn about themselves and their world.

By collaborating, you can make therapy a safe place to experiment and discover more about themselves. Although you will start the process of challenging them, a continual goal is to support them in taking the lead, for it is when the children push themselves that one sees the most growth.

Therapy also can give children the experience of meeting a challenge and not failing. After gaining a sense of accomplishment, children may learn to view themselves in a new way. To provide them with the experience of success is an art of occupational therapy. Your training in analyzing children's abilities, watching the subtle nuances of nonverbal language, and adapting activities and the environment allows you to set up the just-right challenge.

Create Challenging and Fun Experiences

It is therapeutic to establish a balance in which the activity is both challenging and fun. The fun element is enticing and motivating. Everyone loves to have fun. The challenge element promotes change and growth. Some children will challenge themselves, but others will not. Children often like to do what they already know is in their repertoire. Staying in their comfort zone guarantees success and provides a predictable outcome. It is riskier to venture into unknown territory and to try something new. You will want to create a spirit of discovery where it is safe to take the first step without worrying about failure.

First, you want to capture children's interest. Next, create an atmosphere in which learning something new is considered fun. Then you have to work with the children to learn what the just-right challenge is for them. This involves finding out what they can already do and then determining how much of a challenge seems right and achievable to the children. If it appears too difficult, many children will not even try. They may be bored with too easy of a challenge.

Part of the art of therapy is figuring out when to challenge and to what degree. If the children are having a hard day or are upset, it may be better to do an activity they find soothing, even if it is simple. On other days, you can encourage children to try something new and difficult.

With some, you may want to start with a very simple and easy activity that will bring success with little or no effort. Gradually increase the level of difficulty. Push children to do as much as possible and take risks. Be aware of pushing too hard because you may lose them. That means that children might become overwhelmed or fearful and just shut down or refuse to continue. At this point, you need to figure out where the breakdown is occurring. Question yourself: Why are the children having trouble? What made the activity look daunting or impossible? Then make adaptations. Encourage them to take a chance and not give up on themselves.

Determine the Format of Services

> **Children might be thinking:**
> *Hmm. What is this?*
> *What do I have to do?*

In the beginning, you need to decide whether the child should be seen individually or in a group. The choice you make is dependent upon the child's needs and your setting. If the child requires intensive one-to-one attention to succeed, then individual therapy may be best. A group can be beneficial for working on play or social skills. Some children learn more from their peer group than from you.

Provide Individual Therapy

Working with children on an individual basis can be done in various settings. Children feel most comfortable in their home and school. In those two places, you have to enter their world and adjust. Therapy at school can range from working together in the class to providing more intervention in a therapy room or other location. The hospital setting is the most foreign to a child.

Individual therapy is more intensive. It is good for children who need physical assistance such as prompts on how to move their body. It may be needed for those with safety issues. Working one-on-one also can be good for teaching a new skill. You can be more responsive because you are able to devote your complete attention to the one child and make quick adjustments.

Fabulous Five: Provide Individual Therapy

- **Work with the children at home.**

   "Jessica often makes a fist with her hands so she doesn't touch things," her mother said. "If she gets pudding on her hands, she runs to the bathroom to wash it off."

   The next week, I brought a tub of beans to the 3 year old's house to help her get used to different textures. "I have a game. The bunnies are lost in the beans. Find them."

   Jessica looked hesitant but started digging.

- **Provide therapy in the children's classroom while sitting next to them.**

   In the classroom, I put my hand out with my palm up and waited. Three-year-old Lucy placed her hand on mine and pulled to get herself off the floor. I pointed to her center, and she waddled over. The other children were connecting a wooden train set and building a train station. Lucy half-sat and half-fell back to the floor and then sat watching the others.

"Hey, Lucy can make a sign for your train station," I said to the group, and they nodded. I wrote the words *train station* and drew short black lines around the paper because I was helping her learn how to cut. I slipped the scissors onto her fingers and adjusted the paper so she could snip on the lines. "Open, shut them," I cued her with each step.

She needed assistance to open the scissor blades but closed them independently. She snipped around the page, creating a fringe for the sign. I handed her tape, and she put the sign on the building.

"Thanks, Lucy," her friends said in response.

- **Consult with the children in the classroom regarding possible strategies.**

"Your teacher said that you work very hard but sometimes you get your letters mixed up."

"Yeah," 7-year-old Shane said.

"What helps you make them right?"

"Sometimes I look up there," he said, pointing to the alphabet strip on the wall.

"That's a great idea! I also have more ideas that have helped other children. Would you like me to show you those?" I asked, and he nodded. "Which letters and numbers are hard for you? You could try writing the alphabet and your numbers if that helps."

He began printing. When he was done, he said, "Letters 'b,' 'd,' and 'c' are the hardest. Sometimes I mix up '9' too."

I demonstrated five different methods involving body cues. Because he was right-handed, I had him make his left hand into a "c" shape and use his hand as a guide. Then I explained more strategies, and he picked the ones he liked.

"What will help you remember to use these strategies?"

"We could put it on my desk."

"Okay, I'll make it for you. I'll put it on an index card and laminate it. Then you can tape it on your desk."

- **Meet in the therapy or clinic room.**

Five-year-old Reed frequently ran into class with his untied shoelaces whipping around his sneakers. "You better tie your shoelaces so you don't trip," I said.

Looking embarrassed, he said, "I don't know how."

Because I worked with him, I knew new motor movements were challenging. I asked him to come to the therapy room. There I taught him a simple way of tying shoes using blue and yellow shoelaces to show the crossing of the laces.

- **Work with the children in a hospital room.**

When I walked into the hospital room, I saw David crying. "I heard you were in the hospital and brought a couple of activities you might like," I said to the 7 year old, whom I saw monthly in the outpatient oncology clinic. "I can see how upset you are. I know it's scary to be here. Let me show you what I have. One project is easy, and if you are ready, one is hard. It's challenging.

His tears stopped as he looked at the coloring book and the car wood kit. "I want to do the car. I'm ready to face the challenge."

Determine and Adapt the Structure of the Group

How the group is structured is dependent upon a number of factors, some you have control over, some you do not. You may have a predetermined amount of time or an already established group that you need to work with. Other times you can design your own group based on the collective needs of all the children.

One influencing factor is whether you will work with the same group members the entire time or need to be prepared for a constant influx of new ones. Once you know the external constraints, such as the length of time you have to work with the children and the size of the group, you need to decide on the purpose. Consider the goals set by the children and what will help this group of children grow. Then decide what level of interaction is desired. You can set up the group so that children only play or participate in an activity parallel to each other with minimal interaction.

A different type of group would require them to interact and cooperate with each other. One simple idea for this group is to limit the amount of supplies such as scissors or glue, which means they have to talk with each other and share. Another option is to split the group into two and then have them take turns being helpers and participants. An additional method is to have one half of the group do one activity and the other half do another, then have them switch so everyone gets a turn. Two other possibilities are to have each member take a turn one at a time while the others wait or have the group work together to complete an activity. Whatever the structure of the group, you have to find a way to meet the needs of all the children.

Fabulous Five: Structure the Group

- **Have the children do the same or a similar activity while sitting next to each other.**

Two preschoolers shouted, "I want that one," and both pointed to the wind-up toy shaped like a monkey. Cindy, a third group member, folded her arms and pouted.

"Everyone listen. I brought a wind-up toy for each of you. You will get a chance to play with all of them. You can play with the toy for a few minutes, then we will rotate. That means everyone will pass it to the person next to them." I emphasized my point by making a clockwise circle with my finger. I placed a small toy in front of each child, and they played for three minutes.

"Rotate," Cindy yelled.

- **Have some children help the other group members and then switch so everyone gets a turn.**

I propped a target with a painted clown against the wall and said to the second graders, "Jimmie, throw the beanbags at the clown. Zeb, you retrieve and throw back the beanbags that fall on the floor. Then we'll switch, and Jimmie will pick them up for you."

Jimmie pitched the first beanbag, which landed 2 feet in front of the target.

"Too short," Zeb shouted.

He threw again, and the next beanbag flew over the target.

Zeb continued his encouragement: "Too long. Now this one should be just right."

- **Have each child take a turn while the others wait.**

"We have a fun game. It's like digging for buried treasure. Reach into the bag and pull out a box."

Six-year-old Carol searched and wrapped her fingers around a 2-inch heart box. "Hey, I found one."

"Inside the boxes are strategies of what you can do to get yourself calm. It's okay to get help with reading. Some of the words are very big."

"These are like fortune cookies." Carol opened and read, "Count to 10 and tell yourself to relax."

"Everyone try that," I cued them.

"My turn," Tony said. He fished in the purple velveteen bag and removed an octagonal box. "Mine says, 'Put your palms on the table and push down.'" After the others applied pressure on the table, Tony turned and said, "I can read your mind."

"What do you think is on my mind?"

"I bet you're thinking how much fun we're having. I know you think that every time we're together."

I smiled and said, "I do have fun with you and everyone else here. You're right, I like being with you."

- **Design different activities for each half of the group and then rotate.**

"Today you have to take turns," I told the four 6 year olds. "Two of you will get to squeeze these funny chickens. When you push the stomach, an egg pops out. I will help the other two print their names for their books. Then we will switch so everyone will get a turn."

Hayden wrapped his hand around the chicken and squeezed. "Look, he's laying an egg."

"Do some more while I help Dane and Gerry." I looked at both of them and gave verbal cues on how to make their letters. When they were done, I said, "Time to switch."

- **Have the group work on achieving one task together.**

"It's exciting; you get to make your very own newspaper," I told the third-grade class at the day treatment. "Let's write down some ideas of what you could put in it."

Children came up with the suggestions of recipes, interviews, sports news, an advice column, jokes, and pictures.

"Wow, we have a lot of great ideas. I'm going to go around the table and ask each one of you to tell me which part you want to do."

"I'm going to be Dr. Jed and answer people's questions," Jed responded.

"I love football. I'm going to write about that," the next student said.

The rest of the group continued to choose their preferred tasks.

Determine the Activity

Children might be thinking:
That's a good idea.
I like that.
Hmm. What do I want to do?
I wonder if I can do this.

Determining what activity to do is an interactive process. When you first start, children might not know what the possibilities are. One way to start is to offer activities that other children their age have liked. Provide choices and offer alternatives if they do not like any of the ideas. Another approach is to find activities that are related to their interests. Often you can discover what appeals to them by interviewing caregivers, observing, and talking with children. You also can suggest an activity or point out what materials are available. Then follow their lead on what they want to do. Once children learn the range of activities as well as their capabilities, they will start to generate their own ideas. Listen to their wishes. If needed, use a playful approach to work with children on expanding or adapting their ideas to make it therapeutic.

Fabulous Five: Decide on the Activity

- **Offer activities that same-aged peers have liked.**

Three-year-old Ariel, holding onto her bright red walker, came into the classroom. It was her first day in the weekly introductory group that was held 3 to 4 months before preschool.

"She is so excited to come to school," her mother said.

On the floor were four different types of puzzles. One had different pets with knobs attached to each piece, one made a farm animal sound when the piece was put in, and another had barnyard pictures hidden under the puzzle pieces. The last one required a fishing pole with a magnet to catch the fish.

"Which puzzle do you want to do first?" I asked, knowing that other 3 year olds enjoyed these particular ones. She smiled and tried to coordinate her extended fingers as she reached for the fishing pole.

- **Suggest an idea based on the children's interests.**

As we talked in the first session, 9-year-old Ivan mentioned that he liked spaceships. "I have a book with different patterns. Let me get that out for you. I know there is one to make a rocket book."

"All right!" he said.

I pulled out the book, copied the pages, and handed it to him. "Here's a pattern for a rocket. Color and cut out this spaceship for the cover. Then write a story."

He colored his rocket gray with red stripes and wrote: *The spaceship is going to the planet Cheese. The other spaceship is going to the planet Peanut Butter. Both ships are carrying crackers.*

- **Suggest an activity and have the children decide how to do it.**

"Let's do an obstacle course," I suggested. Nine-year-old Henry nodded approval. "Come up with three ideas."

"Mmm. Scoot across the room and back, pick up magnets with the magic wand, and crawl to the wall."

"Let me know when you're ready."

With his stomach on the scooter board, Henry propelled himself to the other side of the room. "Made that one," he huffed. Then he rolled the scooter board over to the magnets. He waved the magnetic wand, and the round magnets jumped. "Oh no, you don't," he said as one fell off and rolled. He pushed himself over and scooped it in his hand, saying, "That's sweet." Then he crawled to the edge of the room as fast as he could. "Whew," he said, taking a deep breath. "That was fun. That was like an obstacle course championship."

"Yes, and you won."

- **Provide materials and follow the children's lead.**

"What do you want to do?" I waved my arm around the room and said, "We have a scooter board, one-legged stool, football, spider tops, putty, Halloween finger puppets, and cookie cutters shaped like a ghost, bat, and pumpkin."

Seven-year-old Jeremy went to the table, took the putty, and flattened it with his palm. "I need a rolling pin."

I grabbed a nearby coffee can. "How about this?"

He rolled the can back and forth and then pushed the ghost cookie cutter down on the putty. When he hit an air pocket, a hissing sound came out. "It likes me," he said. After 10 minutes, Jeremy went over to the football.

"What is your game going to be? What is your plan?" I asked.

"I want to just throw the football."

"You're already good at throwing. How could you make it trickier?"

"I could sit on the stool and throw the ball."

"That sounds like a good challenge."

- **Expand on children's ideas.**

Five-year-old Sam looked in my bag and saw my toys. "Can we play with your cars?" he asked.

"Yes, but wait a minute." I quickly thought about how I could make his request therapeutic. "Let's make a racetrack for the cars," I said. I tore off some butcher paper, hung it on the wall, and gave him a short piece of chalk to make the road. By placing the paper upright, Sam would need to use his shoulder muscles and work with his wrist in an upright position. Using a short piece of chalk would help Sam use the finger muscles needed for a normal pencil grip.

When the track was finished, we placed it on the floor and raced our cars. We were both pleased with the activity.

Plan and Prepare Children for What to Expect When Doing the Activity

> **Children might be thinking:**
> *I'm glad you prepared me.*
> *It's good to know how long this takes.*
> *It's good to know it's hard, but I still want to do it.*

Before children start, you need to plan the initial activity and prepare them for what it entails. Once the activity has been chosen, quickly analyze, at least for a few minutes, the different elements and consider what they can do. Figure out ways to create a good match that allows them to succeed. Usually you have to think fast. As the session progresses, continue to watch for what is helping or hindering and make adaptations.

It is also good to prepare children for what to expect. If you know they will need to practice, be upfront and tell them so. Some may expect to do it right the first time and not make any mistakes. By discussing the need for practice, they can adjust their expectations. Also, alert them about difficult or potentially annoying aspects and suggest helpful strategies. When doing projects, especially with younger children, it is crucial to talk about how long it will take. Many young ones expect to leave with a finished product the same day. If it will take longer, prepare them.

Fabulous Five: Prepare Children for What to Expect

- **Prepare children for the need to practice.**

"This takes practice. The first step is to learn how to use these rubber stamps. Watch me." Picking up a stamp of a teddy bear, I said, "Push it on the inkpad. Then press it hard on the paper and lift straight up. Practice first and get the feel of it. It's important to practice so your cards turn out really well."

"This bear is so cute," 5-year-old Belinda said, pressing the stamp on the scrap paper.

"When you are ready, I have good paper for you."

- **Tell children how long the activity usually takes.**

"This dinosaur book has taken everybody 2 to 3 days to do," the occupational therapy student said.

"Not me. I'll get it done today," 7-year-old Nick said.

"Oh no, there's a lot to do. There are dinosaur stamps, coloring, and writing. Take your time and plan for more than 1 day."

- **Prepare children for the difficult aspects of the activity.**

I demonstrated putting dominos upright and said to the group, "These fall all the time. If they get knocked over, put them back up. If you feel frustrated, just take a break or ask for help."

Six-year-old Rob positioned three in a row and whispered to himself, "If I knock these over, I can just do it again."

- **Talk about any aspect of the activity that may be annoying.**

"This game is called Operation. You use the tweezers to take out the body parts, but if you touch the sides, it makes a loud noise. You will perform surgery," I told the preschoolers.

"What's surgery?" Mariah asked.

"It's when a doctor cuts you open and fixes what's wrong inside you, like your tummy." I placed the game pieces in the slots. "Get ready because this is really noisy." I raised my head, and all three children covered their ears with their palms. "Try touching the silver edge so you know what it sounds like." It buzzed, and they jumped simultaneously.

Mariah used the tweezers to pluck the rubber band attached between the knee and the anklebone.

"Is there a rubber band in me?"

"No. This is a game. You have hard bones inside of you."

- **Let children know what strategies help with the activity.**

"This game is called Jumping Monkeys," I said to 11-year-old Mason. "You have to put a monkey on a catapult and shoot it so it lands on the tree. It takes lots of practice to get the feel of it. If the monkey goes too far, either back up or push with lighter pressure." I demonstrated and missed. "I'm pushing too hard. I have to lighten up."

Mason tried and came close on his first try.

"I thought you had it."

"I thought I had it too," Mason replied.

"Keep practicing." At the end of the game, I asked, "What did you think about that?"

"It was fun."

Discover Children's Just-Right Level of Challenge

Children might be thinking:
I like a challenge.
I hope it's not too hard.
I hope it's not boring.
I remember when...and it was easy/fun/hard.

Because one criterion for the educational experience is to create a challenge, children need to understand that concept. Ask if they know the meaning of the word or what the expression "face a challenge" means. If they do not know, teach them and continue to use the word. The next step is to learn what the just-right challenge is for the children. Watch for what they feel is a good test of their skills. Also, observe for what is too overwhelming and leads to children's stopping and giving up. In addition, find out what they consider boring or too easy. Attaining the perfect challenge may be a discovery process for you and the children. Sometimes they are not aware of their abilities and are surprised at the results of their efforts.

Let children know they have to tell you what is right for them. It is your wish that they talk to you whenever the activity is too hard, too easy, or too boring. They have to define what a good challenge is for them (Figure 14-1). For some, it may feel like you are asking them to go to the edge of a cliff. You will want to make it safe for them to try and take a risk. Experiment together to see what they can do, and stretch outside of their normal way of being.

Fabulous Five: Identify Children's Perfect Level of Challenge

- **Discuss and frequently use the word "challenge."**

"Do you know what the word 'challenge' means?" I asked 9-year-old Carly.

"It's something hard, or it's going to be difficult."

I nodded and said, "What do you think it means to 'face a challenge'?"

"It means, 'Are you ready to try something difficult?'"

- **Ask children to tell you if the activity is too easy.**

"I have an idea, but let me know if you think it's too easy. I was thinking you could lie down on your tummy on the scooter board and push with both hands like you are swimming. When you get close to the wall, knock down these bowling pins. What do you think?"

"Yeah. I'll be a human bowling ball," 7-year-old Barry said, laughing.

- **Ask children to make the activity hard for themselves.**

"Make it hard for yourself and not too easy."

"I'm good at trying different things. I'm going to take a risk. It's going to be a huge risk," 7-year-old Willy said as he stacked odd-shaped wooden blocks.

- **Watch for how and when children challenge themselves.**

On the playground, 3-year-old Andy climbed up the spiral structure and reached across the 1-foot gap for the railing attached to the slide. When he could not quite grasp it, he scooted his feet around and made it onto the platform. He went down the twisting slide and ran again to the spiral. The second time, he climbed and tried different positions but was far away from the railing. Andy moved and lunged for the platform, missing it by inches.

I caught him in midair. "Did that scare you?" I asked.

He shook his head and ran right back to the spiral, still motivated by the challenge.

- **Observe for which challenges the children consider scary or overwhelming.**

As I watched 3-year-old Carrie both in class and on the playground, I noticed that she shied away from activities involving a higher level of balance. She wore a fearful look the one and only time she tried the swing. When the teachers and I asked the class to hop, she walked across the room.

"Try standing on one foot," I encouraged her on another day as I held her hand. She shook her head and looked like she was going to cry.

After a few weeks, I showed her my small wooden balance board with a monkey painted on it. "Hi, Carrie. I'm a fun monkey. I want to play with you." She smiled. "Put your hands on the table and then stand on me." I guided Carrie's hands and moved her body onto the board. Keeping her still, I held her hips with firm support. A panicked look flashed across her face. "See how I am holding you. I will not let you fall." I smiled and said in a light tone of voice, "Wow, you're riding the monkey."

Seeing my relaxed face, she smiled back. For a few seconds she gently swayed from side to side, then stepped off. "Thanks for playing with me," the monkey said in my voice.

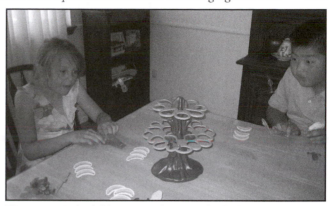

Figure 14-1. Help children create the just-right challenge.

Discover What Children Consider to Be Fun

> **Children might be thinking:**
> *Oh, I like doing this.*
> *Thanks for asking what I like.*
> *I also like this….*

A second criterion of an educational experience is to have fun. Because everyone has different notions about what they call fun, it is your job to start the discovery process. You may begin by directly asking children if they like the activity and what in particular they liked about it. Another approach is to keep a watchful eye on what they typically choose to do and whether it holds their attention. Observe for any nonverbal signs of pleasure, delight, or total engrossment. Also, look for any common elements or threads. For instance, some children enjoy doing any kind of puzzles. Others may like any activity that involves their favorite animal or toy action figure. Find out what children desire and then match the activities to their interests.

> ### Fabulous Five: Discover Individual Notions of Fun
>
> - **Watch for what type of activities the children typically choose and what holds their interest.**
>
> In the first session, 8-year-old Mitchell picked activities involving construction materials. "It looks like you enjoy building," I said.
>
> "Yeah, I like to challenge myself with building stuff."
>
> - **Observe for nonverbal signs of pleasure while doing the activity.**
>
> In class, 3-year-old Pablo fiddled with the six-piece wooden puzzle showing the picture of a truck. The first piece easily slid into the form board, but he struggled with the second one.

"If it doesn't fit, try somewhere else," I said, pointing toward another empty space.

He moved the piece, and it went in. When he finished the puzzle, he smiled and said, "More." He turned it over and independently repeated the same scenario five times.

- **Match activities to children's interests.**

"I went to the aquarium with my dad this weekend," 5-year-old Cooper said in his deep voice. "I like sharks and turtles."

"I have a shark," I said, pulling out a rubber one. "Squeeze him. That helps get your hand muscles strong." He squished the shark with a tight grip.

"I have another idea for a fun game," I said as I went to my cupboard and gathered lobsters, turtles, and fish beanbags. Then I crouched on the floor and unrolled a sheet of blue paper cut in the shape of a lake. After dropping the creatures with a soft thud on the floor, I handed him a wooden clothespin. "Pick up the animals with the clothespin and drop them into the water."

Grinning, Cooper pinched a beanbag and said as he released it, "Here, sea turtle. There you go, little turtle. Go swim to your mommy."

- **Ask children if the activity is fun.**

After burying six 1-inch plastic dinosaurs in thick putty, I said, "Dig out the dinosaurs. They need you to rescue them."

Five-year-old Rick eagerly grabbed the putty, poked his thumb in, and pulled. A T-Rex popped out.

"Is this fun?" I asked.

"Oh yeah!" he said, continuing to dig.

- **Ask what the children liked about the activity.**

"First flatten the putty like a pancake," I said. Five-year-old Fernando placed his left palm over his right hand and pressed. "Here are some pennies. Hide them in the putty." He pushed eight pennies into the putty and rolled it like a sausage. "Now see how many pennies you can find." He dug his thumbs in the putty and pulled out three coins. "You're getting a lot."

"I'm rich," he said.

"Yeah, are you buying me lunch?" I teased.

"No," he said, laughing.

"Did you like playing with the putty?" He nodded. "What did you like about it?"

"It's squishy. It's fun. You can really squeeze it."

Give Directions for the Activity

There are a number of factors to account for when giving directions. First, consider what is happening in the children's lives. For instance, children have a hard time attending if they are hungry or are worried about where they will be sleeping. Second, find out whether they have normal hearing and vision. If not, learn what strategies help. Third, make sure you have their attention and present the directions in a way they can understand.

Capture and Maintain Children's Attention Before Giving Directions

> **Children might be thinking:**
> *What's this?*
> *What am I supposed to do?*

When you are in a group, position yourself so you can see all the children. Address any distractions and gain their attention before starting. Then state the directions. You will find that some focus better if you say the instructions before giving them the supplies. Being lively and intriguing often motivates children to attend. Having animation in your voice also suggests that you are enjoying being with them. Involving children in giving directions is another way to get them to focus on what is being said.

Obtain Children's Attention Before Stating Directions

Before you present directions for an activity, you need to get children's attention. Clear away all distracting items. Avoid talking over loud voices or interfering noises. When there is a quiet moment, then state the instructions. If children are looking around the room, acknowledge what is capturing their attention and then help them to shift their focus to you. One way to pique their interest is to use the word *fun* before stating the directions. Children will often look at you because they do not want to miss something fun. Another way is to playfully call attention to the paper containing the directions. Wait until the children are looking at you, the directions, or the activity before talking.

> ### *Fabulous Five: Get Children's Attention Before Giving Directions*
>
> - **Clear distracting items and then give the directions.**
>
> Seven-year-old Brad broke one Styrofoam packing popcorn into eight pieces. Then he flicked them with his index finger to all ends of the table. I grabbed the trashcan, placed it next to him, and said, "Shoot the pieces in here."
>
> He aimed and shouted, "Score," with each success.
>
> When the table was empty, I put the supplies on it and said, "Time to start group. Everyone take a pencil, paper, and scissors."
>
> - **Avoid giving directions over loud noises.**
>
> "I have something new to show you," I said to the second graders, but my unheard words floated away on a sea of chatter. "I need your attention so we can start." My eyes

scanned the room and rested on each child until quiet ensued. Then I continued, "This is a fun activity. You get to create your own designs with magnets."

- **Acknowledge what is distracting the children and then give directions.**

"The first step is to—" I began to say, but 6-year-old Jack jerked his head toward the door to watch his sister's class as they walked to the art room. "Did you see your sister?" I asked, and he nodded. When the last child passed, I closed the wooden door and resumed giving directions.

- **Use the word *fun* before stating the directions.**

"Bryce, I have something that's fun to do," I said to the kindergartner. I hung a paper with his name written with glow-in-the-dark crayons; closed the door halfway leaving some natural light; and turned off the overhead lights. "Use the flashlight to trace your name."

"I'm going to school at night," he said with a chuckle.

- **Call attention to the paper with the directions on it.**

Five-year-old Gage arched his head, staring at the ceiling. I held the index card containing the directions and waved it in front of his face. He lowered his head and I floated the card in the air, pretending it was a bee. "Buzz, buzz, buzz," I sang. When he shifted his eyes to the card, I said, "The first step is to trace this animal pattern."

State the Directions in a Captivating Way

You may also capture children's attention by making the directions interesting. With younger children, you may want to use props, such as toys or puppets, as a vehicle to provide instructions. When possible, coordinate the prop with the theme of the activity.

Another method for getting children to focus on what you are saying is to be animated in your voice and facial expressions. Incorporate unusual sounds or tones of voice. Avoid using monotone. Instead, use inflection and emphasize different words in the instructions. Singing the directions is another option. Also, vary your gestures and the expression on your face.

Fabulous Five: Make the Directions Interesting

- **Incorporate props when giving a direction.**

For 3 minutes, 6-year-old Adam opened and closed a giraffe whose belly looked like an accordion. I grabbed a similar toy in the shape of a cow. Bouncing the cow on the table, I said, "Hey, Mr. Giraffe, do something with this putty."

Adam pulled the putty toward him and moved the giraffe to the right. "I'm going to make some land for

---

you." Then he turned to me and looked at the cow. "What's he saying now?"

"I can't wait to see you make some land."

- **Use a different or funny tone of voice to highlight directions.**

"This is called a Lite-Brite, and you make fun pictures by poking these colored bulbs in the screen. Then when you turn on the light, they shine." I demonstrated by pinching a yellow bulb between my fingers and saying in a baritone voice, "Push, push, push."

Four-year-old Winslow's face wrinkled into a smile.

- **Incorporate funny sounds as part of the directions.**

"Let me show you how to make a 'z,'" I said to the 5 year old. "Start at the top and go across. Then ZOOP down and across again." Using a clicker in the shape of a bird, I again demonstrated how to make the letter by flying the bird over the letter I had written while stating the same instructions.

- **Use different inflection and loudness on various words in the direction.**

"Your class is learning the letter 'R,' so you are going to make a...." I threw my palms in the air and said with a burst of enthusiasm, "RAINBOW. Put your hand in the middle of the paper and draw a rainbow around your hand."

"I'm going to use every color here," 4-year-old Rita said, pointing to the box of colored pencils. She started to whistle and then sing, "I'm whistling while I work."

"You have a nice voice," I said.

Rita finished the picture and held it in the air. "What do you think, Dr. Clare?"

"Very colorful. I can see you really took your time."

- **Vary facial expressions and gestures when giving directions.**

"Guess what?" I said, wide-eyed with raised eyebrows. The two kindergartners glued their eyes on me in anticipation. "Would you like to learn some magic tricks?"

They nodded, and Skye said, "This is going to be an exciting day."

Using a Jacob's ladder toy, I taught them how to make a penny disappear.

"That's a cool trick," Skye said.

"The next one is a different kind of magic trick. Bury the pennies in the putty. Then dig them out and make them reappear."

Paul pressed the pennies and said, "Look, I'm getting really good at this." He covered the putty over the money. "I did it. All of them are gone."

"Say, 'Abracadabra' and bring them back by pulling them out."

"Abracadabra," he shouted.

Involve Children When Giving Directions

Another method for capturing children's attention is to require a response from them before giving directions. This can be done by making a request for them to show you a sign that they are ready. You may ask them to look at your eyes, say when they are ready, or show you with their behavior. For children who are uncomfortable with eye contact or for whom it is culturally inappropriate, it is better to ask them to look at the activity rather than at your eyes.

A second approach is to direct the children's attention to the activity and have them touch or point to the steps being explained. Incorporating movement helps children become alert. A third way to get attention is to use peers for defining the directions or for demonstrating what to do.

Fabulous Five: Involve Children When Providing Directions

- **Have children tell you when they are ready for directions.**

"Pooh, pooh, pooh." Eight-year-old Petie puffed out his cheeks and tapped them with his index finger.

"Tell me when you are ready for directions," I said.

He stopped his musical serenade and putzed around with the putty for a minute. Then he looked at me and said, "Ready."

- **Say, "Show me you are ready."**

As I opened the game board on the table, 9-year-old Ralph picked at his navy blue sweater. Then he slouched in his chair and slid so low his right hand touched the ground.

"Show me you are ready," I said, and waited in silence. When he raised his body upright and rested his elbows on the table, I said, "The first step is to pick a card."

- **Ask children to take action while you give the directions.**

"This is a mystery picture. Color each number with its own crayon. Everyone point to number one." I waited as five index fingers landed on the papers. "Color all number ones with blue. I'm curious to see what this picture is."

The second graders colored, and when Curt finished, he called out, "Hey, it's a clown."

- **Have a peer give the directions.**

"Peggy has an idea, so she's directing today."

Her pigtails bounced as she hustled and then snuggled in my chair. "Yeah, I'm the teacher. First, you need two pieces of paper."

"Now what?" 7-year-old Sylvia asked.

"Take one of my markers and draw an Easter egg. If you mess up, turn it around."

Sylvia colored and said, "I'm not messing up. I like my Easter egg. There, I drew my egg."

"Now you cut it out and staple them together."

"This is hard to cut through two pieces," Sylvia muttered. Then she jammed the two papers in the stapler. "Slam dunk," she shouted as she pounded the stapler.

"Peggy, thanks for being the teacher," I said.

- **Use a peer to demonstrate the directions.**

I pulled out a container of red putty. Barb turned to Annie, a new member of the group of third graders, and said, "Don't let the putty touch your clothes."

I nodded and added, "Yes, because sometimes it sticks and does not come off." I handed each person a handful of putty and said, "Barb, please show Annie what to do."

"Push down on this and then pinch the edges."

"Why are we doing this?" Annie asked.

"To make our hands strong," Barb said with a smile. "I'm smart today. Oh, I have another rule. We cannot take the toys home."

"You're right," I agreed. "I just share my toys."

Present Directions in a Way Children Can Understand and Remember

Children might be thinking:
I don't get it.
Now it's easier to remember.
Now I understand.
So that's what I am supposed to do.

In addition to having children's attention, you also need to state directions using language they comprehend. Integrating familiar terms promotes a better understanding. Similarly, the use of multisensory directions encompasses all learning styles.

Use Wording and the Right Number of Steps Children Can Understand

When giving directions, it is important to think about the complexity of the wording as well as the number of steps you should describe. Consider the words you will use and the sentence structure. Keep your explanations as simple as possible. As you present the instructions, monitor their level of understanding and watch for any signs of puzzlement. For some, you may want to just say the action word, such as "cut," or use short sentences. For others, you may need to reword the directions or use a simpler sentence structure, especially if they have difficulty with prepositions involving time (e.g., "before" or "after").

Another consideration is to determine how many steps children can remember to follow. If you ask them to remember too many steps, they may become overwhelmed and stop listening to you. It is advantageous, when possible, to show a sample of a finished activity; describe the overall steps in simple, general terms; and then restate just the first step. A sample also facilitates the children's understanding of the purpose of each step. Be sure to speak slowly and allow time for children to process what you said. Also check if they have any questions.

Fabulous Five: Match the Wording and Number of Steps to Children's Level of Understanding

- **Say only the action word.**

"Ah, ah," 8-year-old Pete mumbled as he looked around the room. To help him join his class in making a card, I cued him on what to do by placing an upside-down glue bottle in his hand. I said, "Squeeze," and pointed to the paper. He pushed with his stubby finger, and dabs of glue popped out on the card. I helped him grasp the blue glitter bottle and added, "Shake."

- **Simplify the sentence structure of the directions.**

I looked at 4-year-old Clint, whose chubby cheeks were framed by blond curls, and said, "After you trace the car, then cut it out." His blank expression turned into a baffled look, so I changed the directions. "First, trace the picture of the car. Second, cut."

His blue pencil whirled around the automobile. Then he placed the scissors on his hand and snipped in the air. "I'm cutting the sky," he said with glee.

- **Reword directions if children do not understand or respond.**

I pointed to the *Lion King* book and said, "There are two pictures here. Look at this picture first. Then look at the second one. Look for what is different or missing."

Four-year-old Wendy stared at the page, wrinkling her forehead. Because she looked puzzled, I added, "Find one that is not there. See the bird in this picture?" She nodded. "Now look here. It's gone. There's no bird. What else do you see on this page but not that page?"

She studied the pages with Simba the lion and pointed to a monkey sitting in a tree. "You're right. The monkey is on this page but not on this other page."

"I have a Simba pillowcase and book. I'm collecting Simba."

- **Have children complete the sentence regarding directions instead of answering a question.**

In his preschool classroom, Damien finished coloring the dog with green, yellow, and brown stripes.

"It's a rainbow dog," I said. "What do you have to do next?" He shrugged his shoulders. "You just finished coloring. The next step is to…."

"Cut," Damien said.

- **Show a sample of the finished activity, describe the steps, and then restate the first step.**

Holding a sample, the preschool teacher said, "Today we get to make a reindeer. We will trace your foot for the head, trace your hands for the antlers, add two buttons for the eyes, and glue a curled red pipe cleaner for the nose. So, the first step is to draw around your foot. Do you have any questions?"

"Can we take them home today?" Stan asked.

"Yes."

Fern said, "You know what? I like reindeers."

"I like Santa," Stan said. "He brings presents."

Connect Directions to What Is Familiar

It is easier for children to understand directions when you explain using familiar terms or concepts. One familiar routine that they learn at an early age is to count. Therefore, one strategy is to incorporate numbers into the directions and hold up the corresponding number of fingers. You may start by holding up your index finger and saying, "Number one," and then giving the first step. A second strategy is to use their body as a reference when saying the instructions. A third idea is to weave in familiar objects or actions as part of your explanation of what to do. This makes it easy for them to grasp what you mean. A fourth strategy is to link the directions to their current experiences.

Fabulous Five: Use What Is Familiar When Providing Directions

- **Help children remember by alerting them to the number of steps before giving the directions.**

"You get to make your own terrarium. There are three steps," I said to the 6 year old as I held up corresponding number of fingers. "First, fill the container with dirt. Second, put the plant cutting in the soil and pat it. Third, water your plant."

Tess's nose brushed against the spider plant. "They should call this a tickle plant," she chuckled.

- **Connect the directions to a familiar action.**

"This is a hole puncher. You slide it on the paper and push the button. It's like pushing one of your Hot Wheels cars. Drive it onto the paper."

"Zoom, zoom, zoom," 4-year-old Peter sputtered as he slid the star punch on the purple paper.

- **Relate directions to a body part.**

Three-year-old Tammy held the train wind-up toy with her left hand. Then she turned the knob away from her body, but the train stood still. "I can't," she said, looking to me for help.

"You can do it. Turn toward your tummy."

She made three twists of the knob, and the train tooled along the floor.

- **Link the direction to the children's current experience.**

As we walked down the school hallway, 7-year-old Heather stopped and hugged three friends. She sashayed into our room and squeezed a rubber toy, whose eyes and ears popped out with the pressure. "He's sad," she said, leaning back in her chair and sliding her blue-framed glasses higher on her nose.

"Give him more hugs with your hand," I said, and she resumed squeezing.

- **Refer to objects in the children's lives when giving directions.**

"Today you get to make your own book." I placed three scissors on the table, and the preschoolers slipped them on their fingers. "Wait a minute. First put the scissors back on the table." Three soft thuds echoed as the scissors hit the table. I handed them yellow paper and demonstrated. "The first step is to fold the paper in half. Fold it this way so it's like a hamburger bun." Then I demonstrated folding the paper lengthwise. "If you fold it this way, it's like a hot dog bun."

"Like this, Dr. Clare?" 4-year-old Felicity asked.

"Yes. The next step is to cut on the line."

"I can't see the line very well. I'm not good at cutting on the line."

I used a pencil to trace the line made by the fold, and she snipped across the page.

"Now what do I do?" Ian asked.

"Draw a picture on each page, and then we will staple them together to make your own special book."

Add Movement and/or Touch to Verbal Directions

You need to discover children's learning style before you give directions for an activity. Some learn best through listening, others by doing or seeing. For many, it is easier to follow directions if they are presented in a multisensory manner. This means combining verbal steps with other senses such as touch or movement. For example, you may provide hand-over-hand assistance and take them through the motions as you describe what to do. This allows them to feel the movement needed to start the activity and understand what they are supposed to do. You also may give extra tactile cues to increase comprehension.

Fabulous Five: Add Movement and/or Touch to Verbal Directions

- **Move children's bodies through the motion while giving the directions.**

"We're going to make an 'E' in this salt," I told the four preschoolers. "Let me show your finger how to make the letter, and then you can do it by yourself. Point your finger." I guided Sophie's index finger so she could feel how to make the letter. "Go straight down. Jump up and then make three lines going this way. Your turn," I said, watching as her finger glided in the salt.

After drawing the letter three times, she drew a circle with two dots and a smile. "What do you think? It's me."

"Oh, beautiful," I responded.

- **Use hand-over-hand assistance to demonstrate one step.**

I placed a pipe cleaner in 4-year-old Marisol's left hand and a wooden bead shaped like a horse in her right hand. With my hand over hers, I said, "Push," and guided the pipe cleaner through the bead's hole. Then I handed Marisol a bead shaped like a cow, and she continued stringing on her own.

- **Use hand-over-hand assistance to show a sequence of steps.**

"Look, I have dinosaurs," I said to 4-year-old Tanner, who was nonverbal. I pointed to the cookie cutters and added, "I know you like dinosaurs. Let me show you what to do."

I gently placed my hand on top of his and pushed down on a ball of putty. "Push, make it flat." Then I asked, "Which one do you want?" When he pointed to the T-Rex, I put it in his palm. With hand-over-hand assistance, we pressed the cookie cutter into the putty. "Push again."

I peeled away the putty along the outside edges of the cookie cutter. Guiding his hand, I helped him lift it up. "You did it. You made a T-Rex."

He smiled back at me.

- **Use hand-over-hand assistance to demonstrate the required motion.**

Gently placing my hand over 3-year-old Gene's, I moved our hands above a plastic toy. Pushing down one figure made another one pop up. "Goodbye," I said as we pushed a blue figure down. "Hello," I said when a red one came up. After practicing for a minute, I removed my hand.

Gene began pushing one figure after another while I continued to say the words.

- **Match verbal directions with tactile cues.**

"Today everyone in your class is making a snowman," I said to the preschooler with limited vision. I placed a paper with three circles made with puff paint in front of Pete. "I'm going to touch your hand for 1 minute so I can show you what to do." I gently guided his fingers to feel the raised lines. "Color your snowman. Color inside the circles. Next to your other hand are scented markers."

He chose the yellow marker, sniffed, and said, "Lemon. I like lemon."

Pair Verbal Directions With Visual Cues

Another way to make directions multisensory is to add visual cues when telling children what they need to do. Objects can be used as a cue for the activity. For instance, when children are handed a ball, most will understand that they are to throw it. Demonstrated directions paired with words help children visualize what is entailed. Likewise, use of pictures assists them in seeing and remembering directions. Incorporating numbers helps to organize the steps and delineate the order. Discover what type of directions work best for them and adjust your approach to match.

Fabulous Five: Pair Verbal Directions With Visual Cues

- **Use objects and picture cues when giving the directions.**

  The physical education teacher showed the two 11 year olds pictures of throwing and catching a ball. "Today we are going to play ball. You have to throw and catch the ball."

  Jordan stood in the gym, repeatedly flicking his shirt with his left hand. His classmate, Kent, paced back and forth.

  The teacher handed Jordan the ball as a cue to start. "Throw the ball to Kent."

  Jordan threw it and began tapping his chin. Kent threw it back, but Jordan stood without trying to catch.

  The teacher again placed the ball in Jordan's hand. "Throw the ball."

  Jordan half-dropped and half-threw it toward Kent.

- **Demonstrate when giving verbal directions.**

  "Push here," I said as I pressed the plastic man in the car. The toy sprinted across the floor. "You do it."

  Three-year-old Pedro waddled over, squatted down, and tapped the toy.

  "Push hard," I cued him, making a downward motion with my hand.

  He tried again, and the car zoomed to the other side of the room.

  "Go, car. Go. Oh, oh. He ran out of gas. Push the man again."

- **Draw a picture while saying the steps.**

  Eight-year-old Evan tended to reverse the capital "N" in his last name. I watched him as he drew the first line of the letter correctly, but then he stopped. "The first line is right," I said. "Now jump up to the top of the line. Then go down and across. It's like a slide." I made an "N" and drew a boy swishing down the diagonal line of the letter. "You will know your 'N' is right if the boy can slide down."

  "Oh, I get it," he said with a smile.

- **Use picture cues for each step.**

  "Here are pictures of what you are supposed to do," I told the preschoolers as I pointed to three picture cues at the top of the page. "What is this picture of?"

  "Crayons."

  "Yes, first you color. Then what?"

  Looking at the next picture of scissors, they said, "Cut."

  "And then what?" I asked, pointing to the picture of a glue bottle.

  "Glue."

  "That's right. To make your picture, you color this cute whale, cut out his body and tail, and glue the pieces on the blue paper."

- **Attach numbers to pictures or baskets of activities.**

  When 5-year-old Gabe walked into his specialized classroom, he went to his visual schedule. Next to his name was a pictures symbol of a workbasket. He removed the picture, walked to a table, and attached it to a corresponding one.

  He removed a strip with the number 1 and attached it to the basket with the same number. Gabe took a file folder out of the basket, opened it, and pulled laminated butterflies off the Velcro strip. He then attached each one to the same colored butterfly on the folder.

Assist Children in Learning and Recognizing Their Strategies for Following Directions

Children might be thinking:
I have a good idea.
I know what I can do.
I tell myself….
I'm proud of myself.
I tell my brain, "You're in control."

To be successful in school and at home, children need to be able to understand, remember, and follow multiple directions. For many of those who have difficulty doing so, you can teach them to use cognitive cues. Eliciting or emphasizing their successful strategies can increase awareness. Having them talk about their ideas in a group also allows children to help each other.

Teach Cognitive Cues to Remember Directions

You can help children to learn easier ways to remember directions. One method is to use cognitive cues, which entails having children tell themselves to use a memory strategy. One such strategy is to repeat the directions to themselves. Another is to avoid waiting and do the steps right away. Drawing a picture of the directions or using their fingers that correspond to each step is also useful. In addition, you can collaborate with them in creating a strategy book of the exact words they will use in their self-talk. The use of cognitive cues can be especially beneficial for children who have difficulty with memory or processing information.

Fabulous Five: Teach Children to Use Cognitive Cues

- **Teach children to repeat directions to themselves before taking action.**

Five-year-old Willie wrapped his fist around the animal tongs. To demonstrate the activity, I clicked the ends of another pair of tongs and said, "Put your thumb on one side and your fingers on the other side."

He fixed his fingers; grasped a small, knobby ball; and released it into a blue container. Then he shifted and returned to holding the tongs with his fist.

"How can you help yourself remember the directions?"

"I've got it memorized now," he muttered, switching to the right way. However, as he reached for the third ball, he covered the tongs with his palm.

"One way to remember directions is to repeat them to yourself until you are finished. You can say, 'Use my thumb. Use my thumb....'"

"Use my thumb," he echoed to himself, sliding his fingers into the correct position.

- **Urge children to do the task right away and avoid waiting after directions are given.**

"Put your math papers in your red folders and then take out your spelling words," the third-grade teacher said. Instead of doing what he was asked, Dean tugged on his ear lobe as he dallied.

"Follow your teacher's directions right way," I cued him. "Tell yourself, 'Do it now.' That way you will not forget what you are supposed to do."

He mumbled to himself, "Do it right away. Do it now."

- **Encourage children to draw a picture to help them remember directions.**

"Here's one idea you can use in class," the speech-language pathologist said to the group of second graders. "To help remember directions, draw a picture of what to do. So if your teacher tells you to open the book and turn to page 37, draw a picture of a book and write 37 inside."

"Oh, I get it," Joey said, nodding.

- **Suggest that children use their fingers to help them remember.**

"Listen. You have to color, cut, and then glue the hot air balloon on the paper. How many steps are in these directions?

"Three," 7-year-old Dylan said.

"Use your fingers to remember." I demonstrated by holding up three fingers. "You have three things to do. Color, cut, and then glue."

- **Create a strategy book containing the needed cognitive cues.**

"You get to make your very own strategy book. Strategies are ideas about how to help yourself. What can you tell yourself when you cut?" I asked. "I'll write down what you say. When I cut...."

"Look at the paper," 6-year-old Brandon said. "Watch where I am cutting."

"Hold the paper and scissors with my thumbs up," I added.

"Tell my brain to go slow. Take my time," Brandon said.

"Cut straight and turn the paper."

"And cut on the lines."

Elicit Children's Strategies for Following Directions

When children become more cognizant of helpful strategies, they are more likely to use them. By eliciting children's own ideas for being able to follow directions, you can promote their self-confidence. Explore with children what they can do to enhance their comprehension, memory, and follow-through when they are given directions. Give them a situation and ask what they could do to help themselves. You also can create a situation requiring them to follow detailed directions and talk about any strategies they used. Another way is to pretend you are a child and ask them to tell you what to do. While engaged in activities, call attention to the children's helpful ideas and highlight their creative solutions.

Fabulous Five: Elicit Children's Strategies for Following Directions

- **Ask, "What do you do when you do not understand the directions?"**

In our therapy session, I asked 8-year-old Ella, "What do you do when you do not understand the directions?"

"Sometimes I look at it for a while so I can get the groove of what I'm doing. If I'm reading, sometimes I sound out the word. Sometimes I don't pay attention. If my brain is wacko, I bounce on my specials teacher's ball."

"What do you tell yourself?"

"Okay. I have to work. No distraction. Nothing scary behind me. Everything is quiet and okay."

"Let's think about what else you can do if you do not understand the directions."

"Hmm." She put the tip of her index finger under her chin. "I could ask for help or reread the directions. Mmm. I could ask for the directions to be read and ask friends for help." She paused and then added, "If I come to a long word, I can skip it and then go back and picture what they're saying."

"Those sound like good ideas."

- **Create a situation to elicit strategies for following directions.**

"What is a direction?" the speech-language pathologist asked in our joint therapy group.

"It's when you listen so you can learn," 6-year-old Cecilia replied.

"Teacher tells you something you need to know or do," Chip added.

"We have fun ways to follow directions today," I said. "Look at me and listen carefully, and only do what the direction says." Three pairs of eyes lifted and rested on my face. "There are two pictures. Everyone point to the clown's front. Now point to the clown's back." Three fingers tapped the pictures. "That's right. Now color the buttons purple on the clown's back."

When they raised their heads and looked at me for the next direction, the speech-language pathologist said, "I see you using a good strategy. It helps you if you look at the person who is giving the directions."

- **Pretend to be the child and ask for ideas on what to do to remember directions.**

"In your class, I am having a hard time remembering the directions. What can I do?"

"You can say it in your mind without talking," 11-year-old Ellen replied.

- **Acknowledge children's creative solutions for following directions.**

"Today we are playing a new game," the preschool teacher said, placing four numbered mats on the floor. "When you jump, say the number on the mat."

Three-year-old Anna had a tumor on her foot and could not walk. She watched as the others jumped. Then it came to her turn. She crawled onto the first mat, lifted both arms, and said, "One," as she hit the number.

"What a great idea," I said. "You're jumping with your hands."

She proceeded down the row looking pleased to be participating with her peers.

- **Point out a strategy children used to remember the directions.**

"Go from dot three to four to five," the speech-language pathologist said in our group of first graders.

"Three to four," Jackie repeated until her dots were connected.

"You used a strategy to remember the directions."

"How did her remember the directions?" Hal asked.

"How did she remember the directions?" the speech-language pathologist said. "Jackie kept saying the words until she finished. When I go to the grocery store, sometimes I say what I need to myself so I remember."

"My mom just writes a list."

"That's another great strategy. You can use that one in school too. It may help you remember if you write the directions down."

Help Children Get Started

For children to begin, they have to be aware of their choices and make a decision about what to do. They also need to have the desire to face a challenge and find the activities enticing. Offer the children captivating choices and provide assistance with decision making if necessary. Then help them discover what the just-right challenge is for them.

Call Attention to an Activity, Toy, or Object

Children might be thinking:
Oh, what's that?
I like that.

Some children, especially those functioning well behind their peers, may need extra cues to attend to an activity, toy, or object. Many tend to wander around the room and sometimes will only fixate on a favorite object or motion. To get children engaged, you first have to capture their attention and get them to focus on the activity, toy, or object. One way to do this is to put their hand on it, and often their eyes will follow. You can also use sounds or music. Adding sound effects to an object may gain their interest. Another way is to incorporate the element of surprise, such as using toys where things appear and disappear. Also captivating are cause-and-effect toys in which children's actions results in movement of the object.

Fabulous Five: Call Attention to an Activity, Toy, or Object

- **Place the children's hand on the object.**

"Hi, horse," I said as I gently took 3-year-old Amanda's hand and patted the wooden puzzle piece. I guided her fingers to the small knob on it, and she pulled the piece out.

"Hi, kitty," I said, pointing to the next piece. Amanda pulled the kitten out and continued to remove the other animal pieces.

- **Use sounds or music to gain interest.**

"Aa-ee," 5-year-old Randy repeated as he banged two blocks together. I brought over a toy xylophone and quickly switched a wooden stick for the block in his hand. With my hand over his, we tapped the toy, hitting different musical notes. I removed my hand, and he made music.

- **Add sound effects.**

"Zoom, zoom," I said as I released a plastic car down a ramp. Three-year-old Travis turned his head toward me and came over. I handed him the car, and he placed it on top of the ramp. I continued to make sound effects as he played with it.

- **Incorporate surprise.**

I gently placed 3-year-old Al's hand on the knob of the jack-in-the-box and began turning it. The music played until—POP—the clown jumped up.

Al pushed the clown down, and I helped close the lid. He turned the knob and repeated the sequence.

- **Use toys or activities that incorporate movement.**

Four-year-old Wesley wandered around the room. To get him involved in an activity, I brought over a toy giraffe that was activated by a switch. I pushed the button and the giraffe moved his head to the table. "Look, he's eating."

I put my hand over his and pressed the button one time. The giraffe moved again. "More, please," I said as I made the corresponding sign.

He pressed the button and smiled as the giraffe's head went up and down.

Use Enticing Activities to Get Children Started

> **Children might be thinking:**
> *I want to do that.*
> *I like toys.*
> *I like that a lot.*

One way to get younger children started is to use enticing activities. You can pique their interest by incorporating their favorite toy or object. Playing with a toy in front of them and showing excitement can also capture their interest. Another approach is to point to friends who are having fun. Often if they see their friends enjoying themselves, children will want to participate too. You also can coax them to start by putting toys and/or activities next to them so they can see their choices and do not need to move. Be sure to pick toys and/or activities that children can do independently. That way, once they are engaged, they will experience success and will want to continue.

Fabulous Five: Use Enticing Activities to Get Children Started

- **Incorporate a favorite toy or object into the activity.**

At the beginning of class, 4-year-old Vaughn grabbed a miniature toy train and carried it with him. Later, he still had it when he sat down at the table in the arts center with me. To get him to practice prewriting shapes, I said, "I see you have your favorite train. Let's make a train track for it." I handed him a box of markers and tapped the paper on the table.

He picked a brown marker.

"Make a line this way," I said as I moved my finger across the page.

He made two horizontal lines and, with cueing, made multiple vertical strokes, completing the track. When done, I wound up the train and placed it on the track. Vaughn smiled as it chugged across the paper.

- **Play with a toy in front of the children to get them started.**

In 3-year-old Denise's first therapy group, I brought over a toy and sat down next to her. I pushed one button and a rabbit popped up. I turned the next knob and a puppy appeared. She watched me as a couple more animals popped up. Then she reached for the toy.

- **Show excitement when demonstrating a toy or activity.**

Three-year-old Brock rolled on the floor in the art center. "Brock, I have cars!" I said with excitement as I pointed to car molds. "You love cars. Are you ready?"

He came over to the table and replied, "Ready."

I demonstrated pushing the putty into the mold, saying, "Squish, squash."

"Push, push," Brock said.

"Let's get it out. It's magic. It turned into a car."

Together we carefully pulled, and Brock held it in his hand. "I got car."

"You do. This is fun. Make another one."

He reached for different colored putty and placed it in the mold.

- **Point to a friend having fun.**

Four-year-old Evan sat on the floor in the middle of the center. I waited a few minutes, but seeing that he was not moving, I pointed and said, "What do you want to do? There's the water table. Look at Cameron. He's having a good time playing in the water. Or you can build a train track or play with the farmhouse. You have lots of choices."

Evan thought for a minute and then walked to the water table.

- **Put two choices in front of the children.**

On 3-year-old Sawyer's second day in the therapy group, I guided him to sit between my outstretched legs. He leaned back against me, and I put two toys in his lap. When he touched the steering wheel on a plastic car dashboard, I moved the other toy away. "You want to play with the car. Drive us to the store."

He turned the steering wheel right and left and smiled when he pressed the horn and it beeped.

Assist Children in Making Decision About the Activities

> **Children might be thinking:**
> *What's this?*
> *I'm not sure what I want to do.*
> *I know what I want.*

To be partners, children need to make decisions. For some, it is easy to make a definitive choice. They clearly know what they like or want. Others may be uncertain. When that occurs, explore what is holding them back from making a decision. Consider that they might like all their choices and cannot just pick one. Check if the choices or materials look enticing. It also may be hard for them to choose when they are not sure what each activity entails. Look for signs that they are overwhelmed by too many choices or are questioning their ability. Keep in mind that some need more time to process what you are saying and to think about their options.

To take the first step, you may need to use picture cues or show them their choices. For others it may be better to talk with them and use questions to guide their decisions. Be sure to allow enough time to decide, and address any doubts that they may have.

> ### *Fabulous Five: Provide Children With Choices of Activities*
>
> - **Use picture cues for activity decision making.**
>
> Eight-year-old Cameron jumped up and down while clapping his hands with mounting intensity.
>
> "Cameron, look," I said, pointing to the picture symbols of a puzzle, Play-Doh, and paint. His eyes scanned the three pictures, and he briefly touched the puzzle card. In response, I quickly took out the car puzzle and put it on the table. Seeing it, Cameron sat down.
>
> - **Show children their choices of activities.**
>
> When I went into the hospital room, I put three wood kits on the sliding tray. Ten-year-old Troy sat up, fluffed his pillow, and pulled the tray closer to him. "I brought three choices. You can do a coat rack, toy car, or key rack. If you don't want to do these, let me know and I can get something else."
>
> "I want to do the car," he replied.
>
> - **Use guiding questions to help make the first activity decision.**
>
> Seven-year-old Dustin looked at nine stamps that made different shapes and touched each one. "I have a hard time making decisions."
>
> "First think about who you want to make the valentine for," I said.
>
> He looked at the Winnie the Pooh stamp and said, "Rebecca. I'll make it for Rebecca. She likes Winnie the Pooh."
>
> "Who's Rebecca?"
>
> "My mom's friend."
>
> - **Allow children time to make activity decisions.**
>
> The certified occupational therapy assistant placed the red, purple, green, and blue bingo dabbers upright on the tray attached to the wheelchair and spread them 6 inches apart. "Take your hand and knock over the one you want to use. I know you can do it," she directed, moving Peter's hand to each marker so he could feel how far he would have to move for each choice.
>
> Peter sat still for 2 minutes. Then his shaky right hand moved toward the markers. He hit the purple one, and one second later his hand swung to the left and knocked down the red one.
>
> "I'm not 100% sure you want the purple one." The certified occupational therapy assistant moved the red and purple dabbers to opposite ends of the tray. Seeing Peter's head drop to rest his chin on his chest, she added, "Hold you head up so I can tell what you're saying. Use your eyes

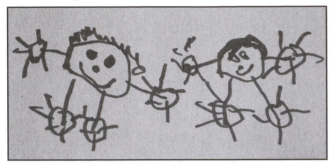

Figure 14-2. Discover what activities make children happy.

too and look at the color you want. Tell me again which one you want to use. Show me with your hand."

Thirty seconds passed, and then Peter pushed the purple marker.

- **Address children's doubts when they are making a decision.**

I pulled four samples out of the craft closet and spread them on the table. There was a small wooden car, a copper tooling design, a leather wristband, and a ceramic mug. "What do you want to make first?" I asked 11-year-old Eli. He examined each activity with his eyes, spending the most time staring at the wristband. When he did not say anything, I said, "Do you want to make a wristband?"

"It looks hard."

"I'll help you," I reassured him. "We'll be partners. We'll make it together."

Incorporate the Fun Factor

> **Children might be thinking:**
> *I like all of these.*
> *I like having fun.*
> *This is a good challenge.*
> *I thought this was going to be hard, but it was really easy and fun.*

The fun factor is an essential element of an educational experience. Children are more likely to become engaged and stay motivated when they consider an activity fun (Figure 14-2). They also are more apt to face a challenge and take risks if they think they are only playing.

To intermingle fun with challenge, find ways for children to experience the pleasurable feeling of success. Build on their strengths, emphasize their talents, and encourage creativity. Realize that children, like adults, highly value personal achievements that are reached without anyone's help. Also recognize that the just-right challenge is rewarding. You will find that some experience fun during the process of the activity. Others, following the completion of an activity, may associate fun with achievement.

Fabulous Five: Weave the Fun Factor Into a Challenge

- **Create a situation or do an activity where children experience success, especially with something new.**

Six-year-old Roy wanted to try the game Perfection. Ordinarily the game requires placing all the pieces in the correct spaces and beating a timer before the board pops up. To ensure success, I said, "Put all the pieces in and then turn the timer on to make them fly."

Roy took his time figuring out the correct placement for each shape. Next, he turned the timer on and grinned when the board popped up, spraying his pieces all over the floor. "Let's do that again," he said.

- **Promote creativity.**

"You can snap these pieces together and make fun monsters."

"Let's see, I have to make the mommy," 4-year-old Madeline said as she pushed the parts together. "I need to make the head. Oh look, this one is the baby. I'm doing good creations."

- **Realize that independent success is fun.**

Four-year-old Mary connected two plastic triangle-shaped pieces together. "I made a diamond. I made it by myself." She added two more pieces. "I'm making a kite. I made it myself. This is fun."

- **Recognize that an achievable test of their skills can be enticing.**

Flipping through a book of mazes, 8-year-old Dominic stopped at a page with pirates and a treasure chest in the middle of the maze. "I want to try this one. It looks hard. I like challenging things."

- **Be aware that a good challenge may be fun.**

Les completed a 10-piece multicolored wooden snake, smiled, and said, "This is a good puzzle."

"Is it fun?"

"Yeah. This is a GOOD puzzle. It's a hard one."

Create a Desire to Do a Difficult Activity

> **Children might be thinking:**
> *I'm not sure I can do this.*
> *Thanks for giving me time to think.*
> *I want to try that.*

The level of challenge children choose is dependent on a number of factors. It is important to realize that saving face and looking good to others is major part of their risk/benefit ratio. They may wonder if the risk is worth it. Also, consider that their past experience will color how they view a new activity. Another factor influencing their desire for challenge is how they feel that day. If they are upset, they may want something familiar and calming rather than taking a chance on something new.

There are many ways to make a difficult activity enticing. One is to present the activity as an option. Children are then free to choose, which also allows them to save face if they think it is too hard. A possible variation is to mention that the activity or toy is really for older children and ask if they would like to try it. What is implied is that if they are able to do it, they are better than children their own age, and if they fail, it can be attributed to the fact that it was really for older children. Further strategies are to have children compete with you, ask them to help you, or use phrases such as, "See if you can…" to motivate them to try.

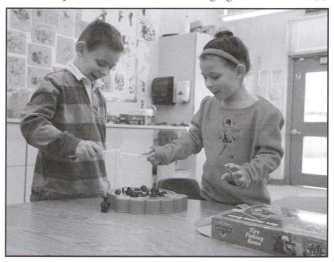

Figure 14-3. Use fun games as part of therapy.

Fabulous Five: Present a Challenge

- **Identify the activity as being difficult and offer it as a choice.**

"Do you want to try something challenging? I have a really tricky game," I asked the third grader.

"Yeah," Jay replied. Using a toy catapult, he sent plastic monkeys sailing into the air and hoped they would land on the brown tree branches. All of the monkeys missed.

"They should call this game Frustration because it's pretty hard," I said.

After 20 tries, Jay finally aimed and landed a monkey on the tree.

"You did it. That's great you didn't give up."

- **Tell children the activity or toy is really for older children but they can try it.**

"This toy is really for older children. You can try it if you want."

Seven-year-old Chris's eyes widened as he eagerly grabbed the spinning toy from me.

- **Have children compete with you.**

Because I knew 6-year-old Kim and Jesse could not remember how to make many of the letters and were reluctant to practice them, I said, "Hey, go to the board. I have an idea for a game." They scooted to the board and turned around. "I'll tell you a letter, and you have to write it. You can help each other. If you both get it right, you get a point, but if the two of you miss, I get a point."

I called out a letter. Each time they did it correctly, they jumped up and down and gloated, "We got a point. We got more than you."

- **Present a challenge as if the children are helping you and doing you a favor.**

I put a top that needed to be assembled on the table. "My friend gave this to me last night. I've never done this, so you'll have to help me figure this out," I told the third graders as I pulled out the directions. "What do you think we are supposed to do first?"

"Put the blue piece on," Bob replied.

"Okay, Bob, you go first. Then, Jarrod, you can put the next piece on."

- **Tell children, "See if you can…."**

Six-year-old Libby straddled a one-legged stool and struggled to keep her balance. As she started to get the feel of staying upright, I handed her a Koosh ball. "See if you can throw this in the coffee can three times in a row."

Make Therapy Fun

Children's lives are geared to having fun. By making therapy enjoyable, they will want to participate (Figure 14-3). One role children like is to be in charge and to dictate what happens. Toys, puppets, and games are desirable because they are familiar ways to play and are automatically associated with fun. Surprises or mysteries are intriguing. The opportunity to win can bring out playful competitiveness. Making gifts, having parties, and celebrating holidays can also be fun.

Incorporate Toys, Puppets, and Games

Children might be thinking:
I love toys and games.
Are we going to play together?
I'm excited.

Toys, puppets, and games are associated with play and hold a universal appeal to children, whereas activities that appear like schoolwork tend to be viewed as serious work and not always fun. Whenever possible, make these items an integral part of therapy. Go to toy stores, thrift shops, and yard sales and think outside the box on how they may be used. One time I found an old-fashioned potato masher. The children were delighted to use it to squish putty and had to use their shoulder muscles to press hard enough. Children also used it to push the putty into the plastic container, which made cleanup fun. Novelty creates interest, so be sure to rotate which toys or games you use. Toy figures or puppets can transform a bland activity into a fun one. In addition, creating a play theme around ordinary items is intriguing.

Fabulous Five: Include Play Objects or Theme

- **Use toys in therapy.**

"What's this?" the second grader asked, looking at a clown on a sting attached to two sticks.

"It's Flying Fred, and he does all kinds of awesome tricks," I replied. "Put your hand on these sticks and squeeze. That makes Fred move, and it makes your hand strong. It's really fun."

"Oh look, he's standing upside-down. Look, now he's doing the splits. I like him doing tricks. I'm getting strong. This is fun."

- **Play games.**

"This game is called Thin Ice. Use the tongs to pick the marbles out of the water. Then put the wet marble on the tissue," I said to 7-year-old Herman, pointing to a tissue stretched tight on a base. "You don't want to break it because then you lose."

"Hi, little marble. I'm doing it safe so the tissue won't break," Herman said. After a few more rounds, he added, "I think it's going to go soon. It might be you. Your turn."

"Not me," I said as I made a successful move.

"Don't be me. Oh no, it's breaking," he shouted as we heard the clanking of marbles hitting the table. "This is a fun time! This is a fun game. I like it when you put them on top and it breaks. Can we play this game again?"

- **Use a toy figure or puppet.**

I brought five animal tongs, a bag of spongy miniature balls, a bowl, and a stuffed animal made to resemble the character Clifford. A group of children gathered around me, including the student who needed to improve her hand strength. We sat on the alphabet carpet, and I said, "Clifford is hungry. Feed him."

The children began using the tongs. "Here you go, puppy," one said.

"Have some more," another child chimed in.

"Yum, yum," I said as I made the dog pretend to eat. At the end of the activity, I said as the puppy, "Thanks for the food. Now I'm going to sleep." Each child hugged the stuffed animal and said goodbye.

- **Incorporate current television or movie characters into the activity.**

Following Cameron's third birthday, he loved singing the birthday song. His favorite television character was Scooby-Doo. One day he ran over to the cupboard and pulled out Legos.

"Let's make a birthday cake for you. What color should we use?" I asked.

"White." He snapped 10 Legos together to make the pretend cake, and I added a small dog figurine on top.

"Look, it's a Scooby-Doo cake. Let's sing 'Happy Birthday' and then blow out the candles."

He danced with excitement as he sang and then blew.

- **Weave pretend play into the activity.**

I put my fingers around a tennis ball that had a slit for a mouth and two dots for eyes. "Hi. I am a ghost, and you know what?"

"What?" 6-year-old Gina replied.

"I eat pennies. You have to put your thumb next to my mouth and push. It'll help make your hand stronger," I said as I demonstrated.

"Hi, Mr. Tennis Ball Ghost. How are you?" She began plunking pennies in the slit. "Mr. Ghost is hungry, so I'm feeding him. See how much he ate. No more. He's full."

Include Novelty, Mystery, or the Unexpected

Children might be thinking:
I like good surprises.
That's new.
You make me laugh.
That was fun.
Let's do it again.

Children are intrigued when you introduce the elements of mystery or surprise into an activity. Their curiosity is piqued by the allure of the unknown matched with the anticipation of something good happening. Incorporating novel objects or activities is also enticing. Rotating them or adding an interesting twist captures their attention. Other ways to create a sense of fun are to incorporate unexpected actions, the unusual use of objects, or magic tricks.

Fabulous Five: Weave in Mystery, the Unexpected, or a Surprise

- **Use ordinary objects in an unusual way.**

The week of Halloween, I brought an old shoebox with a hole on the side. I whispered to the children, "This is a mystery box. You have to put your hand in the hole, find an object, and feel it. Without looking, guess what it is and then write it on your paper."

"I wish I had x-ray vision," 7-year-old Stewart said as he slid his hand into the box. "Oh no, it's squishy."

"That's a body part. What do you think it is?"

"An eye?"

"You're close."

"A nose," he said, then pulled out the slimy flesh-colored object. "I was right."

- **Create an intriguing story.**

I placed an empty bottle on the table.

"What's this? What's this for?" 9-year-old Cassandra asked as she pulled the bottle toward her and sniffed. "It smells like peppermint."

"This is a really fun writing activity," I said. "Some people go to the ocean and put a message in a bottle and throw it into the sea. Sometimes the bottle turns up in Europe. Today we are going to pretend to send a message to children in another country. Write about your life so whoever finds it can know about you."

Cassandra then wrote the following: *Hi. I am 9 and I have blond hair and blue eyes. I am a girl. I have a bird named Tweety. I go to school from 8:10 to 3:00. Then I do homework. I have fish, a bird and a lepord gecko. I like to read and draw and write storys and play games. I like parakeets, dogs, cats, fish and sharks. I go to Oklahoma for the summer. We go to vist our grama and grampa and our nanna and Harly and Jeffy the dog. I mit go to Texas and vist there. Sincerely, Cassandra.*

She drew her parakeet. Then she folded the paper, rolled her message into a tight wad, and wrapped a rubber band around it. She smiled and stuffed the paper in the bottle.

- **Add an unexpected action.**

Holding tongs, 8-year-old Paula grabbed small bunny erasers and dropped them in a bowl. She made the target four times in a row. "This is easy," she said.

I put my hand on the bowl, and just as she was about to drop one bunny, I moved the bowl. "Hey," she laughed.

"I am just making it harder," I said with a chuckle. She picked up another eraser, and I kept moving the bowl in a figure-8. We both laughed as she aimed for the moving target but missed.

- **Use an out-of-the-ordinary approach.**

I handed paper and Popsicle sticks to the two boisterous boys who liked to talk more than write. "Everyone gets a page. Write 'yes' on one paper and 'no' on the other. Then glue them to the Popsicle sticks to make signs."

"Why are we making signs? Is it sign language?" Tim asked, adjusting the glasses hanging on the tip of his nose.

"These are your special answer sticks. When I ask you a question, raise one of the signs. Okay. Everyone write two sentences."

The boys wrote and then shouted, "We're done."

"Now we're going to check your work. Does the first word in your sentence start with a capital letter?" Two *yes* signs appeared. "Did you put a period at the end of your sentence?" Again *yes* signs waved in the air. "Are all your tall letters tall and all your short letters short?"

Hank checked, fixed a small "t," then waved a *yes* sign. "Now it's a yes."

- **Call the activity magic.**

"I have something fun to show you. It's like magic. Do you know how to do magic?" I placed a pink piece of paper on the template and rubbed a blue crayon over the paper and a giraffe appeared. "Try it and make a magic show."

"I can't wait to do this," 6-year-old Jason replied.

Ask Children to Be in Charge

Children might be thinking:
This is great.
I like this.
I like telling everyone what to do.
I like being the teacher.
This is going to be fun.

Children consider it really fun to be able to tell adults what to do. One way to make the activity pleasurable is to have them take charge and direct you regarding what they want to happen. Asking them to be a teacher also allows them to be in charge and accentuates their competence.

Another avenue for children to experience fun is to have free rein in creating the experience. Promote independence in creating their own materials and/or devising their own game. Giving a name to their creations is also gratifying.

Fabulous Five: Have the Children Be in Charge

- **Have children be the teacher.**

"Here is the game you wanted," I said as I pulled out a wooden maze. Seven-year-old Rick had finally mastered how to turn and move each knob that controlled the various parts of the maze.

Chris, a staff member, walked by and said, "What is this?"

"Rick, teach her how to do it."

Rick smiled. "Start here. Tap this knob soft."

Chris followed his direction, and the ball moved to the next step.

"Good job," Rick said. "Now turn this knob. Take the ball through the tunnel. Visualize where you are."

Chris maneuvered the ball through that section.

"You're doing good so far, Chris," Rick said. "Hit this one, but not so hard."

Chris pushed the knob with her index finger. The ball flew and hit the bell, indicating success.

"There you go," Rick said proudly, and I chuckled to myself hearing Rick say many of the phrases I had once said to him.

- **Ask children to create a name for the activity or game.**

The two boys were playing with a red ball on a string that was attached to a bleach bottle cut in half. Tim tried swinging the ball and catching it in the bottle. He caught the ball with every try. Then he tried swinging the ball backward.

"What do you call that?" I asked.

"I call this a dipsy move."

- **Have children tell you what to do.**

Three-year-old Bonnie grabbed the blue Play-Doh. "Help me, Dr. Clare."

"What do you want me to do?"

"Make me a puppy."

"Okay." I made the dog's body and then said, "Here, you do the legs. Roll the Play-Doh in your hands like this." We each added parts, and when it was done, I pretended to be the dog and said, "Hi, Bonnie." She smiled.

- **Encourage children to create their own game.**

"Look around the room. Go ahead and make your own game," I said to 10-year-old Omar.

He spotted a small balance board. "I could stand on this and throw bean bags at the target." He stepped on the board and rocked back and forth. "I'm surfing. I have an idea. It will be two points if the beanbag goes in the hole and only one point if it just hits the target. No points if I miss."

"At what number will you win?"

"Twenty."

"Sounds like a fun and challenging game."

- **Promote thinking about objects in various ways.**

After the two 8-year-old girls squeezed stress balls, I asked, "What else could we do with these that would be fun?"

"Let's throw these squishy balls to each other at the same time. One. Two. Three. Throw."

The two girls tossed their balls and laughed as they tried to keep up with the flying balls.

Provide Opportunities to Win

> **Children might be thinking:**
> *I love to win.*
> *Yea, I beat you.*
> *Let's do more. Let's do this again.*
> *Let's try another game.*

The experience of winning is pleasurable and engenders feelings of success and a sense of accomplishment. When children are the first to finish a race or strategic game, the implication is that they are better or smarter than the other players. The motivation to surpass another is strong when there is a prize or trophy. From children's perspectives, winning is the best.

Fabulous Five: Create a Chance to Win

- **Have a race.**

I placed butcher paper on the easel, and the children drew roads using different-colored chalk. At the beginning of the road, I wrote a letter, and the kindergartners wrote the same letter at the endpoint. Then we put the paper on the floor and lined up five wind-up toys.

"On your mark, get set, go." The wind-up toys began clicking down the roads. One toy in the shape of smacking lips veered to the right and touched a boy's pants. The boy jumped back 2 feet in pretend disgust, and the group laughed.

- **Make the activity a guessing game in which the children know the right answer.**

"Make something and we will guess what it is," I said to 8-year-old Melissa. She molded clay into a shape. "Is it a bird?" I guessed.

"Nope," she replied, smiling.

"Is it a penguin?" another child asked, and Melissa nodded.

- **Let the children beat you.**

At the end of recess, I went out to the playground and found the two second graders, Gwen and Todd. "I'll race you to the door," I challenged them. They sprinted across the field, and I moved slowly. "You won," I said.

"Yeah. You were as slow as a turtle," Gwen said.

- **Have prizes for winning.**

"Today we have a fun game, and there are even prizes. Everyone will get a prize, but the winner gets first pick. There's enough for all of you. We're going to play bingo with letters. When I call out the letter, you have to write it, and then you can put a chip covering that letter on your card. Whoever gets a complete row of letters wins."

"What's the prize?" the 6 year olds shouted.

"I have special pencils. I think you will really like them."

- **Find something in which the children can be a champion.**

In the oncology clinic, we had an ongoing game of Connect Four. Although I really tried to win, 12-year-old Theresa consistently found ways to place four chips in a row before me. Each time she won, she laughed with delight.

Make Gifts, Have Parties, or Celebrate Holidays

> **Children might be thinking:**
> *I love parties.*
> *I like making gifts.*

Children learn that making gifts for others is always appreciated. They discover that it is fun to anticipate the person's happy response and often talk about how the person is going to love the present. It also becomes rewarding when the person smiles and expresses gratitude. Making a surprise gift can create more excitement, although younger children have a harder time keeping it a secret. Many children are used to having birthday parties and equate having a party with a good time. When culturally appropriate, it is also fun to have parties and celebrate holidays. Be sensitive to family beliefs and religious practices.

Fabulous Five: Make Gifts or Have Parties

- **Make cards.**

"I'm making a card for my dad. I'm using his favorite color, blue," 5-year-old Joel said. "I'm making the sky, clouds, and snowflakes. I'm going to do the corners and make it look fancy. My dad lived in another place. I don't know the name of the state. Do you want me to give you a hint?"

"Sure," the occupational therapy student said.

"That girl holds it like this," he said as he raised his right hand.

"Oh, it's the Statue of Liberty. Your dad lived in New York."

- **Make a surprise gift for another person.**

"Do you want to make a surprise for Linda, our secretary? It's her birthday," I asked the second graders, and they all nodded. "What should we make her? I have paper, stickers, and markers for a card, a book, or a picture. Or if you can think of something else and I can get the supplies, we can do that."

"A book. We want to do a book," they said, bouncing in their chairs with excitement.

- **Prepare and have a small party.**

In the first week of November, I announced, "We're going to have a Thanksgiving party, but first we have to get ready. This week we'll make our placemats." The four second graders wove their brown and yellow mats, which were later laminated. The next week they made paper turkeys and printed their "I am thankful for…" lists.

On the day of the party, the children scurried in with excitement. They sat down by their placemats and stared at the cookies, frosting, and sprinkles. "Let's go around and say what you are thankful for, then you can decorate your cookies."

"I'm thankful for my bird, Mommy and Daddy, and my baby fish," Tonia said.

"I'm thankful for my family, my friend Maddie, and nice teachers."

- **Create a special event.**

"Let's make a treasure hunt for Stacey," I said, referring to a staff member.

"Yeah," the group replied. They cut out and made books in the shape of treasure chests and wrote the four clues in them. They hid the present in the bookcase and ran down the hall to get Stacey. "We have a treasure hunt for you," they said with glee.

Stacey came into the room and followed the clues.

"You're getting hot. You're getting cold," they shouted. The children jumped up and down in their chairs as they watched Stacey get closer, and they cheered when she found the prize.

- **Do activities related to holidays.**

At Christmas time, I handed 4-year-old Shiloh a Christmas tree spinner. "Pump this."

As he pumped the knob with his thumb, the tree spun open. Santa appeared, and Shiloh smiled.

Be Fair When Setting Up Activities

From an early age, children have a strong sense of justice. They are cognizant of the degree of fairness or inequality in situations affecting them. They have a keen awareness of who has more or who gets to go first and will remember this information. The children also want fairness regarding waiting time. They do not want to wait longer than anyone else.

When you work with a group of children, you must be conscientious about how you treat each child. Be careful that your actions do not favor one child over another. They are very perceptive when one is receiving more attention or benefits. They usually notice who gets to go first the most and how many turns each person has had. Avoid showing favoritism. Make it a practice to be fair.

Show Fairness and Be Equal

> **Children might be thinking:**
> *I won't get a turn.*
> *They got more than me. I might not get one.*

One way to treat children fairly is to make sure you divide your attention equally among them and especially include quiet or shy ones. Plan activities in a way that allows them to have equal materials, equal time, and equal turns. Promise that everyone will get a turn, and make sure that it happens.

Fabulous Five: Be Equal

- **Give equal time or opportunity to each group member.**

"What do you think we should do today? Color or cut the scarecrows?"

"Color," 7-year-old Wayne said, and immediately started talking about his fun weekend.

"What do you think?" I asked the other two boys.

"Color."

Wayne resumed talking. After a few minutes, I said to Jared and Jose, "I want to hear about your weekends too."

"Me and my sister got new bikes," Jared replied. "She got a big one and I got a little one. It came from a man from an office."

"What color is your bike?"

"Black."

"Jose, tell me about your weekend."

"I went to Michigan. My dad is in Michigan. That's why I'm happy."

"Sounds like everyone had a great weekend."

- **Provide equal attention.**

The first graders were drawing pictures to hang on my new bulletin board. Kris drew an astronaut using red, blue, purple, and green crayons. "Kris, your picture is very colorful."

"Look at mine," Mia said.

"Mia, you have a lot of detail in yours. It'll be so nice to have both pictures on my board," I responded.

- **State that everyone will get a turn.**

"This is a vibrating squiggle pen. It's really fun. Everyone will get a turn. Draw a picture," I told the preschoolers, and I gave stress balls to the children who had to wait.

"Whoa," Sue Ellen shrieked as the pen bounced in her hand. "My hand is getting dizzy."

"Hold it like a pencil," I cued her.

"Now I get it. That's my head, my eyes, my happy mouth, my stomach, my legs, and my foot. There, that's me. Come off."

"Flip the switch to turn it off and then pass it to Mark."

- **Make sure all group members get a turn.**

At the end of our session, I told 9-year-old Tina, "We're out of time, and I know you did not get a turn. So next time, you get to go first. Be sure to remind me because sometimes I forget." She nodded.

The next time we met, Tina announced as she walked in the doorway, "I get to go first."

"You're right."

- **Divide materials by counting so children can see that they each have the same number.**

"Me Ramon," he told me when I walked into his specialized class and sat at his table.

"Hi, Ramon," I replied.

"Me bigger. I'm a big boy."

"Oh, you're growing and getting taller."

"Animals. That one. I want," he said, looking at my animal-shaped tongs.

"Do you want the giraffe, hippo, lion, or elephant?" I asked him. He choose the giraffe, and I offered the other tongs to the rest of the group. To make it fair, I divvied up the animal erasers and counted so everyone could see that they received the same number. Content, they started the game.

When done, Ramon said, "More, more, more."

"You want to play again?" I asked, and he nodded.

Decide in a Fair Way Which Child Will Go First

> **Children might be thinking:**
> *I want to go first.*
> *They got to go first last time.*

You will want to be fair in deciding who will go first or have the first choice. One approach to help a group settle is to have whoever is the quietest go first. You can even use this as an opportunity to include children who are nonverbal because they are often quiet. Other methods are to alternate who goes first or, in a larger group, to have the person who was last automatically go first in the next activity. You also can set up the activity to allow more than one child the chance to have first pick. A possible variation is to ask the group for ideas on how to decide who goes first. If they do not have any suggestions, teach them ways to decide that involve luck, such as tossing a coin or the rock, paper, scissors game. Once children have strategies, you can ask them to decide among themselves.

Fabulous Five: Determine Who Will Go First

- **Start with the person acting the best and go around in a circle.**

I put colorful building blocks on the floor and said to the group of first graders, "We are going to build a group project. Everyone will get a turn. Whoever is the quietest will go first."

As the group settled, I turned to Hector, who could only speak through communication devices. "Hector is the quietest. Which one do you want us to start with?" I held a different-colored block in each hand. "Do you want red or blue? Look at the one you want."

His eyes shifted to my left hand.

"I see you looking at the blue one."

Then we went around the circle, and each person took a turn. When the structure was completed, the boys beamed with pride.

"Let's do another one," they shouted, and Hector's body shook in agreement.

- **Alternate who goes first or have the child who was previously last have the first turn.**

"Because you were last yesterday, you get to go first this time," I said to 5-year-old George.

"My brother always lets me go last." As he picked a toy, he continued, "Mommy won't let me buy the house with my money. The houses around here are expensive."

- **Divvy up first pick.**

I handed 5-year-old Darren the larger board because he tended to write large letters. "Hey, he got the big board the last time," Pete protested.

I slid the box containing four different colors of markers to Pete and said, "Then you get first pick of the markers." Appeased, he grabbed the purple one and began drawing.

- **Teach a strategy involving luck for deciding who goes first.**

"Dr. Clare, I want to go first," 4-year-old Mary said.

"You two decide who gets to be first." When they could not agree, I said, "Let me teach you one way to work it out. It's called rock, paper, scissors. We say, 'One, two, three,' and then make your hand into a rock." I made a fist. "Or keep your fingers straight to make paper or cut with your fingers to make scissors. Scissors cuts paper, paper covers rock, and rock flattens scissors."

From then on, they used this strategy to decide.

- **Ask the group to decide who goes first.**

"Who should go first?" I asked.

"I want to go first," 7-year-old Fallon said.

"No, me," Fiona yelled.

"How can we work this out?" I asked, raising my palms in the air.

"Hmm, you could pick a number between 1 and 10, and whoever is closest gets to go first," Fallon said, and Fiona nodded in agreement.

"Sounds like a good solution."

Help Children Take Turns

> **Children might be thinking:**
> *I might not get one.*
> *I won't get a turn.*
> *They got more turns than me.*
> *I want to play with this longer.*
> *I don't like sharing.*

There are a number of ways to facilitate orderly turn-taking. You may use a prop as a signal. For instance, you may tell children that whoever is holding the toy microphone is the one who gets to talk. Going around in a circle lets children see when their turn is coming. This method is predictable and appears fair. You can use a timer to establish equal time per person. Also, encourage them to negotiate and figure out a fair way for turn taking.

Fabulous Five: Take Turns in the Group Activity

- **Use props to indicate whose turn it is.**

"What strategies have you learned that make it easier for you to get your work done?" I asked the group of third graders. "When you get the microphone, tell us your idea."

I handed Drew a toy microphone. "Look at your neighbor if you are not sure what to do," he said, then passed the microphone to Seth. I wrote down all their ideas: Sit up strong, not slumpy. If too much is on your desk, clean it off. Stretch. Move your pencil away if you keep playing with it. Stretch out words with your fingers and brain.

"Thanks, everyone. These are great ideas. I'll share them with the other groups too."

- **Go in a circle so children can see when their turn is coming.**

"When is it my turn?" 4-year-old Amber asked, looking at the tiger-shaped stress ball.

"First Corky, then Christian, then you," I said, pointing to each one in the circle. "Everyone squeeze the tiger six times, then pass it to the next person."

I started to count, and Corky said, "I want to count. "One. Two. Three. Four. Five. Six," and handed the ball to Christian.

"Annie, you're next. I like it when we share. That way everyone gets to play."

- **Use a timer for turn-taking.**

"Let me have some," 6-year-old Walt said.

"No," Tad yelled, encircling the new toy and pulling it toward him.

"What can you do so you both get a turn?" I asked.

"We can use a timer," Walt suggested, grabbing a gel timer off my desk.

- **Have children negotiate with each other for a turn.**

"Dr. Clare, I want a turn," 4-year-old Caitlin said.

"Did you ask Keegan?"

"No," she replied, then turned to him. "Keegan, I want a turn."

"Let me do one more, then I'll give it to you."

- **Assist the group in finding solutions for turn-taking.**

"I want to play the I Spy game," 11-year-old Greg said.

"But I want to do the treasure hunt game," Luke replied.

"How can you two work it out?" I asked.

"We don't know," they responded, shrugging their shoulders.

I grabbed a piece of paper, wrote the number one, and asked, "What are some solutions?"

"We play my game this time and his game next time," Greg said.

"Okay, that's one idea. What's another solution?" I asked as I wrote the number two.

"We spend half the time on one game and the rest on the other," Luke chimed in.

I wrote the number three. "We could play another game," Luke added.

"I want number one," Greg said. "I want to play my game today."

"If you pick that one, you will both still have to decide which one to play," I replied.

"Let's do number two then," Greg said, and Luke agreed. "I have a watch. We'll do 15 minutes for mine and 15 for his."

"Sounds like you worked out a good plan."

KEY POINTS TO REMEMBER

- Create learning experiences with the elements of challenge and fun.
- Identify children's needs and then determine whether to see them individually or in a group.
- Involve children in determining what activity to do.

- Discuss what children's notion of fun is and what a just-right challenge is.
- Prepare children if the activity is difficult or takes a long time.
- Obtain children's attention before giving directions.
- Keep directions simple and use words they understand.
- Maintain children's attention by being animated and playful when stating directions.
- Pair verbal directions with visual cues, movement, or touch to increase understanding.
- Identify strategies for remembering directions.
- Help children get started by capturing their attention, using enticing and fun activities, helping them make a decision, and creating a desire to face a challenge.
- Make therapy fun using toys, puppets, and games and incorporate the elements of novelty, mystery, or the unexpected.
- Make therapy enjoyable by letting children be teachers, providing opportunities to win, making gifts, having parties, and/or celebrating holidays.
- Be fair when setting up activities and determining who goes first.

REVIEW QUESTIONS

1. Name five ways you can structure a small group.
2. Young children will expect to finish a project in one session. True or false.
3. Children will persist at an activity if the challenge factor is just right for their abilities. True or false.
4. Why do children like challenges?
5. What children consider as fun varies among individuals. True or false.
6. You do not need children's attention before giving directions. True or false.
7. If children are ignoring you when you give directions, it may be because they do not understand the words you are using. True or false.
8. Name five ways to call young children's attention to an activity, toy, or object.
9. Children who are nonverbal can make decisions about their activities. True or false.
10. Children are not aware when group members get more materials or turns. True or false.

Help Children Face Challenges

CHAPTER OVERVIEW

This chapter is a continuation of the discussion of the fourth dimension of the collaborative frame: working with children to co-create educational experiences that are challenging and fun. Children in therapy have often failed in the past and as a result may be hesitant to try challenging activities. I describe ways to get them to take the first step, continue their efforts, deal with mistakes, and not give up. There also are additional strategies for when children have to wait and for providing inconspicuous assistance, thus allowing children to save face.

CHILDREN'S DESCRIPTIONS OF WHAT THEY THINK YOU SHOULD KNOW

Dr. Clare: "How can therapists convince children to try something hard or new?"

Kurt (age 12): "Make them feel comfortable, tell them they can do it, and compliment them."

Sally (age 11): "Tell them, 'If you do this, we can play a game afterwards.'"

Cora (age 9): "Tell them, 'Try it once, and if you don't like it, you don't have to do it.'"

Torrie (age 8): "Say, 'Try it and see if you like it or not.'"

Megan (age 9): "Tell them to try new things and practice."

Dr. Clare: "How can therapists help children stay with a hard activity?"

Melissa (age 9): "Tell them, 'Never give up.'"

Corbin (age 10): "My mom and dad say, 'Calm down, take your time, and go step by step.'"

Scott (age 11): "Tell them, 'Don't give up what you start or you'll always be giving up.'"

Ken (age 10): "I like a really easy thing in the beginning and then a real challenging thing at the end."

Dr. Clare: "When it was hard, what made you stay with it?"

Ken: "Because it was fun."

ASSIST CHILDREN TO GET STARTED, CONTINUE, AND NOT GIVE UP

Facing challenges can be risky. Often you will need to provide support and encouragement to help children start, continue, and not quit. With each child, there is a discovery process regarding the just-right level of support. There is a fine line between helping and taking over. Too much help implies you do not believe they have the ability. Too little help can result in failure.

Curtin, C.
Strategies for Collaborating With Children: Creating Partnerships in Occupational Therapy and Research (pp. 301-323).
© 2017 SLACK Incorporated.

Encourage Hesitant Children

Children may hesitate to start for a host of reasons. They may lack confidence in their abilities, be afraid of failing, or worry about being embarrassed, especially if others are watching. Others may have high expectations and believe they have to be perfect. On the other hand, some have low expectations of what they can do. They cannot picture themselves being successful.

It is important in these situations to examine children's beliefs about themselves, especially their self-talk. Help them to consider that they may actually be able to do the activity by stopping any negative self-talk and adjusting their expectations. You may want to offer help to build confidence. When children are anxious, you can also provide verbal prompts to encourage them to begin.

Address Self-Confidence

> **Children might be thinking:**
> *I'm not so sure I can do this.*
> *You want me to do this? Are you kidding?*
> *I wonder if I can do this.*

The messages children tell themselves affect their motivation to try something new and stay with it. If they have experienced failure in the past and attributed it to being their fault, they will most likely convince themselves not to even try. When they continually replay the "I can't do this" message in their head, they develop a defeatist attitude. Because they think they will be unsuccessful, they tend to believe, consciously or unconsciously, that it is better not to even try. In their eyes, what is the point of taking a chance when they can only envision disappointment?

Make it part of your practice to discover and address children's beliefs. Recognize helpful self-talk, and assist them in changing any negative messages by saying, "Listen to what you are telling yourself." Then provide alternative statements that they can say to themselves. For some, you may want to challenge their beliefs by telling them that they really do not know the outcome until they have tried. Offer encouragement by saying, "Give yourself a chance to try...."

> ### Fabulous Five: Address Children's Beliefs About Their Abilities
> - **Point out helpful messages the children say to themselves.**
>
>   "I'm going to keep doing this till I get it," 5-year-old Gerald said.
>
>   "Good for you. It really helps when you say those words to yourself."
>
> - **Say, "Listen to what you are telling yourself" if children make negative comments about themselves.**
>
>   As I started to draw a maze on the board, 6-year-old George whispered to himself, "This is hard. I can't do this."
>
>   "George, listen to what you are telling yourself. You are telling yourself you cannot do it before you have even tried. It's like riding a bike. It takes practice. Do you think it helps if you keep saying, 'I can't do this'?"
>
>   "No."
>
>   "Tell yourself, 'I can do this if I try.'"
>
>   The next week, George came to the table, looked at the writing activity, and blurted, "This is hard." Two seconds later, he said, "I mean, I can do this if I try." He glanced up, smiled at me, and said, "I caught myself."
>
>   "That is so good."
>
> - **Point out to children when they have a habit of saying they cannot do something but, when they try, they actually can do it.**
>
>   Five-year-old Steve surveyed the carpet covered with plastic eggs. Using tongs, he gathered all the eggs and brought them to the table.
>
>   "Okay, open the egg, take the paper out, and write the letter that's on the paper," I said.
>
>   He folded his arms, sank in his chair, and said, "I hate writing. I can't do this."
>
>   "Just try it," I replied. He opened one and copied the letter. I said softly, "I wonder what letter you will get next?" He continued. At the end of the session, a staff member walked past us. I waved to her and said, "Hey, Linda. Come look at this writing."
>
>   "Wow," Linda said.
>
>   "Yeah, look how good this is. You know it's puzzling." I wrinkled my brow and raised my arms. "Whenever I ask Steve to write, he says he can't do it and that he hates it. Yet look how good he can write."
>
>   Steve looked at Linda and smiled proudly.
>
> - **Ask children how they know they cannot do the activity if they have not tried.**
>
>   Five-year-old Janice looked at the game of balancing wooden blocks and said, "I can't."
>
>   "How do you know you can't do it if you haven't tried?" I challenged her. "Tell yourself, 'I can do it.'"
>
>   A surprised look popped on her face, and she took her turn.
>
> - **Tell children to give themselves a chance.**
>
>   At the children's hospital, 11-year-old Ruben was learning from the dietician how to plan meals. He picked a recipe from the American Diabetes Association cookbook and came to the kitchen in the occupational therapy department to prepare the meal. He turned on the stove,

but then looked at me and said, "I've changed my mind. I don't want to do this."

"You can do this. I know you are just learning how to cook. Give yourself a chance to learn, especially while I can help you."

With a little more encouragement, he started. When the lunch was finished, he went back to the unit and told the staff he had a fine lunch.

Show That You Will Help

> **Children might be thinking:**
> *Oh, I don't know.*
> *Is it hard? Is it fun?*
> *Will you really help me?*
> *You really think I can do this?*
> *Maybe I'll try if you will help me.*

Some children are too worried or fearful to get started. They may think the activity looks too hard and have self-doubts. You can help them take the first step by showing that you will work with them. Your actions will demonstrate your support. Some do better if you start the activity. Then you can ask them to join you or take turns. If children want your assistance, reassure them that you will pitch in if needed. You may want to tell them you will watch them try and only help if they require it. Continually convey your belief in them.

> ### *Fabulous Five: Be Supportive When Children Hesitate*
>
> - **Start the step and ask children to help you or to finish it.**
>
> "Let's make a pizza," I said. Seeing 6-year-old Scott's hesitant look, I started by flattening the putty on the table with my palm and pinching the edges. "What do you like on your pizza?"
>
> "Pepperoni," he said.
>
> "Will you help me?" I asked, and he nodded. I handed him a ball of putty. "First roll this putty into a snake, and then use the scissors to cut it into small pieces for the pepperoni. Then you can squish the pepperoni like I did and put it on the pizza."
>
> He squeezed the putty in his right palm and then started rolling it.
>
> - **Take turns.**
>
> "Let's try making this," I said, pointing to a picture of a dog.
>
> "I can't," 3-year-old Rod said.

"Just look at the picture and find the piece to match. We can take turns. I'll start." I picked up a rectangle shape and put it on the base for the leg. "Find one just like this for the other leg." We continued taking turns until it was finished. "What is the dog's name?"

"Patches," Rod said with a smile.

- **Provide reassurance that you will help if needed.**

Four-year-old Madeline stared at the stencil of a fox. "Will you help me, Dr. Clare?"

"I will show you what to do. Then I want you to try it on your own first. If you need help, I will help you."

- **State your belief that the children can do the activity.**

Three-year-old Pauline tried pushing the upside-down puzzle piece into place without success.

"I can't," she shouted after only one attempt.

"Yes, you can," I said in a reassuring tone of voice, rotating the wooden puzzle piece upright but off to the side of the hole. "Try again."

This time she slid the piece into place and smiled.

- **Tell children you will watch them try and you will be there for assistance.**

"Help me, Dr. Clare," 4-year-old Justin said, holding up two plastic parts.

"Let me see you try it. I'll watch you. If you need me, I'm here."

He pinched the yellow peg tightly and tried to push it through the hole. After about 10 seconds of struggling, the peg popped in place. "I did it," Justin said, sounding surprised.

"You did do it. You didn't need my help."

Nudge Hesitant Children to Take the First Step

> **Children might be thinking:**
> *I can't do this.*
> *This looks hard.*
> *I might make a mistake and look stupid.*
> *No way.*
> *I don't know....*
> *These look boring.*
> *I don't like those.*
> *I can't decide.*

There are times when you will need to nudge children to take the first step. You can give them a push to begin by offering words of encouragement, promoting realistic expectations, and suggesting strategies. Sometimes it only takes a little nudging for them to try.

Use Words That Encourage Trying

Some children need words of encouragement to get them to try a new or difficult-looking activity. Telling them to "just try" or "try one" is one of the best ways to get them started. Avoid saying, "Can you…" because they most likely will say, "No," and stop. Let them know that they may like it if they give themselves a chance to try. Similarly, tell them they may like the activity after they have practiced and are more successful at it. Others will often try if they know something fun will follow, such as playing a game. It also helps others to know that if they try and do not like it, they will not be pressured to continue.

Fabulous Five: Use Words That Encourage Trying

- **Say, "Just try" or "Just try one."**

Eight-year-old Sara took one look at the cursive letter "a" and put her head down on the table.

"I brought salt to practice in. Just draw the 'a' once in this salt tray." I moved the salt in front of her.

She raised her head and said, "I can't."

"Watch me." I made the letter with my finger. "Just try one," I encouraged her.

She slowly placed her finger in the salt and tried to make the letter.

- **Say, "Try it and see if you like it or not."**

"We are making shapes out of shaving cream," the preschool teacher told the class. She went to the tables and put one squirt in front of each child.

Three-year-old Colt stared at it without moving. His classmates placed their palms on the table and began spreading the shaving cream.

"Try it and see if you like it," I encouraged him.

He gingerly put his index finger in it and slowly moved it around.

- **Tell children, "Try something new and practice. You may find out it is fun."**

Ten-year-old Dawn looked her choices of different crafts. Usually she only liked to color posters, but this time she stared at the leather wristband.

Responding to her hesitant look, I said, "I see you thinking about that. Try something new and practice. You may find out it's fun."

When she agreed, I gave her a scrap piece of leather to practice. A few minutes later, she reached for her wristband and stamped her name surrounded by miniature hearts.

- **Say, "If you do this, we can play a game afterward."**

To entice 4-year-old Sean to attempt a cutting activity, I said, "First try making this whale picture, then we can play a game."

"What did you bring?"

"It's a fishing game. You have to catch fish while they are moving and their mouths open and close. But first do the picture and then we will play the game."

He picked up the scissors and began cutting.

- **Tell children, "Try once, and if you don't like it, you don't have to do it."**

"Today we get to make fish out of cinnamon roll dough. After we make them, we get to eat them!" the special education teacher said.

I helped 6-year-old Jessie roll his wheelchair to the table. Knowing he was hesitant to touch different textures, I said, "Just try making one. Then if you don't like it, you don't have to do any more."

I rolled the dough into a snake, and with just his fingertips, he crossed the ends, making the fish shape. As I placed it on the wax paper, I said, "You did it. You made your own fish."

Offer Ideas That Will Help Hesitant Children Get Started

One way to get children started is to offer helpful strategies. You can emphasize that they do not have to be perfect; they just have to try their best. Another way to help them along is to suggest they try an easy method first and make it harder later. If they look overwhelmed or distracted, ask what the first step is. This can help them focus and limits their thinking about all the steps involved. Some may do better if they stop and visualize themselves being successful before trying. Others may begin if you enlist the help of the group to discover alternative and positive thoughts.

Fabulous Five: Offer Ideas That Will Help Children Get Started

- **Tell children they do not have to be perfect; they just have to try their best.**

"We're going to make rainbow letters," I told 4-year-old Collin. I printed his name with large letters. "Pick a marker and trace over the letters. Then do it again with another color."

"I can't," he said, grabbing my hand to put on his. "You do it."

"Collin, you can do it without my help. Just try your best. It doesn't have to be perfect."

He hesitated for a minute, but then reluctantly tried.

- **Suggest to children to try an easy way first and then try a harder way or activity.**

Four-year-old Samantha lifted the plastic monkeys out of the barrel. She held one and connected the next monkey by its arm. Then she put it down and connected two more.

"Do it the easy way one more time. Then try it a more challenging way. Keep hooking them by holding on to the top monkey and make one really long chain," I suggested.

She started hooking three together. "This challenging way is hard. Oh no, they fell."

"I know it's challenging."

She hooked four together. "Oh, I got it!" she said with a pleased look.

- **Ask children, "What do you do first?" or "What is the first step?"**

"Write your name and the date on the top of the paper," I said.

"I'm having a bad dream today. Someone pinch me and wake me up," 8-year-old Patrick said. "Fine, I'll pinch myself. Now I'm really waked-up."

"I'm glad you're awake now. So what's your first step?"

"My name." He hung his pencil over the edge of the desk and tapped it until it flung in the air. He caught the pencil, then settled down to write.

- **Have the children visualize themselves successfully completing the activity.**

"Before you try writing this letter, visualize yourself making it just like I did. Close your eyes. Picture yourself making this letter."

After concentrating with his eyes shut, 8-year-old Max wrote the letter with success. "I think cursive is like the letters are holding hands."

"That's a nice way to think about it. Make sure there is a space between them so they have room to breathe."

- **Ask other children in the group how they get themselves to try something new or hard.**

"I can't do this," 9-year-old Mel shouted as he looked at the writing project.

"I know it looks hard," I said, then turned to Lenny. "How do you get yourself to try new things?"

"I just tell myself, 'I'm going to do this.' And I do it. That's how I learned new tricks on my bike."

Promote Continued Effort and Attention

When children face a challenge, they often encounter a moment when they question if they can finish or succeed. At this juncture, they may become distracted, start rushing, or talk about quitting. Help children get over this hurdle by providing encouragement and strategies for regaining their focus and sustaining their effort.

Assist With Waiting

> **Children might be thinking:**
> *Hurry up!*
> *I'm bored.*
> *I want to do this now. I don't want to wait.*
> *What else can I do?*

One life lesson children have to learn is how to help themselves wait. Encourage them to identify what works for them and then increase their repertoire of strategies. In the group setting, be fair regarding the amount of time each one is required to wait. Make the group successful by minimizing wait time and adapting the activity when needed. It is beneficial to keep the entire group engaged by giving them ideas of something to think about or do. Also, urge indecisive or slow-moving children to go faster when their actions are affecting other group members.

Be Conscientious About Waiting Time

Because waiting tends to be boring, limit the amount of time you ask children to be patient. When planning an activity, think about ways to minimize how long they have to wait. If possible, have all the materials ready and organized so they can begin immediately. You also can ask for a helper to pass out materials. Make it a habit to state your appreciation to anyone who is waiting calmly. It also helps to talk about how hard it is to wait with nothing to do. Reassure group members that you will not forget them and will make sure they get a turn or get what is needed. If you find that the whole group is becoming restless while they wait, incorporate movement.

> ### Fabulous Five: Be Sensitive About Waiting Time
>
> - **Minimize waiting.**
>
> "We're going to make letters in a really fun way!" the occupational therapy student said. She went around the first-grade class, putting dabs of shaving cream on every desk.
>
> Shantelle became bored while waiting and started smearing it all over her desk. By the time the class started to write, her shaving cream had disappeared. "I need more please," she yelled.
>
> - **Recognize children who are waiting patiently.**
>
> I sat on the floor in the center full of blocks and began building a tower.
>
> "Can we help you?" the two preschoolers asked.
>
> "Sure, but we will have to take turns." As one added a block, I frequently said to the other, "You're doing a good job waiting."

When the tower was finished, I said, "Okay, go ahead and knock it down."

The two boys laughed as the tower tumbled to the floor.

- **Acknowledge that waiting can be difficult.**

"Hurry up. You're taking too long. My marker will dry out and I'll have to throw it in the trash," 4-year-old Cecilia complained as Sean passed out papers.

"I know that sometimes it's hard to wait," I said. "Try taking deep breaths until you get your paper."

- **Tell waiting children you will not forget them.**

"What color do you want, Dan?" I asked, fanning out four colors of paper.

"I want blue," Benny blurted as he jumped out of his seat.

"Wait a second. You're next after Dan. I won't forget you," I replied, and Benny sat back in his chair.

- **Give movement breaks to younger children who have been sitting for a long time.**

While I gave directions, the three 6 year olds wiggled in their seats, their shoulders bouncing from side to side. "Before we start, it's time for a stretch break," I announced in response. "Everyone march in place like me." The three stepped in place as if they were in a parade. "Next, everyone put your palms on the table and push down as hard as you can."

"Look how strong I am," Jesse said.

"I see," I said, smiling. "Okay, break is over. Time for our writing project."

Change the Activity or Encourage Children to Go Faster

When one group member cannot make a decision or tends to move in slow motion, nudge the member to take action. Point out how their friends are waiting. You can even use a visual cue such as a timer to set a time limit. If you find that the activity is too hard, make adaptations, such as changing the rules of a game. Or, if the group has to wait too long for one person, change one aspect of the activity to create quicker turn-taking.

Fabulous Five: Ask Children to Go Faster or Adapt the Activity

- **Nudge indecisive children to make a decision.**

Eight-year-old Michelle stared at the game pieces. "Hmm," she sang as she tried to make a decision.

"Hurry up, you're wasting our time," Caleb yelled.

"Pick quick so we have more time to play the game," I said.

- **Tell children who are moving slowly that their friends are waiting.**

"It's really boring here," 6-year-old Chelsea said as she waited for Cameron, who was half-heartedly trying to snag a fish with the magnetic fishing rod.

"You're saying that you're tired of waiting?"

"It's taking so long."

"Cameron, get one. Your friends are waiting. They want a turn too."

- **Use a timer to speed up children who are taking too long.**

"We're waiting," the group said to 7-year-old Kira.

"I can't make up my mind."

"I have a timer. You need to pick before it runs out," I said, flipping over an egg timer.

"Okay, I want the green tongs."

- **Change the rules to limit waiting.**

"The rules say you have to get the number six to start." I read on the box top.

The three preschoolers rolled the dice, waiting to get the right number to start. After two times around the circle with no success and seeing them squirm in their seats, I changed the rules. "Jose, keep rolling the dice until you get the number six."

- **Change the game or activity.**

"Pick up 10 little rabbits, then pass the tongs to the next person," I said.

Four-year-old Morgan wiggled in her chair as she waited and then announced, "I have an idea. Let everyone do just one."

"So you want to change the game?" I asked, and she nodded. "How about everyone does five. That way you don't have to wait so long. You can pick up five rabbits pretty quick."

Give Children Something to Do While Waiting

If a group has to wait too long, they will often become irritated. Some may start to wander around the room. Others may take out their frustration on their peers. To keep children engaged, it is wise to give waiting members something to do. You can provide an idea for them to think about until it is their turn. You also may want to direct them to do simple movements or use pretend play. An additional approach is to suggest or offer another activity to do while waiting. Placing children in the helper role is also effective.

Fabulous Five: Have Children Do Something While Waiting

- **Tell children to think about what they will do when their turn comes.**

"First draw a box, then make a letter 'A' with a white crayon," I told the three preschoolers. When they finished, I added, "The next step is to paint over your letter. You'll see your letter, it's really cool. The paint doesn't stick to the white crayon marks. I only have one paintbrush so you'll have to take turns. It's Christine's turn to go first. Al and Greg, while you are waiting, think about what color of paint you will use when it's your turn."

- **Ask children to do small movements while sitting.**

As I rummaged through the cupboard looking for the game they had requested, I directed the 5 year olds who were sitting at the table, "Wiggle your fingers. Now wiggle your toes. Cross your arms. Now cross your ankles."

They giggled but were sitting still when I returned to them.

- **Have waiting members do a pretend action.**

"It's getting boring," 5-year-old Delany said as she waited for Leila to finish cutting.

"While you are waiting for the next step, here are some pretend marshmallows," I said, motioning toward her. "Put these in your mouth and chew until it's your turn."

Delany puffed out her cheeks and chomped her invisible food.

- **Suggest or give waiting group members another activity to do.**

I handed 7-year-old Cindy a large magnet with silver metal stars. "Try this, it's fun."

"I want to do that," Ester said.

"You'll get a turn too. While you're waiting, here's a martian. Squeeze him with one hand and see if you can make his eyes pop out." After a few minutes, I said, "Time to switch."

Ester passed the martian to Cindy and said, "Do this while you're waiting, and use one hand."

- **Ask waiting children to be helpers.**

"I need something too," 8-year-old Eric said as he waited for his classmate to finish coloring.

I interpreted his statement to mean that he wanted something to do, so I said, "Would you please put these scraps of paper in the trash?"

"Okay," he replied, using the side of his hand to sweep the pieces into the trash can.

"Thanks. You're a great helper."

"Sure. I'm a nice kid."

"You are nice."

Explore What Children Can Do to Help Themselves Wait

When children become impatient while waiting, ask them for ideas on what they could do to help themselves. Another option is to ask the group for any suggestions. If children are unable to figure out a strategy, you can always describe one you use to remain patient. Relaxation techniques such as deep breathing can be used anywhere. Let children know that they can ask if it is possible to get more supplies or do something else.

Fabulous Five: Help Children Identify and Learn Strategies for Waiting

- **Ask children to problem solve how to help themselves wait.**

Carol clutched the sides of her chair and made the chair hop.

"I can see that's it's hard for you to wait," I said to the 8 year old. "What would help you right now?"

"I can get my beanbag pillow and put it on my lap," she said, and went for her weighted lapbag.

- **Ask the group what they can do to help with waiting.**

Seven-year-old Jeremy raced around the room, tapping various objects on the desk.

"Please sit down and wait for me to get the game," I said.

He slid onto the chair but started punching his head with alternating fists as if he were beating a drum.

"Stop. I don't want you to get hurt," I told him with a caring tone of voice.

"Yeah, you could hurt your head," his friend added. "Your brain could stop thinking."

"What can you do to help yourself wait?" I asked the group.

"Put your hands in your pockets," Krista said, who was usually in constant motion.

"I count one to three. That's enough for me," Reba replied.

- **Tell a story of what you do when you have to wait.**

"I hate to go last," 6-year-old Sam said.

"We have to take turns."

"I can't wait much longer. It's been 2 minutes. It has been a long, long time to wait."

"You know what I do when I have to wait? I count how many people are ahead of me. Count to yourself how many people until it's your turn."

- **Tell children to ask if there are any more supplies or if they could do something else while waiting.**

"Don't you know I'm getting really sleepy?" 6-year-old Sergio said, his head rested on his fist.

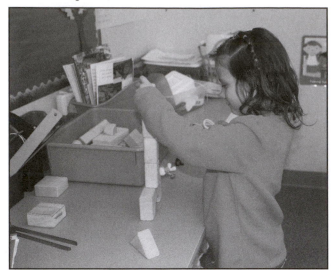

Figure 15-1. Acknowledge children's efforts.

"You have some choices to keep yourself awake while you wait for your turn. You could ask if there are any more or if you could do something else."

"I wait by playing make-up games in my mind," his friend added.

- **Teach relaxation techniques to use while waiting.**

"Hurry up. I don't want to spend my life here," 5-year-old Dee said.

"I have an idea to help with waiting," I said. "Try this. Take a big breath. Now hold your breath. Count to five in your head. Breathe out and relax."

Dee puffed out her cheeks and then blew.

Encourage Children to Continue

Children might be thinking:
I'm tired of this.
It's too much.
I can't do all that.

Once children are engaged in an activity, they often need encouragement to continue. Many respond if you recognize their effort and talk about their successes. The use of supportive sayings and phrases as well as setting a goal can make a difference. Others may need to change their self-deprecating thoughts or be provided with options.

Acknowledge Effort and Recognize Success

One way to prevent them from giving up is to recognize how hard they are trying and mention any successes, even small ones (Figure 15-1). This can be done verbally or with a culturally appropriate gesture. Also, stating your belief in their abilities can be supportive. Validate their accomplishments using detailed and specific feedback instead of general statements. Another strategy is to recognize their unique talents or original discoveries by telling them, "You are the first one I have seen…" and then stating what you have observed.

Fabulous Five: Give Ongoing Encouragement
- **Acknowledge effort and highlight times when children did not give up.**

Using her index finger, 5-year-old Pattie tried to make the toy ants flip into the plastic container shaped like a pair of pants. Twelve times, she missed.

Finally one went in the pants, and I said, "You did great! Even when it was hard, you did not give up. Good for you."

- **Make statements reflecting your belief in them.**

"I hate writing," 5-year-old Deb said at the beginning of the school year.

For the next 3 weeks, she practiced making letters with putty, licorice strings, salt, and aluminum foil. "You are making these letters just right," I frequently commented. After she mastered the 26 lowercase letters, I said, "You'll be so good at writing words."

"I'm getting better at writing. It's getting nice," she responded.

- **Give a nonverbal and culturally appropriate signal of success.**

Seven-year-old Sherrie sanded and stained a wooden mug rack. Then she twisted the first hook in, but it went crooked. "Oh no," she said, unscrewing it. She tried again, this time with success.

Smiling, I gave her a thumbs-up, signaling success.

- **Be impressed with accomplishments or progress.**

To help 8-year-old Darla improve her hand functioning, I gave her two green Chinese medicine balls. "Roll these around in your palm and use your thumb to push them."

With each attempt, a ball fell on the ground. After three tries, she finally developed a rhythm with her thumb. The balls chimed as she rotated them in her palm.

"Wow, you learned that really fast," I said with a smile.

- **Say, "You're the first one to…."**

Six-year-old Peter flattened the red putty on the table and pressed a Halloween plastic figure into the putty. The face of a grinning goblin appeared.

"What a great idea. You're the first one to think of that."

Keep the Challenge at a Just-Right Level

To continue to maintain that just-right level of challenge, you will have to make adjustments. Grade the activity by making changes so that the children can continue to succeed. You can vary the amount of support, the type of materials or utensils, the number of steps, and/or the type of activity. When the activity is at the just-right level, it becomes a rewarding and pleasurable experience. Children are then able to learn about their abilities and are motivated to try more.

Fabulous Five: Maintain the Challenge at the Just-Right Level

- **Monitor and adjust the difficulty level.**

"Throw the ball to me," I said to 7-year-old Sienna. She threw the 3-pound weighted ball, and I tossed it back. It slipped through her outstretched hands.

After three misses and seeing her dejected look, I moved so close I could almost hand it to her. I lightly tossed the ball again, and it landed in her arms. "Good catch," I said, and she smiled.

- **Change the amount of your support.**

"For Halloween you get to make your own jack-o'-lantern," I said to the group of third graders in the specialized class. I handed each child a paper plate and orange tissue paper squares. I set cups of glue and paintbrushes on the table. "Paint the glue on the plates. Then pinch and roll the tissue paper," I said as I demonstrated. "Next use tweezers to put the orange pieces on."

To help Dustin get started, I said, "Let me show you how." I gently placed my hand over his as he held the tweezers. We did the first five pieces together, and when I removed my hand, he continued. He placed 10 more pieces and then dropped the tweezers.

Thinking that his hand might be getting tired, I handed him a wooden clothespin. "This is easier to use. Try this." When he picked it up, I again did hand-over-hand assistance to manipulate it. After two tries, he pinched it on his own and continued until he covered the plate.

Later the class added black eyes, a nose, and a smile. When his teacher came over, Dustin smiled and gave it to her.

"I like your jack-o'-lantern," she said. "Can we hang it up in the class?"

Dustin nodded and pointed to where he wanted it on the wall.

- **Change to a different activity to keep children challenged.**

Seven-year-old Eli swung on the platform swing and pitched beanbags at a tower of cardboard bricks. "Put them back up again," he yelled at me. After knocking them down five more times, he began to look bored.

"Let's make this harder," I said. "I have some targets. Do you want the astronaut or the clown?"

"The astronaut."

I set up the target and said, "Aim carefully and see if you can get the beanbags in his mouth."

Eli resumed swinging. Concentrating, he focused on the target and threw.

- **Match the right number of steps to the children's level.**

Four-year-old Lucy had limited vision and tended to fling anything placed in her hand. One day I brought a large animal puzzle with half-inch wooden knobs attached to each piece. I placed the puzzle on an upright slant board. Sitting next to Lucy, I guided her elbow so that her hand was directly over the knob. "Take it out," I said. She pulled the piece out of the board. I took it and placed it on the table. She then reached for another one.

When all the pieces were out, I handed her one at a time to put back in.

- **Maintain success level.**

Whack. Whack. Three-year-old Lillian hit the plastic ball, and it rolled to the bottom of the toy boat. *Whack. Whack. Whack.* Three balls followed. When none were left on top of the boat, she walked away.

The next day, as soon as she started hammering, I took the balls from the bottom and replaced each one on top of the boat. She continued playing for over 3 minutes.

Use Phrases and Questions to Promote Continuation

The use of certain phrases or questions is helpful to give children the message that they should carry on with whatever they are doing. The phrases, "You're so close," or "You're almost finished," imply that a successful ending is near and it is definitely worthwhile to continue. Like a cheerleader, you can use the phrase, "Keep going," to offer moral support and to encourage children not to give up. Saying, "More, please," and "What are you going to do next?" indicates that more action is needed. Your choice of words can influence children's actions.

Fabulous Five: Incorporate Wording That Encourages Children to Continue

- **Say, "You're so close."**

Janet pushed the head of a plastic frog, and it flipped into the air. The first five frogs went everywhere but the target. With each attempt, I said to the 4 year old, "Oh, you're so close." Finally, one flipped into the target.

"Yes," Janet said as she raised her arms up in victory.

- **Say, "You're almost finished."**

The 8 year old pulled a wooden key rack out of the craft closet. "Madison, the first step is to sand this. Make sure you go the same way as these lines. This is called wood grain. Keep sanding until it is super smooth."

Madison sanded for 1 minute. "I'm done," she said.

I ran my hand over the wood and felt a few rough spots. "You're almost finished. It just needs to be sanded a little more right here."

- **Acknowledge that the children are doing well and say, "Keep going."**

In the first-grade classroom, Chenelle scribbled with wide strokes over the picture of a map.

"Take your time and do your best," I said. She slowed, using smaller strokes and coloring within the lines. Three minutes later, I told her, "Oh, your picture is almost done. I like the colors you used. You are doing well staying in the lines now that you slowed down. Keep going."

Two minutes later, she slid her finished paper toward me and said, "Look how good I colored. I tried my best like you said."

- **Use sign language while saying, "More, please."**

"We're going to make dirt. It's pretend dirt because you can eat it," the teacher said.

Eleven-year-old Julian jumped up with excitement and began tapping his shoulders.

"Aa-ee," 5-year-old Farah screeched, shaking her head side to side.

"I know, it's fun. Keep watching. Ready?" The teacher put four brown cookies in a zipped bag and smashed them with her hand. Everyone squealed with delight. Then she gave each child his or her own bag. "Squish it. Keep smushing it."

I moved Farah's hand to the bag, and she pounded the cookies three times. I used sign language as I said, "More, please." Farah resumed pounding.

"We're going to turn our dirt into mud. It's still pretend," the teacher said. Everyone mixed chocolate pudding. To finish, they filled their cups with pudding, put cookie crumbs on top, and added a candy worm.

- **Ask, "What are you going to do next?"**

Swinging on a platform swing, 9-year-old Travis raised his right arm and aimed for the cardboard brick blocks 2 feet away. His first release of the ball was a direct hit. One by one, he easily hit all eight blocks.

"What are you going to do next?" I asked.

"Move the blocks back," he replied. "That will make it harder."

Use Enticement to Promote Continuation

You can create incentives to continue by highlighting children's competencies and urging them to show off more of their talents. You also may want to suggest that they experiment and see what else they are capable of doing. Another incentive is to identify a goal, made by either you or them. Then challenge them to see if they can achieve it. Because a goal has a set limit of a certain number or certain amount of time, this often appears more attainable than an unknown quantity. Asking children to beat their own record is an additional way to promote interest in continuing an activity.

Fabulous Five: Create Incentives for Continuing

- **Say, "You were so good at... try these."**

Twelve-year-old Greg completed a 2-inch copper tooling of praying hands and gave it to the oncology nurse. "I want to do another one."

I pulled out the more detailed 6-inch molds and said, "You were so good at your last one. Try one of these bigger ones."

He studied his choices and picked the antique car.

- **Ask children to experiment and see how much or how many....**

"I have a timer. Do you want to use it to experiment and see how many beanbags you can get in the target?"

"Yeah," 6-year-old Ezekiel replied.

"How much time should we say?"

"Two minutes."

"Ready, set, go."

- **Provide a goal as enticement to continue.**

When 5-year-old Walter walked in the room, he saw 10 shamrock erasers, bamboo tongs, and a white wicker basket on the table. "Use the tongs to put the shamrocks in here. There's only 10 of them," I said, moving the other 20 erasers to my side.

He pinched the tongs, grasped the shamrock, and released it into the basket. "I did it." On the next one, he lost his grip and dropped the eraser on the floor.

"Try getting the shamrock from your chair. Rescue him," I encouraged him.

He extended the tongs and retrieved it. "I keep saving them."

"You're just like a lifeguard. Would you like to do more?"

He nodded and said, "More erasers, please."

"This time see if you can do 20."

"I bet I can."

- **Have children set a goal.**

"In this game called Perfection, you have to match the piece to the same shape on the board. When the timer goes off, the board pops up. You have to be fast."

I turned on the timer, and 7-year-old Joel reached into a pile, grabbed one, and rushed to put it in the board. *Tick. Tick. Tick.* Four more were placed. *Tick. Ding.* His five pieces flew in the air.

"You put five in. How many do you want to try and get in this time?" I asked.

"Ten," he said, lining the pieces up for easier access.

- **Ask children to beat their record.**

Four-year-old Keri started swinging on the platform swing. Standing on her left side, I handed her a beanbag in the shape of a frog. She grabbed it with her right hand and crossed her midline in the process. "Throw this frog back in the water," I said, pointing to a hoop on the floor.

She threw eight, but only four went in the hoop.

"You got four that time. Try again and beat your record."

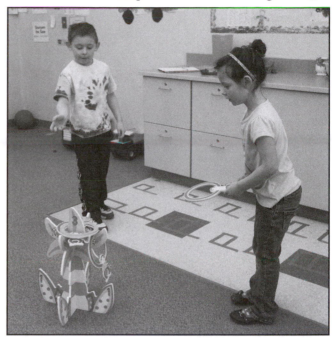

Figure 15-2. Encourage children to keep trying.

Help Children to Not Give Up When Doing an Activity

> **Children might be thinking:**
> *This is too hard. Oh, forget it.*
> *I'll never get done.*
> *I can't do it.*
> *I give up.*
> *I need a break.*
> *Can you help me?*

While doing an activity, watch for signs that the children are about to quit. Continue to listen to their self-talk and observe for frustrated looks. To encourage children to persist, you can help them change their self-talk, make completing the activity appear feasible, or suggest options for dealing with frustration or fear of failure (Figure 15-2).

Change Children's Thinking About Giving Up When Doing an Activity

When children begin to have a pessimistic attitude, challenge their thinking. Help them to change their thoughts in a way that supports their efforts versus focusing on failure or difficulty. One way is to ask what others in their life have told them when they were facing a hard challenge. Another approach is to point out a successful part or aspect of their activity and encourage them to use that as a model. You also may want to highlight the fact that if they did it once, they could do it again. This implies that they have the potential to finish and success is a real possibility. For others, have the children tell themselves, "It just takes practice," or "Just think about the first step." This helps children shift from thinking about quitting to thinking about what they need to do to continue to be effective.

> ### *Fabulous Five: Shift Children's Thoughts About Quitting an Activity*
>
> - **Ask what other people have said when the children are doing something hard.**
>
> "What does your family tell you to do when something is hard?" I asked the group of second graders.
>
> "One time I went snowboarding, and it wasn't as much fun as skiing," Trevor said. "My uncle said you have to try it three times. The first time is awful. The second time is awful. The third time you start to figure it out."
>
> - **Identify one part children did correctly and use it as a model.**
>
> "You just make two hills," I said to the kindergartner as I demonstrated an "m."
>
> Melinda practiced writing the letter in the air and then on aluminum foil. The first letter was right, but then she began to push too hard and the foil ripped. "I can't do this."
>
> "Look at this letter here," I replied. "You did it just right. Make more like this one."
>
> - **Highlight to children that if they did it once, they can do it again.**
>
> Four-year-old Kira held the yellow fishing rod as the snapping magnetic fish circled the toy pond. "Fishies, don't worry. I'll save you." She snagged one and then threw her rod back. "Come on. Get on. I'm trying to get the purple one, and it's not going on."
>
> "You caught one. You'll catch another," I said.
>
> "Oh, I got the purple one." The fish connected but then dropped off her hook. "No, no, no. Get back here. Got you, purple," she said, kissing it.

- **Emphasize that the activity takes practice.**

I pulled out a bag of bendable shapes called Zots and Dots. "Make whatever you want," I said to the group of 7 year olds.

"I can do it," Olivia said. "I learned quickly."

Cassidy bent one piece. "Look, it's an 'L.'" Then she tried to make a circle, but it kept popping open. She grunted, "Nnn. I'm not good at this."

"Keep doing it and you'll learn it," Olivia said

"Tell yourself, 'It takes practice,'" I said.

Cassidy continued and finally made a crown. "I'm a princess. I'm going to look in the mirror."

- **Encourage children to just think about the next step.**

"You get to make your own flip book," I told the group as I held a model. "When you put it together, you can flip through the pages and it makes a movie."

Six-year-old Winston colored one page and then said, "I don't want to do this."

"Does it look like a lot?"

Winston nodded.

"We're not finishing these today. Just think about coloring the pictures today."

Make Completing the Activity Appear Feasible

Sometimes children get overwhelmed and do not always think about what changes they can make. They may tell themselves that the activity is too hard, too long, or too much. Initially you may need to help them start over so they can try again. Another option is to identify one specific action they can take that will make a difference. Teach them to focus on one step at a time versus the whole activity. You may want to relate this lesson to those who climb mountains. Instead of constantly looking at the top, climbers often think only about the next step. To make the activity appear more feasible or achievable, you can say just one step or only show the portion of the work to be completed. The use of a timer is another strategy that lets children know that the amount of effort required is time limited and thus worth continuing.

Fabulous Five: Make Completing the Activity Appear Achievable
- **Help children start over.**

The orange puzzle required getting eight silver balls to nestle in u-shaped crevices. Cupping the puzzle in her palm, 8-year-old Jane guided seven balls into the right places. With only one ball left, she jerked the puzzle and all the balls came loose. "Here, you do it," she said, handing it to me.

"That's frustrating to be so close to getting it. I'll get it back to where you were," I replied.

After three balls were in place, Jane said, "I'll do it now." It took 4 more minutes to finish, and she smiled with her success.

- **Suggest one action to take to make the effort successful.**

I hung a paper on the wall. "This is an alphabet maze. Start at 'a' and go to 'b.' Then keep going."

Six-year-old John rushed and went outside the line. "I keep messing up."

"It's not a race," his classmate answered.

"Go slower and take your time," I said. "Then you will do better."

- **Say only one step at a time so the activity appears achievable to children.**

I handed 3-year-old Carey a picture of a romping Dalmatian puppy outlined with holes. "This is called lacing. It's like sewing." As I demonstrated, I continued, "You go up through one hole and down through the next, then pull the lace tight."

Carey shoved the string down one hole. She stared at the next hole, looking lost. "It's too hard."

"We'll do it together," I reassured her. I started giving one-step directions. "Go up." When she finished that step, I said, "Now go down." She started to go in the wrong direction, so I blocked the space with my finger. "Go the other way."

"I'm lacing," she said with pride.

- **Show only the portion of the activity to be completed.**

Seven-year-old Noah cut out a book in the shape of a whale, and I wrote down the story he dictated. In the next session, I placed his story on the table for him to copy. When he came to therapy, he saw the paper with four lines of writing. His hands flew to his cheeks, and he said, "Not all that."

"I know it looks like a lot, but you just copy the first two lines today," I said, covering the other two lines with a white piece of paper.

- **Tell children you will use a timer to indicate how long to do the activity.**

"Look for the hidden objects in the picture and circle them. Find the chair, house, and squirrel," I said to the preschoolers. They hunted and hurriedly circled.

"Now what, Dr. Clare?" Cecilia said.

"Color the picture."

"Man, my hand will get tired."

"I'll turn this timer over. Just color until the timer stops." I flipped a pink gel timer, and it started to drip.

"I want to be done, Dr. Clare."

"Add more color to your picture. Keep going until the timer stops. The girl in your picture is saying, 'Please color me.'"

She resumed coloring and said, "What does the boy say?"

Rosa, who was seated next to her, responded, "He says, 'I need color.'"

Suggest Options That Prevent Giving Up While Doing an Activity

When children want to stop in the middle of an activity, suggest different options they can try. Tell them it is fine to take a break and then try again. You may need to offer ideas on how to salvage their work. Another approach is to give them two choices of what they can do. Talk with them about their concerns and their desire to stop. Then you can make changes or ask the children how they could handle the situation.

Fabulous Five: Talk About Their Options That Prevent Giving Up Doing an Activity

- **Tell children it is okay to take a break if they feel frustrated.**

Six-year-old Vinnie tried to print the first letter of his name but it ended up looking like an "L." "That's not right," he said as he erased it. After three more attempts, he did it correctly. "I'm good at the 'i.'" Then as he started the "n," he ripped the paper and grimaced.

"It's okay to take a break," I said. "We can tape the paper. It might be easier if you do your picture now and finish your name later."

- **Acknowledge frustration and encourage to continue.**

Using a dowel, 6-year-old Kristy tried to make a "w" in clay but made a "u." "Ugh," she said, throwing the dowel on the table. "Stupid hand. It never obeys me. It does it wrong every time."

"It's frustrating when you don't get it right even though you're trying hard. You're just learning printing. Everyone makes mistakes when they first learn something new." I drew the letter with a yellow highlighter. After she traced it correctly, she smiled.

- **Give children two choices to take if the activity gets too hard.**

"Put your tummy on this red ball, and I will hold your legs. Then put one hand on the floor and use your other hand to throw the balls in the basket. If your arm gets tired, you can take a break or switch arms."

Five-year-old Bill reached, scooped a beanbag, and flung it in the basket. It bounced off the wall, and he caught it. "Try again," I prompted.

- **Help children identify a reason for wanting to stop and change the level of difficulty.**

"Charles, try to catch the tennis ball with this Velcro mitt." As we volleyed back and forth, the 6 year old caught the ball only once.

"Let's do something else," he said.

"Is it boring or too hard?"

"It's just that I can't catch. Let's play something cool."

"Let's move closer to each other. That will make it easier. Just throw it two times. Then we can do something else."

Charles smiled when he caught the next throw.

- **Ask how an activity or outcome could be changed if the children are upset with results.**

Eight-year-old Katie looked at Lynn's card. "Yours is better than mine. I don't like mine."

"What could you do to your card so you will be happier with it?"

"I could start over."

"Okay, and what will you do differently this time?"

"I will just use the star stamp."

Maintain Focus and Effort

> **Children might be thinking:**
> *I want to get this done fast.*
> *I want to be first.*

Some children are easily distracted by what is happening around them. They may need extra cues to shift their attention back to the activity. You may also see children rushing to complete a task or project. Address the reasons for rushing and encourage children to do their best.

Sustain Attention or Interest in the Task

To help children maintain or regain their focus on the activity, it helps to capture their attention. This can be done with physical prompts such as tapping or pointing to the activity. Verbal cues (e.g., "Keep drawing") or asking a question about the activity can also be effective. If children are starting to look overwhelmed, define a specific amount to complete for that day. Another way to motivate children to continue is to discuss the benefits of finishing.

Fabulous Five: Help Children Maintain Their Focus on the Activity

- **Tap or point to the paper or activity to cue children to attend.**

Seven-year-old Sally printed one sentence, then said, "Tomorrow we're going on a field trip."

"Where are you going?"

"To see the friendly giant."

"What's the friendly giant? Is it a play?" I guessed.

She nodded. "There's actors."

"That should be fun." I tapped her paper as a cue to shift her attention back to her writing.

Her classmate, Sue, stopped printing, glanced at Sally, and said, "Less talking, more writing. That's what my mom says."

- **Use verbal cues to encourage concentration on the task.**

"I'm going to make a rainbow fish," 5-year-old Annette said as she started to draw in her classroom journal. She colored with a yellow pencil for 10 seconds. Then she put the tip of the pencil in her mouth and started taping her puffed-out cheeks.

"Keep coloring," I encouraged her.

She colored for another 15 seconds, then stopped. She lined the pencils on the table and rolled them back and forth.

"Color a little more," I said, and she added blue to the fish scales.

Ten seconds later, she said, "My hands are really, really tired. They need a rest."

"Take a rest and then add more color to your beautiful fish."

- **Ask a question about the activity to help children refocus.**

"How many do you have left?" I asked when Dean stared at the door.

The kindergartner shifted his head back to the math activity and counted the pennies. "Five."

- **Define an area or number to be completed and use a countdown.**

Six-year-old Mallory held the colored pencil as her eyes followed two children across the room.

"Start coloring," I prompted.

She colored the sky blue for 5 seconds, then looked around the room.

"More coloring, please. Just do four flowers."

As she colored the flowers, she said, "Three more. Two more. One more. Zero. There, I'm all done."

- **Give reason why they need to continue.**

"Are we doing anything else?" 6-year-old Ashley asked.

"Let's get this card done first because you said you wanted to take this home today. If we have time, then we can do something else."

Prevent Rushing

Children rush to complete an activity for a variety of reasons. They may be nervous about how much time they have to do it or want to finish it that day. Some may not like it, think it is too hard, or want to do something else. They think that the faster they go, the quicker they will be done. If they see other children doing another activity, they may worry that they will not get a chance to participate. Others rush because they are trying to beat someone.

Let children know how much time they have to finish. You may need to mention the consequences of going too fast. When they start to rush, try to figure out why and talk about it with the children. Often by addressing their worries, they will slow down. For some, you may need to tell them it is not a race. Compliment those who are taking their time and doing their best.

Fabulous Five: Stop Children From Rushing

- **Tell children they have a lot of time.**

"I can cut fast," 6-year-old Sharon said as she sped across the page.

"We have 30 minutes. You have lots of time. You don't need to hurry," I replied. "Go slow with the scissors."

- **State the possible consequences of rushing.**

Five-year-old Alan spent 10 minutes coloring the picture for his mother. Then he grabbed the scissors and began cutting in fast motion, snipping off the corners of his drawing.

"Slow down. You've worked hard on this. If you rush, you might make a mistake. Take your time to cut so it turns out good for you."

- **Acknowledge why children are rushing.**

"I think you are trying to rush because you see everyone else is finished," the certified occupational therapy assistant said.

"But I'm behind," 4-year-old Jackie said as she colored her flower picture.

"It's all right. We'll wait for you. We will not start the game until you're done."

- **Tell the group it is not a race.**

"Color these puzzle pieces, match them to the number on the page, and then glue them."

Six-year-old Isaiah began scribbling. "I'm ahead. Nobody can catch up with me now."

"We're not racing. It is better to do your best than to go fast."

- **Give a compliment to whoever is taking their time.**

"I see you are taking your time, and it shows," I said.

"There's no need to rush when you have a bunch of time," 5-year-old Jasmine said.

"We have lots and lots of time," Keith added.

"Yeah, we don't have to hurry. We're doing pretty good," Jasmine said.

Teach Children How to Handle Mistakes

Often children become upset if they make a mistake. A common reaction is to quit. Help them learn other options besides quitting. One way is to change their thinking that mistakes or failures cannot be fixed. A second alternative is to change their perceptions of incompetence and the corresponding negative self-talk. A third alternative is to encourage them to seek help and/or problem solve how to fix it.

Reframe Thinking About Mistakes as a Failure

> **Children might be thinking:**
> *See, I can't do it.*
> *This is too hard.*
> *I don't want to do this.*

When children make mistakes, they may think their project is ruined and their effort wasted. To help change their thinking, you can discuss how the error can be fixed. You can suggest they make it look like they planned it that way or consider it as practice and start over. If the mishap is minor, mention how it is easily rectified. Point out that everyone makes mistakes and everyone has to fix their work. Teach them to view mistakes as an opportunity to learn how to make things work better and how to proceed in the future.

Fabulous Five: Reframe Thinking About Mistakes as a Failure

- **Say, "Make it look like you planned it" when a mistake is made.**

The heart-shaped hole puncher slipped just as 4-year-old Caitlyn pushed down. "Oh no," she said.

"You know what? You can make this the back of your card. If you punch stars around this, you can make it look like you planned it."

- **Convert the mistake into being "just practice" or an experiment.**

Five-year-old Lea pressed the rubber stamp on the red inkpad and then on her paper. When she lifted the butterfly stamp, she looked at the blurry upside-down figure and said, "It's no good."

"That's okay," I said. "This part can just be practice. You can turn your paper over for your good one."

- **Mention that the mistake is minor.**

As we practiced the letters made like the letter "a," 10-year-old Rosa made the letters "d" and "g" in molding sand without problems. She tried to make a "q" but drew the loop in the wrong direction. She slumped down in the seat with a dejected look. "I'm no good at cursive," she said.

"Rosa, you only made one small mistake," the occupational therapy student said. "Look at how you did all these other letters right."

She tried again and was pleased with her effort.

- **Mention that other children fix mistakes too.**

Mary Ellen made a mistake and erased it. Georgia goofed too but started to grit her teeth and grunt.

"Just fix it like Mary Ellen did," I said nonchalantly. "Just erase it."

- **Describe the mistake as being a learning experience.**

Kerry, a first grader, flattened the blue putty with his palm and buried six shamrock erasers. His thumbs tore the putty apart, and the erasers reappeared. "I have an idea," he said, pushing the yellow Koosh ball into the putty.

"Oh, that makes cool designs in the putty," I said, rubbing my index finger over the rough terrain.

Then Kerry buried the Koosh ball. However, the putty had softened, and only parts could be pulled away. A panicked look crossed his face.

I took the putty-covered ball and gave Kerry another toy. As I gradually pulled off small bits of putty, I said, "I didn't know this would stick like this. I guess we both learned that when putty gets soft, it's hard to get off."

Teach Helpful Self-Talk to Deal With Mistakes or Failure

> **Children might be thinking:**
> *I can't do this.*
> *I give up. I'm done.*
> *No more.*

Some children may think mistakes are a reflection of their incompetence. They may tell themselves that they are stupid or a failure and the task is impossible for them to do. Let children know that what they say to themselves is important. Encourage them to use self-talk that is helpful. Often you will need to give the exact words and have them repeat them. If they are feeling frustrated after making mistakes, tell them to say, "I'm frustrated, I need a break," or "I can ask for help if I need it." If they have a history of giving up, give them these words before they even start: "If this doesn't work, I'll try something else." You can also tell them to say, "It's not working. Try a different way," or "It's okay, I can fix it or do another one."

Fabulous Five: Promote Helpful Self-Talk to Deal With Mistakes or Failure

- **Tell children to say, "I'm frustrated, I need a break."**

Four-year-old Clint traced the letters of his name on his name strip. Then he made the "l," but it was crooked. He erased and tried again, but with the same results.

"Ugh," he said through gritted teeth, pushing the paper away. "I can't do it. You do it."

"Clint, say, 'I'm frustrated. I need a break.'"

He repeated the words. I put a stress ball on the table, and he played with it for a few minutes.

"Okay," I said. "Try again. I know you can do it."

- **Have children tell themselves, "I can ask for help if I need it."**

Five-year-old Ally had weakness in her upper left side. During recess, she walked over to the monkey bars. She tried once but fell on the wood chips. She went back but only stood on the platform looking dejected.

"Try again," I said. "And tell yourself, 'I can ask for help if I need it.'"

She reached for the bars, swung for a minute, and said, "Help me, please."

I held her and gently lowered her to the ground. After a few more tries, she was able to do it.

- **Have children tell themselves, "If this doesn't work, I'll try something else."**

When I walked into the preschool classroom, 5-year-old Victor was making a mask and asked his teacher to tie string in the holes on the side. When the string came out, he turned to me and asked, "Can you get a stapler?"

I agreed and brought it to the table. Knowing that he became easily frustrated and not sure if the staple would hold the string, I said, "Now tell yourself, 'If this doesn't work, I'll try something else.'"

He stapled it and the string held when he put the mask on.

"You had a good idea to use the stapler. It really worked."

- **Tell children to say, "It's not working. Try a different way."**

Seven-year-old Seth slammed the lever in the game, and the plastic fly flew past the frog's mouth. He slammed the lever again and overshot the mouth again. "I can't do this," he said, scooting away from the game.

"Tell yourself, 'What I am doing is not working. Try a different way.' Now get closer and try pushing more gently."

He moved toward the game and practiced pushing the lever with different pressures until the fly flew in the mouth of the frog. "I did it," he yelled.

- **Have children tell themselves, "It's okay. I can fix it or do another one."**

As 4-year-old Micah cut out a sports car, he accidentally snipped off the hood. He jumped up and left the table.

I followed him. "Micah, say, 'It's okay. I can fix it. I'll use tape.'"

He repeated the words and headed back to the table.

Help Fix a Mistake and Promote Problem Solving

Children might be thinking:
Do you think that will fix it?
I guess I could do… to fix it.
I fixed it!
I'm glad that I fixed it, and I'll keep going.

After children make a mistake, you can help them continue by salvaging what is left. Adapt the activity so they do not have to look at the mistake. Always bring extra supplies so starting over is an option. That way they do not have to end in failure. Be aware that undoing or erasing a large section can be overwhelming or upsetting. They will often think they will not get it done. In that situation, you could repair the area so children can proceed or suggest starting over with new materials. Let them know you are there to help if needed, but also encourage them to problem solve what they can do to change the mistake. Then ask them to choose when they will fix the mistake, which implies that they will at least attempt to redo or repair their work.

Fabulous Five: Fix a Mistake

- **Salvage what is left after the mistake is made.**

Five-year-old Geena attempted to make the number 3 with a purple marker but drew it backwards. She grimaced and said, "That's not right."

"Let's turn it into a cat." I connected the lines and added a face, whiskers, and ears. "Here's a way to remember how to make the number 3." I pointed to her left arm and said. "Put your arm on the paper and draw the 3 toward your arm." I demonstrated, and she copied with success.

- **Be aware that undoing or erasing a large section can be overwhelming or upsetting.**

"You're going to weave your own placemats for the Thanksgiving feast," the occupational therapy student said to the second graders. She demonstrated the weaving to Kelly and Rachael.

As she talked to Kelly, Rachael wove six strips all wrong. When she turned toward Rachael, she saw the mistake. "Oh, Rachael, you need to fix this." Seeing the look of panic on Rachael's face, she added, "I will take these out and help you put them back in. You need to do this so your mat does not fall apart."

- **Adapt the activity so children do not have to look at the mistake.**

Nine-year-old Ross ripped a hole in the paper when he pressed too hard with his pencil. He threw the paper across the table. I intercepted the flying paper, creased it, and tore off the hole-ridden top half. I handed him the bottom half as a fresh start. "Try again," I said, and he picked up his pencil.

- **Give options on when to fix a mistake.**

As 8-year-old Erika made her valentine, she printed the "e" upside-down. "The 'l,' 'o,' and 'v' are just right, but the 'e' goes like this," I said as I printed the letter. "Do you want to fix it now or after you have drawn your picture?"

She began erasing and printed the letter correctly.

- **Have children problem solve how to fix it.**

Six-year-old Tony tugged on his class assignment that was partially under a book, and it ripped.

"What can you do?" I said.

He rolled his wheelchair over and grabbed the tape dispenser off the teacher's desk.

Help Children Save Face When Getting Assistance

To some degree, everyone, including children, care about what others people think and have a need to be viewed in a positive way. Children like to be treated as special, yet they do not want to be viewed as different from other children. They especially do not want others to say they are stupid. Saving face is when you help someone look good when things are not going well. This means when providing extra help, especially in a group situation, it is done in a way that avoids embarrassment.

Present Help in the Least Noticeable Way

Children might be thinking:
I don't want to look stupid.
Someone might laugh at me.
Don't make me look bad.

When you need to provide assistance, be thoughtful about your approach. Consider how children might feel about receiving help. Another factor is the group dynamics.

In some groups, children will worry about fitting in. With those factors in mind, choose a strategy that addresses the children's needs.

Avoid Embarrassing Children When Providing Assistance

It is crucial to avoid embarrassing children in front of classmates or friends when giving assistance. If possible, approach them when others are not around or looking. Avoid singling them out or calling attention to your actions. Often you can adjust an activity without the children or others noticing. There is an art to this. You have to be aware of who is watching and make adaptations quietly so no one pays attention. Another approach is to make the adaptations look acceptable and appealing to others.

Fabulous Five: Avoid Embarrassing Children When Giving Assistance

- **Approach children when peers are not watching to provide assistance.**

During the last 2 weeks of school, Daryl's parents met with the special education team and asked for my involvement. The next day, I watched for a moment when 11-year-old Daryl was alone and then approached him. "Hi, Daryl. My name is Dr. Clare, and I'm an occupational therapist. I am the one they talked about at your meeting yesterday. I know your body is going through changes, and I have ideas on ways to make your life easier at school. Are you more tired in the afternoon?" I asked, knowing that his endurance was declining due to his progressing muscle weakness.

"I'm tired all the time."

"I have one idea. It's a clipboard that is on a slant that would hold the book up and make writing easier. Is that something you want to check out, or would you prefer to wait until next school year?"

"What does it look like?"

"Do you want me to bring it so you can look at it?"

"Yeah."

"I'll show you tomorrow."

- **Avoid singling out children.**

I entered the kindergarten class to screen Erich's sensorimotor skills and joined him and three other children at the table. I watched him color and cut, and I observed the other children as well. Because he slumped in his chair and his teacher said he was often fatigued, I also wanted to see if he had low muscle tone. I did not want to embarrass him, so I said, "Can I check everyone's muscles and see how strong you are?" They all nodded. I moved around the table gently feeling the children's biceps. "Wow, good strong muscles," I said, and all the children smiled.

- **Avoid calling attention to your assistance.**

At the day treatment, the group of third graders traced and cut out bookmarks. Then they copied from the board and printed on the bookmark five things they could do to get calm when mad. I quietly handed Celina a paper with the list for her to copy, knowing she tended to lose her place as her eyes moved from the board to her desk.

- **Present help as a group need.**

The first graders made their valentines but needed to write *Happy Valentine's Day*. I wrote the words and placed the paper on the table because I knew Lynn would have to copy it.

"I don't need it," Julie said.

"I don't need it too," Lynn said.

"Valentine is a long word. I'll just leave it here," I said.

Lynn pushed the paper across the table but kept it within eyesight. Julie started writing, and Lynn subtly looked up and copied from the paper without Julie noticing.

- **Make the activity or strategy look fun or appealing to other children.**

Knowing that 4-year-old McKenna had limited vision, I brought a package of Wikki Stix to her class. The plastic strings could be made into letters, allowing her to feel the shape. "You can use these for everyone who is at McKenna's table," I told her teacher. When I returned, McKenna and her tablemates were smiling as they used them to make letters.

Provide Assistance in a Subtle Way

There are ways to provide subtle support and help children save face when you know an activity might be hard. You can sit or stand next to whomever will need the most help. This allows you an opportunity to nonchalantly slip in extra cues, directions, or aid. You also may make subtle adjustments in the activity without calling attention to your actions. For some, you may want to talk casually about being a team, which means they are not expected to do the task or activity alone. An additional method to save face is to prevent failure from occurring. When you are certain that children are likely to fail, figure out ways to help them succeed.

Fabulous Five: Provide Subtle Help in the Least Noticeable Way

- **Stand or sit next to the child you know will need extra help.**

The preschool teacher told me at lunch she was planning to do a cutting activity while I was in her class. An hour later, I came in the classroom, pulled up a chair, and purposely sat next to 3-year-old Quentin. I knew he was still learning how to manipulate scissors. I said hello and talked to all the children at his table.

He struggled to put his fingers in the scissors and ended up with the blades facing him. I gently repositioned the scissors and helped him make the first cut. "The scissors are like an alligator," I whispered. "You want the mouth to be away from your tummy." As he snipped, I looked around the table and helped other classmates.

- **Talk casually about being a team, which means you have to work together.**

Pam tried to push the stapler through the thick paper with no success.

"We're a team, so we have to work together. You use two fingers and I'll do the same. We'll press together," I said. "Ready? One, two, three, push." The staple slid through the papers. "Your book is done."

- **Weave in extra cues nonchalantly.**

"We're going to learn about animals," the preschool teacher told the class of 4 year olds. "Get your listening ears on, and I'll tell you what to do." When the class quieted, she continued by pointing to a sample worksheet. "Circle the animals in each row and then color them."

I sat next to Latoya, thinking she would probably need extra help. She stared at the paper with a lost look on her face.

I pointed to the first picture. "Is that an animal?"

She nodded with a smile.

"Circle it. Only circle animals."

She continued now that she now understood the directions.

- **Repeat one step at a time after giving all the directions.**

Because I knew 5-year-old Roberto had difficulty with motor planning, I sat next to him as the group made holiday cards. After the teacher gave the set of directions, I told him one step at a time. "Start cutting here," I said, then glanced around the table making comments about each person's work. When the first step was completed, I gave Roberto the next one. The other children did not seem to notice that I was helping him.

- **Make subtle adjustments.**

Seven-year-old Dan began a three-part obstacle course as his friends watched. He crawled around chairs like a commando, jumped over ropes holding one foot off the ground, and balanced while sitting on the one-legged stool. As he tried to keep his balance, he aimed a blue-and-white football for a white box placed 5 feet away. Each time he threw, the ball only went 3 feet.

I subtly moved the box closer, and on his next try, the ball landed in the target.

"Touchdown," Dan shouted.

Say That Everyone Needs Help

> **Children might be thinking:**
> *Oh, this is hard for everyone?*
> *That makes me feel better.*
> *I'm relieved I'm not the only one.*

It is important to give children the message that everyone needs help with something. You want to emphasize that getting assistance is a normal part of life. To help convey this message, tell a story about a time you needed help or talk about the support one of their heroes required. At the beginning of an activity, you can tell children that you are helping everyone. What you do not need to mention is how much assistance you are providing. Another face-saving strategy is to say the activity or task is hard for all children.

Fabulous Five: Give the Message That Everyone Needs Help With Something

- **Tell children, "Everyone needs help with something. It is okay to get help."**

When Mark's mother saw me in the hallway outside her son's third-grade class, she said, "I just wanted you to know that Mark asked me if he was stupid. He's feeling bad that he can't write and keep up with his classmates."

"Thanks for telling me," I said, and explained how his difficulty with motor planning made the process of learning handwriting so laborious. I reassured her that once he learned the movements and directionality of the letters, it would become automatic and easier.

I saw Mark that day, and as he played with clay, I said, "You know, just because something is hard for you and takes longer to learn than other kids, it does not mean you are stupid. Everyone needs help with something. No one is perfect. It's okay to get help. Once you learn these letters, it will be a lot easier to write. It's like when you learn to swim. It's hard at first but after you practice, it gets easy."

Although he did not say anything, he looked at me with a slight smile.

- **Tell a story about when you needed help.**

Ten-year-old Tim started feeling bad about himself because he needed therapy, so I told him, "When I was in college I had a hard time understanding physics, and I had to get extra help. It really made a difference." He looked at me with gratitude in his eyes.

- **Talk about how children's heroes are not perfect.**

Eight-year-old Jeremy threw a blue Koosh ball at a basketball hoop while trying to balance on a one-legged stool. "Oh, I missed," he said five times in a row. He curled his lip, looking teary-eyed.

"You know, basketball players don't get every shot either. They spend hours training, and their coaches help them too," I reassured him. "Let's move closer." His next throw was a success.

- **Tell children you are helping everyone with the activity.**

"Here, let me show you how this works. You hold both handles and spin 10 times, then pull. That way the Orbiter will spin." I knew Alec would struggle and need extra help, so I put my hands over his and demonstrated. "This is tricky, so I have been helping everyone learn how to do this."

- **State that the task or activity is hard for all children.**

The occupational therapy student brought supplies for the kindergartners to decorate the gingerbread cookies. She held a frosting tube and said, "These are hard to squeeze, even for big kids. I will help everyone."

"These are easy for me to squeeze," Bert bragged.

"Actually a lot of kids have used these. They are almost empty, and it's harder to get the frosting out. They are hard for everybody."

Use Yourself as a Role Model

> **Children might be thinking:**
> *I'm surprised that was hard for you.*
> *Even older people get stuck sometimes—it's not just me.*

Use yourself as an example to let children know that no one is perfect. Mention your own shortcomings and that you are always learning no matter what age you are. This can help shift children's thinking from "I'm a failure," to "I'm just learning." You also can show them that you make mistakes too. Telling a story about a time you did not do well can be comforting, especially if told right after a moment they failed. In addition, saying the activity is hard for you can be reassuring.

Fabulous Five: Discuss Your Life Experiences

- **Mention your own shortcomings.**

When 8-year-old Kurt wrote four words, they all overlapped with no space between them. He looked at his work and threw himself back in his chair.

"It's frustrating when you make mistakes even though you are trying so hard. It's time to go anyway. We'll work on making that easier for you."

As we walked back to his class, he asked, "Next time will you bring the mystery box?"

"Sure. I hope I remember. Sometimes I forget. My memory is not always good."

"Well, just write yourself a note," he said.

"That's a good idea."

- **Let children know you are still learning, even as an adult.**

As 10-year-old Justin struggled with writing, he sighed with frustration.

"This is hard," I said. "Just give yourself a chance to learn. I know how you feel. I'm learning Spanish, and it's really hard for me. For some people it's really easy for them to speak a new language, but not for me. I keep telling myself to practice and I will get better."

- **Make a mistake on purpose to demonstrate that everyone makes mistakes.**

In the occupational and speech therapy group, the four first graders played the game Simon Says.

"Simon says draw a triangle with a blue marker," the speech-language pathologist said.

Everyone drew on the easels.

"Raise your hand."

Shelby raised her hands, and the other three children laughed.

"Oops, we didn't say 'Simon says.' That's okay; everyone is learning how to play." A few minutes later, the speech-language pathologist made a mistake on purpose.

"Oops," I said, "listen for the words 'Simon says.' See, we teachers make mistakes like everyone else."

- **Tell a story about a time you failed.**

Seven-year-old Shane sat on a platform swing and tried to throw beanbags into a target. After five missed tries, he looked upset.

"That's okay," I said. "I have a hard time playing baseball. The last time I played I struck out."

Shane nodded and smiled.

- **Comment on how the activity is hard for you too.**

As Cheryl maneuvered a silver marble through a maze, it slipped into the first hole. "I'm no good at this," she said, her voice filled with frustration.

"This game is hard for me too. It takes a lot of practice," I replied.

Attribute Difficulty to Reasons Other Than Children's Ability

---

Children might be thinking:

That was really hard.

I guess I need to practice to be good.

If I practice some more, I can get better at it.

Another approach to help children save face is to talk about the difficult aspects of a task or object. What you are implying is that the problem is related to the object or task, not their ability. You also can let them know that sometimes you have to get a feel for how something works. Point out that if it is their first time, they need to practice. Being unsuccessful in their first few attempts does not mean they cannot do it. In addition, if they are the first person in a group to try, they do not get the opportunity to watch others figure out what works. Help children learn that instead of thinking they cannot do it, they should tell themselves that it just takes practice.

Fabulous Five: Refer to the Difficulty of the Activity or the Need for Practice

- **Talk about the challenging aspects of the task.**

Seven-year-old Henry sketched himself wearing blue jeans and a football jersey. He outlined his face. "Oh no. The nose is too big," he said in a self-depreciating way.

"It is always hard to draw yourself," I responded, "because the only way you can see yourself is in a mirror."

- **Relate the problem as being a difficult object or game.**

Seven-year-old Sydney put her palms on the footprint hole punch. She pushed two times with no success.

"That may be a two-person hole punch," I said.

"Yeah," she agreed, and she allowed me to help her do it.

- **Discuss the need to get a feel for the activity.**

Eight-year-old Mickey created a tower with four magnets, but the next three magnets dropped off his structure. "Everything is falling down. I'm no good at this."

"With these magnets, you just have to get the feel of it to figure out which ones work. Some are too heavy for the top."

- **Refer to the difficulty as being a lack of practice or needing to relearn.**

In the fall, 7-year-old Roger asked me to bring back a maze he had done in the spring. He twisted the knobs, maneuvering a steel ball and trying to avoid obstacles. Each time he ended up in the holes, he grimaced and tightened his shoulder muscles.

"You haven't done this in a long time. It will get easier the more you do it," I said.

- **Attribute the difficulty to doing it for the first time or being the first person to try.**

As the group watched, I handed a wooden toy with a matching small ball attached by a string. "Hold this in your hand, toss the ball in the air, and see if you can catch it."

After four tries, he was still unsuccessful.

"It's always hard to be the first one," I said. "This toy takes a lot of practice."

Make Adaptations to Save Face

Children might be thinking:
I don't look different from my friends.
Others are doing the same thing.
Hey, I can do this.
That's better.

To ensure success and avoid the repercussions of failure, make adaptations as needed. One way is to provide various options within the activity that enable everyone to participate. Another idea is to make the changes part of the activity. If children notice that something is different, you can always mention that you needed it that way. The focus on you suggests that you are the one with a problem, not the child. You also can help children reframe their thinking that adaptations make them look bad. Rather, you can talk about the adaptations being special and make the changes desirable to others.

Fabulous Five: Use Adaptations

- **Design adaptations for children and integrate into the activity.**

Before the group of second graders started, I thought about how Lori's limited vision made it difficult for her to read small print. I also knew she did better if there was a color contrast between the paper and the table. So I covered the table with black paper and enlarged the written directions on the white paper for everyone in the group. When the group arrived, Lori followed all the directions for making a holiday card using stickers.

- **Provide options for the group that includes one you know the children can do.**

"Today I brought Boggle. Shake the can, let the dice drop on the table, and look for words. Then you can do it two ways: you can write the word or just the first letter of the word."

Seven-year-old Kip shook the container and spilled the lettered dice onto the wooden table.

"I see the word *tea*," Kandace said, printing the word. Kip, who struggled with writing, wrote the letter "t."

- **Attribute an adaptation or simplification to your need.**

Because I knew 8-year-old Taylor was sensitive to noise, I left the timer that clicks in the box when we played the maze game. As we were putting the game away, he saw it and asked, "How come we didn't use this?"

"Because it's too noisy," I said. "It hurts my ears."

- **Refer to adaptations as being special.**

"Here's really cool paper. The lines are raised, which makes writing easier," I told 7-year-old Suzanne, who had limited vision.

I left a pad in her class, and when I came to see her the next week, she said, "I need more of that cool paper." I gave her some. Suzanne wrote one word, stopped, smiled, and said, "See how all my letters are on this line."

- **Make the adaptation desirable.**

Shannon had hand tremors and wrote best when her paper was stabilized in a clipboard. When I talked to her fifth-grade teacher, she said, "I think Shannon hesitates to use the board because she doesn't want to look different from the rest of the class."

"Maybe it would help to have clipboards available to the other students too," I suggested.

When I came back the next week, the teacher said the children now considered it a treat to use a clipboard, and Shannon had started using hers.

Teach Children How to Deal With Losing

Children might be thinking:
I hate losing.
No fair.
He/she cheated.

It is natural for children to have the desire to win. For every winner, however, there is a loser. This means that at the end of a game or race, there is the possibility of conflict if the children do not know ways to deal with losing. Some children may yell, "No fair," and accuse the winner of cheating. Others may see the experience as being another sign of their incompetence and may not wish to play again.

Because winning and losing occurs throughout the journey of life, you will want to help children iron out their differences and, at the same time, learn a life lesson on how to lose gracefully. Build upon the children's strengths by discovering what strategies or solutions have worked for them in the past. You may assist children to broaden their repertoire by enlisting the wisdom of the group members. Use the experience to create the notion that handling losing in a constructive way may actually make them better and stronger.

Fabulous Five: Identify Strategies on How to Deal With Losing

- **Ask children what they would tell a younger child about losing, and then remind them of their wise advice.**

"What would you tell a little kid about losing?"

"To believe in himself and he'll do better. Winning is important, but losing gives you a lesson in patience," 10-year-old Rodney said.

Five minutes later, when Rodney lost a race, he yelled, "That's no fair."

"Remember your wise words about losing," I said.

- **Ask, "What can you tell yourself when you lose?"**

When 6-year-old Katy lost the Operation game, she folded her arms and pouted.

"What can you tell yourself when you lose?" I asked her.

"Hmm. It's okay to lose. You can just do it again."

- **Ask the group about their tips on how they deal with losing.**

Chad looked miffed when he was the last one to finish the dice game. I turned to the group of second graders and said, "How do you help yourself if you lose?"

"I just say, 'Calm down, it's only a game,'" Dusty replied.

"It doesn't matter if you win or lose. I tell my brother that too," Adam added.

"I tell myself not to yell or scream. It's not like it's going to be the end of the world or hurt you if you lose."

Then Dusty offered, "My mom says it doesn't matter if you win or lose. It's how you play the game, except in Las Vegas. Then it's very important that you win."

- **Have the group write a story about how to deal with losing.**

"I need your help to write a story," I said to the group of 8 year olds, showing them a page with missing words. "First I need three names."

"Rebecca," Jane said. "She's my best friend."

"Clare," Colton said, smiling at me, and then Candy added her own name.

"Let's start the story. Once upon a time, Rebecca, Candy, and Clare played a game called…. What was the game?

"Count the pennies," Jane replied.

"When Candy won, she shouted…. What did she shout?"

"Hurray!"

I continued, "Clare became upset because she lost. 'It's okay,' Rebecca said. 'You can just…. What could she tell Clare? You can just….'"

"Wait awhile for your turn to win," Candy said.

"What else could she tell Clare?" I asked.

"Tell her that people lose all the time and it's okay. Play again and you might win the next time."

- **Talk about how you handle losing.**

"When I lose at games, do you know what I do?" I asked 6-year-old Gus.

"What?"

"I tell myself, 'It's all right. I hope I have better luck next time.' Or if the game takes practice, I try to figure out ways I can be better."

Finish With Success After a Challenge

Children might be thinking:
I did it!
Wow, I'm doing good.
I'm getting better.

When children are struggling and giving up hope, try to figure out a way to help them succeed. Observe closely to identify what the problem is and what could be done differently. Then you can say while demonstrating, "Oh, there is a trick to this. Do it this way." You also can ask them for possible solutions. Another approach is to change the rules of the game, modify the activity, or adapt the last step. Do this in a subtle manner. Then make it a big deal that they succeeded.

At the end of a challenge, it is important to have most children finish with a successful experience and to review their progress. This allows them to get a sense of achievement and creates a desire to try again or do more. It also becomes an opportunity to emphasize their strengths.

Fabulous Five: End With Success

- **Analyze what the children are doing wrong, tell them there's a trick, and show or tell them what to do differently.**

Ten-year-old Alex held the Velcro mitt upright like a catcher's mitt. Sophie and Alex tried to catch the tennis ball, but the ball kept ricocheting off the mitt.

"There's a trick to this," I said. "You have to hold the mitt with your palm up like you are holding a plate and throw the ball softly. Then it will stick to the Velcro. That seemed to work for other kids."

They changed their hand position and were successful when they threw.

- **Identify the source of difficulty and encourage children to think of solutions.**

Five-year-old Bart bounced into the room and saw a blue homemade card and various hole punchers on the table.

"I thought it would be nice to make your own holiday card. Today we'll use these hole punchers, and later you can write inside the card. This one makes stars. You hold it in your hand, slide it on the paper, and squeeze. You'll punch the green paper, and then we'll put it over yellow paper so you can see your designs."

"My mom will love this. This is going to be the greatest card." Bart started punching stars in the paper. "This is easy," he said. He then slid the Christmas tree punch on the paper and positioned it under the stars. His thumb turned white as he pressed the button, but nothing happened. "I can't do this," he complained.

"This one is harder, so it can be frustrating. What could you do to push harder?" I asked.

He stood up, straightened his elbows, and pushed the button down with all the weight of his palm. *Click*. The tree popped out.

"Standing up is a great idea!"

- **Change or simplify the rules.**

Everett walked in the room wearing a navy blue Colorado Avalanche sweatshirt. His eyes widened with delight when he saw the hockey game on the table. I demonstrated and said, "To make the hockey players move, pull these rods back and forth. Then twist the knobs on the ends of the rods to make them turn."

Everett practiced moving two players, but his problems with motor planning became evident as he struggled to hit the puck. To make the game more successful, I quickly changed the usual rules of keeping the puck in motion and wrestling it from each other. "We will each take a turn. You shoot it to my side, and I will wait. Then I will shoot it back." I slid the black puck next to Everett's player so all he had to do was spin the knob.

He flicked the rod, and the puck sailed across the board. "I did it," he said with a surge of joy.

- **Modify the activity.**

Six-year-old Sierra tried picking up 1-inch knobby balls with bamboo tongs, but her fingers kept slipping off the tongs. She dropped the tongs on the table, snatched four balls, and bounced them.

I quickly grabbed an empty coffee can and said, "Here, see if you can throw them into this can. See how many points you can get."

She aimed and easily landed each ball in the can.

- **Adjust the last step to ensure success and end on a good note.**

Five-year-old Fawn held the magnet under the board but struggled with maintaining the man upright on top. "I don't want to play this game. It's dumb."

To end with success, I moved the man 3 inches from the end of the maze and said, "Take him home."

She moved through the maze and finished the course. "You did it!"

KEY POINTS TO REMEMBER

- Address children's beliefs about their abilities, show you will help, and encourage them to take the first step if they are hesitant to start.

- Be sensitive to how long children have to wait and, if needed, change the activity or encourage others to go faster.

- Give children something to do while waiting and/or teach them strategies to prevent impatience.

- Encourage children to continue by acknowledging their effort, keeping the challenge at the just-right level, and using supportive words or enticements.

- Prevent giving up by changing children's mindsets, making the activity appear doable, and/or offering possible options.

- Promote sustained attention and prevent rushing by addressing the reason for a lack of focus or desire to rush.

- Teach children ways to deal with mistakes by reframing thoughts of failure, using positive self-talk, getting help, and/or problem solving.

- Help children save face by providing inconspicuous assistance and/or telling them that everyone, including you, needs support.

REVIEW QUESTIONS

1. Children's beliefs about their abilities affect their self-confidence. True or false.

2. A kindergartner stares at a 10-piece puzzle of animal shapes. He looks at you and says, "I can't." What can you say or do?

3. Why is it better to let children try on their own before you give help?

4. Why is it better to say, "Try…" instead of asking, "Can you…?"

5. The longer children have to wait, the more likely they will do something that gets them in trouble. True or false.

6. Pointing out what children are doing wrong will encourage them to continue. True or false.

7. Creating a just-right challenge is key to having all children experience success in therapy. True or false.

8. What are three encouraging statements you can say when children want to quit?

9. Name three ways to help children regain their focus on an activity.

10. Older children do not mind getting a lot of adult assistance in front of their peers. True or false.

Create Smooth Transitions

CHAPTER OVERVIEW

The purpose of this chapter is to illustrate ways of generating smooth transitions between sessions and between activities. When you let children know what to expect by developing a routine and preparing them for changes, it is easier for them to adjust. Therefore, visual ways of showing a schedule, the passage of time, and transitional cues are described. Additionally, to assist children in moving effortlessly from one activity to another, there are strategies for incorporating a unifying theme, modifying transitions, and creating a sense of flow.

CHILDREN'S DESCRIPTIONS OF WHAT THEY THINK YOU SHOULD KNOW

Dr. Clare: "During the day, do you like knowing what is going to happen next? How does that help you?"

Olivia (age 12): "Yes, it helps me to know. Then I know what to get prepared for and what to grab."

Mateo (age 11): "It's good to know where you're going. Then I know what to plan for."

PREPARE, PREVENT, AND IMPROVISE

Making transitions effortless for children requires you to prepare them for changes, prevent breakdowns, and improvise as therapy progresses. The challenge is to assist them in handling change and often waiting. With careful planning, vigilance, and responsiveness, you can guide children from one activity to another with ease.

Assist With Transitions to a New Place

Children might be thinking:
I'm sad.
Will my mom or dad come back?
I'm scared.
I don't know what is going to happen.
I don't know these people.
I'm excited. There are lots of toys.

When children transition to a new place, such as preschool or kindergarten, they often feel a mixture of excitement, hope, and fear. They may be excited to finally go to school like an older sibling or family member. They may start to think of themselves as being big kids; as one preschooler told his family, "I'm not a baby now." They hope they will like it and have fun. Yet, on the first day, fear can

Curtin, C.
Strategies for Collaborating With Children: Creating Partnerships in Occupational Therapy and Research (pp. 325-351).
© 2017 SLACK Incorporated.

set in. Being with new people and not knowing what will happen can be scary. It also may be their first time away from their family.

One way to help children with changes is to create a transition book. Take photographs and write a short story about where they will be going, who they will meet, and what will happen. This strategy prepares them and allows them to picture the new place. You can also have children watch while you acknowledge their feelings by writing a story and drawing figures. This empathetic gesture can be soothing. For some, involving them in a fun activity alleviates their fears. For others, you may need to play with other children in front of them and give them the choice to participate. An additional strategy is to ask them to teach you about something they know or enjoy. Children appreciate and respond when you reach out to them, recognize their feelings, and assume a nurturing and comforting approach.

Fabulous Five: Assist With Transitioning to a New Place

- **Create a transition book.**

When 3-year-old Matt stopped coming to preschool, we had a meeting with his mother. She said he did not want to come but then suggested changing him to the afternoon session. Because I had taken pictures of him previously, I made him a transition book. I wrote the following and attached corresponding photos:

I am coming to preschool in the afternoon.

I will see my teachers Mrs. B. and Miss K.

My teachers are happy I am coming to school.

I will make new friends.

I get to play in new centers. I can be a firefighter in centers.

I have a new talking machine.

I get to play with trucks on the playground.

I have fun at school!

- **Write a story about their situation while children watch.**

In the middle of the school year, 3-year-old Skye's parents brought her to preschool and left. Sitting next to her at a round table, I took a piece of paper and drew a line down the middle. On one side I drew a picture of a crying girl that resembled her and said the words as I wrote them, "I am sad. I miss my mom and dad." Skye stopped crying but continued to whimper. I said as I wrote on the other side, "My new friends like me. My friends like to play with me. School is fun!" Then I added children's faces. As I drew, some of her classmates joined us.

"I want to be Skye's friend. Draw my face," Josh said.

I made a smiling face with curly hair. "Skye, here is your friend, Josh."

"Make me. I want to be her friend too," four other children shouted.

Skye began to smile as she looked around the table.

"Do you want to take this home?" I asked. "It has pictures of all your new friends." She nodded and put it in her backpack.

A 4-year-old girl accompanied her and held Skye's hand as they sat with the class for the good morning song.

- **Use a visual timer to show when the caregiver will return.**

"Nana, help me," 3-year-old Don cried in despair after his grandmother dropped him off on his first day at preschool.

"You're sad to say goodbye to Nana," I said in a soft and caring tone of voice. Then I brought him toys I thought he might like.

He continued crying inconsolably for 10 minutes and repeating, "Nana, help me."

The preschool director came over to him and asked, "Do you want me to call Nana?" He nodded and stopped crying.

I brought over a visual timer and moved the knob until the red was at the 45-minute mark. "When the red is gone, Nana will be here."

"Nana come back?"

"Yes." For the next 10 minutes, he stared at the timer. When his classmates began playing in the centers, I said, "Let's go play."

"I'll just sit here," he replied, tapping the table.

"You could draw a picture for Nana." When he nodded, I said, "Let me show you where the paper and markers are." I scooted his chair 2 feet to join his classmates. I also moved the timer so he could see it.

He scribbled on the yellow paper, periodically checking the time. Seeing the other children make shapes, he said, "I want Play-Doh." When I handed it to him, he turned his back to the timer and began playing.

- **Involve in a fun activity.**

When 3-year-old Tony's mother left him for his first day in our Beginning therapy group, he started sobbing. He walked with us over to the rug where the other children were. Tony found a corner, slid down on his knees, put his fist in his mouth, and continued crying.

The special education teacher brought over a musical toy and activated the song. Tony stopped momentarily to watch but resumed crying 10 seconds later. I brought over a toy boat with four balls on top and demonstrated hitting the balls with a hammer. I offered him the hammer, but he shook his head. The sobbing continued.

"I have something fun to show you," I said, putting my hand out with my palm up. He reached for my hand, and we walked over to a water table. The tears stopped. He put his hands in and splashed, making waves.

- **Ask children to teach you about something they know or enjoy.**

Three-year-old Cooper cried on his first day in preschool. I attempted to soothe him by bringing over a variety of toys, but he turned his head away. "Wow, you're wearing a superhero shirt," I said, and I found the corresponding toy. "I know this toy transforms into different shapes. Do you know how to do it?"

He stopped crying and nodded.

"I don't know how to do it. Could you show me how?"

He took the toy out of my hand and manipulated the parts, changing it into a different figure.

- **Play with other children in front of them and give them a choice on whether to join.**

When I walked in the door, the preschool teacher pointed to the crying child and asked, "Can you help Miguel? It's his first day. He speaks Spanish."

I went over to the 3 year old and said, "Tu está triste. You're sad." He kept sobbing. I brought over magnetic blocks, put two pieces together, and handed him a square.

He shook his head, pushed the piece away, and continued to cry.

A classmate joined us, and I started to play with the peer. I used exaggerated facial expressions and movements, looking goofy. The other child laughed. Miguel stopped crying as he watched us, then smiled.

Create a Routine and Prepare for Changes

When children know what to expect, it decreases the possibility of confusion and frustration. Consistency of a routine provides familiarity and stability. Let children know what the therapy routine will be. Be open to making adjustments depending on their needs and wishes.

Establish a Routine and Schedule of Activities

Children might be thinking:
What are we doing?
What is going to happen?

You can create a sense of flow by defining what the therapy routine will entail. You may want to develop routines regarding starting and/or ending activities and the session. Show children, using objects, photographs, or picture symbols, the activities and their sequence. By showing time in a visual manner before a transition, you give them notice of an upcoming change. Such a forewarning allows them to anticipate and mentally prepare to shift their attention and actions.

Decide What the Routine Will Be

The type of routine you create depends on the children's goals and your setting. You will need to create a more structured routine if you (a) lead a large group or an entire class and (b) have to bring the supplies to them. If you are itinerant and working with a small group or individuals, you may choose to bring four or five preferred activities and let the children choose. You can tell them the purpose for being together and have them decide what they want to do.

Another option is for you to consistently bring activities within the same two to four general categories each time. For instance, you could always start the session with hand-strengthening or movement activities. If you have a designated space for supplies and equipment, you could set up the room and allow children to choose freely.

Fabulous Five: Decide What the Routine Will Be

- **Create a structured routine.**

In the children's hospital, the dietician and I sat with five children of different ages who had diabetes. On the kitchen table in the occupational therapy clinic was a cookbook by the American Diabetes Association. "The purpose of our group is to help you learn how to manage your diet so you can stay healthy. As a group, we are going to plan a meal using this cookbook, and then you actually get to make it," I said, pointing to the kitchen.

The dietician carefully explained how to keep their diet balanced using the right number of exchanges with different types of food. "This cookbook is great because next to each recipe, it gives the exchanges," she told them.

The children looked through the pages and decided to make pizzas with English muffins as the main dish. The dietician worked with them on planning the rest of the meal.

"All right, tomorrow we will have a pizza party at lunch time," I said. "Get ready to have some fun."

- **Have the routine include four or five activities and let children choose.**

At the beginning of the session, I showed 4-year-old Demetrius the four activities I brought. "Today you can paint a picture, cut out a car, make a dinosaur picture, or do puzzles. What do you want to do?"

Pointing to a template of a T-Rex dinosaur, he said, "I want to do that one."

I attached paper on top of it and put both in a clipboard. "Now rub the crayon on it."

As Demetrius rubbed, the head appeared.

"It's like magic," I said. "See how it's popping out. Do some more. He's missing his body."

When he was finished rubbing, he showed his teacher and then put it in his cubby to take home.

- **Define the purpose of the group and have children decide on activities.**

"The purpose of our group is for you to work together. You can do any activity using whatever we have in the department," I said to the children, who were hospitalized.

At first the children thought about crafts, but one child saw the people puppets lining the counter and said, "Let's do a puppet show." Everyone agreed.

"What should our puppet show be about?"

"Being in the hospital," Frank said.

"Yeah," the group echoed.

"Okay, pick the puppet you want to use," I suggested.

There was a moment of silence. The children's heads swayed left to right as they examined each puppet. Lisa jumped up and grabbed the doctor and little girl puppets. "Let's use these," she said. Everyone nodded.

"The next step is to write the script. What happens to this little girl in the hospital?" I asked. "What is she feeling?"

"When I came in the hospital, I was scared," one 10 year old said. "I thought I would get a shot."

"When I came, I didn't know what was going to happen," another child added. After describing their first day in the hospital, the group wrote the storyline for the show.

"Who is going to be the doctor?"

"I don't want to be on stage," a younger child said nervously.

"That's okay. You can help make the posters for the show. That's really important too."

"I'll be the doctor," Frank said, and Lisa agreed to be the little girl. The next day, the group painted posters, designed a stage, practiced the script, and named the show *A Day in the Hospital*. Two days later, the production was ready. Fifteen people, including nurses, psychologists, family members, and other children from the unit, waited anxiously to see the show.

Frank, acting as the doctor, visited the little girl in bed. "How are you feeling?" he asked.

"Good," the girl said.

"That'll be $100."

The audience laughed at his humor. The show was such a success that the group decided to repeat it that night.

- **Use general categories to define the routine.**

"This group is called Kids Helping Themselves," I told the third-grade class in the day treatment. "We are going to share ideas and do different activities to learn all kind of ways to help yourself, especially ways to keep yourself calm and alert." Referring to *How Does Your Engine Run?* (Williams & Shellenberger, 1996), I continued, "Like a car engine, you want to get your body just right, not running too fast or too slow. You also will create your own book of what works for you. This will help you remember. My plan is to make this group fun.

"In our group:

1. We will start by having you tell us if your body is going too fast, too slow, or just right.

2. Then we will squeeze stress balls and count to 10. I have all kinds of fun ones.

3. We will practice a strategy. It will be either one you already found works for you or a new one.

4. Then you will complete one page by drawing or writing in your strategy book.

5. We will do some kind of activity involving drawing or making something."

- **Set up the environment and let children choose the activities.**

Because I shared a room with other professionals, I rolled a cart containing supplies and children's drawings from the occupational therapy department to the pediatric oncology clinic. I covered the walls with the children's pictures and put out paper, crayons, markers, stencils, and scissors on a side table. On the floor and against the wall, I spread out toys, puzzles, magnetic blocks, a toy doctor's kit, and craft projects.

After explaining therapy, I pointed to all the choices and asked 5-year-old Kiefer, "What would you like to do? If you want to make a picture, we can hang it up."

He walked around the room, looking at all his options. Then he grabbed paper and markers and started drawing.

Establish a Routine for Beginning and/or Ending Activities and the Session

Depending on the children's needs, you may want to create a predictable routine. Some may need a routine for the beginning of a session, one for the ending, or both. Others, especially younger children, may benefit from starting and/or stopping activities in the same way. One way for them to learn the routine is to have a peer look at a visual schedule and announce what is next. Often children enjoy being helpers and telling others what to do. A consistent method for switching activities leads to a more orderly and smooth transition.

Fabulous Five: Develop a Routine Within the Session

- **Establish a beginning routine.**

Three year-old Trent, bundled up in his winter coat, entered the classroom and ran past the coat rack.

Stepping between him and the class, I blocked his way. "Take your coat off, please," I said, pointing to his picture above the coat hook. After he hung it up, he started to run again. "Say goodbye to your mom," I prompted him.

He turned around and went back. "Kisses, kisses," he yelled, holding his arms out.

His mother hugged and kissed him.

"Now join your friends," I said with a smile.

- **Start the activity by having a classmate look at the visual schedule and announce what is next.**

After the preschoolers picked up their centers, they came to the rug and sat down. "Elias, you're our helper today," his teacher said. "Tell us what is next."

He went to the edge of the easel that contained a vertical strip of picture symbols. Elias moved the wooden clothespin from the picture of children playing to the next picture of children reading books. "It's time for buddy reading," he announced. The children then picked books and described to a friend what they saw in the illustrations.

- **Start and end the session the same way.**

When 5-year-old Neil came into the occupational therapy clinic, I helped him sit on a small bench facing a mirror. While sitting behind him, I placed my hands on his hips and watched his expression in the mirror.

"First we have to take your shoes off," I said as I loosened the Velcro straps. "Pull off."

Taking a full minute to get his hand to touch the shoe, he pushed it off his foot and repeated the same action on the other foot.

"Next you have to get your socks off," I said, moving the sock to the middle of his foot. I waited as his hand jerked back and forth as he aimed for the sock. Once he reached it, he pulled. After getting the other sock off, I said, "Are you ready to play?"

He raised his head with a big grin.

"Yes, you are. You worked hard. It's time to have some fun."

At the end of the session, he struggled but succeeded at pulling his socks and shoes back on with help. "You're getting better at this," I said, and he smiled.

- **End activities the same way.**

During the occupational therapy student's first week in the specialized preschool program, I said, "When it is time to stop and transition to another activity, we do the same routine throughout the day. The teacher rings a bell and we show the children this." I pointed to a strip containing the numbers 1, 2, and 3, followed by a stop sign picture. "We say, 'One, two, three. Stop!' Then we sing a clean-up song. A few minutes later, when they are done, we give them a picture cue of where to go next. During center time, the children always rotate clockwise to the next center. Having this routine has really helped."

- **Create an ending routine for the session.**

"It's time to go," I said to 3-year-old Sarah. She threw herself on the floor of the occupational therapy clinic and began crying. Everyone glared at me to see what I was doing to her. I coaxed her to the hospital elevator, and she again collapsed on the floor and resumed crying. The others in the elevator stared at me. "I know it is hard to stop when you are having fun," I said, and she finally stood when the door opened to her unit.

The next day I created a routine. At the end of the session, I said, "Say, 'Bye-bye, bear.'"

Sarah waved at the 3-foot stuffed bear. Then we went over to the other end of the clinic where therapists were working with adults recovering from strokes. Sarah waved goodbye to each one. The men and women smiled and waved back.

"Let's go to the elevator so you can push the button," I said.

"Me push, me push."

Once on the elevator, I said, "Let's go see the fishies." We stopped at the aquarium outside the unit and waved to the fish. "Say, 'Bye-bye, fishies.'"

"Bye-bye," she said, then calmly walked into the unit.

We followed this routine every session, and she proceeded to the unit without a problem.

Use Objects, Photographs, or Picture Symbols to Represent Activities in the Schedule

You can help children prepare for changes by creating a visual schedule. Seeing objects, photographs, or pictures of upcoming activities helps children picture the sequence of what will happen next. For those who do not understand that symbols represent activities, it is better to start with an object they can see or hold. You may, for instance, hand them a ball to let them know it is time to go to the playground. Next, you would have them carry the ball as a transitional object.

Another variation is to make a list of activities and attach a small object to each activity on the list. This way the children can also feel the order of what will be happening. This can benefit children with limited vision. The next level would be to make a schedule using photographs of the child doing the activity. A more abstract level would be to use photographs of representational objects. For example, a photograph of a pencil and paper would indicate that it is time to write. The most abstract level would be the use of visual symbols for each activity. For example, a picture symbol of musical notes would represent a music class.

You can involve children in learning their schedule. One way is to have them remove the picture of a completed activity and then look at and/or take the picture of the next activity. Another way is to put photographs or pictures symbols of the activities in sequence and place them on a ring or on a Velcro strip in a small book. Children can remove or flip through the books by themselves. Being able to see what will happen often quells children's anxiety.

Fabulous Five: Use Objects, Photographs, or Pictures to Represent Activities in the Schedule

- **Use objects to represent activities in the visual schedule.**

"It's time to go outside," the teacher in the specialized classroom announced.

I knew that it was 3-year-old Dakota's second day and that she was nonverbal. I showed her a card with picture symbols of the swings and a slide. She threw herself on the rug and began screaming.

"Do you need help?" the teacher asked me.

"She doesn't understand the picture symbol. Could you get her coat for me?" I asked. "I think she'll know that putting her coat on means going outside." As soon as I handed her the coat, she stopped crying and put it on.

- **Display a sequence of photographs of the child doing of each activity in the visual schedule.**

Three-year-old Peyton consistently did not watch as his teacher reviewed the picture schedule for the day. He often turned his back away from the board and patted a friend sitting next to him. The two boys would then start laughing.

To help keep his attention, the special education teacher took photographs of him in each activity. The next morning, Peyton held a cardboard strip of his photographs and looked at each activity as the teacher described the schedule.

- **Display photographs of the sequence of each activity in the visual schedule.**

At first, we showed 3-year-old RJ the picture symbols of the class routine. He did not look at or respond to the cards.

"I don't think he understands the symbols," the speech-language pathologist said. She then took photographs of each activity and attached them with Velcro to a board.

"RJ, here's what your class is doing today," she said, pointing to the pictures. "Look, first you play with toys.

When it is time to stop, take this picture off and look at the next one. It is opening group."

RJ watched, and from then on, he moved the card after each activity was completed.

- **Check an individual strip containing picture symbols of upcoming activities.**

"Let's see what is next," the certified occupational therapy assistant said to 10-year-old Terry. Together they walked over to the wall in his classroom that contained his visual schedule. He pulled off the picture symbol of a slide.

"Look, you get to go to recess," she said.

He put on his coat, went to the door, and waited with his classmates.

- **Have children carry pictures of the activities on a ring or in a small book.**

"James looks lost when we change activities," his kindergarten teacher said. "He needs assistance to follow the others."

To help him understand, the special education teacher made pictures of all the activities. She put them in sequence on a ring and gave them to James. He liked fingering through them, and he quickly learned to look at the pictures for where to go next.

Show Time Visually

Younger children have a different sense of time than adults. An adult may say, "Wait a minute," and think that is reasonable, whereas for a child a minute may seem more like an hour, especially if there is nothing to do. For some, it is helpful to show a visual representation of time. This assists in teaching about the concept of time by showing the passage of minutes before making a change and eliminates an abrupt ending.

You may show time in a concrete manner through a number of ways. First, you can make a strip and have the children pick a favorite character or object. Often they will choose a superhero or movie figure. Then add five pictures of the object or person to the strip. Another alternative is to add the numbers 1 through 5 to the strip. A picture or number would be removed for each minute prior to the change in activity.

A second option is to use an egg, gel, or visual timer. With a visual timer, a red area decreases as each minute passes. The dripping of gel or sand from the timer's top to the bottom also shows time moving on. Another method is to hold up your hand with your fingers spread to indicate five minutes and count down.

Fabulous Five: Show the Passage of Time in a Visual Manner

- **Use a strip showing five pictures to represent time.**

"We're going to put pictures on here," I said as I pointed to a white board with five pieces of Velcro attached. "What do you want the picture to be?"

"A pirate," 3-year-old Erik responded.

I made five pictures of a pirate and put them on the Velcro. "You have five pirates. When they are gone, you will go to the writing table."

As Erik played, I gained his attention before removing one pirate every minute. When there was one picture left, I said, "One more pirate and then you go to the table." At the end, I added, "No more pirates. It's time to go to the table." Erik stopped and joined his classmates.

- **Use a strip showing five numbers to represent time and have a picture of the next activity at the end.**

"We have a new student," the preschool teacher told me. "He's never been in school and cannot talk. He cries a lot. Yesterday when I played the clean-up song, he kept playing at centers. I tried to help him, but he started screaming and ran under the table."

I thought that he probably did not want to stop playing because he did not know what was next. The next day, I brought a homemade strip showing numbers 1 through 5 and a place to put a photograph of the next activity. All were attached using Velcro. Five minutes before the end of centers, I showed Arthur the strip with a photograph of a book about trucks.

"Five more minutes then we read books," I said as I removed the number 5. In response, he crawled under the table. I joined him on the floor and continued to show him the strip and remove the numbers as time passed. "One more minute, then we read your truck book. You like trucks."

The teacher played the clean-up music, and I pointed to the picture of the book. Arthur crawled over to the rug, where the books were. I quickly pulled out the truck book and placed it in his lap. He started turning the pages as his classmates joined him.

- **Use a visual timer to show the passage of time.**

The preschoolers played with puzzles and construction toys for the first 10 minutes of class. "It's almost time to clean up. Could you set the timer?" the teacher asked me.

I slid the knob on the device until the red under-layer showed and the top layer lined up with the number 5. "Five more minutes until you have to clean up," I said, pointing to the timer. I moved it to where everyone could see it and added, "When the red is gone, we will put the toys away."

As each minute passed, the top layer moved and the red portion decreased. "Two more minutes," I announced. When the red disappeared, I pointed to the timer and told the group it was time to stop.

- **Incorporate a gel or egg timer.**

I placed a 4-minute gel timer on the table and flipped it over. The blue gel dripped on a wheel, making it spin. The three third graders watched. Because they did not like to write, I said, "We are going to work on your pop-up books for a short time. I'll turn the timer over. Keep writing your story until the timer stops. Then we'll play a game."

- **Hold up your hand or display a paper hand with the five fingers spread apart to indicate the time left.**

"Five more minutes," the teacher announced, showing 3-year-old Tyler her hand with her fingers spread apart.

He continued to play with the tiger puzzle.

"Two more minutes," the teacher said, showing two fingers.

Tyler yelled out, "No music, no music," knowing the clean-up song was coming.

"When you hear the music, the puzzle pieces go in the box," the special education teacher said.

"One more minute," the teacher called out to the group, holding up one finger.

"The pieces go in the box when the music plays," the special education teacher cued Tyler again as she demonstrated putting in a few pieces.

"Clean up, clean up, everybody clean up," the song played.

Tyler pouted and hesitated, but then threw the puzzle in the container.

Show the Sequence of Activities

In addition to having a visual schedule, you can show and review the sequence of activities in various ways. Before starting, you can point to a picture and say what will happen that day. You may simplify the schedule by only showing two pictures: a picture of the current activity and a picture of the next one. One variation is to make a numbered list of the order of activities. To show completion, you can point to the list and erase the words as each activity is finished. Another way is to have children mark a box on a checklist or remove pictures from a visual schedule.

Fabulous Five: Show the Sequence of Activities

- **Discuss the sequence of activities within the schedule.**

"Today is February 14th," the preschool teacher said. "Let's count the days." The class clapped their hands as they said each number.

"I'm going to check our message for the day," the teacher said as she went to a small red mailbox attached to her easel. She pulled out a slip of paper, smiled, and read, "We are going to have a Valentine's Day party." The children repeated the words as she wrote them on the board.

"Let's go over the schedule." She pointed to the visual schedule of the classroom activities. "We did opening group," she said as she pulled the card off the Velcro strip. "What's next?"

"Centers," the class shouted.

"Then?"

"Small groups."

"Next?"

"Outside time."

"Then?"

"Party!"

- **Use a board showing the current activity and the next sequential one.**

The two preschoolers in the specialized program put thick wooden beads on a pipe cleaner. In the last 3 minutes of our small group, I pulled out a board with the picture symbol of our group at the table and a second picture of children playing in the centers. "Now you are in our small group," I said, pointing. "Next you go to centers."

- **Make a numbered list of the activities.**

At the beginning of my time with 3-year-old Ella, who was nonverbal, I held up a dry erase board with the numbers 1, 2, and 3 listed. Then I drew a picture next to each number as I said, "Number one is to color a butterfly. Number two is to do a puzzle. Number three is to feed the bear."

I placed a cup of 1-inch crayons on the table and attached a piece of paper and a stencil of a butterfly to a clipboard. When Ella finished, I pointed to the board and erased the first line. Then I put out two animal puzzles with knobs on each piece. As soon as Ella touched one, I moved the other puzzle off the table.

She cupped her palm around the large knobs and pulled. With assistance, she slowly push the pieces back in.

Again I pointed to the board and erased the second line. "Next is the bear." I put out a plastic bear that had previously contained honey. I emptied the plastic sticks inside the bear onto the table and demonstrated feeding the bear.

Ella grasped the bear with one hand and, using her index finger and thumb, dropped the plastic pieces into the opening in the bear's head. Enthralled, she maintained her focus on it until all the pieces were gone.

I pointed to the board and erased the last line. "We're all done. It's time to go."

- **Use a checklist of the schedule.**

In the small, specialized class, I made a laminated sheet listing the four activities with corresponding picture symbols. Each one was in a basket. In front of each item on the paper was a check box for the children to mark when they were done.

"Here's what we're doing today," I said to 4-year-old Danny, and he flapped his hands in response. "Number one is to cut. Number two is to draw. Three is to do a puzzle and four is to play with Play-Doh. When you're done, put a check in the box."

The first time he used the checklist, I provided hand-over-hand assistance in making the check. The second time, he made the mark by himself.

- **Remove pictures or erase words of completed activities.**

I joined the ongoing group of third and fourth graders in the specialized program that was led by the speech-language pathologist. Throughout the school year, she had created a consistent routine. My role was to identify possible strategies to help meet the children's sensory needs so they could attend and participate in the group. First the children were given the cue, "Check your schedule." Following the prompt, the children would walk over to their individual Velcro strip containing pictures of the activities for the day and select the picture of the group. The next step was to sit on the carpet next to their name tag. Chase slid on his weighted vest, which I had given him. Derrick reached for his weighted lapbag.

"Look here," the speech-language pathologist said, pointing to three words on the board. "Today we are going to do a story, a song, and a movie." As each activity was completed, she erased the corresponding word.

Make Adaptations to the Routine or Transitions

Children might be thinking:
How much longer do I have?
Thanks for letting me know about the change in our schedule.
You're making sure I'm successful.
It's a lot better now.

Although you may have an established routine, there will always be times when changes are necessary. Preparing children for unusual events or schedule changes gives them time to adjust, which makes for an easier transition. Discovering the right mix of activities can aid in transitions. For children who have difficulty with the current routine or transitions, make adaptations so they can be successful.

Prepare for Changes in Routine

For many children, telling them at the last minute about changes creates anxiety. A variation in the routine is often upsetting. To teach children flexibility and to prepare them, it can be helpful to use a card with a surprised-looking face as part of a visual schedule. Talk about what will happen and when. You also may want to create a story with photographs outlining what to expect and what to do.

Fabulous Five: Assist Children in Getting Ready for Change

- **Talk about what will happen when there is a major change in the routine.**

"Today there is an evacuation drill, and we will be going to the building on the next street," the preschool director told me. "Plus, the teacher is sick, and there will be a substitute for her."

After all the children arrived and were seated, I told them, "We are going for a long walk. It is like a fire drill. It is practice. Nothing is wrong. You are safe. We will go up the street, up the stairs, and into a big building. We will be with the big kids. We will keep you safe. Remember when we walked to the grocery store? You did super good at staying in line, and you used your walking feet. Do that again. You also have to stay quiet so you can hear the teachers talk. There will be a lot of kids, and if everyone talked, it would get too loud." I covered my ears and added, "If it's too noisy, it would hurt your ears. I know you will be really good at walking and being quiet."

The preschoolers followed my directions and stayed calm throughout the drill.

- **Review the visual schedule showing when the change will happen.**

"Today we are doing something different," the teacher said, pointing to the corresponding pictures. "As usual, we will have opening group and I will read a story." She pointed to a picture symbol of multiple children and said, "Then we are going to a school assembly in the gym. We will be with all the older kids and learn about ways to eat healthy." Pointing to the next picture on the schedule, she continued, "When the assembly is over, we will go to the playground."

- **Show a special card to indicate any surprises or changes.**

"Let's look at our schedule. We have a nice surprise," the preschool teacher said to the class. She stood by the visual schedule and pointed to a card with the word *surprise* on it and a picture symbol with a matching facial expression. "We get to go to the kindergarten room to see real baby chicks that were just born."

- **Create a photo book of what to expect.**

The preschool classes rode the bus to the local pumpkin patch. Thirty children spread out, running from one pumpkin to another, looking for the perfect size. After choosing their pumpkins, the teachers put their names on them and told the children to put them in the truck. When the truck was full, it drove back to the school. Seeing their pumpkins disappear, some children cried.

The next school year, I created a photo book for the teachers to read to their class with the following story: *We are going to the pumpkin patch. Some children will go in cars. Some children will ride the bus. We will see animals. We will walk through a maze. We will pick a pumpkin and the teachers will put our name on it. We will put our pumpkins in a truck. The truck will take our pumpkins back to school. We will go back to school and get our pumpkins.*

The children went 2 weeks later, and no one cried when the truck drove away.

- **Make a story about what to do when there is a change.**

Three-year-old Jason had come mid-year to the preschool and began to adjust to the routine. To help him with a new event, I wrote the following story and attached photographs from the previous year on each page:

On Thursday, we are going to have a real pilot come here. His name is Pilot Pat.

My friends from the other class will come to my room.

I will sit with my friends while Pilot Pat tells us about airplanes.

I will be quiet so my friends can listen. I can hold my squishy ball.

I get to sit on a chair just like a real plane. I like planes!

For 3 days, we read the words to him as he turned the pages of the book.

Use the Right Mix of Activities to Aid With Transitions

As you work with the children, you need to analyze how transitions are going for individuals and for the group. Watch to see what is working and what is not. Think about the different elements of the activities and consider the following questions:

- What is the best way to start and create an easier transition?
  - Start with challenging or with easy ones?
  - Start with sitting or movement activities?
  - Start with excitatory or calming activities?
- Also consider motivating factors such as:
  - Is there a good combination of challenging and fun activities?
  - What activities do they avoid?
  - Do they need movement to stay alert?

- ○ Does the next activity have any enticing elements?
- ○ Will they participate in a nonpreferred activity if followed by a preferred activity?
- Another consideration is children's reactions during transitions.
  - ○ Do children lose their focus when they need to change to a different task?
  - ○ Does their attention wander if the activity goes on for too long?
  - ○ Do they become upset when they have to stop an activity?

As you ask yourself these questions, identify what kind of transitions are the hardest for the children. Make the needed changes, such as adding more movement or ending with a calming activity. Keep trying until you find the right mix.

Fabulous Five: Find the Right Mixture of Activities

- **Have a fun activity after a challenging one.**

Four-year-old Jessica colored a picture of a flower. "I kinda got it out a little," she said when she went over the line.

"That's okay," I replied.

"Boy oh boy," she said as she moved to the petals. "It's getting harder. I don't feel like coloring anymore."

"Just finish one petal. You can finish the rest next week. What would you like to do next?"

"It's hard to decide. Oh, I see something I like," she said as she looked in my cupboard. "I like this game. It's good fun." She pulled out a game called Mr. Mouth, which involved catapulting bug-shaped plastic strips into a moving frog's mouth.

- **Use a preferred activity after a nonpreferred one.**

Every chance 3-year-old Kellen had, he gravitated toward the toy phone. He pushed the number buttons, creating his own tune, and stared at the flashing lights. Then he giggled and repeated the sequence. When given crayons or markers, he would make marks for two seconds and then drop them on the table.

To mix more challenging with more fun activities, I showed him a picture symbol of coloring and a toy phone. "First, you color. Then you play with the phone." I gave him markers and stencils. When he stopped, I made the sign for "more" and encouraged him to continue until the shape was covered in color. Once done, he reached for the toy.

- **Determine if and when movement is need in the routine.**

During our monthly planning meetings, one teacher said, "Our morning class is mostly very young boys. It's been challenging to get them to settle down."

"It might help to weave more movement activities throughout the day," I suggested. "Try to avoid long periods of sitting." The team then talked about possible movement activities that matched their current fall theme.

- **Match the level of difficulty in challenges with children's preferences.**

In the first session, 3-year-old Akeisha sat on the therapy mat and cried if her body moved slightly to the right or the left. Before the second session, I thought about how to get her comfortable with movement and interested in objects or toys. *I'm going to start where she is comfortable, and she just has to sit*, I thought.

When Akeisha came, I brought out a switch that was attached to a vibrating pillow. While she sat still, I placed her left hand on the pillow and pushed the switch. She made her happy humming sound. After a minute I stopped until she made her annoyed sound, letting me know she wanted the pillow to vibrate again.

I pushed the switch again. A few minutes later, I moved the pillow just a couple of inches away. She reached for it with her hand, which required her to maintain her balance as she tilted her body to the left. Her happy humming sound resumed as she felt the vibration of the pillow. In the following sessions, I always started with an easy activity, and after she was comfortable, I would gently increase the level of challenge.

- **Determine whether it is better to end with a movement or sitting activity.**

"What do you want to do first?" I asked 5-year-old Jim.

He grabbed the scooter board, positioned himself, and flew down the ramp, knocking over cardboard bricks. After a few more times, he ran over and crawled into the net swing.

"You look like Superman," I said.

He started spinning by pushing himself with his hands on the underlying mats. I set up a tower of cardboard bricks and held beanbags in front of him. Jim stopped spinning and reached for one.

"Hey, Superman, see if you can knock this over and save the town."

He swung forward and threw the beanbags. As the session progressed, he became more excited and ran between activities. To help him settle before leaving, I put Legos on the table. "Check these out," I said, and Jim raced over. His movements slowed down as he played and we talked about his favorite activity for that day. From then on, I always ended the session with a quiet, sitting activity.

Change One Aspect of the Routine or Transition

Transitions between activities can be challenging and stressful. At times, there is more noise and commotion. For children who are struggling, start by observing and analyzing what might be causing the breakdown. Do their sensory needs or sensitivities create difficulties? Does their attention wander during transitions? Does it take a lot of effort to move?

Consider changing one aspect of the routine or transition. You may want to change the amount of movement required or decrease the amount of sensory stimulation during changes. For some, you may want to teach children to use calming sensory strategies prior to transitions. Another option is to limit the number of transitions, minimizing how many times they have to stop and start. Others benefit from changing their placement or having them do the routine at a different time than others.

Fabulous Five: Change One Aspect of the Transition

- **Change the amount of movement required between activities.**

At the beginning of the school year, the preschool teacher designed her opening group to include activities alternating between sitting and moving. In November, the teacher told me, "We have a new girl. Her mother carries her in. She walks like a toddler and moves really slowly."

As I watched 3-year-old Danielle walk, she waddled to the group with her legs far apart. She half-fell, half-plopped down. Then it took her 3 to 4 minutes to get up. At the end of the day, the teacher and I talked.

"It's really hard for her to get up and down," I said.

"I saw that."

"Would it be possible to change opening group a little so she doesn't have to move so much?"

"Yeah, I could do that. Maybe I'll do more songs and finger plays and then dancing."

"That would be great."

- **Have children do the routine at a different time from others.**

When the kindergarten teacher opened the door, a swarm of children came into the room. Everyone rushed to hang up their coats, bumping Nick along the way. He growled as he took his coat off. Nick joined the group but continued to look agitated. Within the first hour of class, he had three incidents of dropping to the floor and crying when upset.

At the end of school, his teacher, mother, and I talked about his day. "I think there's too much commotion and noise," I said. "I saw that he's getting upset when he's bumped. It's too much for him. It's sensory overload."

"Could you bring him 5 minutes early?" his teacher asked his mother, and she nodded. "Then he could hang up his coat and sit down before we let anyone else in."

"That will make school more comfortable and help him start the day being calm," I added.

"I think that will help," his mother replied.

The next day, he started the new routine and did not cry at all.

- **Change children's placement during transitions.**

As the preschoolers stood in line, the child at the back shoved the one in front of him. A domino effect followed, causing many, including Jake, to get bumped.

"Hey," Jake screamed, "stop that!" He swung his arm toward the girl behind him.

Because I had seen Jake be sensitive to being touched, the teacher and I later discussed the situation. We agreed that he could be either the door holder or the last one in line to carry out the toys.

The next day, Jake smiled as he held the door.

- **Minimize stops and starts if transitions are hard.**

In the spring before children started preschool, 3-year-old Hunter came to our Beginning group. On his first day, Hunter ran into the room and fingered every object he saw. He continued at full speed. When I enticed him with a toy, he finally sat on the rug with the other children. When it was time to pick up the toys, he jumped up and again began zooming around the room.

After the children left, we talked. "Once Hunter was sitting," I said, "he paid attention. But every time we stood, he wanted to leave the group and run around the room." The staff decided to put all the sitting activities together and decrease the number of transitions.

- **Decrease the amount of sensory stimulation during transitions.**

Dante and David jumped on the merry-go-round and squealed with delight. "Push," Dante yelled, and the paraprofessional gave a thrust.

I watched the boys and told the surrounding staff of the specialized program, "They are having so much fun and really enjoy spinning. But be aware, spinning can wind children up. I know sometimes they get agitated in the afternoon. When you go back to class, this would be a good time to dim the lights and play soft music."

When the class reentered the darkened room and heard classical music, the boys calmly sat down at their desks.

Make Therapy Flow

One aspect of therapy not often talked about is the need to make the session flow from one activity to another. You can create a natural transition if you make changes at the end of an activity or game. This prevents a feeling of being disjointed or jarring. You also develop a sense of flow by building a bridge interconnecting actions, conversations, and activities. Another option is to use a unifying theme, such as having all the activities related to farm animals. By making therapy flow, you will provide smooth transitions.

Wait for Natural Breaks to Make Changes

> **Children might be thinking:**
> *What else do you have?*
> *What should I do next?*
> *Can we keep playing games?*
> *What's next?*

A good time to make a change is at the natural ending of the activity. A natural break has a defined and clear ending. Children will expect to do something else and will be more open to moving on. Waiting for this type of ending makes it easier to shift because you are not stopping in the middle. It is not abrupt. You can create this type of break by limiting how many supplies you put out for the activity. In addition, you can identify which step will be completed that day before moving on to something else. Another good time to change is after everyone has had a turn.

> ### *Fabulous Five: Transition After a Natural Break*
>
> - **Shift after completing an activity or project.**
>
> "Put the magnet that looks like a man on top of this board," I said as I demonstrated. "Then put the other magnet under the board and move the man through the path."
>
> Six-year-old Trent adjusted the magnets and began the course. As he bumped into the raised edges of the path, the man tipped over. Trent grimaced but realigned them and continued. "I did it," he shouted when he reached the end.
>
> "Do you want to try another board with a different path or do something else?"
>
> "Do something else."
>
> - **Wait until the end of the game.**
>
> "I brought this really fun caterpillar. He dances!" I pushed the button, and the upright toy caterpillar with 10 outstretched hands wiggled. "You have to use the tongs to put the marbles in his hands while he's moving. It's tricky."
>
> The group of 3 and 4 year olds giggled as they tried and often missed.
>
> When each hand held a marble, I told the group, "Next you get to play with putty."

> - **Shift to another activity when supplies run out.**
>
> "What's this for?" 6-year-old Isabelle asked as I handed her a wooden clothespin.
>
> "This is for our game. You pinch the clothespin, pick up the spider rings, and put them in this black kettle. We can pretend to make spider soup."
>
> "Here, I got three. I'm going to get more."
>
> After she plucked seven more, I said, "All the spiders are gone. Do you want to stir the soup and taste it?"
>
> "No," she replied with a smile. "Spiders taste yucky. I want to do the tops next."
>
> - **Change after finishing one step.**
>
> "For Thanksgiving you get to make your very own turkey. First color the turkey. Then cut out the feathers and glue them on. Today we will just color, and next week you can add the feathers."
>
> When the group of 3 year olds finished the first step, I said, "I have two games we can play. Do you want to do an Operation game or a fishing one?"
>
> "Fishing!"
>
> - **Change after each group member has had a turn.**
>
> "We are going to go around the circle," I said to the preschoolers on the rug. "Everyone will get a turn. This is a martian. When you squeeze this toy, his eyes and ears pop out. Use one hand and squeeze it as hard as you can."
>
> "I'm strong," Nate said as he tightened his grip around the toy.
>
> After all the children had a turn, I said, "The martian is tired. He's going to take a nap. Next we get to do a game called Don't Spill the Beans."
>
> "Yea, I love games," 4-year-old Erik said.

Create a Bridge

> **Children might be thinking:**
> *You're using my idea.*
> *You noticed what I like.*
> *You listened.*
> *We talked about that last time. Doing this reminds me of….*
> *You bring up what I care about.*

One way to make therapy flow is to create a bridge from the children's actions, conversations, and/or experiences to therapy. There is a seamless transition when you follow the children's lead and build upon their current actions. You can also make verbal connections relating the activity to children's life experiences. An additional method is to tie together various conversations.

Follow the Children's Lead

It is easier to create a bridge when you start with the children's interests or expand on their ideas. One way you can connect is by joining children wherever they are located. Instead of asking them to join you, you go to them. For instance, if they are sitting on the floor, you would do the same. You can always either bring an activity with you or expand what they are doing. Another way to connect with children is to suggest ideas and expand their play using an object they are holding in their hands. You could also propose to add another element to their action sequence. In addition, you could offer ways to increase the complexity of their current actions or activity.

By allowing children to initiate, you immediately learn about their interests and show respect by not discounting their ideas. Your actions show children that you want to be in a partnership and not have everything adult directed. It is okay to add new ideas because then children can build on what you suggest. Doing so can promote their imagination and foster creativity. Increasing children's sense of control in what they get to do will increase their motivation to continue. Finally, show your enjoyment of their personalities by using their words or invented names in the next activity.

Fabulous Five: Follow the Children's Lead

- **Join children where they are.**

  Three-year-old Lucas lay on his back on the classroom floor. I brought a blue foam pegboard with multicolored pegs over to him. One by one, I handed him a peg and said in a gentle voice, "Put in."

  He rolled to his side with his head resting on one arm while he placed the pegs with his other hand. After putting a few in, he shifted to sitting and continued filling the board.

- **Expand the activity using the object the child is holding.**

  The teacher placed a bin of Duplos, blocks, and plastic animals on the rug. Three-year-old Jackson grabbed a yellow block and walked aimlessly around the room.

  "Jackson," I said, gesturing toward the bin. "Come join us." When he and another child came over, I added, "Let's make a zoo for the animals." I started making a square-shaped structure. "We need your yellow piece here. Help us."

  Jackson sat down and pushed the block onto the structure.

  "Thanks," I said. "Put more on, please."

- **Add another element to their action sequence.**

  "Do you want to create an obstacle course?" I asked 7-year-old Grady, and he nodded. "Look around the room and tell me what you want to do."

  He pointed to the scooter board ramp and the large cardboard blocks shaped like bricks. "First I'll go down and knock the blocks over. Then I'll crawl through the tunnel."

  "That sounds great."

  After Grady completed his course, I suggested, "Let's make it even harder. What if I make a path with the blocks that you have to zigzag around? What do you think?"

  "I like it."

  "Then, instead of crashing into the blocks, use the beanbags to knock them down. Does that sound all right to you?"

  Grady nodded. He smiled as he went through the course and faced harder challenges.

- **Increase the complexity of their activity.**

  Every day, before 4-year-old Zach began playing with manipulatives, he sat on the floor snipping construction paper into small pieces. One day, I joined him on the floor and brought a toy car. After watching him cut for a few minutes, I said, "I see how you enjoy cutting." I showed him the car and then drew two long lines on another piece of paper. "This car needs a road. Here, cut on the lines." I handed him the paper and he stayed on the lines. We then took turns pushing the car on his new road.

- **Use their words or invented name in the next activity.**

  I showed Wayne a pattern book. The first grader browsed through it and pointed to a picture of two feet. I copied the pattern, and he colored it with various colors. "Write something about your feet. You're creative. I know you will come up with something good."

  He thought for a minute and then said, "The totem pole monster had the ugliest feet ever. They were green, orange, and purple."

  After he printed his sentence, he stapled his pages together and handed the book to me.

  "You did a great job. I really like your story." Then I pulled out a bag of blue and yellow Tangles that could be snapped together and said, "Do you want to make another monster?"

  He nodded and began popping pieces together.

Make Verbal Connections to the Activity

Another way to create a bridge is to make verbal connections during therapy. One approach would be to listen to children and suggest or adapt the activity based on what they are saying. This allows you to gain their attention and tap into their interests. It also shows you are truly listening to them and are interested in what they have to say. A second approach is to make verbal connections between the activity and the children's lives. This is an opportunity to talk about how therapy can be a learning experience that is germane to their life. A third approach is to connect the activity to a holiday or current events. Again, this can make therapy more relevant, meaningful, and fun. A fourth approach is to make verbal statements linking the activities within a session together. This gives you a chance to highlight a common theme.

Fabulous Five: Make Verbal Connections to the Activity

- **Connect the activity to children's conversations.**

"Guess what I'm going be for Halloween?" 6-year-old Sean said.

"What?"

"Superman," Sean said.

"Okay, Superman, I have an idea. Let's get your shoulders super strong." Sean smiled. "Try putting your hands on the floor, and I will hold your feet. Head over to those spider tops. Then use that wooden clothespin to get those spiders back in their home."

- **Make statements that connect the activity to the children's life.**

As 4-year-old Logan cut out a snowman, I asked, "Will you get to play in the snow when you go home?"

"Yeah, I'm going to make a big snowman. My brother will help me."

- **Relate the activity to an holiday.**

Five-year-old Morgan dumped a container of heart-shaped erasers on the table and said, "Hey, it's a mountain."

"A mountain of what?" I asked.

"Valentines."

"Because Valentine's Day is this week, I brought some fun things to do. The first thing is to pick up these heart erasers with chopsticks."

"It's kind of hard. I almost got it," she said as the eraser slipped through. After a few tries, she retrieved them all.

"I brought several hole punchers that make different-sized hearts, so you can make a card if you want. You have to push hard. The paper is thick."

"I'm going to need a little help here," she said. I assisted her, then handed her a glue stick. "This is slippery glue. What happens if my fingers get sticky?"

"You can just wash it off."

When Morgan finished her card, I said, "There is one more fun thing you can do, if you want." I pointed to a heart cut out of bubble wrap that was attached to an easel. "You can decorate it with shaving cream."

As she smeared on the cream and popped some of the bubbles, she said, "I like this."

- **Incorporate current events into an activity.**

"What are we doing today?"

"You're going to the Olympics," the occupational therapy student said to the two boys. "You need to pass the torch to each other until we get to the stadium. Pass this medicine ball over your head to the other person."

The boys took turns lifting the ball over their heads and moving toward the coffee can with a yellow paper flame.

"It's heavy," Hector said.

"It's not heavy for me," Juan said.

"This is my favorite game."

"This is a fun game."

"We're going through Denver. We're almost there," the occupational therapy student said when the boys were halfway down the hall.

A few more minutes passed and then boys shouted, "We lit the torch."

"You are champs!"

- **Make statements that connect activities.**

Four preschoolers met with a special education teacher, the speech-language pathologist, and me for our social skills group. "I am going to read two books, and then we will play a game. The first story is about Tucker the Turtle," the special education teacher said. She read the story that taught a self-calming technique of stopping, taking a deep breath, and thinking of how to solve problems with friends.

"Put your hand on your tummy," I said. "One, take one breath. Move your hand up. Two, take another breath. Move your hand higher. Three, another breath." Holding up my index finger, I cued them, "Now, blow out the birthday candle."

Then the teacher read a story about a dinosaur who shared his toys.

"Next we have a game," I said. "I brought these fun beanbags. When they hit the ground, they talk! These are my toys, and I'm sharing them with you." I held up a picture from the solution kit showing children sharing. "Ask me with nice words like, 'Could I have the green one, please, or the red one?' Then I will give you that one, and you throw it at the target."

The children took turns and laughed when the beanbags landed on the floor and said, "Oh no."

At the end of the group, I connected the activities by saying, "So when you're mad, be like Tucker the Turtle. Stop, keep your hands to yourself, and take three big breaths. Then, if you are having trouble with a friend, use an idea in the solution kit. One solution is to share."

Connect Conversations to Children's Experiences

A third way to create a bridge is to connect conversations to children's experiences. Throughout the session, ask about their activities. Also mention previous conversations and check how they are doing now. As children are talking, refer to what they have told you in the past. You can also talk about the time you spent together. Comment at the end of the session about conversations you had at the beginning. These connections show children you have listened and remembered what they said. Create a sense of flow by linking different conversations together.

Fabulous Five: Connect Conversations and Experiences

- **Ask children to talk about their experiences.**

"Did you have a good summer?" I asked the 9 year olds in the first therapy session in the fall. They all nodded. "What did you do?"

"I had so much fun. You have to hear this. I played in the sprinklers with Adam."

"I went to the beach. We found a shell as big as my dad's hand."

"I went riding for a long time. I rode my bike around a lot of houses."

- **Refer to a memory from a previous session.**

As 7-year-old Susan drew with different-colored chalk, her hand became covered in the dust. "Oh, I'm getting all chalky," she said, and then laughed at her invented word. "That's a good one," she said, and I smiled.

The next time I saw her, I asked her what she wanted to do. Grinning, I said, "Do you want to paint, draw, or get chalky again?"

- **Make statements that connect what was said or happened in past and present sessions.**

As 4-year-old Lorna colored a picture, she said, "I like princess stuff. I get excited if I eat sugar. My mom said I'm getting my ears pierced when I'm 5. My dad said he's ready for a baby."

"What kind of princess stuff do you have?" I asked.

"I have a dress, crown, and wand."

When I saw Lorna the next week, I asked, "Did you get to wear your princess dress this week?"

She nodded and smiled.

- **Mention a concern from a previous conversation and check in.**

"I know last week you said you were having a hard time," I said to 11-year-old Kaylee. "How are things going in your class now?"

"It's still hard. Yesterday I forgot my reading log. Now I don't get credit."

"That's so frustrating when that happens."

- **Comment at the end of the session about conversations had at the beginning.**

"Your teacher said you're going on a field trip this afternoon," I said to 4-year-old Cooper as we walked to the therapy room. "Where are you going?"

"We are going to the fire station. My mom is coming too."

"It's really nice that your mom can join you. That should be fun."

When our session was over, I said, "Have a good time at the fire station. Tell me about it next week."

Use a Unifying Theme

Children might be thinking:
This is fun.
These activities are connected.

There are creative ways to weave different activities into a cohesive whole. When you use a unifying theme, you make the session flow from one activity to another without feeling disjointed (Figure 16-1). One method to do this is to use the same object, such as tongs, in all of them. Similarly, you can connect a common element, such as vibration, that is present in each activity. Puppets, marionettes, or toy figures are another fun way to create a sense of unity. A theme based on pretend play or children's life experiences is an additional approach for making connections.

Fabulous Five: Unite Activities Through a Theme

- **Keep the same element in all the activities.**

Four-year-old Karl pressed a toy car on a pillow that vibrated. The humming reverberated throughout the room. He turned on a ladybug-shaped massager and placed it on the wooden balance board. The loud rattle echoed. Next, he moved the massager to the car and pretended to give it gas.

Seeing that he enjoyed vibration and to introduce writing utensils, I pulled out a large sheet of butcher paper and a vibrating pen. "Make a road for your car." He reached for the pen, flipped the switch, and made wiggly lines.

- **Incorporate a theme related to children's experiences.**

At a preschool next to a farm, the children often saw horses and cows in the pasture. One day for a joint occupational and speech therapy session, I placed plastic farm animals, a toy barn, and putty on the table. "These animals are hungry," I told the two 4-year-old boys. "Roll the putty in your hands to make their food."

Dustin formed the putty into a ball and said, "Here, Mr. Cow, eat."

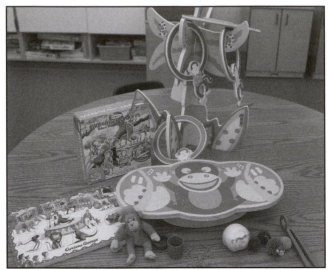

Figure 16-1. Incorporate a unifying theme, such as having monkeys in all the activities.

After a few minutes, I said, "I think the animals are full. Now they need some exercise." I handed the boys some tongs to promote strengthening of their fingers. "Use these tongs to move them."

"Put the cow behind the barn," the speech-language pathologist said to help the boys learn different prepositions. They followed along. "Next, put the cow on top of the barn."

"Watch out for flying cows," I teased. The boys smiled. After a few more directions, I said, "We have one more activity. You get to make your very own farm. First color the grass, sky, and animals. Then cut out the cow, sheep, and pig and glue them on your paper."

Logan made a few marks on the page and said, "I'm done."

"Color some more," I replied. "Make your grass greener." He resumed coloring and finished his picture. "What are you going to call your farm?"

"Logan's farm."

"Dustin, what are you going to call your farm?"

"The happy farm."

- **Use puppets, marionettes, or toy figures to connect various activities.**

I handed bubble wrap to the three third graders. Holding a wizard marionette with wild gray hair protruding out of his pointed hat, I pulled the strings and waved his arms. Pretending to be him, I said, "You have to pop all the bubbles to scare the dragons away."

"Okay, Merlin," Will replied as he touched the wizard.

The sounds of *pop, pop, pop* filled the room.

"Next we're going to make a pop-up book," I said in my wizard voice. I gave them a picture of a wizard brewing a potion. "Color this and then think of your story. I will write it down. Next time you can copy it and finish your book."

After the children told me their stories of the magic potion, they each had a turn with the marionette. They tapped his feet on the table and waved his arm with the magic wand. "I turn you into a frog," Casey said with a laugh.

"I turn you into a hamster," Will said during his turn.

At the end of the session, I made the marionette fly again. "Don't let him touch you," I said. "He might cast a spell on you."

The smiling children made a quick exit.

- **Use a play theme to connect activities and help with transitions.**

"Jared and Ethan, let's pretend you're seals," I proposed.

The second graders grinned in response.

"To do a seal walk, get down on your tummies, put your palms on the floor, and lift your shoulders. Then pull your body with your arms." Pointing to a blue beanbag chair and small fish erasers, I added, "Head to the rock so you can catch some fish."

The two boys scooted across the room, stopping twice to flap their hands. They climbed on top of the beanbag chair and made sounds like seals. "Ar-ar, ar-ar."

"Okay, seals. Time for lunch. To catch a fish, you have to pick it up using a wooden clothespin."

Pinching the clothespins, which strengthened their hand muscles, they picked up six yellow fish erasers and dropped them into the bucket.

"Let's go to the table. I have a real fish snack for you." They plopped down in their chairs. "Line up these goldfish crackers on these two letters. Then trace the letter in the air. After you show me how to make the letter, you can eat the crackers." They followed the directions and soon were nibbling on crackers. "Okay, seals, it's time to go. Did you have fun?"

"Yeah!" they said in unison.

- **Use the same object in all the activities.**

I handed each second grader a clip shaped like teeth. "Pinch the ends and the teeth will open. Pick up the cotton balls and put them in the bowl."

"Yum, yum," they said, laughing as they pretended to eat.

When the bowl was full, I put a wind-up toy that was also shaped like teeth on the table. "Everyone gets a turn. Wind him up. Don't let him eat you though," I joked.

"Did you lose your teeth?" Marisol joked back.

As the wind-up toy came closer, the children took turns squealing, "Aaah, don't bite me."

Then I pulled out a large set of plastic, rubbery teeth that had lettered dice inside the mouth. "Now we get to play a game. Shake the teeth and drop the dice on the table. See if you can make a word, and we will practice printing those words."

Create Seamless Transitions

Making smooth transitions keeps children's interest and motivates them to shift gears. That makes change easier and is not abrupt. Also, involving children in defining when they are finished with the current activity allows for a sense of completion and creates a readiness to move on to the next one.

Ease Into the Next Activity

> **Children might be thinking:**
> *I'm done with this.*
> *I don't want to do this anymore.*
> *This is boring. Can I do something else?*

To make a smooth transition between activities, first watch for any obvious or subtle signs the children want to stop. Be responsive and address their feelings. Enlisting children's help engages them in the process of moving on. Pointing out enticing elements of the next activity also makes it easier for children to change. Another approach is to use transitional objects, actions, or picture. This helps children visualize what is coming next and shift their thinking from what they are currently doing.

Watch for Subtle and Obvious Signs That Children Are Finished

Being in a partnership means respecting what each other says. Thus, in the beginning of therapy, tell children to speak up and let you know when they are finished or want to stop. Then, during activities, watch closely for any nonverbal signs of frustration, restlessness, or boredom and intervene. You may want to offer help, suggest they take a break, or finish it at a later date. For children who are nonverbal, teach the sign language for "more" and "all done" so they have a way to communicate with you. Also be responsive to any statements, such as, "This is boring," that reflect the children's struggles.

For children who stop at the slightest difficulty out of fear of failure, acknowledge their feelings and provide encouragement. They also may need to take a break. You also can tell children what the options for the next activity are and ask them to tell you when they are ready to change. When children feel comfortable telling you they want to stop and you respond, they will be more likely to try harder challenges. In addition, you will learn about their frustration tolerance and can grade activities accordingly.

Fabulous Five: Establish When Children Are Finished

- **Learn children's way of saying they are done.**

  In the specialized classroom, 3-year-old Bailey was given paper and marker. She took the marker and pounded it on the table. When the tip was destroyed and the marker no longer worked, she put her arm on the table and, in one sweeping motion, shoved the paper and marker to the floor. "By-ee," she yelled as the supplies fell.

  Whenever she was done with an activity, she yelled, "By-ee."

- **Watch for nonverbal signs of restlessness or frustration.**

  Holding a tennis ball with two eyes and a slit for a mouth, I said as I demonstrated, "This ghost likes to eat pennies. Try it."

  Six-year-old Trevor squeezed, and the mouth opened slightly. He tapped the ball on my arm and said as the ghost, "I want to eat Dr. Clare."

  "He only eats pennies. I don't taste very good," I replied with a smile. "I'll do a few. Then you do a few."

  When it was Trevor's turn, he struggled. He placed the tennis ball on the table and began looking around. Responding to his signs of frustration, I said, "Here, I'll open his mouth and you feed him the food." After Trevor put three pennies in, I said as the ghost, "Thanks for the lunch."

- **Recognize signs of boredom.**

  In the specialized class, 4-year-old Nan sat in a bean-bag chair and played with a wooden puzzle. When she was finished, she pushed it off her lap, and the pieces scattered around her. She looked at a musical toy.

  "You're done with the puzzle," I said, putting all the pieces back except one. With my hand over hers, I helped her put in the last piece. Then I handed her the toy.

- **Teach acceptable ways of stopping an activity.**

  Juan left his specialized classroom to spend time in the third-grade class. While others were reading to themselves, Juan grabbed a book and sat on a large pillow. He quickly turned the pages, closed the book, and pitched it over his shoulder.

  I retrieved the book and brought over the bin. I handed him the book. "Put it here," I said, pointing. "When you are done reading, put the books in here."

  Juan dropped the book in the bin.

- **State the action children can take to indicate they are done.**

  As 5-year-old Darius tinkered with a set of blocks, he said, "I'm big. I got taller when I was sleeping in my bedroom. There was a tooth fairy in my room."

  "I see you're getting taller," I replied with a smile. Noticing that he was losing interest with the blocks, I added, "If you are done playing with those, put them in this container."

  A few minutes later, he put them away.

Have Children Tell You When They Are Finished

An important part of collaboration is for children to have a say about beginning or stopping an activity. Tell them to let you know when they are finished so you can respect their wishes. For those who are nonverbal, ask them to communicate by using sign language or a communication device. Pay attention and respond to any statements indicating boredom or disinterest. You also can inform them about options for the next activity and have them tell you when they are ready.

Fabulous Five: Have Children Tell You When They Are Finished

- **Tell children to let you know when they want to stop.**

"I have something I think you will like," I said to 8-year-old Ariel. "I brought some different activities today. Which one do you want to start with?"

"I want to do the magnetic board."

As I attached the white board to an easel, I said, "You get to make a monster with these pieces. They are magnets. Be sure and tell me when you are done and want to try something else."

- **Ask children to tell you they are done in sign language or with their communication device.**

The class of preschoolers sat at two tables eating their snack. Three-year-old Parker, who was nonverbal, munched on goldfish crackers. When he finished what was in front of him, I asked him, "Do you want more crackers?" as I moved his fingertips together to sign "more." I continued by pulling his hands apart to make the sign for "all done." "Or are you all done?"

He patted his hands together.

"Oh, you want more. Thanks for telling me," I said, placing more crackers on his napkin.

After a few weeks of practicing both messages, Parker began signing "All done" when he was finished with his food and activities.

- **Respond quickly to any statements reflecting boredom or disinterest.**

"I'm bored," 6–year-old Bobby said as he drew.

"You can stop," I replied. "What would you like to do next?"

"The train puzzle."

- **Give options for the next activity and have children tell you when to change.**

I handed 5-year-old Gina a gel ball containing small plastic snakes.

"I love these snakes," she replied. "I wish my dad would buy this." She continually squeezed the ball.

"There's some buried all the way down at the bottom. I'm going to count to five. I'm strong enough to squeeze the ball to see the snakes."

"I also brought our writing game and the Operation game," I said. "Let me know when you are done squeezing."

- **Say, "Let me know when you are ready, then you can...."**

Five-year-old Drew pulled the red plastic monkeys out of the barrel. He connected their curved arms, creating a chain.

"Wow, that's getting long," I said.

He added a few more, but then the bottom half fell off. After he recreated the chain two more times, I said, "Let me know when you're ready, then you can try the vibrating pen or the tops. They're both fun."

"I'm ready," he replied.

Signal a Change

Giving a signal that there will be a change causes children to shift their attention from the current task. They tend to stop and look or listen to the signal. One fun and playful way to indicate a change is to use a finger puppet or toy figurine to make an announcement. Another way is to use a toy or object, such as a clicker that makes a funny or different sound. Children are usually delighted if you asked them to be in charge of giving the signal. You also can use an action or movement pattern to represent a transition.

A common option is to turn the lights off and back on. This quickly gets their attention and quiets the group. However, use other approaches if any children in the group or class are sensitive to the flickering of lights. Finally, having children change their position (e.g., moving from sitting to standing) is a natural cue that you are going to do something different.

Fabulous Five: Signal a Change

- **Have a puppet or toy figure suggest the change.**

Using tongs, 6-year-old Jan picked up erasers shaped like carrots and placed them in a container. Then she took an eraser and offered it to a toy rabbit. "I'm feeding him," she said.

I put my fingers on the rabbit and said in a falsetto voice, "Thanks for feeding me. Now I want to watch you cut."

"You're full, huh?" she said to the rabbit.

"Yeah, thanks."

Jan followed me as I carried the rabbit over to the table and placed the toy facing Jan's paper.

- **Create a symbol indicating change.**

I brought a wooden clicker shaped like a bird. "Push down on his tail and he chirps. He'll tell you when it's time to stop," I told the kindergartners. They each took a turn making the bird sing.

After they cut out shamrocks, I handed Renee the bird and said, "Click his tail." She smiled and made the chirping sounds. Everyone stopped and looked at me. "Next, you can decorate your shamrock with crayons, markers, or glitter glue."

- **Use an action to indicate a change.**

"Today we are going to switch things up," the preschool teacher said and, with her hands raised, made circles in the air. "We are going to the playground before we do science. Everybody switch it up."

The class waved their hands in the same circular pattern as the teacher.

"Is it okay to switch things up?" the teacher asked.

"Yeah," the class replied back.

- **Turn the lights off and then on to signal a change.**

The kindergartners sat at their table coloring, cutting, and gluing their sheets about the germination of flowers. The volume in the room increased as they all chatted while working. After about 10 minutes, their teacher turned the lights off and then back on. The room became quiet. "Finish up. You have 5 more minutes, and then we go to the library. If you're not done, you'll have time this afternoon."

- **Have children change their position, such as sitting or standing, for a different activity.**

Pierre and Paige played with putty at the table.

Moving to the floor, I said to the third graders, "Come sit on the floor. I want to show you a game."

Entice to the Next Activity

In children's minds, stopping a fun or engaging activity is often viewed as a loss. Encourage thinking about what is ahead versus what they are leaving. You need to make the next activity just as much or more fun, interesting, and appealing than the current one. One way to aid the transition is to let children see what the next activity is or what their future choices are. It then becomes a known versus a vague option. Another way is to mention an enticing element in the next activity. A third method is to use mystery. Mystery is intriguing and attracts interest. Their curiosity will be aroused and their attention will shift. Using a phrase such as, "I know you like…. Check this out," or using the word "fun" in mentioning the next activity is also alluring.

Fabulous Five: Entice to the Next Activity

- **Let children see the next activity before changing from the current one.**

As 4-year-old David was finishing coloring a card for his mom, I put two games on the table and said, "When you're done, you can pick what game you want to play next."

He drew a heart on the page and signed his name on the card. After he examined his choices, he selected a treasure hunt game.

- **Point out an enticing element of the next activity.**

Marie, the music therapist at the specialized program, brought a guitar, a keyboard, a xylophone, castanets, and a microphone. She divided the equipment among the three fourth graders, who were nonverbal.

Todd took the mallet and started pounding on the xylophone with full force. After about a minute, Marie held the castanets in front of him and tapped them. "Try these. You can click them." When he looked up, she moved the xylophone away and quickly exchanged the castanets for the mallet.

- **Use mystery as an enticement.**

"Come sit down here so I can show you what is next," I said, patting the table.

"What is it?" the second graders asked.

"Sit down and you'll see," I said with excitement. "Oh, I think you'll like it."

After they sat, I pulled four musical tops out of my bag and gave one to each child.

- **Say, "I know you like…. Check out…."**

As 4-year-old Jordan played with putty, I said, "I know you like hammering. I remember how much you liked hitting the ice cubes in the game Don't Break the Ice."

"Yeah, that's a fun game."

"Check this out," I said, pointing to a pumpkin. "You get to hammer golf tees into the pumpkin. It's really fun too."

He put the putty away and reached for the hammer.

- **Say, "We need to stop doing this/finish up because we have other fun things to do."**

"You can play with the putty," I told 6-year-old Shane. "What are you going to make?"

"Me. That's my person. Here's my leg. This is me. I'm a superhero."

After 5 minutes of making different figures, I said, "Finish up because we have more fun things to do. I brought a new toy I want to show you."

Shane squashed the putty in the container, and I showed him a new wind-up toy.

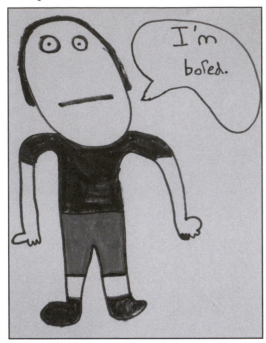

Figure 16-2. Minimize wait times during transitions.

Prevent Frustration or Boredom With Transitions

Children might be thinking:
I don't like to wait.
I like being a helper.

Transitions can be difficult for some children. They may be upset about stopping a fun activity, leery about changing, or unsure about what is next. This can lead to frustration or boredom during the transition. To prevent these unpleasant feelings, especially with younger ones, limit waiting, enlist their help, or use singing and/or movement activities.

Limit Waiting During Transitions

For younger children, especially ones who often wander and do not self-initiate play, keep waiting time minimal. When they indicate disinterest in the current activity, have other options close by and be prepared to be quick in switching (Figure 16-2). They will tend to keep playing if the activity keeps their interest and there is only 5 to 10 seconds of waiting. When they stop, you can hand them another object or toy to capture their attention.

It also helps to analyze what they understand and can do. Then match the activities involving the same type of motion. For instance, if children only drop objects into containers but do not take them out, you could keep handing them different types of objects to put in. To get these children to try something new or different, give them a fun object or toy with one hand while your other hand removes the current one. This 1- to 2-second switch prevents leaving them empty handed and losing their interest.

Fabulous Five: Limit Waiting When Making a Change

- **Eliminate or shorten wait time during transitions.**

While the substitute preschool teacher searched for a book, the class began squirming. Two boys wrestled. I went to the front of the class and asked one of the rough-housing boys, "Tucker, what song should we sing?"

The boys stopped, and Tucker replied, "'Twinkle, Twinkle, Little Star.'"

- **Have options of activities close by and within reach.**

Before center time in the specialized preschool classroom, I put puzzles, wooden lacing boards, wooden beads with pipe cleaners, putty, and cookie cutters next to my small table. Later, the children took turns in the art center where I was stationed. Pointing to their options, I said, "What would you like to do?" When they were done with their first choice, I quickly grabbed two more activities that were within my reach and had them choose another.

- **Bring or hand the next object to the children.**

At the beginning of class, 5-year-old Elliott wandered around the room, alternating between tapping his fingers on his cheek and tapping objects around him.

When he joined his classmates at the table, I brought over a stack of my wooden puzzles. I put an animal puzzle in front of him and took out the pieces. He immediately put them back in. As soon as he was done with one puzzle, I replaced it with another. He continued and stayed focused for the next 10 minutes.

- **Switch activities but keep the same type of motion.**

For the first few days, 3-year-old Wyatt whimpered as he wandered around the specialized class. When shown toys, he pushed them away with his hand and continued circling the room.

I grabbed a yellow plastic shape sorter. In the lid there were three cutout shapes of a circle, square, and triangle. When Wyatt sat in the red wagon at the back of the class, I brought the shape sorter to him. Using hand-over-hand assistance, I helped him drop three pieces in. After that, I handed him the pieces, and he dropped them in the container. When all the pieces were in, I popped off the lid to retrieve them. Wyatt jumped out of the wagon.

Throughout the morning, I tried different toys with him to see what he liked and could do. I noticed that Wyatt stayed focused when putting objects in but not taking them out.

After his teacher and I talked, I went to the resource room and gathered a variety of toys that involve putting objects into them. As soon as Wyatt placed all the pieces in one toy, we would quickly give him another toy requiring the same motion. He then played continuously.

- **Give a new object with the one hand as you move another object out of sight with the other one hand.**

On the first day, 3-year-old Trey walked into the therapy group, flapping his hands. He grabbed a mallet, sat down, and hit a plastic ball into a hole. The ball rolled down the maze. Then he started hitting the next ball on top of the maze. He continued playing with the toy for over 5 minutes.

To introduce other toys he could use the mallet on, I grabbed a small wooden table–shaped toy containing pegs. He could pound the pegs and, when done, turn it over and start again.

As each ball rolled to the end of the maze, I reached with my left hand and moved the ball behind me. The second the last ball rolled down, I moved the maze away with my left hand and with my right hand put the table-shaped toy in front of him. I made the gesture of pounding and pointed to the peg. Trey began hammering.

Enlist Help to Ease the Transition

You can motivate children to change by enlisting their assistance. Because children often enjoy being helpers, you can give them a job when changing from one activity to another. Asking them to be in charge and responsible for a certain task shows that you believe in them, which can be appealing and rewarding. Another way is to ask for a peer's assistance such as holding a younger child's hand or showing the child the way to go. However, make sure the peer is someone the child likes. If you know that children like to clean, ask for their help in getting ready for the next activity. You can also ask the group to carry the needed items for what is next. Obtaining children's help creates smooth transitions and promotes a sense of pride. As always, show appreciation for their efforts.

Fabulous Five: Ask for Help During a Transition

- **Give children a job during the transition.**

Every time the teacher announced that it was time to go inside, 4-year-old Jordan ran away from the group. One day, knowing that his favorite toy was a plastic lawnmower, the teacher said, "Jordan, come here. We need your help. It's going to be your job to take the lawn mower back to our classroom." From then on, Jordan ran and grabbed the mower and proudly pushed it as he walked in line with his classmates.

- **Have a peer hold a young child's hand during transitions.**

Three-year-old Jeff wandered around the playground, walking on his toes and flapping his hands. When the preschool teacher rang the bell, the class ran to the fence to line up. Jeff did not respond.

Then his teacher turned to another preschooler and said, "Kayla, would you please help your friend? Ask him to join us."

Kayla smiled and nodded. She went to him, gently took his hand, and said, "Come on, Jeff." He walked with her without any resistance. From then on, Kayla helped him make the transition off the playground.

- **Have a peer show another child where to go.**

"It's time to go to the tables," the preschool teacher said to the children on the rug. Knowing that MaryAnn had difficulty understanding the directions and liked to be with Kelly, the teacher added, "Kelly, show MaryAnn where to go."

Kelly tapped MaryAnn's arm and beckoned to her, "Come with me," and she did.

- **Ask children who like cleaning to help get ready for the next task.**

On the first day of the Beginnings group, 3-year-old Lucas cried when his mother left. He came to the rug and sat with the other children but backed into a corner and covered his face with his hands. "Here's a fun toy," I said, trying to entice him into hammering balls into a toy boat. He peeked but kept his face covered.

"I have a bubble machine," the special education teacher said to him. Again, he peeked but withdrew behind his hands.

After the others played for five minutes, we said, "It's time to put the toys away." Lucas reached for some blocks with both hands and immediately dropped them in the bin. He continued until they were all picked up. When the other children walked over to the table, Lucas retreated to his corner and covered his face again.

I reached for a wet paper towel and said, "Lucas, you are really good at cleaning up. Could you wipe this table for us?"

He stood up, took the towel, and washed the table. When he was done, he sat down in the chair.

"Thanks! We appreciate your help."

- **Ask a group to work together to help carry items for the next activity.**

"After we finish painting, we get to make an obstacle course. I need your help setting it up," I said, and the preschoolers smiled in response.

When their artwork was finished, I said, "We need to carry the balance beam, tunnel, blocks, and hula hoop out into the hall."

The group scooped up the items, and together we decided on the course. They would walk on the balance beam, jump over the wooden blocks, crawl through the tunnel, and then jump in and out of the hula hoop on the floor.

Use Singing or Movement During Transitions

Transitions go more smoothly for younger children when using singing or movement activities. Parents often hum and sing to comfort and calm them, especially when they were infants. Children tend to view singing as a soothing and pleasant experience. To assist children in making changes, you can make up your own song and sing the directions of where to go next. By repeating the directions in the song, you help them process and remember where they need to go.

Another option is to turn the transition into an activity. You can sing, use songs with finger movements, incorporate animal walks, or even make an obstacle course. Activity-based transitions help children let go of thinking about what they are leaving or worrying about where they are going. Instead, children focus on the current activity.

Fabulous Five: Use Singing or Movement During Transitions

- **Sing where to go.**

On the first day, the preschoolers in the specialized class headed to the bus. One child repeatedly dropped to the floor, another cried, and another tried to run away from the group. It was chaotic.

The next day, I made up a song. "To the bus, to the bus, to the bus," I sang as we walked down the long hallway. "Oh, we must, we must, we must—go to the bus." The other staff joined in, and the children listened as they continued walking.

- **Use songs with finger plays for younger children who are waiting during transitions.**

While the preschool class sat on the rug and waited for the others to join them, I started singing, "Five little monkeys jumping on the bed…." and made the corresponding finger motions. The children sitting in the circle started singing. We continued until all the children sat down as the teacher joined us.

- **Sing during the transition.**

The preschool class had to walk past the older children's playground to reach theirs. During the first week of school, to help the 3 year olds keep walking I started singing, "The ants go marching one by one…." The staff smiled and joined in this familiar song. The children began to march, and continued until they reached their area.

- **Create an obstacle course during transitions.**

To create a smooth transition and develop the preschoolers' motor skills, once a week I created an obstacle course in the school hallway. After the class went to the bathroom, they went through the course twice before returning to their classroom.

"Step up on the stepstool and jump down with two feet," I told them. "Next, walk on the balance beam. Then jump with two feet on the four plastic circles. You can do it!"

The children quickly moved through the course, focused on keeping their balance.

- **Use a transitional movement.**

"After opening group, when we go to the tables, Rick keeps running around the room," the preschool teacher told me. "He wants us to chase him. Transitions are the hardest time for him."

We talked about ideas, and I suggested, "It might help him if you have the whole class do a movement like a bear or crab walk to the tables."

When I checked back the next week, she said my idea worked. Rick liked doing different animal walks.

Use Transitional Objects, Pictures, or Actions

> **Children might be thinking:**
> *Oh, what's that?*
> *What do you have? What is it?*
> *I like fun things.*
> *I'm back.*

To assist children in shifting calmly from one activity to another, it can be helpful to incorporate transitional objects, pictures, or actions. You can use objects and pictures as concrete representations of the next activity. Holding an object and/or seeing a picture increases the likelihood of children understanding and remembering where to go or what to do. Transitional actions can decrease the noise level and create a bridge between children's current actions and what is next. These types of supports are especially beneficial for children who are visual thinkers, have difficulty processing information, or are learning a new language.

Incorporate Transitional Objects

A transitional object is any item that assists children in moving from one activity to another. When they, especially young children, are able to hold something in their hands, they are better able to stay focused and make a change. One way is to hand children something that will be used in the next activity and ask them to carry it. If they are already holding or playing with an object, replace it with one representing the next activity. Another way is to show them an object they like that will be used in the next activity. Encourage them to follow you as you carry it to where you want them to go.

You also can use a transitional object when children hesitate to join a group or wander away. This can be something in which they currently show interest or can hold. Have them bring the object or activity over to where their peers are. You can suggest that they show it to a person in the group. Another approach is to bring an object to them that everyone else is using. This may capture their attention, gain their interest, and facilitate joining their peers.

Fabulous Five: Use Transitional Objects

- **Have children hold an object or toy during transitions.**

When 3-year-old Jeremy started preschool in February, he cried during transitions. I thought that it might be even more difficult for him to stop playing at recess. Because his mother had told us he loved to play with cars at home, I put two toy cars in my pocket. When it came time to stop, the teacher gave a 5-minute warning, and I showed Jeremy a picture symbol of the next activity. A few minutes later, the class began lining up, and Jeremy immediately began to cry. I pulled a shiny red car out of my pocket and showed it to him. "Let's get in line, and then you can hold the car," I said, pointing to his friends. He came with me and quietly walked inside holding the car.

The next week, he started riding the school bus. He held the car in his hand while on the bus, and even learned to keep it in his backpack during the school day.

- **Hand children an object that will be used in the next activity.**

The six preschoolers in the specialized program sat around the teacher. She read a story about a curious monkey. Then the class sang songs with corresponding hand motions, "Five little monkeys swinging from a tree teasing Mr. Alligator…." Next she called Billy and handed him a piece of paper with the outline of a tree and his name on it. "Take this paper to the table." He held the paper with two hands as he walked over and sat down.

After all the children were seated, I said, "You get to make your own fall tree. Here's yellow, orange, and red paper. Cut them into small pieces to make leaves and glue them onto your tree."

- **Show children an object they like that will be used in the next activity and carry it to where you want them to go.**

In the specialized program, 4-year-old Drew crawled under a table, yelling. Remembering how in our last session he liked the white plastic alphabet board, I went to get it. The last time, he had used the magnetic wand, and as he had traced the letter, small magnetic balls popped up. When done, he used his index finger to push the magnetic balls back down. He had sat for the next 10 minutes, mesmerized with this activity. Recalling this incident, I brought the alphabet board over to show him.

"No!" he screamed at me.

Then I showed it to a teacher, and Drew watched. A few minutes later, he stood with his hand outstretched. Holding the board within his eyesight, I moved to our table. Drew followed, sat, and began making letters.

- **Use an object the child is holding to transition back.**

"Jay's mother moved, so he will be coming to your pre-school. He does better if he carries a transitional object between activities," his previous school therapist told me.

On his first day, 3-year-old Jay walked in the room and looked at the different centers. He ran to the dollhouse and moved doll furniture. Then he went to the block area, grabbed a plastic hammer, and pounded on the wooden blocks. A few minutes later, he moseyed over to the art center.

"Look," I said, pointing to the children on the rug. "It's time to join your friends."

Jay threw himself on the floor and rolled around. Next, he reached toward a box containing colored plastic lenses. I took the box and pulled out blue and yellow ones and handed them to Jay. "Take these with you to the group."

I stretched out my hand and he took it. We walked together. He plopped down in the beanbag chair and held the yellow lens to his eye as he watched the teacher point to the calendar.

- **Have children show or give the object of interest to a person who is in the group.**

While her classmates did a science experiment, 3-year-old Leila wandered away from the group. She went into a center and fiddled with a toy figurine. I joined her and said, "Oh, you found a princess. Show your teacher that princess."

Leila went back to the group and handed the toy to her teacher.

"That's a pretty princess. We're glad you're back with us. Have a seat," the teacher said, patting the chair and handing Leila a magnifying glass.

Leila sat down and peered through the glass.

Use Pictures, Drawings, or Pointing to Assist With Transitions

When transitioning from one activity to another, realize that some children need additional visual cues. Photographs and pictures are easier to understand than words. You can promote an orderly change by handing children a photograph or picture symbol of the next activity and having them carry it to that location. You also could show the photograph or picture symbol and mention an enticing element of the next activity.

Another approach is to draw a picture of the next activity and give it to children to carry. Having them draw a picture to bridge their current interest and the next activity is also an option. Pointing to where friends are and what they are doing can be helpful. You may want to emphasize how their peers are having fun.

The use of pictures, drawings, or pointing requires minimal words. This decreases the amount of sensory stimulation during transitions. After practice, they also can learn to use visuals to move independently. Helping children understand the sequence can prevent uncertainty and frustration.

Fabulous Five: Incorporate Pictures, Drawings, or Pointing to Assist With Transitions

- **Hand children a photograph or picture symbol of the next activity to carry with them.**

The preschoolers sat on the rug and sang a song with corresponding hand motions. "The wheels on the bus go round and round…." When the song ended, the teacher said, "Everyone go to the tables." The group divided in two and sat down.

During her first two days, 3-year-old Abby stayed on the rug and cried when the class made this transition. Realizing that she did not understand what was happening, the speech-language pathologist made two picture symbols of a child sitting at a table. She taped one symbol on the table where Abby was supposed to sit.

On the third day, when the music stopped I handed Abby the picture symbol and walked her over to match it to the one on the table. From then on, whenever we would give her the picture, she immediately joined the others.

- **Show a photograph or picture symbol of the next activity and mention an enticing element.**

The preschool teacher of the specialized class gave a five-minute warning before the end of recess. Before it was time to go, I told the occupational therapy student, "If you tell them it is time to stop, many of them will get upset and cry. Instead, show them a picture symbol for snacks and tell them it is time to eat a snack and get a cool drink."

A few minutes later, the teacher rang the bell. The occupational therapy student walked over to Arthur, showed him the picture, and said, "It's time for a snack. It's hot out. Let's get a cool drink. Come on."

Arthur calmly followed her.

- **Draw a picture of the next activity and give it to the children.**

Three-year-old Cooper placed small plastic bears on the dots of the math sheet and then counted.

"That's right," the teacher said. "Now do the next row." When he was done, his teacher asked, "Do you want to go to science or blocks?"

"Science."

On a small piece of paper, she drew a stick figure of him chipping through plaster to find a dinosaur egg. As she drew, she said, "Here is Cooper at the science table. Cooper is using a little mallet to find a dinosaur egg."

Cooper showed the picture to his friend, put it in his pocket, and went straight to the science table.

"Wow," I said to the teacher, "drawing a picture really helped him."

"Yes," she replied. "I found that I was fumbling through the picture symbols to find the right one. By the time I found it, he was already out of his seat. It's easier and faster to draw."

- **Have children draw as a transitional activity.**

Three-year-old Silas examined the container of cocoons and budding butterflies. "It's time to go to your tables," his teacher announced. His classmates quickly moved to their seats and were given boards for drawing shapes. "Silas, come join us," his teacher said.

He continued to look at the butterflies and did not budge. The special education teacher brought a board to him. "Draw a butterfly," she said with a smile. Silas took the board and made two circles and a line. "Oh, let's go join your friends and draw some more." He responded by carrying the board to the table.

- **Point out where their friends are and what they are doing.**

At the end of the group movement activity, 4-year-old Duncan threw himself on the floor and began kicking the shelf. The teacher moved the shelf while she told the rest of the class to go to their tables. Duncan continued kicking and shouting, "I want a break."

"Okay," I replied, then quietly waited close to him. After a few minutes, I whispered, "Look at all your friends. They are drawing their plants. I think your seed grew into a plant. Let's go see."

He stood and calmly walked over to his teacher.

Use Transitional Actions

Transitions are often noisy and chaotic. To facilitate a calm and peaceful change, help the group become quiet. You can have them imitate your actions or participate in a pretend game or action. Doing the motions and merely mouthing the words of a familiar song may also lead to quiet.

To aid in changing, you also can use children's current actions as the transition. Do this by creating a bridge between their current interest and the next activity. Another option is to build on their actions by adding to or slightly changing what they are doing. You can help children handle change by making the process less stressful.

Fabulous Five: Use Transitional Actions

- **Have children quietly imitate your actions during a transition.**

"Do what I'm doing," I said as I stood in front of the line of preschoolers. The teacher was gathering stragglers before taking the class to recess. "Everyone be an airplane," I said as I raised my arms.

All the children's arms popped up, and they quieted down.

"Now be a bird." I waved my arms up and down as if flying.

The children responded silently again.

"Thanks," the teacher said when she came to the doorway, and then proceeded to lead the class outside.

- **Build on children's current actions to make a transition.**

Three-year-old Shelton stood at the water table and continually poured water on his left hand. After about five minutes, I quietly moved a water toy next to his hand. The water splashed off his hand onto the toy, making a wheel spin. Shelton moved closer to the toy and began pouring water directly into it.

- **Do the motions and mouth the words of a familiar song to quiet a group during transitions.**

"Today is Wednesday, September 1st," the preschool teacher said as she pointed to the calendar. Two children rolled on the floor, and three others chatted with each other. Three-year-old Rudy rocked side to side. With every change in activity, the noise level increased.

As the week progressed, the teacher taught three songs with corresponding finger movements. They sang the songs every day.

The next Monday morning, the class became restless. The teacher said, "Follow me."

The children's heads turned toward her. The teacher did the hand motions and mouthed one of the familiar songs without making a sound. The class became quiet and imitated her actions.

- **Use children's current action as a transition.**

Seven-year-old Mitzi lifted the yellow flashlight off the desk, flipped the switch, and scanned the room with the light.

"It's fun to play with flashlights," I said. "Bring it to our table and shine it on our game."

As she walked closer, the circle of light expanded.

"Thanks for helping us see our Operation game better. Mitzi, you go first."

She placed the flashlight on the table and grabbed tweezers for the game.

- **Use pretend games or actions during transitions.**

"We need to be quiet when we're walking to the library," the kindergarten teacher said to the children standing in line. "Everyone catch a bubble and put it in your mouth."

Following the teacher's movements, they reached high, pretended to catch a bubble, and puffed out their cheeks after bringing their hand to their mouths. The class quietly proceeded down the hall.

End the Current Activity Before Moving on to the Next One

Children might be thinking:
I guess I have to put this away before we move on.
I need to stop doing this.

Closure of the current activity before moving on to the next has a number of benefits. First, it is a defined ending, which helps children maintain focus on one activity at a time. You can have children determine when to stop by asking how many times they want to do something before doing the next thing. You also may want to tell them, "You need to stop… so you have time to do…." Second, when you are working in small areas (e.g., on a table), putting away materials makes room for something new and eliminates clutter. Clearing off a space also limits the amount of visual stimulation, making it easier for children to pay attention and stay organized. Third, asking children to clean up as a sign that they are finished gives a clear message that they are ready to move on. Finally, by asking them to put things away while you gather supplies or get the next activity ready, you can promote working together to expedite a faster transition.

Fabulous Five: End the Current Activity Before Moving on to the Next One

- **Ask the children how many times they want to do… before doing the next activity.**

"This is called a zoom ball. You hold these two handles, and I'll hold the other two. When you pull your hands apart, the ball will travel on the strings to me. Then put your hands together, and I will send it back to you."

As we learned to coordinate our movements, the ball zipped back and forth with rhythm. After about 5 minutes, I said, "How many more times do you want to send this ball to me before going to the table to build?"

"Ten times."

"Okay," I said, counting out loud as the ball flew my way. "Time to go to the table. Check out these magnetic tiles. You can build all kinds of shapes with them."

"I'm going to build a house."

- **Ask children to clean up as a sign that they are finished.**

After building with blocks, 7-year-old Ken stood and wandered around the room.

"Are you finished with these?" I asked, and he nodded. "Then please put the blocks away and decide what you want to do next."

- **Tell children, "You need to stop… so you have time to…."**

"Do you want to do the reindeer puzzle, the snowman puzzle, or both?"

"I want to play both," 6-year-old Curtis replied, and then pointed to the Operation game. "Then that game." He picked up the snowman puzzle.

"Look for corners," I cued him.

"Here it is. I knew it," he said as he popped a corner piece in place.

"You're good at these."

"I've been practicing at home." He quickly finished and then reached for the next puzzle. "I don't need any help on this one. I think I can do it." He manipulated a piece and said, "Nope," when it did not fit. He tried another. "Gotcha," he said when it slid into place.

When the puzzle was complete, I said, "You were right, you did it all by yourself. It's time to stop doing puzzles so you have time to play the game you wanted."

- **Tell children you will get out the next activity while they clean up.**

The group of 5 year olds used their index fingers to make letters in the trays full of blue sand. After about 5 minutes, Jorge asked, "Can we play the fishing game?" The others nodded.

"Sure," I replied. "Everyone pour the sand back into the container. While you are cleaning up, I will get the game out of my cabinet."

- **Talk about how cleaning up will make room for the next activity.**

I placed two magnetic bases on the table and spread out metal stars, marble-sized balls, and shapes. "Today you get to play with lots of magnets. You can make whatever you want with them," I told the two 6 year olds.

They eagerly connected the pieces. When they were done with their designs, they tugged hard to take the pieces off the base.

After a few minutes, I said, "Let's pick up everything so we can make room for some games." After they cleaned the table, I showed them two choices. "In this one, you take a magnetic wand and move a ball through a maze. In the second one, you take the magnetic wand to move these black slivers to give the man hair, a beard, or a mustache. If you want, you can play with both of them."

KEY POINTS TO REMEMBER

- Create a predictable routine so children know what to expect.
- Have routines to end activities or sessions.
- Develop a visual schedule using objects, photographs, or picture symbols to display the sequence of activities.
- Show the passage of time in a visual manner for younger children or those who are visual learners.
- Modify the routine or type of transition when needed.
- Prepare children for changes.
- Create a sense of flow in the therapy sessions by purposely making connections.
- Make smooth transitions by responding to children's cues and asking them to tell you when they are finished.
- Alert children about a change by using a signal.
- Prevent frustration or boredom during transitions by limiting waiting, enlisting children's help, or using singing or movement.
- Use transitional objects, pictures, or actions to help children change from one activity to another.
- End the current activity before moving onto the next one.

REVIEW QUESTIONS

1. Why is it good to prepare children for changes?
2. A preschooler wanders away from the group. Name at least three approaches you can use to help him or her rejoin the group.
3. Children dislike routines because they are boring. True or false.
4. It is easy for children to leave one activity without knowing what is next. True or false.
5. All children like to start with a sitting activity before doing a movement one. True or false.
6. When children transition within groups or a class, the amount of sensory stimulation increases. True or false.
7. Name three ways you can create bridges for a sense of flow within a session.
8. Why incorporate a unifying theme in your session?

9. Children will not always tell you when they are finished. True or false.

10. It is easier for younger children to transition when they see or hold onto an object or picture representing the next activity. True or false.

REFERENCE

Williams, M. S., & Shellenberger, S. (1996). *How does your engine run? A leader's guide to the Alert Program for Self Regulation.* Albuquerque, NM: TherapyWorks.

17

Promote Therapeutic Endings

CHAPTER OVERVIEW

It is important to help children end the sessions and end therapy on a positive note. Alerting and preparing them before stopping the sessions is vital. In this chapter, there are strategies for providing verbal and physical cues to signal the time to stop, making cleanup simple and fun, developing ending routines, and using props or games to define an ending point. In addition, there are ideas about emphasizing children's strengths at the end of the session, monitoring their progress, and updating the plan. When therapy comes to an end, a crucial process is putting closure on the relationship. Also included are ways to reminisce, review what happened and the progress made, and say goodbye.

CHILDREN'S DESCRIPTIONS OF WHAT THEY THINK YOU SHOULD KNOW

Dr. Clare: "What should therapists say to kids or do when it is time to stop?"

Lupe (age 10): "Let them play, then say, 'One more, that's all,' because kids like playing!"

Kim (age 10): "I think real nicely ask them to please put that thing down."

Kris (age 11): "Tell them you will bring it back and hopefully you can play longer."

Dr. Clare: "When therapists have to leave or say goodbye, what should they say or do on the last day?"

Jim (age 9): "Let us draw a picture. I love drawing."

Sam (age 10): "She could have us play a game or play the most favorite game us kids like."

Ben (age 11): "Tell the kid, 'Have fun, keep writing, and don't give up what you start,' because that's what you tell me and it works!"

CREATE THERAPEUTIC ENDINGS

The endings of a session and of therapy need to be thoughtful and planned processes. Stopping a session abruptly tend to be upsetting for children. To be respectful of their feelings, it is wise to prepare them regarding time limitations and an endpoint. As your time together ends, like closing a book, facilitate reflection on the competencies, changes, and lessons learned (Figure 17-1).

Prepare Children Before Ending a Session

When it is time to end the session, be sure to prepare children beforehand. To signal that it is time to stop, you may want to (a) use verbal, visual, or physical cues; (b) define a specific endpoint; or (c) use words, phrases, or songs. Also, make the cleanup as simple and fun as possible. This is necessary because cleaning up means the end of playing.

Curtin, C.
Strategies for Collaborating With Children: Creating Partnerships in Occupational Therapy and Research (pp. 353-374).
© 2017 SLACK Incorporated.

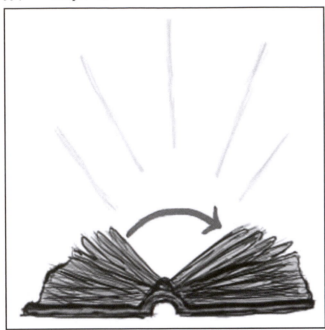

Figure 17-1. Like closing a book, create therapeutic endings.

It is often associated with chores and may be thought of as drudgery. In the last few minutes, check with the children regarding their perception of the session. Getting their feedback will help you make future adjustments. Remember to provide your view on how they did with a special emphasis on their competencies and progress.

Alert Children Before Ending a Session

> **Children might be thinking:**
> *I don't want to stop. I'm having fun.*
> *It's time to clean up.*
> *It helps to know how much time I have left.*
> *I have this many left to do.*
> *I like songs.*

When children are engrossed in an activity, they may feel sad, angry, or frustrated that they have to stop. They are enjoying themselves and having fun. For some, with no guarantee that what is after therapy is also fun, they may think it is just better to continue. Others may balk at stopping if they do not know what is next.

It is critical that you prepare children and give ample notice before ending to allow them to mentally shift from what they are doing to leaving. Consider that in addition to giving verbal cues, some children will need extra visual and/or physical ones. Younger children may also do better with songs or music indicating it is time to clean up. Others may need a defined endpoint, such as saying, "Build your last tower, and then it will be time to go." It also might be necessary to be explicit, such as showing a picture of what happens after therapy.

Give Verbal and/or Visual Cues to Indicate That It Is Time to Stop

Children know what to expect when cleanup is a regular part of the routine. They will tend to respond when they are told to put things away. Many children also do better when given a five-minute and then a two-minute warning before ending. For children working on long-term projects, alert them to how much time they have left. Knowing their time limitation helps them judge how much they can get done. Being prepared allows for a gradual adjustment to stopping and helps them pace themselves. Letting them know what is next aids the transition. In addition to talking about where they are going, you can help children understand and remember by showing a photograph or pictures of what is coming next.

Fabulous Five: Prepare Children Before Ending the Session

- **Make clean-up time part of the routine.**

"It's cleanup time," I announced, which I did at the end of each session.

"Hey, where's the rubber band for this box?" 3-year-old Nancy asked.

"Are you sitting on it?" I replied.

She stood and saw it on her chair. "That's delirious," she said through her laughter.

"That is hilarious. It's very funny."

- **Announce when there are only 5 and then 2 minutes left to the session.**

The preschool class sat on the rug as they played with a variety of toys. "Five more minutes," their teacher announced.

One set of boys stacked plastic pieces together. "Look, I made a robot," one said to his friend.

"Two more minutes," the teacher said. She looked at the boys and asked, "Is that a long time or a short time?"

"Short time."

"You're right." She waited and then said, "It's time to put the toys away."

- **Identify time limitations.**

Seven-year-old Wayne pulled out the Wedgits building blocks and the pattern book.

"We only have 5 minutes. You have time to make one design, and then we'll need to stop. I'll bring the blocks back next time so you can do more." Wayne opened the pattern book and picked one of the hardest. "Save that one for next week," I said.

"I can do it," he insisted.

"I believe you can do it. I'm worried about the time. Your mom and your sisters are waiting for you."

"I can do it," he repeated, and began building with little success.

"It's hard to do a tricky one when you feel rushed. Give yourself a break and save that one for next time. Make your own design." I put the pattern book away, and he built a seven-tier structure. "That is very cool. I like this one even better than the one in the book." He grinned in response.

- **Talk about what the next activity is after the session.**

As 4-year-old Lance finished cutting a butterfly he had colored, I said, "When you're done cutting, it will be time to go back to class." Referring to the visiting librarian who read new books and used puppets and storyboards, I added, "I heard Miss Mary is coming. She is so good at reading stories. I think you will enjoy her."

- **Show picture symbols of what they will be doing after the session.**

Four-year-old Liam, who was nonverbal, held the magnetic pencil. As he traced the lowercase letters, small magnetic balls popped up. After going through the alphabet, he used his finger to push the tiny balls down. He repeated this sequence multiple times.

"Five more minutes.... Two more minutes.... Time to clean up," the teacher announced.

When Liam did not stop, I showed him a picture symbol of the playground. "It's time to stop. We are going outside."

He grabbed the picture and stood up.

Provide Physical Cues for Stopping

Physical cues can be useful in giving the message that it is time to stop. One cue is to turn off the lights. When the room darkens, they understand they cannot continue. Make sure, however, that there is enough light to see how to get out of the room! If you are sitting at a table with them, another cue is to stand up. This implies an ending. Other ideas include using an object associated with cleaning or stopping. For instance, handing children a towel suggests that it is time to take their hands out of the water table and wipe them. Also, placing storage containers next to them also is a hint to clean up. Finally, picking up and putting away items not being used eliminates the temptation to continue. Physical cues are easier for children to understand than words.

Fabulous Five: Give Physical Cues to Stop

- **Turn off the lights to convey that it is time to leave the room.**

Collin curled into a ball on his chair and faced the wall as the rest of the group exited the room. "Time to go," I prompted him. When he did not budge, I turned off the light and started to walk out the room. He stood and followed.

- **If you are sitting at a table, stand up to indicate that it is time to stop.**

The certified occupational therapy assistant gave each of the four third graders a pointed dowel rod and a baking tray covered in clay. "Use the dowel rod to make the letters of your name." She went around the group and helped them form the letters correctly. After all had practiced, she said, "Go ahead and draw pictures in the clay. Draw whatever you want." She sat and watched them make cars, superheroes, and buildings.

When it was time to leave, she said, "Make your last drawing, then it will be time to go." Then she stood up and, as the children finished, took their trays and dowel rods. They headed out the door.

- **Move storage containers next to children as a cue to stop.**

I slid the plastic container for the putty toward 11-year-old Mario.

"I just need to finish my pizza," he said.

"When you're done, squish it in here."

He flattened the putty, added small rolled balls for the sausage, and pretended to take a bite. Then he stuffed it in the container.

- **Use an object to cue children to stop.**

"Haley cries during transitions and flaps her hands when she's excited," her preschool teacher told me on the second day of school. "When she's upset, you can see red and white wrinkles on her forehead. She makes sounds but no words yet."

During center time, Haley went to the water table, took a cup, and poured water over her left hand. She alternated between doing that, pushing her hands down on the bottom of the table, and dropping plastic fish into the water.

When the teacher announced there were two minutes left, I grabbed a picture symbol of the next activity showing children dancing. I went over to Haley and used sign language to indicate stop. I showed her the picture card of dancing children. "Next we are dancing."

Haley continued playing in the water. I went for a towel, thinking it would be a good physical cue to indicate stop. I thought she would probably understand that a towel is for wiping hands. When I showed her the towel, she took her hands out of the water and allowed me to help her dry them off. I showed her the picture again, and she walked with me without crying over to the large group.

- **Begin putting away any pieces of the activity or game that children are not using.**

The group spun 20 tops one after another. As each top stopped, I scooped it in my palm and put it in the container.

"Which top do you think will go the longest?" I asked.

"This little green one," Gina said.

"The blue one," Billy said.

When the green top stopped, Billy shouted, "Yes." Then he handed me the last one.

Use Words, Phrases, or Songs to Signal a Time to Stop

By using certain words, phrases, or songs, you can give children cues to stop. Words like *last* (e.g., "This is the last one") or *finish* (e.g., "Put your finishing touches on") indicate an ending is near. You can also use sayings, such as, "We all won that game. Everyone say, 'Hip, hip, hooray!'" Another way is to incorporate rhymes or songs. In many preschool classrooms, a specific song is picked as the music to indicate cleanup time. You can make up your own song using words like "It's time to go in," and applying them to a familiar tune. Repeating the song until the children do what you are requesting helps them keep the message in mind.

Fabulous Five: Choose Words, Phrases, or Songs to Indicate Stopping

- **Use the word *last* as a verbal cue to stop.**

"What's the last thing you are going to make with the magnets?" I said to the two third-grade boys.

"Guess what I'm doing. I'm making a castle," Andrew said.

Brian connected three circles and said, "Look. It's a snowman."

I smiled and said, "You both have good ideas. I can't wait to see what you create next time." I stood to leave, and they followed me out the door.

- **Tell children to put on last or finishing touches.**

Six-year-old Priscilla immersed herself in painting the sky on her plaster plaque. She rested her elbow on the table and dabbed on blue paint like an impressionist painter.

"In a few minutes, it will be time to go," I said. "Put on your last touches. You can finish it tomorrow."

- **Use a saying to signal the end.**

When we were out of time playing Don't Spill the Beans, I said, "It didn't tip. Say, 'Hip, hip, hooray!'"

The first graders threw their arms above their heads and shouted, "Hip, hip, hooray!"

- **Use songs or rhymes to help younger children stop playing.**

To help the preschoolers stop playing in centers, the teacher created a routine incorporating songs and rhymes. I watched her start by saying, "Before we go to wash our hands, everyone make a circle and sit down. When I call your name, jump over this block. We're pretending it's a candle." She placed a cylinder-shaped wooden block in the middle of the rug. She looked around the group and said, "Nate, it's your turn.

"Nate, be nimble, Nate, be quick," the teacher chanted, and the class followed her lead. "Nate jumped over the candlestick."

He leaped over the pretend candle. "I did it!" he said with a smile.

The teacher smiled back and replied, "Now go wash your hands for lunch."

- **Make up a song about it being time to stop.**

When 4-year-old Mason did not want to leave the playground, I made up a song and began singing it.

"It's time to go in. It's time to go in. High-ho the cheerio, it's time to go in." He recognized the tune and began to follow me. I kept repeating the song until we reached the door.

Define an Endpoint

When children know a defined endpoint, they can mentally prepare for stopping an activity. By knowing an exact number, they can adjust their expectations. Using this approach avoids surprising children by stopping abruptly. Rather, the transition is predictable and gradual. One way to give a concrete marker on when to stop is to tell them that after completing a certain number of items, steps, or actions, it will be time to go. You also can tell them how many minutes are left and ask what or how many items or steps they want to do.

Using a countdown method can be quite effective. For example, tell them what you are doing and say the number out loud with a minute pause between each number. The end of the game is also an endpoint. You can tell children that when the game is done, it is time to leave. If the game is not over near the end of the session, for a quicker ending change the rules of who will win or say everyone won. Knowing the time frame helps children feel prepared and often prevents power struggles about when to stop, especially when they are enjoying the activity.

Fabulous Five: Define an Endpoint

- **Tell children to stop after a certain number of items, steps, or actions.**

Five-year-old Cooper sat cross-legged on a balance board. Eight plastic fish with open mouths were scattered around him. I put a white bowl on the floor and said, "When you catch your fish, put them in here."

He flicked his wrist and cast his line. His body wobbled when the board tipped to the left, but he maintained his balance. "I've been fishing with my dad. I caught a big fish."

"I could tell by the way you used your fishing rod."

One by one, he hooked the fish and dropped them in the bowl. "Can I do it again?" he asked.

"Sure, we have time for you to do it one more time. After you catch all the fish, we will go."

- **Tell children how much time is left and ask what they want to do for the last activity.**

"We have 10 minutes left, so think about what you want to do for these last few minutes," I told 6-year-old Rich.

"I want to make a picture for my mom."

"I have some stickers you can use, if you want. Be sure to print your name. You're getting good at doing that."

- **Use a countdown and then say, "Time to…."**

In the center set up as a car wash, 3-year-old Collin dunked the plastic truck in soapy water. He squished a sponge in his hand and scrubbed the toy. Next, he rolled the truck back and forth, creating waves in the water.

"Five more minutes," the teacher announced, and when the time passed, she put on the cleanup music. As his classmates put items on the shelves, he continued playing.

"It's time to stop," I cued him, but he kept rolling the truck. "I'm going to count to three, and then you will need to stop. One," I said, and waited a full minute. "Two…. Three. It's time to stop and join your friends on the rug. We're going to sing our goodbye song." Collin stepped aside, wiped his hands on a towel, and went to the rug.

- **Have children define a number or how many steps left after being given a time frame.**

"We have 5 minutes left," I said to 7-year-old Jonas as he sat on the platform swing. "How many more blocks do you want to knock down with the beanbags?"

"Six."

I spread out six upright cardboard blocks and handed Jonas a handful of heavy beanbags. He aimed and hit one after another.

"Bullseye. You did it," I said. "You knocked them all down." I held the rope of the swing and said, "It's time to stop."

- **Change the rules of the game or activity for a quicker ending.**

"This game is called Thin Ice," I said to the 6 year olds in the last 10 minutes of our session. "Use the tongs to put these wet marbles on top of the tissue." I pointed to a tissue stretched tightly across a frame. "When the tissue breaks, all the marbles will fall, and it will be time to go."

They took turns dropping the marbles.

"Wow, it's not breaking," I said, realizing I had used a more expensive and stronger tissue. When all the marbles were on and the tissue was still holding, I said, "It didn't break. We all won. No one lost. Go ahead. Poke it because it's time to leave."

Three hands jabbed it, and the marbles crashed down to the base.

Provide Hope for Playing or Doing the Activity Again

> **Children might be thinking:**
> *I don't want to stop.*
> *I want to do this again.*
> *Are you sure I'll get to play with this again?*
> *I'm glad you are bringing it back.*

Children may not want to stop an activity if they think it is their only opportunity to do it. To assist them in coming to an end, validate their feelings and acknowledge that it is difficult to stop when they are having fun. Offer to take a picture of their creation so they can rebuild it at a later date. You can also promise to bring the item back (and, of course, be sure to remember to do so). Ask if they like what they are doing and if they would like you to bring it back. Answering your question helps them shift their thinking from their displeasure at stopping to the hope of doing it again. Another option is to tell them you will bring a similar item next time. If a child within a group barely had time to play, promise that he or she will go first when you return. It is easier for children to stop when you provide reassurance that they will get another opportunity.

Fabulous Five: Give Hope for Playing or Doing Activity Again

- **Ask children if they would like you to take a photograph of their creation.**

"Look what I made. It's a castle," 4-year-old Juan said to me.

A minute later, the preschool teacher played the music and sang the cleanup song. Another child ran over and grabbed one of the tiles off the castle.

"Stop! Don't," Juan yelled.

"Would you like me to take a picture so you can show your mother and you can make it again?" I asked.

He nodded. After the photograph was taken, he dismantled it and put the pieces away.

- **Promise to bring the item back and do so.**

"If you want, you can make cards today. I brought different hole punchers," I said to the second graders. "Keep them in the middle of the table so you can both use them."

As the two girls worked on the cards, Amanda grabbed a snowflake hole puncher and sang, "Oh, oh, snow, snow. Snowflakes everywhere." She struggled to slide it onto the paper and said, "Hey, get in there. Now I'm going to make lots of snowflakes."

Lucinda started singing, "Decorate, decorate, rate, rate."

"We only have five minutes left," I said.

"Oh no, I'm not finished," Lucinda replied.

"Please don't rush now. I promise I will bring your card and all the hole punchers when we meet."

The next time I came, I followed through on my promise.

- **Ask, "Would you like me to bring this back for you?"**

Near the end of the session, 7-year-old Ava smiled as she made designs on the Lite-Brite.

"We only have a few minutes left," I said.

"But I don't want to stop."

"Do you like playing with this?" She nodded. "Would you like me to bring this back?"

"Yeah. Pinkie promise?"

"I promise," I said as we hooked our little fingers together.

- **Offer to bring a similar item next time.**

"Whoa, come back," 5-year-old LaToya said as she tried to catch moving plastic bugs with her tongs.

"Bedbugs is a fun game," I said after she plucked all the bugs off the vibrating bed.

"Can I play again?"

"I'm sorry, but we are out of time," I replied. "Next time would you like me to bring another game like this one?"

She smiled and nodded.

- **Say, "Next time you get to be the first person to play with it."**

In the last 10 minutes with the group of third graders, I put a new game on the table. "This is a fun maze. Move the knobs and see how far you can move the ball without falling into the holes."

Three group members practiced and reached the number 10. When Drew tried, his ball repeatedly fell in the second hole. Because it was time to leave, I said to him, "You didn't get as much time to practice as the others. Next week, I'll make sure you are the first person to play with it."

He nodded and pushed the maze toward me.

Make Cleanup as Easy and Fun as Possible

Children may balk at cleaning up if they do not want to stop playing or if the job looks overwhelming. To engage them, try to make the process as easy and as much fun as possible. To do this, you can set up an activity to minimize the mess and make it simple to put items away. In addition, create a helping mentality that everyone helps and that by working together, cleanup will go faster. You can also use familiar endings that are easy to understand, such as saying goodbye to a doll. Using props makes cleanup a game and can transform a difficult situation into a fun time.

Make Cleanup Easy

> **Children might be thinking:**
> *At least cleanup is not too much work.*
> *That was easy.*

It is better to keep cleanup as simple as possible. If it is easy, children will be more motivated to participate. Plan ahead to minimize the work involved. Having pictures on the shelves where things go promotes an orderly process. Depending on your space, you may want to put away items after each activity so it is not overwhelming. This also prevents losing parts or having items get stepped on or broken.

Because cleanup is a necessity, it is important to include children. Involving them teaches responsibility and ownership of the space. You may need to show them how. For instance, you can hand the child one item at a time and point to where it goes. If you think they may get overwhelmed, clean up most of the items but save a few for them to finish. That way they are helping, but there is a quick ending. They also can see the results of their efforts. Do what you can to make cleanup fun and enjoyable.

> ***Fabulous Five: Simplify Cleanup***
> - **Figure out ways to keep cleanup simple.**
>
> "I want to do shaving cream," 4-year-old Cody told me during center time in his classroom. To minimize cleanup, I put a tray on the table, pumped three squirts of shaving cream on it, and added a few drops of green food coloring.
>
> Cody swirled his finger, making interlocking circles. He smoothed the shaving cream with his palm and then created more designs. When he was done, I told him, "Just take the tray to the sink and wash it off." I turned the water on for him, and the tray was quickly cleaned.
> - **Use picture cues to indicate where items are stored.**
>
> To help decrease the amount of visual stimulation in the preschool classroom and to make cleanup easy, I

talked with the teacher about adding picture cues. She liked the idea, and I offered to help her take the photographs and tape them on the shelves. The next day, I watched the children stack the blocks on the shelf, matching the taped photograph. At the end of cleanup, all the shelves were neatly organized.

- **Hand children one item at a time to put away.**

"Everyone clean up," the kindergarten teacher said.

Mark flapped his hands while sitting next to the cabinet. I showed him a corresponding picture symbol and sat behind him. I put one cardboard block in his hand. With my hand over his, we pushed the block into the shelf. After assisting him with few more, I handed one to him. "Put it away." He grabbed the block and put it on the shelf. I continued handing them to him until all the blocks were off the floor.

- **Have children do only the last step of cleanup or put away the last few items.**

Three-year-old Connor sat on the rug in the block area. First, he pulled out a bin of wooden blocks and dumped them all out. Then he grabbed the bin of Lincoln Logs. He tipped it until the contents spilled, covering his legs. As he reached for another bin, I intervened. "Let's put some of these away first," I said as I picked up a majority of the Lincoln Logs. I left five pieces for him and moved the bin to Connor's lap. One by one, I handed him the last piece. "Put this in," I cued him and pointed where. He easily dropped them in the container.

- **Make cleanup fun.**

"Today we get to draw in shaving cream," I told the four preschoolers.

"Yea!"

"I know, it's fun."

They flattened their palms on the table, and the shaving cream oozed through their fingers. Drawing with her finger, one said, "Look, it's me," and pointed to her figure.

"I'm making superheroes," another said.

When they were done, I told them, "I have a cool trick to show you for cleaning up. Turn the paper cup upside-down and make circles on the table. The shaving cream will stick to it."

Use Familiar Endings

Children might be thinking:
Bye-bye, baby doll.
Bye, toys.

To assist younger children with stopping an activity or session, use familiar routines. For instance, children learn at an early age that when someone leaves, they are to wave

and say, "Bye-bye." They equate those words with an ending. You can use those same words by having them say goodbye to toys or creating a farewell play scenario. They also understand that when it is time to go to sleep, they have to stop what they are doing. Hence, another approach is to enter their play and encourage the children to put the toys or objects down to sleep. These ideas make stopping part of their play.

When children have something to take with them, it is often easier and less stressful to leave. For many children, a familiar routine while visiting relatives or shopping with their families is to leave with something in their hands. By using approaches similar to their life experiences, children will better understand and adjust to stopping.

Fabulous Five: Use Familiar Routines for Endings

- **Have young children say, "Bye-bye [name the object]" and wave.**

"This puppy is hungry," I said and tapped the head of the red stuffed animal. "You have to use the tongs to pick up these cotton puff balls and put them in the bowl."

After the two preschoolers filled the bowl, I had the puppy pretend to eat them. When it was time to leave, I said, "Say, 'Bye-bye puppy. See you next week.'"

They waved and in unison said, "Bye-bye, puppy dog."

- **Create a goodbye play scenario.**

When it was time to stop, I flattened a piece of putty inside the storage container and made a groove for the figure that 4-year-old Josiah was holding. "He needs a pillow," I said. Josiah rolled a ball, placed the figure on the makeshift bed, and put the pillow under its head. I said, "Good night. Have a good sleep."

"Good night," he said and then added the lid.

- **Give young children the words to say goodbye.**

As the rest of the class put away the toys, 4-year-old Ricky picked up a toy phone and pressed the buttons. "Who are you talking to?" I asked.

"My grandma."

"Say, 'Good-bye, Grandma.' Tell her, 'My teacher is reading a story and I have to go.'"

He repeated my words, hung up, and headed over to the group.

- **Have the toys or object pretend to sleep.**

As the cleanup music played in the preschool classroom, I saw 3-year-old Jessica cradling a baby doll. "It's time for the baby to go to sleep," I said, pointing to the doll bed.

She gently placed the baby down and covered it with a blue blanket. "Go to sleep, baby."

- **Give children something to take with them.**

As the mother of the 4-year-old twins stood at the preschool doorway, she said, "Bob and Brad, it's time to go."

Brad ran toward her, but then he veered to his right. I tried to block his way and pointed to his mother. Brad ignored me and raced into the center that was designed to look like a post office.

I followed him and quickly grabbed a piece of paper. "Let me write you a letter that you can take home." He stood by my side and watched. I said the words as I wrote, "Bye, Brad." Then I drew a heart and added, "Dr. Clare likes you." I handed it to him. "Take this home."

He went to his mother, waving the letter in his hand. His mother breathed a sigh of relief. "Thank you," she said gratefully, and they all went out the door.

Use Props or Games to Define the Ending

> **Children might be thinking:**
> *I can beat you if we race.*
> *I like winning.*

The use of props or games to end an activity or session changes the focus from feelings of loss to feelings of fun. One enticing game is to suggest the children race against you. This promotes a quick cleanup of items. Because a race has a defined winner, this creates an opportunity for them to beat you. Let them win and they will be very happy! You also can make putting things away part of an activity or game. For instance, you can call a box a garage and ask them to roll the toy cars into the garage. Incorporating puppets, figurines, or toys is another playful approach to signal an ending. An out-of-the-ordinary strategy is to attach a stop sign to a Popsicle stick and have one child wave it to announce to the group that it is time to stop. Children like having the chance to be in charge and telling others what to do. Making cleanup time fun eliminates their resistance to stopping.

> ### *Fabulous Five: Use Props or Games to Define the Ending*
> - **Make it a race to put materials away.**
>
> "See if you can beat me," I challenged 7-year-old Sally and began scooping up small animal figurines.
>
> She stuffed 10 tiny animals in her palm, shoved them in the bag, and said, "I won."
> - **Make cleanup a game or part of the activity.**
>
> "Save the dinosaurs," I said. "Bring them home."
>
> Kyle plucked the dinosaur erasers out of the putty using a clothespin and dropped them into the bag. "Don't worry, I'll get you." Then he dropped one and missed.

"Oh no, save that guy," I said, pretending to be distressed.

He rescued the last one and released it in the bag. "Now they are safe and sound."

- **Use puppets or figurines to end the session.**

At the end of the session, I picked up a blue mouse finger puppet. I slipped it on my index finger and said in a squeaky voice, "Goodbye. Adios. See you next week."

Pauli put a purple bird puppet on her thumb and said back, "Goodbye."

- **Create a card with a stop sign on it.**

Bob flattened the putty, looking enthralled. Knowing he would not be pleased to stop, I handed him a Popsicle stick with a picture of a stop sign on it. "Wave this to let the group know it's time to leave."

Within seconds, he stuffed the putty into the container and waved the stick. "Time to stop. Let's go. Let's go," he announced, looking especially pleased to be telling his classmates what to do.

"I'm out of here," his friend replied, heading for the door.

- **Use toys to signal the end of the session.**

At the end of the group session, I handed Rico a toy microphone, which echoed when he talked into it. "Say, 'Time to go.'"

"Time to goooo."

Their voices reverberated as the children took turns with the microphone and then left.

Create a Helping Mentality

> **Children might be thinking:**
> *You think I can really help.*
> *I feel important.*

While ending the session, you can create a mindset that everyone, including you, will work together to clean up. You can let children know that if everyone pitches in and helps, cleanup will go faster and easier. Create a sense of community by promoting the mentality that we help each other. Talk about how rewarding it can feel to help one another. Rather than demanding children do it all, present it as a partnership and a kind gesture on their part.

Make cleanup a normal part of the routine with the expectation that everyone contributes to putting things away. You can mention how it benefits them, such as making sure all the parts of a game are put away and will be there for them the next time. You might want to mention that one of their strengths or competencies is needed. Giving the group choices on what to clean up or divvying up the job also increases motivation to cooperate. You also can use this approach if children have to wait or if they have finished before the others. A bonus is that being helpers is a good opportunity for them to get special attention. Additionally, it is easier to stop if there is a clear ending of the activity, project, or game.

Fabulous Five: Help Each Other

- **Mention that cleaning up benefits everyone.**

After we finished playing the Operation game, I said to the second graders, "Please help me get all the pieces in the box so we don't lose them. That way I'll have them for you the next time we play."

- **Mention that their strength or competence is needed to clean up.**

"Cody, Max," I said as I waved to them and pointed to the floor. "I need your big muscles to carry these blocks to the shelves."

The preschoolers ran over and carried the container of blocks. "Give it some muscle," Cody said to Max. "That's what my dad says."

"Thanks a bunch," I said when they were all finished.

- **Tell children you need their help to clean up and ask what they want to do.**

Looking at the table covered with putty, rolling pins, cookie cutters, plastic knives, and empty containers, I said to the 4 year olds, "We have a lot to clean up. I need your help. What do you want to put away?"

"I'll get the putty," Preston said.

"I'll get the cookie cutters," Colton said.

"Thanks!" I replied. "I'll put the rest in the cupboard."

- **Ask children to help you.**

"I need your help. Could you please put the scooter board on its side against the wall?" I asked.

Serena slid her stomach onto the board and, using her palms, scooted over to the storage space. She stood up, tipped the board sideways, and said, "All set."

"Thanks so much."

- **Divvy up the putting away of materials.**

"It's like magic," I said to the group of 5 year olds. "Put the template under the paper, turn the crayon sideways, and rub. Voilà, a picture comes out. Pick the one you want to do. There are lots of templates and different colored crayons."

As the group created their pictures, I encouraged them, "See how they're popping out. Be sure to push hard." When the group finished, I said to them, "I'll collect the templates. Could you please gather all the crayons and put them back in the box? Thanks."

Provide Closure to the Session

Children might be thinking:

What are we going to do the next time? Are we doing the same thing?

What new games will you have?

What else are we going to do?

Are we done?

I liked doing….

Thanks for saying nice things about me.

At the end of the session, it is wise to spend time reflecting on what happened while you were together. Because children learn what to expect in the first session, purposely save a few minutes and create a routine that incorporates processing. Talking with them gives you an opportunity to discover what piqued their interest, as well as their views of themselves.

Ask them what they liked the best that day or what their favorite part of therapy was. Doing so will let you know what they enjoyed and help you tailor future activities to the children's preferences. End on a hopeful note. Mention what you saw as their strengths. Tell them that what is challenging today may be easier next time, especially with practice. Ending on a positive note helps them embrace the idea that therapy is a safe place to try something new.

Additionally, in the last few moments, outline what they can expect for the next session. It is reassuring for them to know what is going to happen. All of these areas can often be discussed in a brief two- to three-minute conversation. Taking time to reflect and review the session prevents the sense of an abrupt ending. Rather, providing closure helps children feel content just like they do when they finish a story and shout, "The end."

Fabulous Five: Provide Closure to the Session

- **Ask children at the end of the session what they liked best.**

Seven-year-old Caleb tossed a weighted ball, rode a scooter board through an obstacle course of cardboard bricks, and started a rocket book. At the end of the session, I asked him, "What did you like best today?"

"The scooter board."

"I noticed you were really good at pushing yourself through the path without knocking down any of the bricks. That's hard to do."

- **Ask children what their favorite part of the session was.**

"Pick two animals," I said to 4-year-old Micah as I pointed to a variety of stress balls. He picked a cow and a frog and began squeezing them as he counted. "Your hands are getting stronger," I told him, and he smiled. "I also brought a fun puzzle. You have to cut the pieces and glue them. It makes an animal."

He cut the strips and arranged them in the correct order. "Hey, it's a squirrel."

"You did great figuring those pieces out. What do you want to do next? The caterpillar game or throw beanbags at the dog target?"

"Caterpillar game." With tongs, he tried to drop plastic balls onto the moving caterpillar's hands. "I dropped one."

"Keep trying, you'll get it." I replied. We chuckled as he would get one on and then drop the next. When done, he went to the beanbags. "Now I want to feed the dog."

"Get those beanbags in, and then it will be time to go. Give the dog tons of food."

As we walked back to his class, I said, "You spent time with lots of animals today. What was your most favorite part?"

"The caterpillar game."

- **Tell children what impressed you.**

"Whew, that's hard," 6-year-old Jake said as he tried to make the letter "s" and it came out backward. He tried again, and it looked like a wet spaghetti noodle. "I'm never going to give up until I do a good 's.' There, that's much better."

At the end of the session, I said, "I was really impressed with how you kept trying to make that 's' and you told yourself not to give up. And it worked. You made a beautiful one."

- **End the session on a hopeful note.**

Holding a toy, 4-year-old Jake stepped onto a balance board that had a monkey's face painted on it. I held the board still and then moved my hands to his side. "Do you feel my hands?" I said. "I will not let you fall." At first his body trembled, but then he began playing with the toy. Ever so slightly, he started shifting his weight from side to side. I gradually moved my hands an inch away from his body and he maintained his balance.

As we talked at the end of the session, I said, "Wow, you rode on the monkey. It's hard to keep your balance when the board is moving, but you did it. Next time it will be even easier."

- **Talk about what to expect for the next session.**

At the end of the first session, I said to 6-year-old Cara, "Next time we meet we'll squeeze more stress balls to make your hands stronger, work on your writing, and then play a game. I saw that you really liked the Mr. Mouth game. You were good at getting the chips into the moving mouth. Would you like me to bring that back?"

"Yeah, that was great fun."

Review Progress on a Regular Basis and Update the Plan

It is essential to monitor children's progress in therapy. This multifaceted process involves getting a plethora of information from various sources, including children. Continue to identify changes seen in each session, recognize progress made over time, and update the plan for therapy.

Obtain Children's, Caregivers' and Teachers' Perspectives Regarding Progress

> **Children might be thinking:**
> *I'm getting better.*
> *I feel proud of myself.*

To know if therapy is being effective, you need to solicit feedback from children, caregivers, and teachers. Their perspectives are important sources of information. When you hear what they have to say, you will discover whether therapy is on the right track or if adjustments need to be made.

Obtain Children's Perspective on Their Progress

In the last few moments of the session, take time to briefly review what happened and elicit children's perspectives. Ask them what they did well in the session or within a group. This type of questioning promotes thoughtful reflection on and an increased awareness of their strengths. Another benefit is the shift of their thinking from what they cannot do to what they can do.

In addition, acknowledge children's efforts when they report progress. Highlight the times they successfully challenge themselves and discuss the benefits of taking risks. For some, you may want to encourage them to show or tell another person about their progress.

> **Fabulous Five: Obtain Children's Perspectives on Their Progress**
> - **Ask, "What did you do well today?" at the end of each session.**
>
> "Cut out the whale," I said. Five-year-old Earl's eyes wandered around the room as he cut one side in two seconds. Seeing the jagged edges, I cued him, "When you cut, keep your eyes on the paper and go slow."
>
> Then he started cutting the next side. "I'm telling my brain to go slow," he announced.
>
> "That's great."
>
> He finished cutting and then glued the whale on the paper. Picking up a blue crayon, he said, "I'm making a blue whale." His hand swung in broad strokes, and he overshot the whale's body and accidentally colored the waves.

"There's an easy way to fix that. Just color the water with a darker crayon," I suggested.

Earl reached for a navy blue crayon and covered the light blue marks.

At the end of our time together, I asked, "What did you do well today?"

"I told my brain to go slow, and I colored in my mistake."

"You fixed your mistake so well that I can't even see it."

- **Have children identify what they did well in the group.**

"So what is one thing you did well in our group?" I asked.

"Chair push-ups," 11-year-old Angel replied.

"It was great when you came up with the idea that everyone should do push-ups when some kids were bouncing in their chairs."

"I'm doing them in class when I get hyper."

"It must feel good to know ways to help yourself," I said, and he grinned.

- **Listen to children's comments and acknowledge their effort.**

"Look, Dr. Clare, I did this button all by myself," 3-year-old Kiera said as she pointed to the top of her sweater.

"That's great! Buttons are hard to do."

- **Check in at different times.**

"My revolution is to do my homework in cursive," 9-year-old Nancy said.

"So that's your New Year's resolution," I replied and turned to the rest of the group. "What are your resolutions?"

"To be nice to my sister."

"To practice modeling because I want to be a model."

- **Have the children show or tell another person about their progress.**

Four-year-old Brandy printed her name on the Magnadoodle and correctly made the "y" for the first time. "I did it!"

"That's right," I said. "Go show your mom."

Brandy ran to her and said, "Look. It's my best. I made it myself."

Her mother smiled and said, "That's a good one."

Then Brandy slid the knob to erase it. "Goodbye."

Obtain Caregivers' and Teachers' Perspectives

Gather information from various caregivers and teachers regarding children's progress and discuss highlights with each child. Talking to others and getting their feedback gives them and you an opportunity to learn how therapy is affecting their lives. You can then learn what is happening when you are not at their home, school, or community.

To involve caregivers and keep children informed, start a conversation about progress when all are present. Ask questions that focus on strengths. Guide discussions on different ways to continue the momentum. Elicit concrete examples, especially following vague comments such as, "They are doing well."

If it is not possible for everyone to be together, you can relay caregivers' and teacher's compliments and stories. Tell children what strengths and achievements were discussed. Obtaining information from a variety of sources provides a richer picture of the children's progress.

Fabulous Five: Obtain Caregivers' and Teachers' Perspectives

- **Start a conversation with children, caregivers, and teachers regarding their progress.**

"What progress have you seen? What is Dwayne doing well?" I asked the 4 year old's mother.

She turned to him and replied, "He's using his words to get what he wants now."

"I told my brother to stop calling me names," Dwayne added. "I use my words. But he doesn't always listen."

"I've also seen you use your words when you're mad," I added.

- **Ask the caregiver and/or teacher about progress in the presence of the child.**

With the 6 year old standing next to me, I asked his teacher, "What progress have you seen with Josiah?"

She smiled at him. "You're doing much better at recess. When I blow the whistle, you come right in. You listen the first time and you're following your schedule. You're being a good student."

- **Relay a compliment a caregiver or teacher made.**

"Your mom told me you are more responsible at home. She said that you are cleaning up your room without being asked."

Five-year-old Mateo smiled and said, "Yeah, I'm getting good at putting my toys away now."

- **Share a specific story a caregiver or teacher told you regarding progress.**

"Could you please tell me about one time when you have seen progress with River," I said to the 12 year old's mother.

"It used to be that I would always have to ask him what assignments were coming up. Well, on the way home Friday, he said, 'I have a writing assignment that I need to do and it's not due until next Thursday.' This is progress because he told me about it ahead of time instead of the night before. By telling me on Friday, he had time to work on it over the weekend."

When I saw River the next day, I retold the story, and he smiled.

- **Tell children highlights regarding information obtained from a questionnaire or meeting.**

Before meeting with 8-year-old Danielle's parents, the special education team gave a questionnaire to her teacher and parents. After the meeting, I told her, "Your parents and teachers said a lot of good things about you. I hear you are prepared for class and turning in your homework."

"I brought my homework home last night," she said.

"I also heard that you are now raising your hand and asking questions when you don't understand."

Provide Your Perspective on Children's Ongoing Progress

> **Children might be thinking:**
> *Thanks for making me feel good.*
> *Wow, I'm doing good.*
> *Next time I'll do even better.*

In addition to eliciting children's, caregivers', and teachers' perspectives, it is important to provide your view of their progress. Often you can identify the small changes that are not recognized by others. After getting others' views at the end of the session, mention something, even if it is small, that indicates change. You can share what you see as specific differences and contributing factors as therapy progresses.

Identify Factors Contributing to Children's Progress

When you notice positive changes, talk with children about contributing factors. Instead of just saying, "Good job," describe in detail exactly what they did and what supports they used. Emphasize how their efforts and practice made a difference.

Clarify which strategies seemed to work the best. For example, mention times when they gave themselves a chance to try something new or did not give up. When children get this type of information, it is easier for them to repeat their actions and continue to experience success.

> ### Fabulous Five: Give Detailed Descriptions of Changes
> - **Attribute progress to children's efforts.**
>   Using her right hand, 5-year-old Jill picked up her limp left hand and placed it on top of her paper. She began to draw a picture of her family.

"I remember when it was hard for you to hold the paper still," I said. "But now you are so good at using your helper hand. That really makes a difference. You're holding the paper, and that makes it easier to draw."

- **Comment on an achievement.**

"We are starting to make your books about workers in our community. When you're done, you will be taking it home," the preschool teacher told the class. "Today, color, cut, and glue these pictures on your book cover."

I watched as 4-year-old Lane followed his teacher's three-step directions and accurately cut on all the lines. Then I said, "Lane, you did everything your teacher asked. And look how good your cutting is now. That's great! You have a good start on your book."

- **State the successful strategies that helped children make progress.**

Three-year-old Eli made three cuts on the darkened line. He sped up, veering off the line and ripping the paper.

"Tell your brain to go slow," I said. As he snipped, I repeated the words "Go slow," and he stayed on the line. When it was time to leave, I said, "When you slowed down, your cutting was really good. Keep telling yourself to go slow."

- **Point to the positive results when children give themselves a chance to try something new.**

"I'm not doing that. It's wet," 5-year-old Wade said when he saw the gold putty.

"It may look wet, but it's not. It's just shiny. Try touching it once," I said.

He rubbed his index finger over an inch of putty and said, "Oh, it feels okay." Then he buried six silver balls in the putty. "It's like a treasure. We're pirates, and we have to find Black tooth's treasure."

In the last few minutes of the session, I said, "I saw that you liked the putty. It's good you gave yourself a chance to try something new even when you were not sure about it."

- **Describe a specific situation when the children did not give up.**

Amie removed her ceramic mug from the mold, and as she tugged on the handle, it came apart. "It's no good," she said, looking forlorn.

"Wait a minute, I'll teach you how to fix it," I said, and guided her through the steps of patching.

When the mug came out of the kiln the next day, she raised it with pride. "You did great. Look, you can't even see where it broke. This time you fixed it and didn't give up. All your hard work paid off," I said, and Amie beamed.

Use Positive Wording or Phrases to Contrast the Past With the Present

Another way to emphasize progress is to use wording that contrasts the past with the present. Some children are not always cognizant of the gains they have made. To increase their self-awareness, be sure to provide a detailed description of the differences. It can be reassuring to them to hear that their efforts and hard work are paying off.

Fabulous Five: Use Positive Wording to Indicate Progress

- **Say, "I see how hard you are trying, and it is getting a little easier/better to do…."**

"This is a memory game," I said. "Turn two cards over at a time and try to get matching pairs. To start put your tummy on this big ball and walk on your hands. Then pick up the cards."

Seven-year-old Ramiro placed his stomach on the therapy ball and walked with his palms, picking up two set of cards. After getting each set, his body dropped to the floor. "It's okay to take a break if you want," I said. "This is hard to do."

"I'm going to rest and think about which card I should take. I almost got it. My hand started to get tired." After a minute, he restarted, and this time he collected four sets.

When he stopped, I said, "I see how hard you are trying, and it's getting a little easier to stay on the ball while you are playing the game." He nodded.

- **Say, "I remember when… and now you…."**

Four-year-old Ricky sat still at the table, focused on a fish puzzle. He used a fishing rod with an attached magnet to catch each fish. "I remember when you could only do one puzzle and then you had to get up and move around. Today you have done nine puzzles and are staying with this hard one. You have really become good with puzzles and keeping your mind on what you are doing. That's great."

He smiled. "I like puzzles now."

- **Point out, "Look what you can do now" and mention one detail.**

Four-year-old Janice had a tumor on her right foot. She could get out of her wheelchair but needed assistance getting back in it. "I can't," she said when encouraged to try.

To help her figure out what to do, I took photographs of her doing each step of getting in. Pleased to be the star in the photographs, she began trying. The photos also let her teacher and paraprofessional know each step.

When I returned the next week to her school, Janice waved at me and said, "Dr. Clare, watch me." She pulled herself up from the floor, pivoted her body, and eased into the wheelchair seat. She grinned.

"Wow! Look what you can do now. That's so great that you can get in the wheelchair all by yourself."

- **Say, "You have worked very hard and it shows."**

On the children's psychiatric unit, 10-year-old Sharon chose to do a wooden box. "I'm going to make this for my mom. She can use it for her jewelry." For the next week, she carefully sanded, stained, and polished it. When it was done, she held it up and smiled. "My mom is going to love this."

"You really took your time on the jewelry box and didn't rush," I said. "You worked very hard and it shows. I think your mom will love it too."

- **Mention, "That used to be hard for you, but not anymore."**

Every day the preschool class transitioned from the bathroom in the hall back to their classes. On the days I was with them, I brought out a step stool and four plastic circles into the hallway. "On the way to your class, step up on the stool, jump down, and then keep jumping on the circles," I told the group.

The first time 4-year-old James tried, he was so uncertain and unstable that I needed to hold his hand. In the second month, he started jumping down, but paused before jumping on each circle. Finally, in the third month he completed the jumping activity without help.

"I can jump fast now," he said and beamed.

"You must feel proud. Jumping used to be hard for you, but not anymore."

Provide Immediate Feedback to Children Who Are Younger or Nonverbal

If you are working with younger children or those who are functioning well below their age level, it is important to provide immediate feedback on their progress. Hearing instantaneous feedback helps them make the connection that their effort has positive results. Instead of waiting to comment in future sessions, highlight their progress in the moment.

Show your excitement nonverbally for their achievement and pair it with one encouraging word such as "Yea!" or "Wow!" They may even join you and clap with delight at their success. You also can tell them to "Look at…" and point to what they have accomplished. Other ways are to say, "You are doing good," or "You did that all by yourself." Emphasizing their progress provides motivation to continue.

Fabulous Five: Give Immediate Feedback to Younger Children

- **Use one word such as "Yea!" with nonverbal signs of excitement.**

Three-year-old Karen tried to put a star-shaped block into a square hole. She then tried jamming it into a triangle-shaped hole. When her third attempt was successful, I said with a smile, "Yea!"

She clapped in response, pleased with herself.

- **Tell children, "Look at…" and point to what they accomplished.**

I placed a wooden dog-shaped bead in 3-year-old Eric's left hand and a pipe cleaner in his right hand. I guided his hands together to help him slip the bead on. He then continued adding beads without help. When the pipe cleaner was full, I took it from his hand, held it up, and pointed to it. "Look what you did. You put all of the beads on."

- **Say, "You're doing good."**

In the specialized program, 4-year-old Logan grabbed a pair of preschool scissors. I slid the scissors on his fingers, opened them, and slid the paper in.

"Whoa," he said as he closed the scissors, making one cut.

"More, please," I said. "You are doing good." I helped him open the scissors again.

"Whoa," he said as he made another cut and smiled.

"You like cutting."

- **Say, "You did it," and state what they achieved.**

For a month, 4-year-old Connor sat on a tricycle and pushed it with his feet. "Put your feet on the pedals, and I'll help you," I prompted him. For the next 2 weeks, I moved behind him and pushed as he practiced steering and keeping his feet on the pedals. Then one day I gave him one push, and he continued on his own. He circled the playground and kept going. When he stopped, I said, "You did it! You rode the tricycle all by yourself without any help."

- **Tell children, "You did that all by yourself."**

The first week of preschool, 3-year-old Marvin's grandmother took his coat and hung it on the hook. The next morning I attached a photo of him above his hook. When he arrived, I pointed to the coat racks and said, "Find Marvin."

He found his picture and touched it with his index finger.

"That's right. It's you. It's Marvin. Now hang up your coat."

He shoved it on the hook and it stayed.

His grandmother and I grinned. "You did it all by yourself," I said, and he smiled.

Update the Plan for Therapy

> **Children might be thinking:**
> *I made progress.*
> *Now I want to get better at….*
> *Now I want to work on….*

To keep track of progress, collect a variety of data. Include children in the process and use visual representations of their changes (Figure 17-2). You can collect samples or photos of their work and ask children to compare and contrast their improvement. They can be involved in graphing the frequency or achievement of their goals. Using props makes the process more fun. For instance, you can ask them to move a bar on a paper thermometer to indicate their judgment regarding how much help they still need and the level of their progress. Seeing the results of their efforts can provide a sense of achievement and give them hope that more change is possible. It also can create a desire for more challenging and fun experiences.

> ## Fabulous Five: Review and Update the Plan for Therapy
>
> - **Review the general purpose of therapy.**
>
> The first week of school, 11-year-old Darian and I walked to the therapy room for the joint occupational and speech therapy group. I said, "Mrs. H. and I are doing groups together this school year. You'll be with Dawn."
>
> "Yea, no boys! Dawn and I have a lot in common," Darian said.
>
> "Yes," I said. "You're both nice."
>
> She smiled and said, "We both have disabilities. I have sensory integration dysfunction, and Dawn has a hard time talking."
>
> "So you are working on being able to move your body better, and she's working on speaking better."
>
> - **Compare samples of the children's work as evidence of progress.**
>
> "Write a sentence about something you like," I told 7-year-old Sal at the evaluation.
>
> He printed *I like my dog.* The letters in his words overlapped, and the words ran together.
>
> A month later, I showed Sal his first writing sample and placed it next to a page he had just written. "Look at the difference. What do you see?"
>
> "I'm better at putting my finger between words."
>
> "Yeah, you are good at putting spaces between the letters and the words. They are not on top of each other."
>
> - **Have children use props to identify their progress.**
>
> To check on 8-year-old Leticia's progress, I pulled out a homemade paper thermometer with the various levels: Need Help, Doing Okay, Getting Better, Good, Great, I've Done It! "This is a good time to see how things are going. It helps me to know how you see yourself doing."
>
> She moved the lever to Getting Better and said, "It's getting easier for me to put my clothes on."

"Do we need to change our goals or do anything different?"

"No. It's okay."

"You have worked really hard and it shows."

- **Ask children what they would like for new goals.**

In the first week of school, I said to Chris, a third grader, "I have been talking with kids about…."

"Their goals?" she replied. "I know my goal for this year. I want to be a better artist and do the computer better."

- **Discuss progress and identify a new plan for therapy.**

"Here's a sample of Ken's writing," the special education teacher said. Ill-formed letters dotted the page, with no spaces between the words. Next to the jumble of letters, his fourth-grade teacher had written, "Too messy."

I turned to him and said, "You did all that work to write it. However, it doesn't help if your teacher can't read it." I brought out a page of his cursive writing. "Which one is easier to read?"

"I see what you're saying," he replied. "The cursive is better."

"You know cursive. How come you are still using printing?"

"I forget. When I go to write, my hand does printing."

"Do you see that when you use cursive, you automatically put spaces between the words and your letters are clearer? I understand it is hard to change a habit. And it may be hard if you only do cursive part of the time. I know you told me you want to get faster at cursive. It would be easier to change your habit if you do cursive all the time. Are you ready to do that?"

He nodded.

"When do you want to start?" I asked.

"Monday."

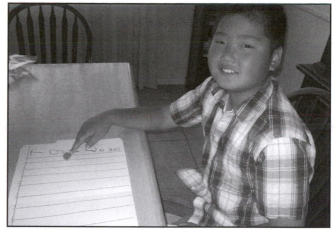

Figure 17-2. One option is to use the visual of a football field to mark progress.

End Therapy

Just as important as a good beginning to therapy is a good ending. Like writing a book, the first chapter of intervention needs to be engaging to get the person involved and create a desire to continue. Similarly, in the last chapter of therapy, you have to create closure. This entails tying events together, summarizing what happened, wrapping up loose ends, and making sense of the time by conveying the moral of the therapy story.

There are various reasons for stopping therapy. You may be leaving your job, children may be discharged from the hospital, or they may be changing schools. For some, therapy is no longer warranted due to the progress made.

You have a responsibility to create a healthy ending and put closure on the relationship. This means helping everyone, including you, acknowledge that your relationship is coming to an end or will change. A second consideration is to assist children in dealing with their feelings. With any type of ending, there are various feelings associated with this change. It is common for you, children, and their caregivers to be sad that your time together is over. This is especially true for those with whom you have developed a close bond or connection. You may feel sad that you will no longer get to enjoy the children's personalities and will miss seeing them continue to grow. The children and caregivers may experience sadness because you will not be present on a regular basis to support them.

Be sure to review the changes that occurred in therapy. This is an opportunity to talk about what you have learned from each other and express your wishes for them in the future. It is a time to openly discuss what you appreciate about the children. Because therapy involves creating educational experiences together, you also will want to highlight what the children learned and, just like a story, emphasize the moral. Common themes are "Always give yourself a chance to learn," "Don't give up," and "When you have to learn something new, just try."

Going through this process of reflection is imperative for you as much as the children and gives you an opportunity to learn about yourself. For instance, during my first year as a therapist in a psychiatric hospital, I worked with a teenager who had just come out of a catatonic state. At the time, she was in a special care unit because she was out of touch with reality and angry. In occupational therapy, she chose to do a leather project and started following all the steps. Suddenly, she took the wooden mallet used for stamping and began hitting her arm.

"Please stop, you are hurting yourself," I told her.

"I don't care," she screamed back at me.

"Well, I do care," I answered back in a calm but firm tone. "Please stop."

She put the mallet down, and we went back to her unit. For the next 5 years, she returned to the acute care hospital for short stays whenever she had psychotic episodes. Then it came time for me to change jobs. When we said our goodbyes, I talked about what I would remember about her. I was surprised when she said, "I will miss you. I remember you said you cared."

Make time to end on a positive note and create a good ending.

Prepare for Departures

> **Children might be thinking:**
> *I'm sad you're leaving.*
> *Why are you leaving?*
> *Did I do something wrong?*
> *I don't want you to go.*
> *I'm not sure what's going to happen.*

When you know you will be leaving, give children notice regarding your last day. Tell them ahead of time so they can mentally and emotionally prepare for your departure. Some children may be surprised or shocked to hear the news. Timing is a factor. For instance, children are accustomed to change at the beginning of each school year because that is when they get new teachers. They will be surprised if you leave midyear. For children who have had multiple losses, such as many foster children, your leaving may bring back memories and feelings associated with other people exiting their lives. Consequently, they may feel more upset, sad, or overwhelmed than you would normally expect.

Children usually have no choice if they are the ones to leave a situation. For instance, caregivers decide if the family is moving. Doctors decide when they are to leave a hospital. Children may have a range of feelings regarding the change. They may feel excited about a new adventure, sad about saying goodbye, and maybe upset to leave their friends. Some may feel indifferent, shocked that it is happening to them, or scared about the unknown. Help children deal with whatever feelings they may have.

Talk About Your Leaving

You may want to give them the reason you are leaving. If you know who will replace you, give them that information too. They often will worry about who is taking your place and may wonder if the new therapist will be mean or nice. Consider having a group make a welcome poster or card for the new therapist. Avoid making promises that you cannot keep, such as saying you will come to see them again when that may not be possible. Finally, reminisce, share your feelings about saying goodbye, and acknowledge the children's competencies and progress. Keep in mind that sometimes the hardest children to work with are the ones who teach you the most about yourself. Be grateful for what you have learned from your time being with them. For all children, wish them well in the future.

Fabulous Five: Talk About Your Leaving

- **Prepare the children for the last time together.**

I told Bill about my departure a week before my last day. The 6 year old folded his arms, pouted, and began stomping his feet. "I don't want you to go. Why do you have to leave?"

"It's sad to say goodbye, and sometimes it makes you mad when someone leaves. I'm sad to go too, and I will miss you."

On my final day, Bill's mom came to the school and took a picture of the two of us. He handed me his home-made card and a scented green velvet pillow with a heart etched in it.

- **Give the general reason you are leaving.**

The occupational therapy student glanced around the group and said, "I was here to learn how to be a therapist. Dr. Clare was my teacher. I'm sad to leave, and I will miss you. Now I'm going to work in a hospital so I can learn more."

"I don't think you'll like it there because there's lots of blood," 6-year-old Fred replied. "I'll miss you too."

- **Help the children prepare for someone new.**

When I had to change schools, I told the children about my leaving and said another therapist named Audra would take my place. "Let's make her a welcome poster," I suggested. I covered the chalkboard with butcher paper. Then I gave them markers, crayons, stamps, and vibrating pens. Shaun made a "w" and filled it with stars. Each child printed another letter with a unique design.

"What is she like? Is she nice?" Shaun asked.

"She's very nice. I think you'll really like her," I said and continued to answer all their questions.

On Audra's first day, she smiled when she saw the poster. Each child proudly pointed to the letter he or she had drawn.

- **Avoid making promises you cannot keep when saying goodbye.**

I handed 7-year-old Martin a goodbye card and said, "I'm sad about leaving. I will miss you." Seeing his frown, I responded, "Are you sad I'm leaving?"

He nodded. "Maybe I'll cry in my room. Maybe I'll see you sometimes. Maybe I'll see you at the gas tank."

"I don't want to promise you when I'm not sure. I'm so glad to have the picture you drew. Even though I will not see you, I won't forget you."

- **Share your feelings about leaving them.**

"I am going to another school, so I will not be here next year," I told the third grader in day treatment. "When you come back after summer, there will be someone new. I am sad to say goodbye. I will miss you."

In our last time together, she handed me a card:

Dear Dr. Clare, I will miss working in OT with your big laugh and your funny faces. I guess I got mad sometimes but I still liked you and I will remember you always. Your friend, Maria

Help Children Address Feelings if They Are the Ones Leaving

It is helpful for you to check in with children regarding their feelings about changes. Ask questions about their future and what they know. Explore how they are feeling and validate the normality of their feelings. Discover if they have unanswered questions and ask if they want to write them down. If you can, help them get the answers or encourage them to talk to those with the information. Also to help them deal with their feelings, talk to them about what they will miss and what they are looking forward to. Sometimes just having a caring adult to talk to is beneficial.

You may want to encourage them to make a transition book of their successful strategies. They can give such a book to their new teacher. Similar to the situation where you are leaving, reminisce about your time together, highlight the children's strengths, and review the progress made.

Fabulous Five: Help Children Process Feelings About Their Departure

- **Ask questions about their future.**

"I am getting a new cat when we move into our new house."

"Have you seen your new home?" I asked, and 8-year-old Kyle nodded. "What do you think about it?"

"It's good. I've already made a new friend."

"It's nice to know you'll have someone to play with. Have you seen your new school?" Kyle nodded again. "What's it like?"

"It's a good school. Good teachers, good students, good everything."

"I'm glad you're feeling all right about it."

- **Inquire how children feel about the changes.**

"What's happening?" I asked 7-year-old Josiah.

"I'm moving. My parents bought a new house."

"How do you feel about it?"

"A little sad because I'm going to miss everybody. At least I'll be able to call my friend, Bob, and I'll have the same phone number. I'll live close to my cousins, but I'll miss all my teachers. I've known them for a long time."

- **Help children prepare a list of questions if needed.**

"We're moving," 11-year-old Brianna said. "I'm going to a new school. I'm not sure what it's going be like."

"Do you have questions about it?" I asked. She nodded. "What are you wondering about or worried about your school? Sometimes it helps to write down questions that you could ask your parents or the school staff. Do you want to do that?"

Brianna then wrote the following:

Will other kids be mean to me?

Who is my teacher?

What kind of schoolwork do we get? Is there a lot?

Is there a lot of homework?

Is everyone friendly?

How will I know where to go?

- **Discuss what the children will miss and what they are looking forward to in their new place.**

"What will you miss about preschool?" I asked 5-year-old Jenna at the end of the school year.

"I will miss you. You do good stuff."

"What did I do?"

"You helped people and you helped people get stronger."

"I will miss you too. What will be good about going to kindergarten?"

"I get to learn science. I get to learn math. One plus one equals two."

"That's right. What else?"

"I get to play in the big place. That's what my cousin calls the playground."

"You will be on a different playground with big kids."

"And I get food at school."

"You will get to eat in the lunch room with all your friends. There are a lot of good things about kindergarten."

- **Have children make their own transition book of their successful strategies.**

The week after 9-year-old Joe told me he was moving, we talked about making a book to show his new teacher. He wrote the following and drew matching pictures of himself:

I am best at math.

I like to do art second best.

Sometimes I wiggle so I use strategies. I can push my palms together. I can do chair push-ups. I can do wall push-ups. When I do these it makes me stop wiggling.

"What do you think about your book?"

"I never thought I could write a book all by myself with only a little help with spelling."

"You worked hard on it. This will really help your new teacher get to know you."

Assist Children in Saying Goodbye

> **Children might be thinking:**
> *I'm sad to say goodbye.*
> *I'm excited about my new school/home.*
> *I'll make new friends.*
> *Will I ever see you again?*
> *Thanks for teaching me.*
> *I'll remember you the rest of my life.*

At the end of therapy, bring closure to relationships, especially long-term ones. Talk to children about accomplishments, and celebrate their last day. For many, you might want to make a goodbye card for them. If you are leaving, another idea is to have them write in or draw a picture in your autograph book. Reminiscing is another important step.

Celebrate Achievements and Make the Last Day Special

When children no longer need therapy, you may want to refer to the ending as a graduation. They are stopping because they are doing so well. Older children understand that graduation is a special event. Some children like getting certificates as recognition of their hard work.

Celebrate their achievements, and make their last day a special one. Ask what their favorite activity is and use it in the last session. In situations where you bring supplies to therapy, be sure to check with them ahead of time. On their last day, you might want to let them choose all the activities.

Fabulous Five: Celebrate Their Achievements and Make the Last Day Special

- **Refer to the ending as a graduation—they are stopping because they did so well.**

In the middle of the school year, 8-year-old Lindsay had met all her goals.

After talking with her parents, teachers, and Lindsay, we all agreed that she was doing well in class. She no longer would have an Individualized Education Program. Before stopping therapy, I talked to her about her progress. "Now that you are able to keep up with your work in class, you do not need the extra help," I said with a smile. "It's time for you to graduate from OT, and in two weeks it will be our last time together. It will be your graduation. Congratulations!"

Lindsay smiled. "Thanks."

- **Make the last day a special one.**

"Today is a special day. As we've talked about, you have done so well that you do not need to come to our group. Congratulations!" I said to 7-year-old Geneva.

"Because this is your last day, you get to go first in our activities."

"I can't wait until it's my lucky day," her friend said.

At the end of the session, I gave Geneva a homemade goodbye card and let her pick a pencil.

- **Give children a certificate.**

"Congratulations! You have worked very hard," I said to 7-year-old Christina. "You have been a great helper. I enjoyed being with you." I showed her three preprinted certificates. "Pick the one you want."

She chose the one with the smiling honeybees. I printed her name on it and handed the certificate back to her.

"Wow, I get an award," she said with a smile as she fingered the paper.

- **Have children tell you their favorite activity and bring it for the last session.**

"This is a really fun game called Don't Spill the Beans. We will take turns," I said. "Use these tongs to put beans on the lid of this swinging pot. Be careful. Whoever tips it over loses."

"Hey, there are spider and skeleton rings in the beans," 6-year-old Kellen said.

"I added those for Halloween. You can put them on the pot lid too."

"I like this game," he said as we played.

A week before our last session, I asked him, "Because next week is our last time together, what would you like me to bring?"

"That bean game," he replied. "That's my favorite one."

- **Let children choose the activities within the room for the last session.**

"Because today is your last day, pick whatever you want," I said to 4-year-old Duncan.

He looked around the therapy room and reached for a car puzzle. Duncan took the rod with an attached magnet at the end of the string and fished for each car. When all the pieces were out, it took a while for him to figure out where they went back in.

"What's next?" I asked.

"You have lots of puzzles. I'm going to do another one," he said, but instead reached for a fishing game.

Using a plastic rod, he tried to catch moving fish as they opened and closed their mouths. When he kept missing, I said, "Stop swimming away, fish."

"Look, I got a red one." After catching all the fish, he said, "Now I want to do one of the puzzles again." He went back to the one with the cars.

At the end of the session, I said, "What was your favorite thing to do today?"

"The race car puzzle."

"It was tricky to put the cars back in, but you did it." I gave him a homemade goodbye card and added,

"Duncan, what I'll remember about you is how you tried everything even when it was hard, and you were a great help when we were cleaning up."

He smiled.

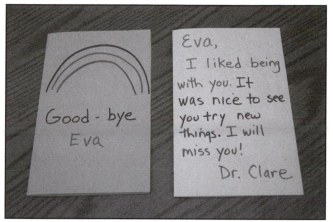

Figure 17-3. For some children, you may want to make a goodbye card.

Use Cards, Drawings, or Small Gifts to Say Goodbye

When you are leaving, you can help children say goodbye. One way to do this is to have a mutual exchange of gifts. On your part, you can give them a goodbye card, in which you describe their strengths, their accomplishments, and how you feel about leaving them (Figure 17-3). For some children, you may want to give a small symbolic gift that reflects your work together and their new beginnings after your parting. Another gift you can give is a book of photographs showing the time spent with each other.

To assist them in saying goodbye to you, one option is to create an autograph book. Ask them to a draw a picture of themselves or write a message on a page. As they do, inquire about what they liked about therapy. Write down what they say as they draw. Then you can put all the pages together in a book.

Fabulous Five: Help Children Say Goodbye

- **Give a goodbye card.**

I worked at an elementary school one day a week for 3 months until administration hired a therapist named Irene. When I was due to leave, I made cards for each child, including two second graders named Melinda and Sue. I was surprised at the end of the school year when the teacher sent me this story written by Melinda:

Clare has black long haire and green eyes. I liked Clare but the worst thing she did was leave us with Irene. The thing we do best is play games and do glue but Clare is still my favorite teacher. I still think Irene doesn't have to be so strict and so does Sue. She can be nice but Clare is nicer. I hope she remembers me. I still have the card she gave me. I hung it up on my wall to remember her. But Irene is my teacher now. I miss Clare a lot.

- **Give children a small symbolic gift.**

On my last day of therapy, I handed 10-year-old Chris a gel pen and a homemade card that said the following:

Dear Chris,

You are very special. It has been a joy to work with you. I am happy that now you can write and everyone can read it. Your hard work made a difference! I will miss you. Dr. Clare

"You have a lot to be proud of," I added.

"I have come a long way," he replied.

"Write a lot. You have good things to say."

"I'm thinking of keeping a journal over the summer."

"You have a real gift with words, and you are very wise. You always had good ideas, but it took so long to write. Plus, no one could read your work, which made it frustrating. Now you can write well."

"Thank you for the gel pen."

"You're welcome. Use it. You have many wonderful things to say."

- **Have children draw a picture of themselves.**

In our last session, I said to 7-year-old Jeff, "Would you draw a picture of yourself? That would be very special to me and I will have that to remember you."

"What are these?" Jeff said as he pointed to his picture.

"They're eyes," I replied, knowing that was his way of engaging me.

He continued to draw. "What are these?"

"They're tears. Are you sad that I am leaving?" I asked, and he nodded. "I'm sad to say goodbye to you too."

- **Create an autograph book.**

"Here's an autograph book," I told the occupational therapy student during her last week of fieldwork. "Have each child draw a picture and write something if they choose. Do this in your last session. It will help the children adjust to the change. It's also nice for you to have a book of memories."

The next week, when she saw the group of third graders, she said, "Remember that I said I was leaving. Today is my last day. I sure will miss you. Dr. Clare made me this goodbye book. I would love it if you would write or draw anything you think I would like to remember you by. Be sure to write your name on it too."

"I'm drawing a rainbow heart. I'll really miss you," Tina said.

- **Create a goodbye book with pictures of your time together.**

After working intensely with all the children in a specialized preschool program, the occupational therapy student wrote the following story and attached photographs:

Spending time with Ms. Megan.

We shared meals at the table together.

We spent time learning and playing in centers.

We played outside with our friends.

Playing outside is fun!

We listened to our teachers when they read books with us.

We sang songs and dance together.

I had so much fun playing with everyone and getting to know you. I liked watching you play nicely, and work hard at drawing and cutting. You are all very special and I will miss you!

Your friend, Ms. Megan

After she left, the book was placed in the rack with the other books. The children frequently read it and talked about missing her.

Reminisce, Review, and Share Feelings

After talking to children about their feelings, spend time reminiscing about your time together. Think back: Were there any humorous situations? What was the most fun? Did you learn something from them? Was there anything special about these children?

If you're going to miss them, let them know. Share what you feel comfortable saying. Be sure in your discussion to highlight the children's competencies and the gains they made. Finally, encourage children to continue to use what they learned in therapy. Emphasize that you believe they have the ability to do it on their own or will know how to get the help they need.

Fabulous Five: Recall and Review

- **Reminisce and discuss what you wish for the children in the future.**

On Tate's last day at the day treatment, the staff and all 18 children circled around him. The social worker stood and said, "We'll go around and each of you tell one thing you remember about him and one wish you have for him."

"I remember when you helped me with my math. Good luck at your new school," 8-year-old Ernie said.

"I remember you played every day with me on the swings. I hope you make lots of friends," Abby added.

Tate grinned. "Thanks."

"I remember how you always offered to help other kids," I said. "My wish for you is that you will continue to stop and think when you are frustrated and keep giving yourself a chance to learn something new."

The next staff member said, "I remember how you worked really hard in gym to jump rope, and now you can jump 50 times. My wish is that you will remember what you have learned here."

Tate beamed in response.

- **Talk about missing the children.**

"I'm not coming back to this school. We're moving to Minnesota," the third grader told me.

"I know your dad is there and you've talked about wanting to see him. I'm glad you will get to be closer to him, but I will miss seeing you."

- **Share your thoughts and feelings.**

After spending time together, at the end of our last session I told 5-year-old Ashley, "I'll remember how kind you were with everyone in the group and always willing to help them."

She smiled.

- **Highlight the children's strengths.**

"I may be going to another school next week but I'm not sure," 7-year-old Joe said.

"That can be hard when you don't know if you are changing schools." He nodded. "If that happens, I'll be sad to see you go and will miss you. I like being with you. You are so nice. You share and help others."

"I'll miss you too. It was fun."

- **Encourage children to keep making progress on their own.**

On my last day with a second grader named Molly, I gave her a card with the following message: *Have a good summer and good luck at your new school. I enjoyed working with you. I think you are very special. Remember to keep using the strategies (ideas) to help with writing. Dr. Clare*

I read the message to her, and we reminisced before saying goodbye. Later, when I walked down the school hall, Molly's classmate stopped me and said, "That was a very sweet card you gave Molly."

Have Children Evaluate Services

Children might be thinking:

Thanks for asking.

I liked….

I think you should….

It would be better if you….

You could try more….

It is important to have children evaluate the occupational therapy services. This gives them the opportunity to analyze their experience and provide useful feedback regarding what worked and what did not. By giving them a voice, you have a chance to learn more about yourself and better ways to work with children. Because children are experts on their own lives, use this time to gain from their expertise. This will help you become a better therapist and provide more meaningful intervention. It is enlightening to learn about their perceptions of you. You can also learn how therapy affected their lives and what therapy meant to them.

Possible questions to ask at the end of therapy include what they liked, what went well, and/or what helped them the most. Inquire what they think therapists should know when they work with children. Ask for their suggestions on how to improve therapy and make the time together better. If possible, have another adult talk to them about their experiences with you in therapy. Finally, end the session on a positive note and wish children well.

Fabulous Five: Have Children Evaluate

- **Interview children about their experiences with you.**

"What did you like about being with me?"

"All the games we play," 6-year-old Mason replied. "Doing handwriting. I'm getting really, really good at printing."

"What should therapists know when they work with children?" I asked.

"Be really nice. Make it fun. Pay attention to them and see if they are doing things right or wrong."

- **Inquire what went well overall.**

"What went well this year during our time together?" I asked the second graders.

"We learned how to get along with each other and our friends."

"We learned how to share."

"We made each other laugh, and no one made fun of me."

- **Ask what ideas children have for improving the group or individual time together.**

"What ideas do you have to make our group better for others?" I asked a group of third graders.

"Buy new games that will help us learn more."

"We can do spelling words in cursive."

"Draw letters in the air more often. That really helped me."

"Have a model of the letters so you don't have to take time to write them for us."

- **Have another adult talk to children about their experiences in therapy.**

The certified occupational therapy assistant went to the children's psychiatric unit and interviewed three 10-year-old boys. She asked what they thought about me and wrote down their responses.

"She has lots of personality. She doesn't let you bring out artwork until you are finished. She wants you to do your best," Cedric said. "She's a really nice person."

"Nice personality," Steve told her. "Doesn't let you give up and makes you do your best! She can handle us getting mad real good. She doesn't let you throw stuff."

"She's real nice," Jeremy said. "She helps you with things."

- **Share positive feelings.**

Six-year-old Sean had difficulties with coordination and struggled with multiple tasks. After 2 months of intervention once a week that included many successful experiences and a focus on his strengths, Sean asked for paper. He made a heart and drew the two of us inside.

"I really like being with you too," I responded.

Then the last week of school at the end of the session, he said, "Turn around. I have a surprise for you. Don't look." Behind my back, I could hear him drawing on the board. "Okay, you can look."

As I turned around, I saw a heart inscribed with "I love you."

I smiled and replied, "You are very special to me too."

KEY POINTS TO REMEMBER

- Prepare children before stopping the session.
- Use verbal, visual, or physical cues to give children notice of the limited time left.
- Incorporate words such as *last* or *finish*, or define an endpoint to alert children that they will be stopping soon.
- Make cleanup easy and simple.
- Use familiar goodbye scenarios with younger children.
- Incorporate props or games to make cleanup part of the play.
- Promote a mindset that everyone helps clean up and that their participation is appreciated.
- Put closure on each session by quickly reflecting on and talking about what had happened.
- Involve children, caregivers, and teachers in monitoring progress and updating plans.
- Provide your perspective and information regarding progress, and emphasize present and emerging competencies.
- Prepare children beforehand for the end of therapy.
- Review what occurred in therapy, share feelings, and discuss lessons learned.
- Let children know what you appreciate about them.
- Ask children to evaluate their time in therapy and provide suggestions to make it better.

REVIEW QUESTIONS

1. Children do not mind stopping an activity abruptly. True or false.

2. What can you do if a young child does not stop an activity when asked?

3. A clear endpoint (e.g., giving a time or number limit) helps children mentally prepare to stop. True or false.

4. One reason children do not want to stop an activity is that they do not know when they can do it again. True or false.

5. Children are more willing to clean up if it does not look like too much work. True or false.

6. To provide closure, what questions can you ask children at the end of a session?

7. Saying, "Good job," lets children know about the progress they are making. True or false.

8. It is important for children, caregivers, and yourself to have closure in the last session. True or false.

9. Name two possible feelings children who have bonded with you may have about stopping therapy.

10. It is too difficult for all children to evaluate their experiences in occupational therapy and make suggestions. True or false.

18

Methods to Enhance Children's Participation in Research

CHAPTER OVERVIEW

If adults want to respect and learn from children, doing research with them is required. What becomes challenging for researchers is *how* to engage children in the process and elicit their perspectives. In the past, researchers mainly interviewed caregivers and teachers. Many believed it was either too difficult or not possible to obtain children's perspectives, especially young ones. Consequently, they did not even try.

Following the 1989 United Nations Convention on the Rights of the Child and a philosophical shift, those in academia began to recognize children's competencies. They began to think creatively to discover fun and innovative ways to involve them. They explored different methods and thought about what children would consider understandable, easy to respond to, and enjoyable. This chapter describes these verbal, visual, and activity-based techniques that have been used in research studies with children.

WHY INVOLVE CHILDREN IN OCCUPATIONAL THERAPY RESEARCH?

Occupational therapy is a profession that is committed to being client centered. This requires having research that includes clients' perspectives and knowledge to inform our theories and practices. In addition, researchers demonstrate respect for clients' human rights by partnering with them, especially children and those with disabilities.

Davis (2009) summarized five other theoretical positions that justify children's involvement in research. First, children's services can be improved by including their perspectives of professionals. Second, with their input, their services can become more efficient and hence more cost effective. Third, the development of social policies that include their views can enhance their rights and participation. Fourth, because children have a different point of view and understanding from adults, they can be valuable contributors to generating a more thorough knowledge base, especially regarding childhoods in different cultures. Fifth, participating in research can be a learning experience for them, which may lead to the development of new competencies. For instance, following the completion of her study, one 9-year-old co-researcher said, "Doing the research helped with my confidence. I was quite shy, but I stood in front of people at the conference and told them about the research" (Kellett, 2010, p. 201). Children have the opportunity to learn that their views will be taken seriously and their participation may help other children. Some realize they can be change agents, valuable counterparts of their own and other's lives.

Although doing research *with* instead of *on* children can be challenging, an open and creative mind makes it feasible. Having a repertoire of methods enables occupational therapy researchers to include children as participants.

Curtin, C.
Strategies for Collaborating With Children: Creating Partnerships in Occupational Therapy and Research (pp. 375-398).
© 2017 SLACK Incorporated.

WHAT ARE PARTICIPATORY RESEARCH METHODS?

When conducting studies with adults, researchers commonly use methods such as observations, interviews, questionnaires, and experiments. These also may be used with children. The addition of other methods, such as drawing and photography, often leads to even richer data and a greater understanding of children's perspectives and their worlds.

Participatory methods are the means by which researchers obtain children's views and knowledge about their thoughts, feelings, and experiences. In the past decade, there have been many innovative ways of engaging children, maintaining their interest, and eliciting their voices. Examples of verbal methods are interviews with props, informative conversations during walking tours, and focus groups. Some visual methods may include photography, drawing, video diaries, or mapmaking. Examples of activity-based methods are the use of puppets, games, collages, and construction projects. Each generates different data, and they are often combined, such as pairing photography with interviews. They can be used in quantitative and qualitative research. The choice of methods is based on the research question and children's abilities and interests.

One challenging aspect of these methods is the increased time and issues involved in the collection and analysis of the data. Children need to be involved in analysis to clarify the meaning of their images. Because they have more control over what is communicated, they may not directly provide information regarding the research question. The use of visual images raises more ethical considerations in terms of getting consent, confidentiality, and ownership of the data. Furthermore, it can be harder to convert data into a written text needed for publication and dissemination.

The benefit of participatory methods is that it allows the researcher to use children's preferred avenues of communication. When researchers use these methods, they are adapting to the children's style of communication instead of expecting them to adapt to adult ways. By matching their style, it is easier for children to understand and respond in a manner that is familiar. Use of these methods supports a strengths-based approach because they are matched to the children's current competencies.

Incorporating these different types of methods provides more options for learning from children who have limited verbal skills. Many methods, such as drawing or photography, allow children extra time to respond and select what they want to say, which eliminates the pressure to reply immediately. The power is shifted to the children because they have more control of how and what they communicate. Making a drawing, for example, is more open-ended than answering a direct question. Children find research methods with a "doing" component more enticing, fun, and motivating.

Another advantage is that a combination elicits a greater range of information. Visual images, such as drawings or photographs, convey different information from words alone, including feelings that are difficult to speak about. Thus, researchers are likely to gather more comprehensive data.

Children may need these methods, Punch (2002) maintained, due to their lack of experience being in a research situation with unfamiliar adults, their marginalized role in society, and their different language and cognitive skills. She argued that participatory research methods are good for adults too. Instead of calling them child friendly, she suggested calling them participant friendly.

BASIC PREMISES TO USING PARTICIPATORY METHODS

1. Children's knowledge is as valuable as adults' knowledge. Their knowledge contributes to our understanding of children and childhood and needs to be incorporated into our theories, practices, and public policies.

2. Children's competencies, language skills, and attention span need to be viewed as being on a continuum and not based on age alone.

3. Not all children will like all methods. For instance, there are children who do not like to draw. It is best to have options so that they can choose the most comfortable method(s).

4. The use of a variety of methods will generate different and complementary types of information.

5. Most of the visual and activity-based methods require children's descriptions and explanations to clarify their meaning and interpretations.

6. It is a researcher's responsibility to find and, if necessary, adapt the methods so children can be successful in their participation.

7. Occupational therapists can apply their expertise in adapting activities to their research methods so that children, including those with disabilities, can participate.

HIDDEN AND TAKEN-FOR-GRANTED INFLUENCES

It is easy for researchers to think that their way of seeing the world is shared by everyone else. At the beginning of a study, however, they need to recognize the influence of their, caregivers', and children's culture, history, world view, and theories. These hidden and often taken-for-granted aspects are major factors in any research.

Sociocultural and Historical Influences on the Research

In a study with refugee children (Oh, 2012), one child took a picture of sandals. When asked about her picture, she talked about the time when her village had been attacked. She escaped with her family in bare feet because she did not have her sandals. Her simple picture represented a time in her life and the history and culture of her family, village, and nation.

In Barker and Smith's (2012) study of children's views of their afterschool clubs, they asked them to take photographs of what they liked, disliked, or wanted to say about their experiences. The researchers observed how the children had to negotiate with the adults about which adults would or would not be in the photos. These lengthy and influential negotiations were not visible in the children's photos. The researchers also noted that photos of school spaces were restricted to places the adult allowed the children to go. They highlighted the necessity of recognizing and acknowledging that sociocultural factors are inseparable from the methods. Hence, when using participatory techniques, researchers have to be cognizant about maintaining a broader historical and cultural perspective.

Influence of the Researcher's World View and Theoretical Orientation

In any study, researchers' world views and theoretical orientations influence all aspects. One factor is their beliefs regarding how knowledge is constructed, which reflects how they incorporate a certain paradigm, such as positivism or social constructionism. Another factor is the researchers' application of their discipline's theories. Their way of thinking affects the determination of the research questions, consideration of the best research methods, and interpretation and presentation of the results. Other influential factors are their life experiences and views on childhood, development, and children's competencies.

For example, occupational therapists using a social construction paradigm and their client-centered theory would consider the children's participation essential. To add to evidence-based practice, they might ask a research question such as, "What are children's perspectives on how therapists helped them?" They would involve them in choosing research methods, such as interviews, drawing, or photography, and engage them in the different stages of the research process.

Each paradigm and theory guides researchers in generating different kinds of knowledge. One paradigm and theory alone cannot satisfactorily explain all the complexities of children, childhood, and development; multiple ideologies and methods are needed (Burman, 2008). It is important that researchers identify their theories and recognize how they affect their studies.

Meanings Associated With Places

Another influencing factor is the location of the research. Children attribute meanings and expectations to particular spaces. For instance, they know they have to act differently at school than they do at home. Some may be more relaxed being interviewed in their homes. Some spaces have a negative connotation. Children may think they are in trouble if a researcher interviews them in a principal's office. When Phelan and Kinsella (2013) interviewed children in their homes, they found that the children equated sitting at the kitchen table with schoolwork. On their second visit, the children choose to sit on the floor. Therefore, researchers will want to be thoughtful about the research space and ensure the children are comfortable, such as having the right-sized furniture and privacy.

METHODOLOGY, METHODS, AND MIXED METHODS

Based on their research question, researchers have to make decisions regarding their methodology and related research methods. As defined by O'Reilly and Kiyimba (2015), methodology is "the particular research approach grounded in a particular school of thought" and methods are "the practical means by which data are collected" (p. 3). In qualitative research, for example, one methodology would be grounded theory and one method would be interviews.

Although there are debates whether two different paradigms can be combined in one study, some have assumed a practical and pragmatic approach. They have incorporated mixed methods in their study. The term *mixed methods* has come to have different meanings and definitions. Kara (2015) described different ways this term has been used. She contended that it referred to a study that mixes (a) paradigms (usually quantitative and qualitative), (b) theoretical perspectives, (c) researchers from different professions, and/or (d) methods within a methodology or paradigm.

Use of this methodology is increasing, and there are now detailed descriptions of different types of mixed methods designs and guidance from the National Institutes of Health (Fetters, Curry, & Creswell, 2013). The research question is the key for knowing if a mixed-method approach is desirable. The benefits of a combination are that different methodologies and methods can complement each other, resulting in more comprehensive and in-depth research findings. Researchers have incorporated this research design for instrument development, enhanced understanding of intervention, case studies, and participatory research to promote social justice (Fetters et al., 2013).

The challenges of mixed methods are that it requires knowledge and competence in each method used, takes more time, and increases the volume of data. It often involves an interdisciplinary team, requiring good communication and negotiation skills for dealing with (a) group dynamics, (b) differing philosophies, and (c) decisions regarding the integration of different data sets. An example of a large, multidisciplinary, multitheoretical, mixed-methods study is described in Goelman, Pivik, and Guhn's (2011) book, *New Approaches to Early Child Development: Rules, Rituals, and Realities.*

The Researcher's and Children's Roles

Assuming a client-centered and strengths-based approach in research requires the development of a partnership with children. The researcher's role is to guide the process or support children as they conduct their own studies. There is a continual belief in children's competencies and the recognition of their expertise. The children's roles vary and may include being an advisor, participant, or co-researcher.

Researcher's Role

When using participatory methods, the researcher's role is nontraditional and nonauthoritarian. The researcher is responsible for guiding the research process. The researcher starts by letting children know that he or she has a different role from most adults, such as caregivers and educational staff. This is important because children are used to teachers asking questions when they already know the answers. They learn that to be a good student, they need to guess the right answer. Unless they are told otherwise, they will naturally expect to do the same when a researcher asks them questions. Also important is that the researcher conveys the message that he or she will genuinely listen to children, value their perspectives, and be open to learning from them.

Mandell (1988) captured this unique relationship by advocating that researchers adopt the "least adult role," shown by their words and actions. Sitting at the same level as the children, they would participate in their activities and try to enter the children's worlds. They would avoid assuming an authoritarian role, such as setting limits, unless children's safety was at risk.

In response to criticisms that children will still view a "least adult" as an adult (due to their size and their understanding of society's roles), Christensen (2004) proposed that researchers be "unusual" adults. Instead of trying to take on the status of a child, she proposed maintaining an adult status but letting go of traditional adult ideas, ways, and roles. The researchers would convey their serious commitment to understanding the children's perspectives and experiences. In her research, she avoided assuming an "I am in charge" role; instead, she began by observing them to learn their ways and then copying their actions. When talking with them, she was careful not to interrupt and waited until they were finished.

Corsaro (2015) adopted this same type of role in his research with Italian and American preschoolers. When he joined them, he would sit quietly and wait for them to react to him. This allowed them to control their interactions. The children learned that he was a different kind of adult and responded by naming him "Big Bill" (p. 52). Lowe (2012) let them know she was there to learn by saying that she had "forgotten what it was like to be a child." To which one child responded, "You need some help... cos [sic] you are so old" (p. 272).

Children are often mystified and surprised when researchers display unusual adult behavior. When Mandell (1988) played in the sand pit with them, the children asked, "Who are you?" Some will test to see if the researchers will correct them or resolve conflicts. For example, Fine and Sandstrom (1988) described a situation where a researcher observed children getting in trouble and did not react. One child yelled out, "What's wrong with you, mister, aren't you going to report us?" (p. 53).

When including children in studies, researchers need to use kid language and open body language and consider the message their clothing conveys. Another way to reduce the adult-child power difference is to sit or stoop to the children's eye level. Researchers need to be flexible and willing to adapt to children's communication styles and explore and respect the meaning of silence. A nonjudgmental attitude is also a requirement.

Children's Roles in the Research Process

Collaborating with children in research can take many forms. Children can be (a) on advisory boards or in reference groups, (b) participants in the study, or even (c) co-researchers. Different factors can affect a researcher's decision of how to involve them. Children have a choice if they want to participate, which can depend on their interest and the required time commitment. The research question, the context of the study, and practicalities all play a role. The researcher's skill in communicating with children, including those with disabilities, is another factor. Moore, Saunders, and McArthur (2011) contended that one level is not necessarily better than another—what is important is that the children's involvement was meaningful to them. This was evident in my study (Curtin, 1995) when 10-year-old Tony reviewed the tapes of his interviews and commented on how he felt like a real professional.

Children's Advisory Boards or Reference Groups

At this level, children are consultants for one phase, multiple stages, or throughout the entire study. The group provides assistance in developing and/or giving feedback in pilot studies, instrument development, interviews questions, data collection, data analysis, and dissemination. They help researchers do the following:

- Understand children's perspectives
- Use appropriate wording
- Make the research interesting, enticing, and fun
- Involve children in analyses
- Identify ways to disseminate the research findings, especially to other children

One example of children's involvement in instrument development is Charles and Haines' (2014) study. They had 93 children and young people assist in the creation of a new measurement scale. They ranged in age from 11 to 16 years old. The presentation, format, and content of multiple instruments were analyzed. Next, they constructed a five-point scale entitled *The Measure of Young People's Participation in Decision-Making*, which they contended children could understand and easily respond.

In a second example, children acted as consultants throughout the study. Moore et al. (2011) used a reference group of children when they wanted to learn about children's experiences of being homelessness. In this case, the group recommended that adults versus peers do the interviews due to the sensitive issues related to being homeless and their knowledge of how to handle strong emotions. One group member said, "There's a lot that goes on for homeless kids, hard stuff and they need to be able to talk about it… They need someone who can listen, who can deal with it" (p. 261). The researchers followed their advice.

Children as Research Participants

In the role of a research participant, children are viewed as vital informants. Various research methods, which are described later in this chapter, are used to elicit their perspectives, understandings, and experiences. They often have a choice of the data collection method, such as the use of drawing or photography. In such cases it would be necessary for them to provide their explanations or interpretations of their visual or activity-based images.

Children as Co-Researchers

In this role, children are seen as equal or primary researchers, with the adult researcher as a partner or mentor. With guidance, the children become partners and/or lead the research. They work with researchers in identifying the research question and collecting, analyzing, and disseminating the data. In some studies, they are the ones to interview and collect the data from their peers.

Another variation is for children to be responsible for all stages of the research with adult support. Kellett (2010) argued that one reason children are not thought of as primary researchers is that they (like many adults) have not had the necessary training. To rectify this situation, Kellett (2010, 2011) and other professionals developed an educational and mentorship program to help children learn research skills. The children decide on their research questions and, with guidance, collect and analyze their data. Their findings are published on the Open University's Children Research Centre's website (http://childrens-research-centre.open.ac.uk) in the United Kingdom. Some of their results have been published in academic journals and disseminated through presentations.

For example, in one child-led study, 11-year-old Manasa researched her experience of a being child whose father used a wheelchair (Kellett, 2010). She examined three modes of transportation: train, bus, and sidewalks. She conducted observations, maintained a research dairy, and wrote a life narrative of related memories. Her research highlighted the personal effects of the inaccessibility of these transportation modes. For instance, she recounted one incident of going to the movies with her father, but the bus passed them by when the driver saw her father in a wheelchair. Consequently, they were late to the movie. She presented her results to the government's transportation department, and changes were made. The authorities added ramps to more buses, changed bus driver training, and started placing an escort seat next to the spaces for people in wheelchairs. In this case, the child became the advocate for the adult.

STAGES OF RESEARCH

There are ways to involve children in all stages of research. Often simple adaptations, such as using kid language and adding picture cues, can facilitate children's understanding and engagement. This section includes ideas for making research child friendly from start to finish.

Decide on the Research Question

Maintaining a client-centered approach requires researchers to consider whether the research is important and of value to the client. Hence, they need to take into account whether their research question and corresponding study will affect children's lives. In addition, is the study worthwhile for children to invest their time and energy? It is helpful to ask children what they think is important to study. One 10-year-old co-researcher emphasized this point: "Children see things differently to adults. I think if an adult had done this research, they wouldn't have got the same responses. They wouldn't have asked the same questions" (Kellett, 2010, p. 201).

To apply a strengths-based approach, researchers' questions would concentrate on (a) what promotes instead of hinders development, and (b) learning about children's competencies and adaptations. Moyson and Roeyers (2012) found that previous studies on siblings of children with disabilities had focused on maladjustment. They were careful to word their research questions and interview guide more neutrally, which elicited a balance of positive and negative feelings.

Determine Risks Versus Benefits

As described earlier in the chapter, there are multiple benefits to involving children in research.

One risk to consider is whether the research topic has the potential to bring up upsetting or painful feelings. If this is a possibility, researchers can ensure there are supportive adults or counselors available before starting. Moyson and Roeyers (2012) addressed this concern when designing their research. After their interviews with the siblings, they purposely spent time playing with them to give the children an opportunity to talk about any upsetting feelings. (For detailed descriptions of ethical issues, see Alderson and Morrow's (2011) *The Ethics of Research With Children and Young People*; Richards, Clark, and Boggis' (2015) *Ethical Research with Children: Untold Narratives and Taboos*; and Sargeant and Harcourt's (2012) *Doing Ethical Research With Children*.)

Provide an Information Leaflet

To enable children to make an informed decision, they need a description of the study and required commitment. An information leaflet is used to convey these important details about the research in a way children can understand. By giving this information before the study, children have time to think about their questions, talk with their caregivers, and decide if they are interested in taking part. The leaflet needs to be in kid language and tailored for different ages. Also recommended is to attach photo(s) of the researcher(s) and supplement the form with pictures, clip art, and/or graphics (Twycross, Gibson, & Coad, 2008). It should be in children's native language, if possible, and written with the use of personal pronouns, such as "I," "we," and "you" (Alderson & Morrow, 2011). The format can provide a summary of the research process by (a) listing questions with the answers or (b) including simple statements.

Researchers have relayed the information in leaflets, booklets, comic strips, and videos (Clarke, Boorman, & Nind, 2011; Twycross et al., 2008). Loyd (2012) created a booklet that contained picture symbols matching each word, which could be used with visual learners. Include details on the following:

- Researcher (s)
- Purpose of the research
- Amount of time and their involvement
- Methods or activities
- Risks and benefits
- Handling of the results
- Contact information

In Alderson and Morrow's (2011) leaflet, for example, two questions they wrote were, "Could there be any problems for me if I do take part?" and "Will doing the research help me?" (p. 93). Another important element is to tell them that their participation is voluntary, they can stop at any time, and what is said will remain confidential. To ensure the leaflet is child friendly, have it looked at by a children's reference group.

Obtain Informed Consent to Participate

It is essential to get the consent of both caregivers and children. Although only the caregivers' written permission is legal, ethically children need to agree as well. Providing consent entails the following three aspects: (a) understanding the information about the research, (b) making an informed decision, and (c) giving an indication of agreement, which is usually a signature (Gallagher, Haywood, Jones, & Milne, 2010).

For children who are not able to give consent, their assent is required. O'Reilly and Parker (2014) defined consent as children "actively communicating" their willingness to participate and having the needed capacity to make that decision. They defined assent as the child complying with or implying agreement to engage in the research (p. 45). Age is not the best criterion for children's ability to consent; children's competences vary and are based more on their context and experiences (Groundwater-Smith, Dockett, & Bottrell, 2015). A further contributing factor is the researcher's ability to talk with them and provide information in a way they can understand.

Cocks (2006) argued that researchers needed to shift from assessing competence before seeking consent to considering consent as a process of obtaining verbal and nonverbal agreement to participate. She maintained that, in research, adults' judgments regarding competence have hindered the inclusion of children with disabilities. Hence, even children who may not understand the research process will have an opinion regarding whether they want to be involved. This opinion may be expressed verbally or through their actions. It is important to note that children's verbal and nonverbal agreements need to clearly indicate yes (Phelan & Kinsella, 2013). In addition, obtaining consents is an ongoing process. Sargeant and Harcourt (2012) had younger children give their permission by writing "OK" next to their names. Each time they met, children printed OK in a different color if they wanted to take part. Researchers also need to respond to any actions suggesting children want to stop.

Similar to the information leaflet, it is best if the consent form is easy to understand and visually appealing and has pictures or graphics (Lambert & Glacken, 2011). Include the information that they have a right to stop at any time, and if a personal safety issue arises, the researcher will talk to them first and then talk to others and get help. The consent process can be made fun. In one study, researchers (Kumpunen, Shipway, Taylor, Aldiss, & Gibson, 2012) created a storyboard containing pictures and phrases of different stages of the research. As they read the phrases that had missing words, the children filled them in with representative pictures. Children then made happy or unhappy faces to convey their feelings about participating. For older children, they created a word search related to the research. Children were asked to define the terms, which were explained if they did not know them. Afterward, they decided whether they wanted to sign a consent form.

During the consent process, children have been asked what signal they wanted to use to indicate their wish to take a break or to stop (Kumpunen et al., 2012). In other studies, they were taught to say, "Pass" if they did not want to answer any questions or hold up a red stop sign card to stop and a yellow card for a break or to skip the question (Alderson & Morrow, 2011; Twycross et al., 2008). O'Reilly and Parker (2014) had children circle yes or no to four questions. They asked the children whether (a) the research was explained, (b) they asked all their questions, (c) they knew it was okay to stop any time, and (d) they were happy to take part (p. 46). In other studies, children have indicated their permission on consent forms by (a) signing their name, (b) printing "OK" or "Happy," or (c) circling one of three figures that showed a thumbs-up, a neutral face, or a thumbs-down (Dockett, Einarsdóttir, & Perry, 2012; Groundwater-Smith et al., 2015; Sargeant & Harcourt, 2012).

TYPES OF PARTICIPATORY RESEARCH METHODS

A wide range of creative and participatory research methods can be used with children. The following are descriptions of various types of verbal, visual, activity, and online methods. Also included are examples of studies demonstrating how each method has been used. Although these studies come from a variety of professions and countries, they provide ideas that can be applied to occupational therapy research.

Participant Observation

Participant observation is an informal and indirect method of discovering children's perspectives. It is often used to complement other participatory methods. Observations provide researchers with information about children's worlds, including an opportunity to hear their natural conversations.

Researchers typically see events through an adult lens. They have a choice. They can switch to viewing the actions and events through a child's lens. In a study of early interventions services with two children with Down syndrome,

Paige-Smith and Rix (2011) assumed a child's lens by recording all the events in the first person as the child (e.g., "I threw the ball," instead of "The child threw the ball"). Taking this perspective provided them with greater insight into the children's roles in the interactions.

It also is beneficial for researchers to apply a strengths-based model by ensuring their observations include a focus on competencies. Bluebond-Langner's (1978) ethnography with hospitalized children with cancer is a good example. She found that although the children knew they were dying, they maintained a mutual pretense of normalcy for the sake of their parents. They were savvy in adjusting their behavior to meet the adults' coping needs.

(For more guidance on this method, see two classic references: Spradley's [1980] *Participant Observation* and Fine and Sandstrom's [1988] *Knowing Children: Participant Observation With Minors.*)

Verbal Research Methods

Common research methods that rely on verbal responses are interviews, focus groups, questionnaires, surveys, and vignettes. The advantage of verbal techniques is that they provide an opportunity to gather and analyze in-depth data often quicker than the visual and activity-based research methods. Children can participate in all of these methods, but some may need adaptations.

Interviews

Interviews are the most direct way to discover children's (and adults') perspectives. When researchers ask open-ended questions, they give children the chance to convey their thoughts and feelings. This method supports learning about their perspectives that may differ from an adult's point of view.

The same principles of good interviewing used with adults also apply to children. The research question becomes the guide to which questions are asked. Questions are scrutinized for clarity and meaningfulness, often tested within pilot studies. The researcher's responsibility is to listen closely, provide thought-provoking prompts, and check for understanding. Creating a nonjudgmental and relaxed climate and location is also crucial.

At the same time, there are different considerations for interviewing children. Researchers need to (a) address the adult-child power differential, (b) clarify that the interview is not a test, (c) ensure comprehension and ease of responding, and (d) prevent boredom. The use of a prop to represent the research topic helps children, especially younger ones, understand the concept. The prop also tends to capture and maintain their attention. Another way to enhance interviews is to use an activity is to elicit more details and clarify what they are thinking. (See Curtin's [2001] article, *Eliciting Children's Voices in Qualitative Research*, for more specific adaptations.)

Examples of Studies Using Interviews

To gain an understanding of children's perceptions of play preferences and experiences, two occupational therapists, Miller and Kuhaneck (2008), conducted 10 interviews with children. They asked the boys and girls, aged 7 to 11 years old, about their choices, preferences, experiences, associated feelings, and the meaningfulness of play. The researchers found that the core component of play was the element of fun. There were other influential factors. One was the characteristic of the activity, such as level of difficulty. One child said, "I always like challenges…not real easy but not really hard either. In the middle so that I'm being challenged but I'm still doing good" (p. 411). Another factor was who they considered playmates, which included siblings, friends, and pets. Additional factors were associated with their age, ability, and gender, as well as the time and location of the play.

In another study, Serdity and Burgman (2012) interviewed 10 children with disabilities about their role as an older sibling. There were five boys and five girls, aged 8 to 11 years. They had different physical, cognitive, and sensory disabilities. The researchers found that the children assumed the roles of teacher, protector, and caregiver, such as supervising their siblings. The children discussed being playmates and friends with their siblings but also described typical conflict situations with them. Personality, gender, and family dynamics appeared to affect their relationships more than their disabilities. The researchers stressed that obtaining these children's perspectives, which highlighted their competencies, contradicted the assumption that they were passive and dependent.

Example of a Study Using Interviews With a Visual Prop

Moyson and Roeyers (2012) studied how siblings of children with intellectual disabilities defined their quality of life. Fifty Belgian children, ranging in age from 6 to 14 years, participated. The researchers conducted three in-depth interviews in the children's homes. In the first interview, they used a timeline and asked the children to talk about themselves and important life events up to the present. The second interview centered on their experiences and quality of life as a sibling. Using a hand-drawn thermometer, the researchers asked them to mark how much they liked being a sibling, with 10 being really liked and 0 being disliked. The third interview explored the meaning of being a sibling. Later, two focus groups were also conducted.

The siblings identified nine domains related to their quality of life. Some of these domains were (1) doing joint activities, such as playing together and being able to help; (2) having a mutual understanding by being an interpreter for others on what the child is trying to say; and (3) having acceptance. One 11 year old said she told herself that her sister "is different, she has other capacities and that's so nice! I really learned to appreciate the things she can do!" (p. 93).

Another sibling stated, "I can understand my brother—a lot of other people don't—even my dad doesn't always understand him" (p. 93).

Example of a Study Incorporating Interviews Enhanced With an Activity

Lingam, Novak, Emond, and Coads (2013) interviewed 11 children and young people, ranging in age from 11 to 16 years. All had a diagnosis of developmental coordination disorder. Individual interviews were followed by small-group ones. To enhance the discussions, clip art pictures were used as prompts if the children became bored, gave short answers, and/or at the end of the interview. In the group they were asked to apply sticky labels to a 10-rung ladder to indicate the importance of the subjects identified in previous interviews, the highest rung being the most important. The researchers found that one common perspective was the participants' emphasis on what they were able to do rather than focusing on difficulties. One said, "I don't think I'd like to change who I am. I wouldn't like to get rid of this [disorder] because it's all part of me like…I'm not ashamed of it because it kind of makes me who I am" (p. 312).

Focus Groups

A focus group involves having a small number of children (four to five is ideal) discuss the topic or issue identified by the researcher (Morgan, Gibbs, Maxwell, & Britten, 2002). The group members are usually the same gender and similar in age. Although depending on the topic, some researchers have used mixed groups.

The merits of this research method are that the children tend to be more relaxed and comfortable with their peers. The conversation is usually casual, and children decide when they want to speak. Group discussion can promote reflection and stimulate the exploration of ideas. The researcher is able to elicit multiple views in a short time, leading to the discovery of commonalities as well as differences in their perspectives.

The drawback of a focus group is that the researcher needs to be a skilled facilitator. The researcher needs to (a) recognize and address group dynamics, (b) ensure everyone gets an opportunity to talk if they choose to do so, (c) prevent boredom, and (d) keep the conversation on topic while at the same time following the children's lead. A second drawback is that children who are shy or quiet-natured may prefer individual interviews. In addition, when a research is about sensitive topics, such as being homeless, some children would prefer a private conversation. And finally, a third drawback is that documenting the discussion can be challenging, especially when two or more children talk at the same time.

To make focus groups more child friendly, researchers have woven activities, visuals, and props into the group session. Some start by doing a warm-up or icebreaker type of activity. Other researchers have incorporated drawing, vignettes, role play with dolls or toys, or the sorting of pictorial or statement cards. Griffiths, Stenner, and Hicks (2014) had the children hold a prop while speaking and later conducted an activity in which children wrote their views on sticky notes. Clark (2011) used a large ruler as a concrete way of rating from best to worst. In one group she had children decide where to place a representative item on the ruler. In another group, as she moved the item on the ruler, the children yelled, "Go," and "Stop," which she reported they enjoyed. Griffiths et al. (2014) ended their groups by letting children choose a game to play.

Example of a Study Using Focus Groups

At the invitation of a school principal, Ren and Langhout (2010) conducted a study of the school's recess and ideas for improvements. Following four weeks of observation, they conducted eight focus groups, with 30 children in total. The children in each group were the same gender and grade level, ranging from second through fifth grade. For the groups, the principal and recess aides identified a variety of students who were viewed as being leaders, followers, troublemakers, and ones who played on the sidelines. Two focus groups also were conducted with the recess aides.

The children identified the problems as being a lack of materials (e.g., basketballs), broken equipment, a lack of organized games, and a need for more space. They suggested obtaining more play materials (e.g., different types of balls), having more recess aides, using an adjoining field next to the school, and getting more age-appropriate and interesting movies for indoor recess. Following this study, these suggestions were implemented by the principal. Of their own accord, older children began organizing games for younger ones. Rather than putting all their efforts on intervention for individual children, the educational staff talked about their realization that children could be resources for identifying problems and developing solutions.

Example of Children Having a Choice of an Interview or Focus Group

Lindsay and McPherson (2011) interviewed 15 children and youth with cerebral palsy about bullying and social inclusion. Because this was a sensitive topic, the participants had the option to be in a focus group or be interviewed individually. Six participated in the focus group, and nine were seen on a one-to-one basis. The participants ranged in age from 8 to 18 years.

The purpose of the research was to learn children strategies for improving inclusion in schools. The children said they wanted classmates to focus on their abilities, not their disabilities. One said, "The number one thing is to teach and let kids know there's nothing wrong with being different and there's nothing wrong with having a disability" (p. 811). The children's strategies to increase social inclusion included (a) increasing awareness and knowledge of disability, (b) letting teachers and classmates know when they are bullied, and (c) developing self-confidence and a peer support group.

Questionnaires

Questionnaires provide a structured and systematic way to collect multiple children's perspectives in a short time period. Children can remain anonymous and those who are shy may prefer this written method (Hill, 2006). Another benefit is that there tends to be a good response rate when administered in the schools (Gallagher, 2009). Additionally, when done at home, children can choose when and where to complete it.

A disadvantage of questionnaires is that it takes time to ensure they are well designed and piloted. The written forms require a certain level of literacy and writing skills, which may preclude some children from responding. If the questions are not clear, the researcher is not there to explain or clarify. If all the questions are closed, such as circling yes or no, children are not able to explain their answers. When the questionnaire is administered at school, children may not feel like they have a choice on whether to participate. They also may become disinterested or bored if there are too many questions or view it as schoolwork or a test.

Questionnaires can be administered within an interview or over the phone. They can be a written form mailed to participants or completed online. Scott (2008) maintained that questionnaires can be modified for children and used for population and longitudinal surveys. One valuable way to make it child friendly is to use children's focus groups to identify the questions. Another option is to have a children's advisory board review and provide feedback. Pilot studies are also beneficial.

The form needs to be short and, according to O'Reilly, Ronzoni, and Dogra (2013), no more than two printed pages. There needs to be only one idea per question, and the children need to understand all the words and what the question is asking. If the content is more complex, O'Reilly et al. (2013) suggest giving an example or using stories of children's characters to further explain. Including contradictory statements is helpful to check if children are providing the same answer for all the questions. Another consideration is to think about the range of children's living situations (e.g., being raised by a single parent or grandparents), when writing questions about parents or families.

It is vital that the form be visually appealing and interesting. Gallagher (2009) suggested including a photo of the researcher(s) to make it more personal. Highly recommended is the use of pictures, images, and/or diagrams and the incorporation of animation in the online versions (O'Reilly & Parker, 2014). If completed at school, it is better to have the researcher, not the teacher, administer it (Hill, 2006). Gallagher (2009) emphasized that to keep the research truly voluntary in a school setting, children should be able to easily leave and have a place to go if they do not want to participate. He also suggested adding as a choice a box with, "I don't want to answer this question."

Example of a Study That Included Children's Involvement in the Development of a Questionnaire

To develop a questionnaire about quality of life for children with medical conditions, Chaplin, Koopman, Schmidt, and the DISABKIDS Group (2008) conducted focus groups with children and parents. To identify the items, focus groups with children aged 4 to 7 years were held in seven countries. This led to the development of 12 questions and a Likert scale using five different types of smiley faces to respond. The faces ranged on a continuum from sad to happy.

Following a pilot study, the 12 questions were reduced to six. An adult, such as a nurse, would assist the children by reading the questions and children pointed to each answer. In addition, a parent's version was developed. The reliability and validity were examined in a field study of 435 children.

Vignettes

The inclusion of vignettes in a study involves having children respond to short, hypothetical stories. The researcher can isolate different factors in each story. A benefit of this method is that children may feel safer talking about a similar person without having to admit they feel the same way.

A disadvantage is that what they think for a hypothetical child might be different from what they would want if they were in the actual situation (Zwaanswijk et al., 2011). Also, the vignette has limited information and often does not describe the physical and social environments and the culture.

Example of a Study Using Vignettes

Zwaanswijk et al. (2011) asked three groups to identify their preferences regarding communication entailing information and decision making for cancer treatment. The first two groups were children receiving treatment for cancer and survivors; both groups ranged in age from 8 to 16 years. The third group consisted of parents. In a previous study, the researchers found seven important factors involved with pediatric oncology consultation. They randomly combined these factors in 200 vignettes.

The participants completed a questionnaire, responding to questions about their 10 individual vignettes. They marked their level of agreement on a continuous line between two points. The researchers determined a score by measuring the distance from one of the points. Overall, 1,440 vignettes were assessed. The results of the study were that the three groups reported generally preferring that (a) parents and children hear about the illness and treatment at the same time and (b) children are involved in the decision making.

Tours

When children give tours of important places in their lives, they are able to point to and describe associated memories and meanings. The tours can be a casual walk, with the researcher recording the children's comments, or may be combined with taking photographs along the way. As they show the researcher around, different spaces and objects often prompt them to talk about connected experiences. For instance, seeing a favorite space on the playground may trigger a memory, leading them to say, "This is where my friends and I…" Thus, being in the actual location makes it easier for them to talk about what they like and dislike and their experiences there. Another benefit of this method is that the children get to move around as they talk, which is especially good for those who have difficulty sitting still.

Example of a Study on the Development of a Walking Tour Research Method

In a planned and funded 5-year study about children's resiliency after trauma, Gibbs, McDougall, and Harden (2013) wanted to develop a respectful and ethical way to involve the children. Following a devastating bushfire in Australia, the researchers wanted to learn from the children about their needs and experiences. After developing the walking tour research method, they planned to first have children give tours of their local areas without inquiring about the fire. The children would then be familiar with the research methodology, and consent would be obtained again before conducting a second tour to ask about the fire, its destruction, and their experiences. Photographs would be taken, converted into cartoon images, and turned into a storyboard. The main focus of the study would be on what factors supported them after the fire.

Visual Research Methods

Researchers elicit different information when they use visual rather than only verbal techniques. Creating drawings, timelines, maps, and spider diagrams allows children to visually represent their perspectives and experiences. Children also tend to enjoy the action-oriented nature of taking photographs, shooting home movies, and making video diaries. The combination of visual methods with interviews has expanded access to children's worlds and knowledge.

Drawing Pictures

Drawing is one of the most frequently used research methods with children. For many, it is a familiar and fun activity that provides them freedom to express themselves. They have time to think about and control what is drawn and can exert their creativity. Drawing increases their adeptness as informants and allows greater ease in articulating their views (Tay-Lim & Lim, 2013). It often is easier for them to convey their understanding of the topic or capture personal meanings and experience in a picture. Some feel safer drawing about their emotions or difficulties rather than saying them. It can be especially beneficial to use drawing with children who are (a) shy or quiet, (b) limited in verbal skills, (c) learning a new language, or (d) from a different culture (Literat, 2013).

Researchers have combined drawing with interviews. They have used this activity as an icebreaker, a prompt to start or refocus the conversation, or to follow-up an interview (Freeman & Mathison, 2009). In studies, children have been asked to draw themselves as well as the following:

- Families and communities
- Experiences of an illness and participation in therapy
- Understanding of a concept
- Relationships
- Daily activities
- Evaluation of services
- Likes and dislikes regarding school (Christensen & James, 2008; Curtin, 1995; Driessnack & Furukawa, 2012; Einarsdóttir, Dockett, & Perry, 2009; Eldén, 2012; Gibson, Aldiss, Hortstman, Krumpunen, & Richardson, 2010; Knighting, Rowa-Dewar, Malcolm, Kearney, & Gibson, 2010)

As a research method, drawing can be used to discover children's meanings and perspectives. The focus is on the process versus the product. There is interplay between talking and drawing; each transforms the other. Their picture stimulates conversation and talking may lead to additions to the picture. There may be self-talk or conversation with the researcher.

The picture that is portrayed is influenced by children's culture, contexts, relationships, and the presence of the researcher. Their interpretation is essential. Otherwise, the researcher may misunderstand what is conveyed. One girl, for instance, drew a picture of a child with one leg. Instead of thinking it was an immature drawing, the researcher inquired about it, and the child explained it was a girl hopping on one foot (Cox, 2005).

One disadvantage of this method is that not every child likes to draw. They may think it is for younger children, they are not artistic, or it is not pleasurable. If drawing within a group, they may be concerned about pleasing their friends and imitate their pictures. If they do not like the results, they may scribble over it. Their artwork may capture painful experiences and bring up difficult emotions.

It is important to keep in mind that they will often want to take their pictures home. The researcher needs to be prepared to scan or take a photo of it, provided the children give permission.

Example of a Study Describing Drawing as a Research Method

To identify the relationships and places children receive care, Eldén (2012) interviewed and asked children to draw their day. Using a framework of concentric circles, she asked them to draw themselves in the inner circle and others in the outer circles. They were told to draw those who take care of them, whom they take care of, and which people were important to them. Closeness was determined by placement closest to the inner circle. Discussion occurred during and after the drawings. These activities allowed them to identify (a) whom they considered family and felt close to and (b) whom they helped, such as younger siblings.

Timelines

Timelines are a way to visually represent a life course. The activity is useful for learning about children's life history. By recording major events, children can relay what has happened to them and shaped who they are. These memorable times often have strong emotions: some happy, some sad. Another option is to have them create a timeline of their daily activities. This provides an opportunity to discover what their life is like and what activities they value.

Example of a Study Using Timelines

To learn about street children's relationships and environments in Kampala, Uganda, Young and Barrett (2001) used four visual research methods. The children created timelines, photo diaries, drawings, and mental maps of the city. As a group, they identified their activities and created representative symbols. Then they drew daily timelines, using the symbols to illustrate their typical day. This led to a discussion of where they went throughout the day, capturing their movements in the city. The children also took photos, drew their usual activities and places, and created maps of where they went and slept in the city.

Mapmaking

Creating maps is a way for children to illustrate the meaning of different places, spaces, and interaction with others. Groundwater-Smith et al. (2015) described five different types of mapmaking that can be incorporated into research. They contended that maps can be developed and used to document (a) common places visited, (b) relationships, (c) social and demographic information, (d) physical locations, and/or (e) children's descriptions along a predetermined route. This method allows children to provide information about their daily lives in a visual manner. In some maps, they also can highlight what they consider as being typical and/or valued places.

Example of a Study Using Mapmaking

Fleet and Britt (2011) had children create a map of the school to identify what they considered important spaces. Three guiding questions were (1) What are important places in the school? (2) What places are special to you? and (3) Why? The maps were made in a variety of ways, with drawings, photographs, tours, and/or stories of each place. A main theme that emerged was that favorite places were connected to where they could be or play with friends. A second theme was that they valued having private, secret, or risky places.

Spider Diagrams

A spider diagram is one tool to represent abstract ideas. The main theme or concept is written in the center circle.

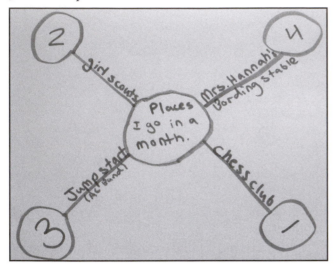

Figure 18-1. "Places I go in a month" spider diagram.

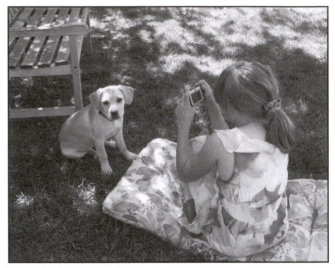

Figure 18-2. Photography as a research method.

Then, similar to spider legs, lines are drawn and related ideas are written on the lines or in small circles placed at the endpoints. One example would be to have the phrase, "Places I go in a month," in the center circle on the page (Figure 18-1). Different activities can be written on the lines, and the number of times they participate are placed in the connecting circles. This method can create a quick visual representation of their ideas.

Example of a Study Using Spider Diagrams

One of the task-based activities Punch (2002, 2009) used in her studies of children's coping skills and their relationships with siblings was the spider diagram. In one study, the group wrote "coping with problems" in the center circle. Then they drew lines, and in the smaller circle, each member wrote one idea of what help them deal with their problems. In another study, they drew their ideas in the small circles. Punch found that the spider diagram increased brainstorming, discussing, and focusing on central features of a theme or concept.

Photography

Photography has been used as a research method in two major ways: photo-elicitation and photovoice (Figure 18-2). Photo-elicitation involves having the researcher or children take photographs and then use those images as the basis of their discussions. Photovoice is a community-based, transformative research method for assisting marginalized groups to create social change (Wang & Burris, 1997).

Clark (2011) has called the use of photographs in research a "virtual passport for entry into the world of the informant" (p. 165). Children's photographs are a tool for learning about their perspectives and experiences as well as what they consider meaningful and significant. Their photographs let the researcher see what life is like from their point of view. As photographers, they can enter into and document places the researcher may not be able to go, such as children's secret places and homes.

Children often enjoy taking photographs because it is action oriented, allows for creative expression, is easy and fun, and does not require reading, writing, or drawing. They have control over which photographs they take and select for discussion and what they say. The interview becomes child led because their photographs direct the conversation (Hill, 2014).

The photographs become a vital visual image that can spark conversations, promote telling life stories, and assist in maintaining attention and interest in the interview (Cook & Hess, 2007). The images tend to convey more details than words alone and can be symbolic representations. To understand the meaning of the photographs, children need to interpret their images. It also is helpful to ask about pictures they did not or could not take. Children become an integral part of the analysis.

Drawbacks of photography are the cost of providing equipment and materials and possible technical difficulties. However, digital photography has made it easier and more economical. This method requires more time than just conducting an interview. In addition, there are more privacy and confidentiality concerns that require extra vigilance and the consent of those in the photographs.

Photovoice, developed by Wang and Burris (1997), involves having a group of marginalized community members identify a concern, define a topic, take photographs, and then use the information gathered to create change. In a study by Newman and SCI photovoice participants (2010), 10 adults with spinal cord injuries took photographs of what helped and hindered them from participating in their community. In addition, they each created a photo-documentary of one day in their lives. The group used their pictures to identify features and structures that enabled or prevented their participation. The information was presented to a state transportation committee and described in newspaper stories, leading to the development of a citizens' advocacy coalition.

Examples of Studies Using Photography

Herssens and Heylighen's (2012) study drew on the expertise of children who were born blind. The researchers, professors in departments of architecture, wanted to learn about the nonvisual aspects of sensory environments. The children, considered co-researchers, were given cameras and asked to take pictures of pleasurable places and materials in their school. They first felt the objects and then placed the lens against them. They liked pushing the button as confirmation the picture was taken. The researcher took notes of what was taken and recorded their comments. The emphasis was on the process, not the product.

Pictures were taken of the elevator for the sounds it made, the herb garden and a kitchen for their smells, and warm rooms. One of their favorite places was a room filled with mats that they associated with freedom of movement. The children emphasized the importance of textures, temperatures, sizes, and contrast between surfaces. The researchers used the information to create design parameters for architects.

In a second example, two occupational therapists, Berinstein and Magalhaes (2009), studied what 16 children living in Tanzania considered to be play. They were given cameras for a week with the directive to take pictures of play. After the photographs were developed, the children selected those they thought most represented play. There was a recorded group discussion about their pictures and what play meant to them.

They found the children to be creative and resourceful, such as creating games with sticks, stones, and dirt. Their play was self-initiated without the encouragement of adults. All of the photographs were of two or more children suggesting they considered play a social versus an individual endeavor. There were multiple pictures related to playing soccer, a highly valued sport in their country. Children were able to collect photographs of spontaneous play within their villages, which the researchers being outsiders would have had difficulty capturing.

In a third study, Doutre, Green, and Knight-Elliott (2013) interviewed six children, aged 11 to 13 years, who took care of parents who had mental illnesses. They asked the children to take photographs of things they found helpful or challenging or that they were proud of. The researchers used the pictures to expand the conversations. The children describe their lives as being "quite hard," but at the same time, they found positives in their situations (p. 35). One said, "It is a good life that I have to like help my mum" (p. 36). Some viewed themselves as being helpful, protective, and brave family members. Others adapted by engaging in activities and developing relationships outside the family. Although their situations were complex, the researchers noted that their views of their lives were "growth orientated" (p. 37).

Participatory Photo Mapping

An interdisciplinary group of researchers, Dennis, Gaulocher, Carpiano, and Brown (2009), developed the participatory photo mapping research method. This approach involves participants taking photographs with the use of a global positioning system (GPS). Afterward, they select the most representative photos related to the topic and participate in interviews or focus groups to discuss the meanings and stories regarding their images. A map is then made integrating information from the photographs, narratives, and GPS locations. The last step is to use the findings to create needed change in policies with decision makers. Participants are partners from the beginning to the end of the project.

Example of a Study Using Participatory Photo Mapping

Dennis et al. (2009) incorporated this approach in their study of a neighborhood's health and safety in a socioeconomically disadvantaged area of Madison, Wisconsin. They partnered with the children and young people, aged 10 to 18 years, who lived in that community. The most frequent image taken was of fried chicken. The researchers learned that the picture represented a fast food restaurant that was welcoming to children and teenagers, and thus a favorite place for friends to hang out. The participants and researchers used the map, which visually summarized the findings, to inform and work with city officials in planning changes. The youth also started giving tours of their neighborhood to local health care providers.

Home Movies

Another visual research method is to have children take home movies. As the "movie producer," they decide what to include or omit to represent their experience. They have the opportunity and time to edit and delete scenes. Because the researcher is not present, they are able to capture aspects of their life that would not have been seen with a stranger in their home. An added benefit is that movies include more information about the environment and the family's actions, talking, and nonverbal language. A disadvantage is that analysis of this quantity of information is time consuming.

Example of a Study Using Home Movies

In a South Korean study by Hwang (2013), siblings of children with autism took home movies to capture their everyday life. Nine children, aged 7 to 15 years, filmed for two weeks. There were 110 episodes recorded in and out of their home. The movies were not shown to their parents.

Afterward, the researcher met with the children to talk about what they had recorded. The researcher first used drawings, finger puppets, and spider diagrams as ice breakers. Then they watched their own movie clips and paused for questions or explanations. In one snippet, the child showed a brother having tantrums late at night and told the researcher, "This is part of my life at everyday night. You may not know how much I need a proper sleep" (p. 451). When the children were asked about the process, one child stated, "I really enjoyed making movies. It was really fun. I wasn't bored at all" (p. 451). Another said, "I liked to do it this way because I could do it my own way. If I was interviewed, how much could you understand about my life?" (p. 452).

Video Diary

A video diary is a novel approach that parallels reality television programs. Children speak into a camera without the researcher being present. They decide what they want to say and are able to review and edit their comments. Some researchers have had children speak into a camera at home, whereas another created a video diary room within a specialized school. This approach requires no writing or drawing. Some feel more comfortable talking to a neutral camera than being in a face-to-face interview. One disadvantage is that the researcher does not get to immediately ask for clarification on their comments.

Example of a Study Using a Video Diary Method

Clarke et al. (2011) created a video diary room as part of their research with teenage girls who were excluded and disengaged from their home school. The girls were often considered troublemakers who frequently challenged authority figures and expressed their views in disruptive ways. They attended an independent school. The researchers provided them with choices of which visual and verbal methods to use. They purposely avoided the direct questioning method. The video diary room was the most popular choice.

The girls reported that teachers often ignored them when they raised their hands, so they tried to figure out ways to get teachers to listen to them. One girl commented, "If they don't listen, I shout, and when I shout, they listen" (p. 774). One of the findings of the study was that the girls were trying alternative strategies not to cause trouble but because they wanted to be heard.

Mosaic Approach

The *mosaic approach* is a "multi-method, strength-based framework for gathering young children's views and experiences of their everyday lives" (Clark, 2010a, p. 116). Developed by Clark and Moss (2001), methods include observations and interviews with children, parents, and practitioners. Children take photos, make maps, and create books containing their drawings, photographs, and comments. A "magic carpet" method involves having children watch and talk about slides of other places, such as park playgrounds. They are often between 3 to 5 years old and can choose what methods they prefer. Similar to creating a wall mosaic, all the different images are compiled to create one detailed image (Clark, 2010b). The children's input is used to create changes. This method has been used to evaluate early childhood services and design their buildings and outdoor spaces (Clark, 2010a).

Example of a Study Applying the Mosaic Approach

A three-year longitudinal study entitled Living Spaces (Clark, 2010a, 2010b) entailed having children, architects, and researchers work together in evaluating and designing early childhood spaces. In one phase, the children gave tours and assembled maps containing their photographs, drawings, and captions. Their maps highlighted the importance of smaller and quiet spaces, lighting, windows, and different types of ceiling and floor surfaces. They took photographs of where they worked, their teachers, and the class rules. The data generated by the children enriched the architects' understanding of children's views, interests, and priorities and was used in the design of indoor and outdoor spaces.

Activity-Based Research Methods

Activity-based methods are similar to children's everyday play. They are familiar with games and building materials. They know what to do with puppets and understand sorting cards. Putting together a collage is like an art project. Many like to make their own creations. Consequently, there is a level of comfort with this approach.

Puppetry

Puppets have been used in a variety of ways in research. Children have talked to a puppet held by the researcher and answered questions. In other studies, children hold the puppet and talk through the puppet. Another approach has been to have two puppets provide opposing statements and children choose which one is more like them.

There are many advantages to incorporating puppets. For children, the puppet is a neutral "person" who listens or speaks for them. Consequently, they find it safer to talk about difficult situations or angry feelings or express what they do not like. Talking to a puppet can be less intimidating because children do not have to make eye contact with the researcher (Aldiss, Horstman, O'Leary, Richardson, and Gibson, 2009). For younger children, this approach is fun and playful.

Epstein, Stevens, McKeever, Baruchel, and Jones (2008) and Aldiss et al. (2009) made the following recommendations. Keep in mind that older children may view puppets as babyish. As long as they have a choice, it can be offered as a research method. Be sure to use puppets that have similar characteristics to the children, such as gender and race. Use of puppets with neutral facial expressions is recommended to allow for a greater expression of feelings. Another alternative is to let the children choose from a variety of puppets with fixed expressions, such as smiles or frowns.

Examples of Studies Using Puppetry

In 2008, Epstein et al. used puppets to elicit children's views on their experiences in a specialized camp for children with cancer. The children had a choice of whether and how to use the puppets. One option was to talk to and teach an "alien" puppet from another planet what it would be like to go to the camp. Two other options were to give their answers through the puppet (which the researcher coded and evaluated on a six-point scale) or listen to two puppets making opposing statements and choose which comment was the most like them.

The appearance of the puppets made a difference. Girls and children with bald heads were more guarded or chose not to talk to a boy puppet with hair. When the puppets were used, the researchers found that the children were more comfortable describing negative camp experiences and provided more ideas for changes.

Aldiss et al. (2009) conducted a study with 10 children with cancer, aged 4 and 5 years. They used puppets to explore their views and needs regarding their hospital experiences. The researcher asked children various questions, such as, "Fizz wants to know what it is like at the hospital you go to," "What is in your room at the hospital?" and "What do you do when you are in the hospital?" (p. 88). The children identified their priorities, saying that it was important to have lots of toys at the hospital (including their own), and to have their "mummy and daddy" nearby.

The next year, these researchers and another colleague (Gibson et al., 2010) continued to study the perceptions and needs of 38 children with cancer. With the 4 and 5 year olds, they used the puppets and similar questions as in the previous study. For the 6 to 12 year olds, they incorporated drawing, and for the 13 to 19 year olds, they held an activity day in a pizza restaurant that included a focus group, peer interviews, spider diagrams, and written tasks.

They found that children made the hospital more like their home by bringing their toys, photos, cushions, and bedspreads. The children talked about being tired and missing their friends, school, and sports. The older children wanted more information about their treatment to address their worries and more direct communication with them. One 12 year old stated, "They speak to mum first; they should talk to me first" (p. 1402). Other older children said that at times they would get overwhelmed and wanted staff to be sensitive to their cues of not wanting to talk.

Sposito et al. (2015) interviewed 10 hospitalized children with cancer who were undergoing chemotherapy. The children ranged in age from 7 to 12 years. The aim of the study was to learn from children the coping strategies they used to deal with chemotherapy. The children made their own puppets and the researcher had extra puppets they made. Holding the puppet, the researcher asked questions like, "What helps you feel better during chemotherapy? And after chemotherapy?" (p. 145).

The children said that knowing about chemotherapy helped them cope. One 11 year old said, "Understanding why I take chemo helps me not to complain about the treatment." Another 11 year old reported, "I prefer knowing what's going to happen so that I can prepare myself" (p. 146). Some children referred to pain-relieving and anti-nausea medication as helping. Other strategies they identified were praying, getting their favorite food from home, massages, playing games, being on the computer, distracting themselves, and participating in the play activities the occupational therapists developed.

Games

Children are familiar with playing games and usually find them entertaining. Unless they have had negative experiences, such as always losing to an older sibling, they tend to equate games with fun. Most games present an opportunity to win, which is enjoyable. Another benefit is that the required turn-taking structures the interaction.

Some researchers have incorporated games when they first meet children to put them at ease. Kirova (2006) purposely chose this strategy to minimize the adult-child power differential by starting as a play partner instead of an adult with authority. She commented on how their time playing together allowed the children to get to know her and develop trust. Others (Curtin, 1995; Einarsdóttir, 2007) have used games to elicit children's perspectives.

Examples of Studies Using Games

The purpose of Kirova's (2006) research was to learn about children's experiences of loneliness. With the help of her young son and feedback from kindergartners in a pilot project, she developed a board game to be used in her study. She named it, "How Do They Feel?" The board contained different paths to the endpoint, and a feeling word was inside each step. The children drew cards that described a character in a common school situation (e.g., being excluded) and identified what the character would be feeling. At the end of the game, she asked the children to pick one feeling and tell about a time they felt that way. She then proceeded to interview them.

In my study (Curtin, 1995), as described in Chapter 2, I created a guessing game to change the interview format. The routine I had developed was to ask questions after an activity, which was effective in the beginning. However, later in the study, the child's answers had become stilted. To change this routine, I developed two games and the child chose the guessing one. With this game, the child was in control of picking the questions from a pile of cards and asking his mother, brother, and me to guess the answer. Because the questions were about his experiences in therapy, he was the only one who knew the right answer. His response conveyed his perspective on therapy. He was delighted to tell us when we were wrong and thrilled that he was always right!

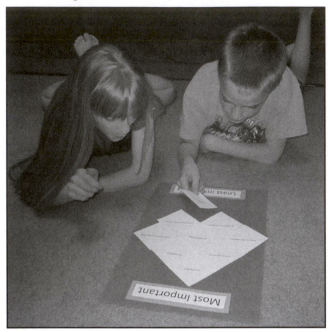

Figure 18-3. Use of a diamond ranking activity as a research method.

Einarsdóttir (2007) also used a game in her study of Icelandic preschoolers' perspectives of their school. She adapted a board game the teacher had made by adding questions, such as what they liked or disliked about school. During their free-choice time, the children could choose if they wanted to play the game. As they played, the teacher read the questions and recorded their answers. The advantage of this approach, Einarsdóttir emphasized, was that it was woven into the student's daily activities instead of being a contrived situation. A bonus benefit was that the students were able to decide whether and when they would participate.

Activities Involving Sorting or Ranking

Activities with sorting or rating help children identify their priorities and relative importance. Manipulating objects such as pictorial cards makes abstract ideas more concrete. This helps them to remember and reflect on the representative picture depicted on the card. Additionally, the activity requires them to consider and decide what they value the most. This clarifies their priorities.

Example of a Study Using Activities That Involved Sorting or Rating

As part of a larger study (O'Kane, 2008), 45 children who were "looked after" (i.e., in foster care) participated in interviews about their roles in decision making about their care. Three different activities were paired with the interviews. In the first meeting, children made their own pocket chart to indicate types of decisions and who decided. On the side were the names of people (e.g., the child, social worker, parent, teacher) and on the top were the major decisions affecting them (e.g., when they saw their parents). The children

used different colored stickers to rate whether they had a lot of say, some say, or no say.

In the second meeting, six pots were used to represent aspects of the review meeting process and labeled with "how much" questions, such as, "How much did you speak?" They had three beans per pot and decided how many beans to put in each one. In a third meeting, they did diamond ranking by placing statement cards into the shape of a diamond with the most important at the top and least at the bottom (Figure 18-3). In this study, the children placed the card with the statement "To be listened to" as the most important. At the bottom of the diamond they placed the card "To get what I want" as being the least important.

Collages

Another innovative activity-based method is to have children make collages related to the research question. They cut out pictures and captions, often from magazines or brochures, to represent their response. The pieces are arranged and glued onto a poster board. Sometimes photographs, drawings, or small objects are attached. For instance, in a study described by Carter (2014), one girl added feathers to her collage and explained that her stomach felt "fluffy and wobbly" before her operation (p. 9). When using this medium, it is essential to have a wide range of magazines and supplies to prevent limiting the children's expression of their views (Mayaba & Wood, 2015). This method is especially well suited for those who are artistic.

Example of a Study Using a Collage

In a study (Malone, 2013) funded by urban developers, children were invited to be project advisors in designing a new community in Australia. Thirty kindergartners and 120 fifth graders participated in two research workshops. The children drew their favorite, least favorite, and dream neighborhood places. The fifth graders also took photographs. Afterward, they completed individual interviews and a survey. In a focus group, they described where they went in their neighborhood and their various activities.

The children analyzed the data, which led to a list of eight child-friendly indicators (e.g., supports play, protects nature, has pathways, promotes learning). Then a small group of children put together a thematic collage of drawings and photographs from the workshop, which became the blueprint for the children's report. The developers wove the indicators into their design and presented the draft of the play space and pathway at a school assembly. Children were invited to a breaking ground event of the new playground. One child said, "I liked that I got to help design it—now it feels like I own it somehow" (Malone, 2013, p. 391).

Activities With Construction Tasks

Building models or completing a project is similar to children's everyday play. They are familiar with the materials, which allow them to focus on what they want to metaphorically portray. Thus, many children may feel more comfortable using this activity-based medium to depict their experiences. One challenge for researchers can be encouraging and guiding them to stay on the research topic.

Examples of Studies Involving Model Making

To ensure a new children's hospital was child friendly, 55 children who were either inpatients or outpatients were interviewed. Lambert, Coad, Hicks, and Glacken (2013) enhanced the interviews by having the children, aged 5 to 8 years, participate in various activities of their choice. In an arts and crafts workshop in the hospital playroom, they were asked to build their ideal hospital that include what they considered the most important rooms.

Later, the rooms were placed on a large campus to establish a blueprint. They were then asked if anything was still needed. The children identified the need for (a) various activities for different ages and genders, (b) entertainment using technology, and (c) spaces to spend time with their family and other children. They recommended having a device with a camera and online access in every hospital room to help them stay connected and see their friends.

Example of a Study Using Construction Materials

Pimlott-Wilson (2012) described the use of three research methods incorporated within her study of children's attitudes regarding their parents' employment. Children had a choice what methods they wanted to use. There were 124 children in the study, aged 5 to 9 years. The first method was the use of Lego Duplos. The children were asked to create a representation of their home and act out the roles of everyone within it. Their depiction showed the family's roles, movement, and frequent visitors. The second method was the use of rainbows and clouds. They filled in positive thoughts on cutout suns and attached them to the rainbow. On raindrops, they wrote concerns or worries and attached them to clouds. The third method was to create a mood board. Similar to a collage, the board contained images and text to portray an experience, such as past events or upcoming changes.

Example of a Study Involving a Construction Project

In addition to interviewing parents and social workers, Winter's (2012) study included 14 children, aged 4 to 7 years, who were in the care of the state. She told the children that she wanted to find out what they thought about their lives. Once they consented, they were given choices of methods; one option was a construction task. She introduced the task as a special box called a "reality box" that they could decorate. The outside was for how they thought others saw them, and the inside was for their thoughts and feelings.

One 5 year old placed lollipop sticks and pom-poms inside and then added, "I'm drawing a sad picture." When asked of what, she responded, "That my baby died," referring to the death of her younger sister. On the outside of the box, she used craft materials to create an image of herself. The researcher later discovered that was the first time she had talked about her sister.

Online Research Methods

One method growing in popularity is doing research online. To obtain children's perspectives researchers may use interviews (e.g., with Skype), questionnaires, or focus groups. There are two ways of conducting the research: (1) synchronous, when everyone talks in real time; and (2) asynchronous, when comments are added when they log in online.

A possible merit of the online approach is that children can be anonymous. With the asynchronous type, children can decide where and when they want to respond. The interpersonal dynamics are minimized; one person does not dominate and they are less likely to feel judged. They get to read and respond at their own pace and may feel freer to be honest and contradict others (Nicholas et al., 2010). There is written documentation of what is said. Additionally, it can be easier for those living in rural areas or those with disabilities to participate. For instance, children who have difficulty in social situations may prefer the impersonal nature of this approach.

Drawbacks are that children need to have computer access and the skills to participate. This may prevent those living in poverty and/or those who do not have computer access from being included. Some may not like the impersonal approach. They may prefer a more personal face-to-face meeting and being able to connect with their peers. Additionally, the researcher cannot read the children's nonverbal behavior, which can offer important information regarding the meaning of their responses.

When Nicholas et al. (2010) compared face-to-face with online focus groups, they found major differences. Those meeting in person talked more and provided richer information. They often added personal stories and contexts to the discussion and expanded their comments based on what their peers said. Those participating online stayed more focused on the topic and responded more to the questions asked versus each other's comments. The online focus groups also allowed children with compromised immune systems to participate. Hence, the two approaches, face-to-face or online, offer different benefits and drawbacks. The researcher will want to choose based on (a) the research question and (b) which one plays to the strengths of the children.

Example of a Study Using an Online Focus Group

Tates et al. (2009) conducted online focus groups with children receiving treatment for cancer, their parents, and child survivors. The children and young people, ranging in age from 8 to 17 years, discussed what they considered good communication by professionals when sharing medical information.

The researchers developed a website for the participants to log in to during a one-week period. Using a topic guide, they posed one question each day about the children's needs, preferences, and experiences. The participants responded, read others' comments, and added their own. The last few days, the children were invited to add their own questions. At the end, they were asked to evaluate this method. Children reported that they liked that it was easy, convenient, and anonymous.

Research Adaptations for Children With Different Levels of Abilities

If the researcher makes adaptations, children with various levels of ability, including those who are nonverbal, can participate in studies. To obtain their perspectives, the researcher first needs to learn how they communicate and their style of learning. Some children "talk" using their facial expressions and actions. Others use informal and formal communication systems, including assistive technology. It is especially important for determining assent that the researcher learn their methods for indicating (a) agreement and happiness and (b) dissent or displeasure.

One adaptation is to prepare children for what will happen during the study. Sloper and Beresford (2014) created a Social Story for children to read prior to their visit. They wrote simple statements and attached corresponding photographs or pictures. Included were photographs of (a) the researcher and her car, (b) pictures symbols of the questions that would be asked, and (c) a picture symbol of what the child would do after the researcher left. Preece and Jordan (2009) gave children and family members a sheet with all the interview questions ahead of time so they would know what to expect.

Another approach to helping children feel comfortable is to spend time visiting with them before starting the research. One researcher played with the child and his dog before asking any questions (Harrington, Foster, Rodger, & Ashburner, 2013). Kelly (2007) asked the children to complete a picture book with her. The book contained information about each other, such as their interests.

Integrating visuals, such as photographs or picture symbols, into the research process is another major adaptation. To increase comprehension, picture symbols can be paired with interview questions. Possible responses can be given in pictorial form, allowing children to point, move, or circle their answer.

In a study by Kramer et al. (2013), they made their survey responses visual. They had a large hand with a thumb up for "really good," the same hand in a smaller size for "good," a small hand with thumb down for "bad," and a larger hand with thumb down for "really bad." For their "how often" questions, they used a completely shaded box for "always," a half-shaded box for "sometimes," and a box with no shading for "never."

Other studies have included nonverbal ways of responding. Wickenden and Kembhavi (2014) had children use stickers or thumb prints as a response. In a study about transition meetings for youth with autism, Hagner, Kurtz, May, and Clouter (2014) found accommodations that helped the youth in the meetings. The strategies included letting them sit away from the group, use sticky notes or Skype to respond, and write answers. One youth made a PowerPoint presentation of his perspectives.

Another adaptation that is beneficial is to keep the time together short, extend the number of sessions, and allow extra time for any activities. Incorporating activity-based and visual research methods can be advantageous. Using young people with disabilities for a reference group, as Morris (2003) did in her study, can guide researchers about the best ways to include children.

Example of a Study Using Nonverbal Ways of Responding

Rabiee, Sloper, and Beresford (2005) conducted a study with children who were nonverbal. The purpose of the study was to learn about their perceptions and priorities regarding their care and support. To identify important areas and issues in their lives, the researchers first interviewed their caregivers and children with disabilities who were verbal. Next, the information was converted into pictorial statement cards to be used for the questions and to represent a range of possible answers. Children could then choose the card(s) that represented their views and place it on a mat as their response.

For example, the researchers asked how the children wanted the doctor to talk to them. Three statement cards were, "'John wants his doctor to talk to him in a way he understands,' 'Adam doesn't want his doctor to talk to him,' and 'Naeem doesn't mind'" (Rabiee et al., 2005, p. 389). Another question was if they wanted their communication system to be faster, include more words, or be used without help and/or wherever they went. The children in the study were able to respond authentically using this method.

Example of a Study Using Visuals to Control the Research Process

Harrington et al. (2013) studied the mainstreaming experiences of young people with autism spectrum disorder. The young people, ranging in age from 12 to 15 years, were interviewed after their parents' interviews. During the consent process, they were given a "stop" card to hand to the researcher if they wanted to terminate the interview (Figure 18-4). Before starting, the researcher sent them a Social Story explaining what would happen.

For the interview, the researcher created a checklist of the three topics. They checked off each topic before moving on to the next one. This visual support was reported to help maintain their attention. Along with their stop card, they also were given a pictorial break card. To answer questions, they had the option of answering by using pictorial symbols of different emotions. One young person who usually spoke with only one to three words used the symbols to express how he felt lonely, sad, and angry when he was bullied at school.

Example of a Study Using Visuals to Convey a Topic or Clarify a Question

Ashburner, Bennett, Rodger, and Ziviani (2013), who are occupational therapists, studied young people's sensory experiences. The three boys, ranging in age from 12 to 16 years, were diagnosed with autism spectrum disorder. When interviewing them, the researchers used visual supports, which were pictures of objects related to each sensation. For instance, when asked about their reactions to sounds, they were shown pictures that included a school bell ringing and people talking. The interviews centered on their reactions to different types of sensations. The researchers found that they preferred predictable, expected, self-selected, and controllable sensations. They were both more aware of and had difficulty filtering background sensations, tended to seek movement, and at times were overly focused on certain sensations.

Example of a Study Adding Visuals to Make Answering Easier

Lindsay and McPherson (2012) conducted interviews and a focus group with children and youth with cerebral palsy. They ranged in age from 8 to 19 years. The purpose of the study was to learn about their experiences of being bullied and excluded. Visual prompts were added, such as providing pictures of the different ways children are bullied. The children circled the ones that applied to them and/or drew their own picture. Next, they were shown pictures of places where bullying commonly occurred. Again, they could circle the picture or draw. Then they were given a page with thought bubbles and asked to think of a related experience and write how they felt. The children reported that they had been called names and had incidents in which they were bullied physically and verbally.

Analysis

Children's involvement in analysis is often overlooked. One of the first ways they can participate is by reviewing the transcriptions of what they said and deciding if they want anything changed. Before starting the analysis, Moyson and Roeyers (2012) followed this step in their study.

Because analysis can be time consuming, it is important to discover if children are even interested (Coad & Evans, 2008). If they are, researchers can involve them at different levels. Children can be involved in coding questionnaires and qualitative studies, as well as selecting important quotes. Researchers can hold follow-up focus groups or interviews to discuss portions of the transcriptions and provide feedback on the analysis (Lahman, 2008). Another level of involvement suggested by Coad and Evans (2008)

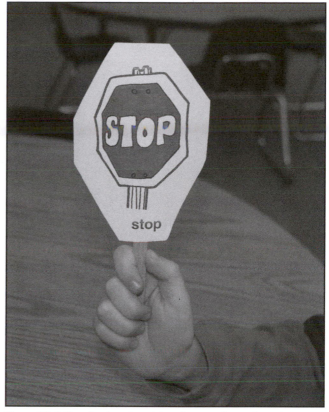

Figure 18-4. Use of a stop sign picture for stopping an interview.

is to train children's reference groups or advisory boards to assist. In child-led research, children should be involved from start to finish of the study.

Examples of Studies of Children's Involvement in Data Analysis

In one study (Alderson & Morrow, 2011), the researcher asked child participants to review her preliminary findings for the accuracy and representation of their views. She created a leaflet for them that summarized the main themes. As the group discussed the themes, one child challenged her findings by pointing out that she left out the theme of tensions between school staff and children. Their feedback was incorporated into the final analysis.

A second example is a study (Ost, 2013) about maintaining safety when talking to strangers online. After collecting the data, the researchers wanted children to draw their own conclusions. The children participated in the interpretation of the data. They identified issues and developed "Fakebook" cards containing the question, "You think you know who you're talking to?" (p. 216). They decided to attach these cards to notice boards around the school.

Dissemination

Dissemination of the research findings can be done in traditional and creative ways. In addition to presenting the information in academic journals, it is important to let children know the key results. The feedback can be in the form of a leaflet, poster, email, or oral presentation (O'Reilly & Parker, 2014). When Kelly (2007) finished collecting her data, she sent a booklet to the children's homes. It contained the key themes of the research findings and children's drawings and quotes. She asked the children to tell their parents, draw, or write their comments on the included colored paper. One child drew her hand with her thumb up to indicate approval. Providing feedback lets children know their voices were heard and made a difference. It can be especially beneficial to include child participants and/or reference groups in deciding how to disseminate the information. They have a unique perspective on how to convey the findings to other children.

Examples of Studies of Children's Involvement in Dissemination

Vaughn et al. (2013) conducted community-based research on preventing youth violence in their area. They considered the community to be partners and collaborated with community leaders, youth, and children. Two focus groups were held. In the first, the children ranged in age from 10 to 13 years, and in the second, they ranged in age from 10 to 17 years. In a discussion about how to disseminate the research findings to the community, the children and youth dismissed the idea of putting the information in newspapers. They argued that others their age often do not read them. Instead, they recommended conveying the information through comics, which led to the idea of animated comics. The messages about preventing violence were then made into digital animation, which was placed on a community Facebook page and included in a yearly community symposium. They also printed posters and placed them on buses. In these ways, the value of children's voices were publicly validated.

Moola, Johnson, Lay, Krygsman, & Faulkner (2015) studied how Canadian children experienced their walking routes. At the end of the research, they held a children's conference, and 40 of the 46 children participants (who were fourth through eighth graders) attended. The children chose which of their images (e.g., photographs, drawings) they wanted displayed. During the conference, they worked with city policy makers and planners on solutions for improving their environment.

SEEK OCCUPATIONAL JUSTICE AND RIGHTS FOR CHILDREN

For children to truly have a voice, their participation and contributions in research need to expand our knowledge base and influence change (Lundy, 2007). They must see that their time and effort was worthwhile. One group cannot represent all children. Therefore, eliciting the voices of many is essential. Also paramount is that occupational

therapy researchers use the findings to increase our understanding of their competencies, improve their lives, and make therapy meaningful. On a broader scale, researchers can work with children to enhance policies, create social change, and ensure occupational justice and rights for all.

KEY POINTS TO REMEMBER

- To be truly client centered, occupational therapy researchers need to include children in research.
- Children's involvement in research has the potential to add to occupational therapy's theories and knowledge base, improve services, and be learning experiences for them.
- Children's knowledge is just as valuable as adults' knowledge.
- When doing research, it is important to consider the sociocultural, historical, political, and theoretical influences.
- Children's roles can include being on advisory boards, being participants, or being co-researchers.
- When given information in a way they can understand, children can communicate whether they agree to participate in research.
- Obtaining children's consent is an ongoing process.
- Verbal participatory research methods include interviews, focus groups, questionnaires, vignettes, and tours.
- Visual participatory research methods include drawing; photography; video diaries; making maps, timelines, spider diagrams, or home movies; and using the mosaic approach.
- Activity-based participatory research methods include the use of puppets, games, sorting or rating activities, collages, and construction tasks.
- Online research is a newer method that is growing in popularity.
- Occupational therapists have the expertise to adapt research methods to allow children with disabilities to participate in the research.
- Children can play a role in data analysis and dissemination.

REVIEW QUESTIONS

1. Name five reasons why it is beneficial to include children in research.

2. What approach did Corsaro (2015) use to give preschoolers the message that he was an unusual adult?

3. Children's ability to participate in research is affected by the researchers' ability to communicate with them. True or false.

4. Researchers can use children's advisory boards to assist with all stages of research. True or false.

5. A child's age is the best determinant for judging his or her competence to participate in research. True or false.

6. Children need to be able to sign their name to give their consent. True or false.

7. Children like focus groups more than interviews. True or false.

8. Researchers need children's interpretations of the data when using visual or activity-based research methods. True or false.

9. It is too difficult for children with disabilities to participate in research. True or false.

10. In child-led research, children are actively involved in all stages of the research process. True or false.

REFERENCES

Alderson, P., & Morrow, V. (2011). *The ethics of research with children and young people: A practical handbook.* Thousand Oaks, CA: Sage.

Aldiss, S., Horstman, M., O'Leary, C., Richardson, A., & Gibson, F. (2009). What is important to young children who have cancer while in hospital? *Children & Society, 23,* 85-98. doi:10.1111/j.1099-0860.2008.00162.x

Ashburner, J., Bennett, L., Rodger, S., & Ziviani, J. (2013). Understanding the sensory experiences of young people with autism spectrum disorder: A preliminary investigation. *Australian Occupational Therapy Journal, 60,* 171-180. doi:10.1111/1440-1630.12025

Barker, J., & Smith, F. (2012). What's in focus? A critical discussion of photography, children and young people. *International Journal of Social Research Methodology, 15*(2), 91-103. doi:10.1080/13645579.2012.649406

Berinstein, S., & Magalhaes, L. (2009). A study of the essence of play experience to children living in Zanzibar, Tanzania. *Occupational Therapy International, 16*(2), 89-106. doi:10.1002/oti.270

Bluebond-Langner, M. (1978). *The private worlds of dying children.* Princeton, NJ: Princeton University.

Burman, E. (2008). *Developments: Child, image, nation.* New York, NY: Routledge.

Carter, B. (2014). How arts-based approaches can put the fun into child-focused research. *Nursing Children and Young People, 26*(3), 9. doi:10.7748/ncyp2014.04.26.3.9.s9

Chaplin, J. E., Koopman, H. M., Schmidt, S., & the DISABKIDS Group. (2008). DISABKIDS Smiley Questionnaire: The TAKE 6 assisted health-related quality of life measure for 4 to 7-year-olds. *Clinical Psychology and Psychotherapy, 15,* 173-180. doi:10.1002/cpp.570

Charles, A., & Haines, K. (2014). Measuring young people's participation in decision making. *International Journal of Children's Rights, 22,* 641-659. doi:10.1163/15718182-55680022

Christensen, P., & James, A. (2008). Childhood diversity and commonality: Some methodological insights. In P. Christensen & A. James (Eds.), *Research with children: Perspectives and practices* (pp. 156-172). New York, NY: Routledge.

Christensen, P. H. (2004). Children's participation in ethnographic research: Issues of power and representation. *Children & Society, 18*(2), 165-176. doi:10.1002/CHI.823

Clark, A. (2010a). Young children as protagonists and the role of participatory, visual methods in engaging multiple perspectives. *American Journal of Community Psychology, 46,* 115-123. doi:10.1007/s10464-010-9332-y

Clark, A. (2010b). *Transforming children's spaces: Children's and adults' participation in designing learning environments.* London, UK: Routledge.

Clark, A., & Moss, P. (2001). *Listening to young children: The Mosaic Approach.* London, UK: National Children's Bureau.

Clark, C. D. (2011). *In a younger voice: Doing child-centered qualitative research.* Oxford, UK: Oxford University Press.

Clarke, G., Boorman, G., & Nind, M. (2011). "If they don't listen I shout and when I shout they listen": Hearing the voices of girls with behavioural, emotional and social difficulties. *British Educational Research Journal, 37*(5), 765-780. doi:10.1080/01411926.2010.492850

Coad, J., & Evans, R. (2008). Reflections on practical approaches to involving children and young people in the data analysis process. *Children & Society, 22,* 41-52. doi:10.1111/j.1099-0860.2006.x

Cocks, A. J. (2006). The ethical maze: Finding an inclusive path towards gaining children's agreement to research participation. *Childhood, 13*(2), 247-266. doi:10.1177/0907568206062942

Cook, T., & Hess, E. (2007). What the camera sees and from whose perspective: Fun methodologies for engaging children in enlightening adults. *Childhood, 14*(1), 29-45. doi:10.1177/0907568207068562

Corsaro, W. A. (2015). *The sociology of childhood.* Thousand Oaks, CA: Sage.

Cox, S. (2005). Intention and meaning in young children's drawing. *International Journal of Art and Design Education, 42*(2), 115-125. doi:10.1111/j.1476-8070.2005.00432.x

Curtin, C. (1995). *Collaborative treatment planning with children* (Unpublished doctoral dissertation). University of Illinois at Chicago, Illinois.

Curtin, C. (2001). Eliciting children's voices in qualitative research. *American Journal of Occupational Therapy, 55*(3), 295-302.

Davis, J. (2009). Involving children. In E. K. M. Tisdall, J. M. Davis, & M. Gallagher (Eds.), *Research with children & young people: Research, design, methods and analysis* (pp. 154-167). Thousand Oaks, CA: Sage.

Dennis, S. F., Gaulocher, S., Carpiano, R. M., & Brown, D. (2009). Participatory photo mapping (PPM): Exploring an integrated method for health and place research with young people. *Health & Place, 15,* 466-473. doi:10.1016/j.healthplace.2008.08.004

Dockett, S., Einarsdóttir, J., & Perry, B. (2012). Young children's decisions about research participation: Opting out. *International Journal of Early Years Education, 20*(3), 244-256. doi:10.1080/09669760.2012.715405

Doutre, G., Green, R., & Knight-Elliott, A. (2013). Listening to the voices of young carers using interpretative phenomenological analysis and a strengths-based perspective. *Educational & Child Psychology, 30*(4), 30-43.

Driessnack, M., & Furukawa, R. (2012). Arts-based data collection techniques used in child research. *Journal for Specialists in Pediatric Nursing, 17*(1), 3-9. doi:10.1111/j.1744-6155.2011.00304.x

Einarsdóttir, J. (2007). Research with children: Methodological and ethical challenges. *European Early Childhood Education Research Journal, 15*(2), 197-211. doi:10.1080/13502930701321477

Einarsdóttir, J., Dockett, S., & Perry, B. (2009). Making meaning: Children's perspectives expressed through drawings. *Early Child Development and Care, 179*(2), 217-232.

Eldén, S. (2012). Inviting the messy: Drawing methods and children's voices. *Childhood, 20*(1), 66-81. doi:10.1177/0907568212447243

Epstein, I., Stevens, B., McKeever, P., Baruchel, S., & Jones, H. (2008). Using puppetry to elicit children's talk for research. *Nursing Inquiry, 15*(1), 49-56. doi:10.1111/j.1440-1800.2008.00395.x

Fetters, M. D., Curry, L. A., & Creswell, J. W. (2013). Achieving integration in mixed methods designs: Principles and practices. *Health Services Research, 48*(6 Pt 2), 2134-2156. doi:10.1111/1475-6773.12117

Fine, G. A., & Sandstrom, K. L. (1988). *Knowing children: Participant observation with minors* (Vol. 15). Newbury Park, CA: Sage.

Fleet, A., & Britt, C. (2011). Seeing spaces, inhabiting places: Hearing school beginners. In D. Harcourt, B. Perry, & T. Waller (Eds.), *Researching young children's perspectives: Debating dilemmas of educational research with children* (pp. 143-162). New York, NY: Routledge.

Freeman, M., & Mathison, S. (2009). *Researching children's experiences.* New York, NY: The Guilford Press.

Gallagher, M. (2009). Data collection and analysis. In E. K. M. Tisdall, J. M. Davis, & M. Gallagher (Eds.), *Researching with children and young people: Research design, methods and analysis* (pp. 65-88). Thousand Oaks, CA: Sage.

Gallagher, M., Haywood, S. L., Jones, M. W., & Milne, S. (2010). Negotiating informed consent with children in school-based research: A critical review. *Children & Society, 24,* 471-482. doi:10.1111/j.1099-0860.2009.00240.x

Gibbs, L., McDougall, C., & Harden, J. (2013). Development of an ethical methodology for post-bushfire research with children. *Health Sociology Review, 22*(2), 114-123. doi:10.5172/hesr.2013.22.2.114

Gibson, F., Aldiss, S., Hortstman, M., Krumpunen, S., & Richardson, A. (2010). Children and young people's experiences of cancer care: A qualitative research study using participatory methods. *International Journal of Nursing Studies, 47,* 1397-1407. doi:10.1016/jnurstu.2010.03.019

Goelman, H., Pivik, J., & Guhn, M. (2011). *New approaches to early child development: Rules, rituals and realities.* New York, NY: Palgrave Macmillan.

Griffiths, R., Stenner, R., & Hicks, U. (2014). Hearing the unheard: Constructions of their nurture group experiences. *Educational and Child Psychology, 31*(1), 124-136.

Groundwater-Smith, S., Dockett, S., & Bottrell, D. (2015). *Participatory research with children and young people.* Thousand Oaks, CA: Sage.

Hagner, D., Kurtz, A., May, J., & Clouter, H. (2014). Person-centered planning for transition-aged youth with autism spectrum disorders. *Journal of Rehabilitation, 80*(1), 4-10.

Harrington, C., Foster, M., Rodger, S., & Ashburner, J. (2013). Engaging young people with autism spectrum disorder in research interviews. *British Journal of Learning Disabilities, 42,* 153-161. doi:10.1111/bid.12037

Herssens, J., & Heylighen, A. (2012). Blind photographers: A quest into the spatial experiences of blind children. *Children, Youth and Environments, 22*(1), 99-124. doi:10.7721/chilyoutenvi.22.1.0099

Hill, L. (2014). "Some of it I haven't told anybody else": Using photo elicitation to explore the experiences of secondary school education from the perspective of young people with a diagnosis of autistic spectrum disorder. *Educational & Child Psychology, 31*(1), 79-89.

Hill, M. (2006). Children's voices on ways of having a voice: Children's and young people's perspectives on methods used in research and consultation. *Childhood, 13*(1), 69-89. doi:10.1177/0907568206059972

Hwang, S. K. (2013). Home movies in participatory research: Children as movie-makers. *International Journal of Social Research Methodology, 16*(5), 445-456. doi:10.1080/13645579.2012.729796

Kara, H. (2015). *Creative research methods in the social sciences: A practical guide.* Bristol, UK: Policy Press.

Kellett, M. (2010). Small shoes, big steps! Empowering children as active researchers. *American Journal of Community Psychology, 46,* 195-203. doi:10.1007/s10464-010-9324-y

Kellett, M. (2011). Empowering children and young people as researchers: Overcoming barriers and building capacity. *Child Indicators Research, 4,* 205-219. doi:10.1007/s12187-010-9103-1.

Kelly, B. (2007). Methodological issues for qualitative research with learning disabled children. *International Journal of Social Research Methodology, 10*(1), 21-35. doi:10.1080/13645570600655159

Kirova, A. (2006). A game-playing approach to interviewing children about loneliness: Negotiating meaning, distributing power, and establishing trust. *The Alberta Journal of Educational Research, 52*(3), 127-147.

Knighting, K., Rowa-Dewar, N., Malcolm, C., Kearney, N., & Gibson, F. (2010). Children's understanding of cancer and views on health-related behavior: a "draw and write" study. *Child: Care, Health and Development, 37*(2), 289-299. doi:10.1111/j.1365-2214.2010.01138x

Kramer, J., Barth, Y., Curtis, K., Livingston, K., O'Neil, M., Smith, Z.,...Wolfe, A. (2013). Involving youth with disabilities in the development and evaluation of a new advocacy training: Project TEAM. *Disability & Rehabilitation, 35*(7), 614-622. doi:10.3109/09638288.2012.705218

Kumpunen, S., Shipway, L., Taylor, R. M., Aldiss, S., & Gibson, F. (2012). Practical approaches to seeking assent from children. *Nurse Researcher, 19*(2), 23-27. doi:10.7748/nr2012.01.19.2.23.c8905

Lahman, M. K. E. (2008). Always othered: Ethical research with children. *Journal of Early Childhood Research, 6*(3), 281-300. doi:10.1177/1476718x08094451

Lambert, V., Coad, J., Hicks, P., & Glacken, M. (2013). Social spaces for young children in hospital. Child: care, health and development, 40(2), 195-204. doi:10.1111/cch12016

Lambert, V., & Glacken, M. (2011). Engaging with children in research: Theoretical and practical implications of negotiating informed consent/assent. *Nursing Ethics, 18*(6), 781-801. doi:10. 1177/096973301

Lindsay, S., & McPherson, A. C. (2011). Strategies for improving disability awareness and social inclusion of children and young people with cerebral palsy. *Child: Care, Health and Development, 38*(6), 809-816. doi:10.1111/j.1365-2214.2011.01308.x

Lindsay, S., & McPherson, A. C. (2012). Experiences of social exclusion and bullying at school among children and youth with cerebral palsy. *Disability & Rehabilitation, 34*(2), 101-109. doi:10.3109/09638288.2011.587086

Lingam, R. P., Novak, C., Emond, A., & Coads, J. E. (2013). The importance of identity and empowerment to teenagers with developmental co-ordination disorder. *Child: Care, Health and Development, 40*(3), 309-318. doi:10.1111/cch.12082

Literat, I. (2013). "A pencil for your thoughts": Participatory drawing as a visual research method with children and youth. *International Journal of Qualitative Methods, 12*, 84-97.

Lowe, R. J. (2012). Children deconstructing childhood. *Children & Society, 26*, 269-279. doi:10.1111/j.1099-0860.2010.00344.x

Loyd, D. (2012). Obtaining consent from young people with autism to participate in research. *British Journal of Learning Disabilities, 41*, 133-140. doi:10.1111/j.1468-3156.2012.00734.x

Lundy, L. (2007). "Voice" is not enough: Conceptualizing article 12 of the United Nations Convention on the Rights of the Child. *British Educational Research Journal, 33*(6), 927-942. doi:10.1080/01411920701657033

Malone, K. (2013). "The future lies in our hands": Children as researchers and environmental change agents in designing a child-friendly neighbourhood. *Local Environment, 18*(3), 372-395. doi:10.1080/13549839.2012.719020

Mandell, N. (1988). The least-adult role in studying children. *Journal of Contemporary Ethnography, 16*, 433-467.

Mayaba, N. N., & Wood, L. (2015). Using drawings and collages as data generation methods with children: Definitely not child's play. *International Journal of Qualitative Methods, 14*(5), 1-10. doi:10.1177/1609406915621407

Miller, E., & Kuhaneck, H. (2008). Children's perceptions of play experiences and play preferences: A qualitative study. *The American Journal of Occupational Therapy, 62*(4), 407-415.

Moola, F., Johnson, J., Lay, J., Krygsman, S., & Faulker, G. (2015). "The heartbeat of Hamilton": Researcher's reflection on Hamilton children's engagement with visual research methodologies to study the environment. *International Journal of Qualitative Methods, 14*(4), 1-14. doi:10.1177/1609406915611560

Moore, T., Saunders, V., & McArthur, M. (2011). Championing choice: Lessons learned from children and young people about research and their involvement. *Child Indicators Research, 4*, 249-267. doi:10.1007/s12187-010-9083-1

Morgan, M., Gibbs, S., Maxwell, K., & Britten, N. (2002). Hearing children's voices: Methodological issues in conducting focus group with children aged 7-11 years. *Qualitative Research, 2*(1), 5-20. doi:10.1177/1468794102002001636

Morris, J. (2003). Including all children: Finding out about the experiences of children with communication and/or cognitive impairments. *Children & Society, 17*, 337-348. doi:10.1002/CHI.754

Moyson, T., & Roeyers, H. (2012). "The overall quality of my life as a sibling is all right, but of course, it could always be better." Quality of life of siblings of children with intellectual disability: The siblings' perspectives. *Journal of Intellectual Disability Research, 56*(1), 87-101. doi:10.1111/j.1365-2788.2011.01393.x

Newman, S. D., & SCI photovoice participants. (2010). Evidence-based advocacy: Using Photovoice to identify barriers and facilitators to community participation after spinal cord injury. *Rehabilitation Nursing, 35*(2), 47-59. doi:10.1002/j.2048-7940.2010.tb00031.x

Nicholas, D. B., Lach, L., King, G., Scott, M., Boydell, K., Sawatzky, B. J.,…Young, N. L. (2010). Contrasting internet and face-to-face focus groups for children with chronic health conditions: Outcomes and participant experiences. *International Journal of Qualitative Methods, 9*(1), 105-121.

Oh, S. (2012). Photofriend: Creating visual ethnography with refugee children. *Area, 44*(3), 282-288. doi:10.1111/j.1475-4762.2012.01111.x

O'Kane, C. (2008). The development of participatory techniques: Facilitating children's views about decisions which affect them. In P. Christensen, & A. James (Eds.), *Research with children: Perspectives and practices* (pp. 125-155). New York, NY: Routledge.

O'Reilly, M., & Kiyimba, N. (2015). *Advanced qualitative research: A guide to using theory.* Thousand Oaks, CA: Sage.

O'Reilly, M., & Parker, N. (2014). *Doing mental health research with children and adolescents: A guide to qualitative methods.* Thousand Oaks, CA: Sage.

O'Reilly, M., Ronzoni, P., & Dogra, N. (2013). *Research with children: Theory & practice.* Thousand Oaks, CA: Sage.

Ost, S. (2013). Balancing autonomy rights and protection: Children's involvement in a child safety online project. *Children & Society, 27*, 208-219. doi:10.1111/j.1099-0860.2011.00400.x

Paige-Smith, A., & Rix, J. (2011). Researching early intervention and young children's perspectives: developing and using a "listening to children approach." *British Journal of Special Education, 38*(1), 28-36. doi:10.1111/j1467-8578.2011.00494x

Phelan, S. K., & Kinsella, E. A. (2013). Picture this… Safety, dignity and voice: Ethical research with children: Practical considerations for the reflexive researcher. *Qualitative Inquiry, 19*(2), 81-90. doi:10.1177/1077800412462987

Pimlott-Wilson, H. (2012). Visualising children's participation in research: Lego Duplo, rainbows and clouds and mood boards. *International Journal of Social Research Methodology, 15*(2), 135-148. doi:10.1080/13645579.2012.649410

Preece, D., & Jordan, R. (2009). Obtaining the views of children and young people with autism spectrum disorders about their experience of daily life and social care support. *British Journal of Learning Disabilities, 38*, 10-20. doi:10.1111/j.1468-3156.2009.00548.x

Punch, S. (2002). Interviewing strategies with young people: The "secret box," stimulus material and task-based activities. *Children & Society, 16*, 45-56. doi:10.1002/CHI.685

Punch, S. (2009). "I felt they were ganging up on me": Interviewing siblings at home. In L. van Blerk & M. Kesby (Eds.), *Doing children's geographies: Methodological issues in research with young people* (pp. 26-41). New York, NY: Routledge.

Rabiee, P., Sloper, P., & Beresford, B. (2005). Doing research with children and young people who do not use speech for communication. *Children & Society, 19*, 385-396. doi:10.1002/CHI.841

Ren, J. Y., & Langhout, R. D. (2010). A recess evaluation with the players: Taking steps toward participatory action research. *American Community Psychology, 46,* 124-138. doi:10.1007/s10464-010-9320-2

Richards, S., Clark, J., & Boggis, A. (2015). *Ethical research with children: Untold narratives and taboos.* New York, NY: Palgrave Macmillan.

Sargeant, J., & Harcourt, D. (2012). *Doing ethical research with children.* New York, NY: Open University.

Scott, J. (2008). Children as respondents: The challenge for quantitative methods. In P. Christensen & A. James (Eds.), *Research with children: Perspectives and practices* (pp. 87-108). New York, NY: Routledge.

Serdity, C., & Burgman, I. (2012). Being the older sibling: Self perceptions of children with disabilities. *Children & Society, 26,* 37-50. doi:10.1111/j.1099-0860.2010.00320.x

Sloper, P., & Beresford, B. (2014). Children who have disabilities. In G. B. Melton, A. Ben-Arieh, J. Cashmore, G. S. Goodman, & N. K. Worley (Eds.), *The Sage handbook of child research* (pp. 245-265). Thousand Oaks, CA: Sage

Sposito, A. M., Silva-Rodrigues, F. M., Sparapani, V. C., Pfeifer, L. I., Garcia deLima, R. A., & Nascimento, L. C. (2015). Coping strategies used by hospitalized children with cancer undergoing chemotherapy. *Journal of Nursing Scholarship, 47*(2), 143-151. doi:10.1111/jnu.12126

Spradley, J. P. (1980). *Participant observation.* Belmont, CA: Wadsworth Cengage Learning.

Tates, K., Zwaanswijk, M., Otten, R., van Dulmen, S., Hoogerbrugge, P. M., Kamps, W. A., & Bensing, J. M. (2009). Online focus groups as a tool to collect data in hard-to-include populations: Examples from paediatric oncology. *BMC Medical Research Methodology, 9*(1), 15. doi:10.1186/1471-2288-9-15

Tay-Lim, J., & Lim, S. (2013). Privileging younger children's voices in research: Use of drawings and a co-construction process. *International Journal of Qualitative Methods, 12,* 65-83.

Twycross, A., Gibson, F., & Coad, J. (2008). Guidance on seeking agreement to participate in research from young children. *Paediatric Nursing, 20*(6), 14-18. doi:10.7748/paed2008.07.20.6.14.c6625

United Nations. (1989). *Convention on the rights of the child.* Geneva, Switzerland: Author.

Vaughn, N. A., Jacoby, S. F., Williams, T., Guerra, T., Thomas, N. A., & Richmond, T. S. (2013). Digital animation as a method to disseminate research findings to the community using a community-based participatory approach. *American Journal of Community Psychology, 51,* 30-42. doi:10.1007/s10464-012-9498-6

Wang, C., & Burris, M. (1997). Photovoice: Concepts, methodology and use for participatory needs assessment. *Health Education and Behavior, 24*(3), 369-387. doi:10.1177/109019819702400309

Wickenden, M., & Kembhavi, G. (2014). Ask us too! Doing participatory research with disabled children in the global south. *Childhood, 21,* 400-417. doi:10.1177/0907568214525426

Winter, K. (2012). Ascertaining the perspectives of young children in care: Case studies in the use of reality boxes. *Children & Society, 26*(5), 368-380. doi:10.1111/j.1099-0860.2010.00335.x

Young, L., & Barrett, H. (2001). Adapting visual methods: Action research with Kampala street children. *Area, 33*(2), 141-152. doi:10.1111/1475-4762.00017

Zwaanswijk, M., Tates, K., van Dulmen, S., Hoogerbrugge, P. M., Kamps, W. A., Beishuizen, A., & Bensing, J. M. (2011). Communicating with child patients in pediatric oncology consultation: A vignette study on child patients', parents' and survivors' communication preferences. *Psycho-Oncology, 20,* 269-277. doi:10.1002/pon.1721

Take the Road Less Traveled

One Last Story and Parting Thoughts

"YOU WON'T FORGET ME."

"What are you good at?"

"I don't know," 7-year-old Homer replied. He slumped down in his chair and stared at the floor.

On his first day on the children's psychiatric unit, Homer tried painting and only mentioned his mistakes. That afternoon in the team meeting, I heard that Homer's parents were very critical of him. The next day, Homer joined our craft group and gravitated to the bin of scrap wood. He hammered all sizes and shapes of lumber into unique designs. At the end of the session, I said, "WOW! Homer, I've never seen anyone build like that. You're very creative."

Each day, Homer continued to experiment and make his own creations. The next week, he used a square piece of red velveteen material to blanket three books, and carefully positioned a spider plant on his new stand. "Miss Curtin, look," he said, pointing to the stand. "Isn't it bee-you-tee-full?"

"It is! You come up with the best ideas."

After a month together, I had to take a day off to go to a conference. When I told the group, Homer made a fist, pointed his index finger at me, raised his thumb as a trigger, and pretended to shoot. Because violent actions were not tolerated on the unit, Homer had to take a timeout. When the group session was over, I walked to Homer's room and sat next to him on his bed. "Why are you in a timeout?" I asked.

"Cuz I shot ya."

"I wonder if you're angry with me because I am going to be gone for a day." He nodded. "Homer, I'm just going away to a school for one day so I can learn. I'm not leaving because of anything you did. I'm coming back." Homer's body relaxed as I spoke.

A month later, I was quitting my job and was concerned about telling Homer the news. He was so upset over my absence for 1 day that I worried about how he would feel about my departure. I told the group I was leaving and was surprised when Homer looked at me and said, "Don't worry, Miss Curtin, you won't forget me because I'm creative."

He was right—I have never forgotten him!

PARTING THOUGHTS

The profession of occupational therapy was founded on a social justice framework. This mindset led to the core and current belief that collaboration is necessary and powerful for creating change. Over the years when we worked with other professions, such as medicine, we followed them down their main road. We would reach a juncture and make a decision: continue along or veer off to a less traveled road that was true to our values and beliefs. We would get off only to gradually drift back on another's main road.

We are at another juncture (Table 19-1). In this book, I advocate for therapists to be leaders on how to create partnerships in therapy and research, especially with children.

Curtin, C.
*Strategies for Collaborating With Children: Creating Partnerships
in Occupational Therapy and Research* (pp. 399-400).
© 2017 SLACK Incorporated.

TABLE 19-1
RECOMMENDED FUTURE DIRECTIONS

CURRENT EMPHASIS	PLUS ADDITIONAL EMPHASIS	RESULT: BALANCE
Therapists' expertise	Clients' expertise (including children)	Expertise shared by all in a client-centered approach
Collaborate with caregivers and teachers	Collaborate with children	Collaborate with all
Focus on the child	Focus on the context	An ecological approach
Collaborate with children who are verbal	Collaborate with children who are nonverbal	Collaborate with all children
Problem-based practice	Strengths-based practice	Identify and build on strengths; address concerns
Quantitative research for evidence-based practice	Qualitative research (for examining why, how, and personal meanings)	Value and use both quantitative and qualitative research for evidence-based practice
Research with caregivers and teachers	Research with children and communities	Research with children, caregivers, teachers, and communities

In summary, in the future:

- Collaborate with children, including those with disabilities, in addition to collaborating with caregivers and educational staff.

- Embrace client-centered and strengths-based theories and approaches.

- Recognize children's competencies, accentuate their strengths, and strengthen their voices in therapy and research.

- Take the road less traveled.

Appendix

Answers to the Review Questions

CHAPTER 1: HISTORICAL REVIEW OF COLLABORATION IN OCCUPATIONAL THERAPY

1. True. Early leaders in occupational therapy deemed it essential that clients be active participants in therapy for treatment to be effective.

2. False. Although there are key elements in collaboration, such as respect for each other's perspectives, how the process unfolds will vary with each group of people.

3. When occupational therapy aligned with medicine, therapists placed more emphasis on the biomedical aspects of therapy, such as focusing on clients' bodies and skills.

4. The four reasons Shannon (1977) gave for the derailment of the profession of occupational therapy were:
   a. Became too reductionistic with the alignment of medicine
   b. Did not adequately address the needs of the chronically ill
   c. Devalued arts and crafts
   d. Viewed the client as a "mechanistic creature" versus a "creative human being" (p. 233)

5. True. The medical model of disabilities considers a disability as an individual health problem and focuses on preventing or curing the disability.

6. The slogan for the disabilities rights movement in the United States was "Nothing about us without us" (Charlton, 1998).

7. Disability rights activists demanded the right to:
   a. Make decisions about their own lives (e.g., regarding their living situation, medical interventions, rehabilitation)
   b. Equal citizenship
   c. An education
   d. Access to public transportation and buildings
   e. Accommodations
   f. A voice in disability theory and research

8. True. Many disability theorists and activists argue that if society eliminated barriers, made accommodations, and accepted differences, they would not be disabled.

9. In the 1990s clinical reasoning study, Mattingly and Fleming found that the humanistic/phenomenological (i.e., a focus on the clients' experiences, values, and wishes) part of occupational therapy practice was often hidden and not articulated in team meetings, notes, and descriptions of the clients.

10. In the 1980s to 1990s, leaders in the field called for therapists to be occupation based and client centered, recognize client's strengths, embrace the humanistic aspects of therapy, address the environment, and change society's injustices.

Curtin, C.
Strategies for Collaborating With Children: Creating Partnerships in Occupational Therapy and Research (pp. 401-411).
© 2017 SLACK Incorporated.

Chapter 2: Theoretical Underpinnings of a Model of Collaboration

1. Four personal qualities children in the study of collaboration believed therapists should have were being nice, being fun, being understanding, and staying calm.

2. The three actions children in the collaboration study said they want therapists to do were talk with them, check to make sure they understand what is being said, and include them in decisions.

3. Children in the collaboration study identified the three crucial elements of activities within therapy. They said activities needed to be fun, based on what they like, and between hard and easy (i.e., a just-right challenge).

4. True. Clients must have a voice in defining the purpose of therapy and throughout the sessions. Using a client-centered approach ensures the meaningfulness and effectiveness of therapy.

5. False. Children are not too young to have a voice in therapy. All children have a view. Therapists need to make accommodations and incorporate their views, which may be expressed through different modes, such as words, actions, nonverbal language, and/or communication devices.

6. False. If therapists learn how clients with cognitive impairments communicate, especially for agreement and dissent, and make adaptations, they can engage and collaborate with the clients.

7. True. It is possible to use a strengths-based approach while working in a deficit-based system. Therapists can maintain a strengths-based perspective in their observations, assessments, documentation, and reporting in team and parent meetings. With a strengths-based approach, therapists build on clients' strengths and address their concerns.

8. False. Clients' concerns (problems) are addressed in a strengths-based approach. However, rather than focusing on fixing problems in the past, the focus is on building on competencies and addressing concerns needed to reach a desired future.

9. False. A strengths-based approach centers on what *promotes* rather than *hinders* development, such as the studies on resilient children. Research studies focus on competencies, adaptation, and wellness.

10. False. Occupational therapy's core values already include an emphasis on promoting clients' self-determination, strengths, and potential. A strengths-based approach is compatible with current occupational therapy practice.

Chapter 3: An Ecological Approach to Enhancing Children's Competencies and Participation

1. False. There is not one model of development that explains every child's development in every culture and country in every time.

2. False. Children have their own thoughts and feelings and are active in their development. They both learn from and influence adults.

3. False. A positivist paradigm is one but not the only paradigm that can be used to generate knowledge. Multiple paradigms and theories are needed to address the complexity of human nature and development.

4. True. The new sociology of childhood and childhood studies share the same core tenets.

5. True. The United Nations Convention on the Rights of the Child (UNCRC) was the first legal instrument to identify children as subjects with rights.

6. True. Children and adults with disabilities contributed to the development of the United Nations Convention on the Rights of Persons with Disabilities (UNCRPD).

7. False. Children's rights allow children to contribute their views. Parents make the final decisions. When children have a voice, parents can (a) make more informed decisions and (b) teach respect for and negotiation of different views. When children have rights, it also ensures that children who are being abused will be heard.

8. False. Occupational therapists need to maintain a broader ecological perspective. They need to focus on children, caregivers, educational systems, communities, and the occupational rights of all.

9. True. Just as important as listening to children is making sure their voices influence decisions and actions. Children need to know and see that their views are taken seriously and are not just tokenistic.

10. Although occupational therapy jobs are very demanding, therapists can choose to address broader issues, even if it is on a smaller scale, such as creating changes within a school. Sometimes small steps create momentum for larger changes.

CHAPTER 4: INTRODUCE YOURSELF AND EXPLAIN THERAPY

1. False. You need to introduce yourself even if children are nonverbal and seem unaware of your presence. Because you never know how much children understand, it is better to assume they comprehend what you say. Tell them who you are and, in a few simple words or with picture cues, say why you are with them.

2. You have been asked by Johnny's second-grade teacher to figure out ways to help him stop having meltdowns when he is in sensory overload. He is especially sensitive to loud and constant noise. You could say: "Hi, my name is… and I am an occupational therapist. I am like a teacher. I work with kids and teachers to help figure out ways to make school more comfortable and easier. I heard that when it's really noisy in the class that bothers you [look for nodding or signs he is listening]. If it is okay with you, we can work together with your teacher to figure out how to make your time at school better."

3. Three possible approaches to use when children are shy or leery of you are (a) to play with others in front of them, (b) to talk with their caregivers and with a smile briefly glance at them (you also might want to wave hello), and (c) to play with a toy in front of them.

4. False. Even if children are not looking at you, assume that they are listening. Always be aware that when children are within earshot, they are listening to everything you say.

5. Children tend to categorize adults as either being nice or mean.

6. Four types of conversations starters are (a) use easy-to-answer questions (e.g., about age, family, pets), (b) acknowledge their individuality (e.g., their choice of clothing), (c) ask about interests, and (d) inquire about life events.

7. False. When you first meet a second grader, she avoids eye contact with you. You do not have to require her to look at you before you continue talking. Be responsive to children's nonverbal language. She may not be looking at your eyes because she is shy, is unsure of you, or feels uncomfortable making eye contact with people. She may have been taught that it is disrespectful to look directly at adults' eyes. Continue talking and watch for other signs that she is listening.

8. Children can tell you their choices nonverbally in the following ways: looking with their eyes, touching with their hand, making a sound or different types of sounds, making head movements, moving toward or away, and/or using sign language.

9. When you asked a 6 year old to draw a picture, he turned his back to you. In response, you can say, "I see you have turned away from me. I think you're telling me you don't want to draw." (Often children will turn around and say, "That's right," and add either, "I'm not good at drawing," or "I don't like to draw.")

10. You see a 10 year old holding the pen in her fist and moving her arm as she writes each letter. You could say, "I see you holding the pen with your whole hand instead of just your three fingers. When you do that, you are using all your finger, hand, and arm muscles. You are using a lot of muscles, which can quickly make you tired when you write."

CHAPTER 5: ESTABLISH A COLLABORATIVE FRAME

1. False. Occupational therapists use the saying "Occupational therapy is a safe place" to let children know they will be physically and emotionally safe when they are with you.

2. You see that a child is getting a shot or having an intravenous line put in (or any other painful medical procedure), and tears are running down the child's cheeks. You could say, "I know shots (or name the procedure) are painful. I can see that was upsetting for you. I'm sorry you have to go through this."

3. True. When you prepare children for what you are going to do before moving them, you are showing respect and consideration. This allows children to mentally prepare for your actions. Be sure to especially think about this when helping children in and out of wheelchairs.

4. The following actions can be converted into strengths:

   Rather than saying children are:

   - Passive, you can say they like to check out people or situations before acting.
   - Distractible, you can say they like to actively explore the environment/what is around them.
   - Opinionated, you can say they are good at saying what they think and are able to express themselves.

5. When you asked children about their strengths, they may feel happy, proud, and/or respected. Some may feel humble or shy. If talking about strengths is counter to their cultural values or beliefs, they may feel uncomfortable.

6. False. If children are unable to answer your question about their strengths, you should reword the question and give an example. They may not have understood what you were asking in your first question. Only change topics if they are showing discomfort.

7. Signs that children think the activity is fun are the following: smiling, laughing, focusing on the activity, making positive comments about it, saying they like it, and continuing their actions.

8. A just-right challenge is when children try something new or hard without giving up and stay focused on the challenge. They remain engaged and perceive that the challenge is not too easy or too hard.

9. True. It is important for children to experience success the first time they are with you. By grading activities, you can enable children to succeed. They will quickly learn that you can help them achieve what they did not think they could do. Success also provides motivation to engage in therapy.

10. Some of the different ways to grade an activity are to change the number of steps, change materials or how the game is played, or vary the amount of assistance you give.

CHAPTER 6: LEARN ABOUT CHILDREN AND THEIR WORLDS THROUGH INTERVIEWS

1. True. Children will often wonder if the interview is a test. You need to tell children the purpose of the interview is to get to know them. Otherwise, they will often wonder if it is a test with one correct answer.

2. False. Some children feel more comfortable answering yes and no questions, such as, "Do you have any brothers or sisters?" When they become more at ease, you can switch to open-ended questions.

3. You can ask children to talk about a certain topic (e.g., their family or friends) by using the following prompts:
   - "Tell me about…"
   - "Tell me everything you can about…"
   - "It would help me to know…"
   - "I would like to know…"
   - "I am wondering how…"

4. False. Although most younger children enjoy drawing, there are some who do not. Have drawing be one of the options for answering your questions.

5. Some creative ways to ask questions in an interview are to use props, toys, games, visuals, or cartoon characters.

6. False. You can ask children who are nonverbal to respond to your questions by using their communication devices or systems, showing you, pointing, or looking at a picture of their answer.

7. False. Instead of assuming children are incompetent, quickly reflect on your role in the interview. Ask yourself the following:
   - How did you word the questions?
   - Were they vague or unclear?
   - Are you using kid language?
   - Did you ask more than one question at a time?
   - Did you try rewording the question?

8. True. When asking questions, you have to observe children's nonverbal responses as well as listen to their words. You have to watch to see if children's nonverbal language matches their verbal answers. For instance, if they grimace while they are saying school is fine, you would explore that topic thoroughly.

9. True. It is not enough to just nod your head to let children know you are listening, In addition to nodding your head, you have to let children know you are listening by making empathetic comments and reflecting back what you hear them saying.

10. It is paramount to put closure on the interview by summarizing the important points the children made because this gives a clear message that you truly listened. These points can then be used in determining the purpose of therapy.

CHAPTER 7: OBSERVE AND PROMOTE STRESS-FREE TESTING

1. "This preschooler is poking at children because he wants their attention and wants to play with them." This sentence is an interpretation because you are providing your own explanation for why the child is poking at others.

2. True. Checking with others allows you to verify whether your observations are consistent. This also helps you learn whether the children's actions were unusual and may be attributed to having a bad day or not feeling well.

3. Four ways small toys or puppets can be used during testing are the following:
   - To give directions
   - To let children play between test items, especially if a change in set up is required
   - To play after completing each test item or after completing a test
   - To make adaptations

4. Children dislike waiting while taking a test because:
   - They may become anxious thinking about how hard the test might be.

- They may get bored or distracted by what is in the room.
- Waiting gives them time to think about something else they want to do or that they prefer to stop the testing instead of to keep trying.

5. It is stressful for children to take tests because:
   - Testing can show what they cannot do, and they probably already know that.
   - They may worry about not doing well.
   - Some want to please teachers and their caregivers.
   - Some worry they will get "yelled at" if they do not do well.
   - They may think others will notice and tease them if they do not do well.
   - Testing may bring back unpleasant memories of past failures.
   - Some children get overwhelmed if they think the testing is going to take too long or be too hard.

6. True. Before testing, examine what distractions are in the room. As much as possible, clear clutter, move, or cover distractions, such as therapy toys. Then guide children to sit in the chair with the fewest distractions in their view. Place the test materials in front of the best chair as a cue for where you want them to to sit.

7. False. It does not help to emphasize accuracy over effort. Focusing on what children did right and how many they did wrong can create anxiety, especially if they're not doing well. Often they will want to give up if they think they are failing. Emphasize that they just try their best. You may want to mention that you see how hard they are trying. Upon hearing those words, children may attempt more test items even if they are not doing well and be less likely to give up.

8. You asked 4-year-old Sam to cut on the thick black line of a circle. He responded by cutting the circle in half. Because he did not follow the verbal cutting instructions, you can help him move his hand with the scissors open toward the circle and make one cut on the line. This time if he continues cutting and stays on the line, he did not understand the verbal directions. If he is concentrating on the task but veers off, it is most likely related to his motor skills.

9. Children need to focus during testing. If they are bouncing in their chairs and it is interfering with their ability to focus and complete test items, take a movement break or change the type of seating.

10. When children refuse to start testing, ask yourself:
    - Did they know you were coming?
    - Are they missing something desirable or fun?
    - Do they feel ill? Have they had a rough morning?
    - Did something happen before they came?
    - Do they understand the purpose for the test?
    - Do they dislike taking tests?
    - Do tests make them anxious?
    - Have they failed tests in the past?
    - Do they like to be in control, especially in uncomfortable situations?
    - Are they worried the test will be too hard or too long?

CHAPTER 8: COLLABORATE TO DETERMINE THE PURPOSE OF THERAPY

1. False. It is not best to think of treatment planning as a problem-solving process. The primary emphasis in this approach is to fix children's problems so they can function better. Strengths-based treatment planning has a different emphasis. This process focuses on building on children's competencies, identifying successful strategies, and addressing desired changes. The focus is more on brainstorming ideas for the future and allows more opportunities to discover solutions that might not be related to the "problems."

2. True. Children who are nonverbal or young can show you what is important to them. You can observe children's actions and nonverbal language to identify what is meaningful to them. This information can be incorporated into determining the purpose of therapy.

3. False. Children are usually aware of what is going right or wrong in their lives. They tend to be very perceptive. They usually know what is hard for them and what they wish was easier. Often their actions demonstrate this knowledge.

4. True. In addition to obtaining caregivers' and teachers' perspectives, you also need to elicit children's perspectives to ensure that therapy is meaningful.

5. False. Asking children, "What do you want for goals?" is not the best way to include them. Although some children understand the notion of goals, it is more child friendly to ask, "What do you want to get better at, learn, or change about yourself?" Another approach is giving a context (e.g., school, home) and asking what is hard for them and what they wish was easier. Even young children will understand and respond to being asked what they want help with.

6. True. The use of creative participation methods engages children and makes it easier for them to communicate their concerns. The use of drawing, visuals, games, or props, such as a toy magic wand, makes the process

more engaging and fun. These techniques reflect your attempt to enter their world instead of insisting they enter the adult world.

7. True. It is easier for children to build on the successful strategies in their repertoire than to learn something new. It is easier because they already know they can do it and this approach emphasizes their current competencies.

8. True. Children's, caregivers', teachers', and your perspectives are equally important. To ensure therapy is meaningful and effective, ALL perspectives must be equally valued.

9. False. Identifying and prioritizing the goals for therapy is not a straightforward process. Often negotiation and prioritization is required to address everyone's needs.

10. When you summarize the plan for treatment, you need to emphasize children's strengths and restate children's, caregivers', and teachers' desired changes; the required environmental modifications; the agreed-upon goals; and the methods for creating the change.

CHAPTER 9: TEACH CHILDREN SELF-ADVOCACY

1. True. For children to advocate for themselves, they have to learn what helps and hinders them. Self-knowledge is critical for being able to advocate for what they need.

2. True. Involving children in deciding on and implementing strategies creates a sense of ownership. When children have input, they will let you know what is feasible and realistic. They will say if the strategy is not something they would do or use. Thus, when they do agree, there is a sense of ownership.

3. False. Children tend to be aware of how they are doing in school. Children see every day if it is easier or harder for them to do what their classmates do. If they are slower, sometimes peers will point that out as well.

4. True. When children figure out their own strategies and solutions, they are more apt to use them. Children are more likely to incorporate the strategies and solutions that they identify.

5. False. Children who are nonverbal can tell you no. They may not use words, but they can tell you through a communication device/system, or nonverbal language (e.g., looking away, dropping their heads, crying, gestures).

6. False. Children do not always want adult help. Children often want to do things independently without any help from adults. Teach children ways to ask for help,

especially if they are nonverbal, so you are only providing assistance when they request it.

7. False. It does not help to always reach for a young child's hand while walking with him or her to where he or she needs to go. Instead of automatically taking a young child's hand, put your palm up and wait for the child to put his or her hand in yours. This allows the child to decide if he or she wants or needs your assistance.

8. True. Being assertive is highly valued in Western culture, and children are expected to learn to speak up for themselves.

9. True. It is helpful to give children the words to use if they continually have problems with peers. They may not know how to be assertive versus aggressive. Hence, it helps to give them the words in the moment, such as saying, "Tell your friend you do not like being pushed."

10. False. It is not easy for children to be assertive. Although many children have the confidence to speak up, for some it takes courage to do so.

CHAPTER 10: BECOME PARTNERS WITH YOU AS A GUIDE

1. False. It is okay to tell children if you have made a mistake. Being honest shows children that everyone makes mistakes. Doing so is especially helpful for children who think they are a failure if they are not perfect.

2. False. You should not berate yourself for what you did wrong in a difficult situation. Instead of berating yourself after a difficult situation, ask yourself, "What did I learn from the situation?" Then identify what you plan to do differently in the future.

3. When a child is screaming at you and calling you names, tell yourself to stay calm. You may say to yourself, "This child is angry and is lashing out. It is his/her issue, not mine. We can talk about this incident later." Afterward, reflect on whether you contributed to the situation.

4. You must follow through on any promises you make because this shows children you are trustworthy. Therefore, only make promises you can keep, and do whatever you said you would.

5. True. You read in the 9 year old's Individualized Education Program that he has hit others, refused to do schoolwork, and tried to run out of the building. You should tell yourself to start looking for his strengths and interests when you first meet him. All children have strengths and interests. Identifying these, especially with his teachers' and caregivers' input, will color your perception of the child in a positive way.

6. Different ways you can show you are a fun person are to be playful, make funny faces, wear fun clothes, use silly tones of voice, play with words, tell jokes or funny stories, joke around, or imitate their actions.

7. If a child criticizes your clothes, you can smile and thank the child for telling you what he or she thinks.

8. True. Children look for signs that you like them. They are perceptive and will observe your nonverbal language, words, and actions to determine if you like them.

9. False. When children are playing, they are very aware of what is going on around them. Although the children may be playing, they will still be listening and notice what else is happening, especially if there is something unusual.

10. If the 7 year old continually refuses to do anything you ask, you can tell yourself, "She has a strong spirit and knows what she wants. That strong spirit will be helpful later in her life. The approach I am using does not seem to be working. Maybe a different approach would be better."

CHAPTER 11: SET RESPECTFUL LIMITS

1. Three-year-old Logan finds a stick buried under the rocks on the playground. He picks it up and starts swinging it, just missing a classmate. You can say, "Stop! You almost hit your friend. Keep your friends safe." As you calmly reach for the stick, say, "Let me help you find a toy that's safe for you to play with."

2. True. You need to tell children the rules before you expect them to comply.

3. False. Tell children what to do when stating rules. It is easier for children to understand if you tell them what they are expected to do versus what not to do.

4. You should use a firm but not harsh tone of voice to tell children to stop an action. A harsh tone can be demeaning, whereas a firm tone indicates that you care about them and mean what you say.

5. True. You get the group's attention and begin giving directions for the activity. Five-year-old Carly turns her back to you, takes a magic marker, and draws on the table. You should have her wipe off the marks with a wet paper towel. Then you should check if she understands the words you used in your directions. If children are not paying attention when you give directions, check to make sure they understand what you are saying. Also, watch to see if they need (1) more time to process the directions, (2) one-step directions, or (3) visual cues, such as picture symbols.

6. True. It is best to prevent children's unwanted actions than deal with them later. When you prevent issues by changing the situation or a removing a problematic object, you can eliminate struggles with children.

7. False. Children respond to nonverbal gestures indicating stop. Unless they are new to Western culture, they understand shaking your head or using hand gestures to indicate stop.

8. False. Often talking louder adds to the commotion. When you whisper, children tend to stop talking so they can hear what you are saying.

9. To avoid having children say, "No," you can say, "It's time to…" or "Try…" instead of "Do you want to…?" The question, "Do you want to…?" implies that the children have a choice and can say no.

10. If children are refusing to participate, you can help them save face by saying, "Oh, you just want to watch." This allows them more time to consider whether to join. It also gives them time to observe others so they know what to do. Later, try to discover the children's reasons for their hesitancy.

CHAPTER 12: TEACH CHILDREN TO REGULATE THEIR EMOTIONS, THOUGHTS, AND BODIES

1. It is important for occupational therapists to have a repertoire of skills for dealing with children's feelings. First, therapy requires children to face challenges. It is common for them to feel frustration or even anger when they experience failure. Second, children are often seen in groups, which can lead to conflict and upset feelings. Third, when children are involved in an activity, they often will bring up their concerns or upsetting situations. Fourth, if children are starting to lose control, therapists need to know how to neutralize the situation and assist the children in returning to a calm state.

2. True. Children's self-control tends to improve when they can say their feelings instead of acting them out. Saying, "I am mad," allows the children to get their message across without hitting.

3. It is vital to discover what went on before children's meltdowns. Children might be experiencing sensory overload and/or reacting to an earlier interaction or upsetting situation. Knowing what happened gives you information about how to prevent a reoccurrence.

4. True. Some children have to be taught how to recognize what others might be feeling. They need to learn

to look for concrete signs of emotions (e.g., changes on a face) to recognize others' feelings.

5. False. Punishment is not the best way to stop unwanted behavior or actions. Teaching children new strategies is a better way to stop unwanted behavior or actions. The use of punishment assumes that the child knows a different way to act, which is not always true. Assume their current actions may be the only way they know how to act.

6. True. Social Stories (Gray, 2010) provide children with the details on how to act in a certain situation.

7. You can cue children visually on what to do by:

- Showing them a photo of the desired action
- Showing them a picture symbol of the desired action
- Showing them a series of pictures indicating the steps to do
- Using a representative object, such as using a trash can to indicate throwing away
- Reading a Social Story with pictures of the child doing each action

8. False. Everyone reacts to sensory stimulation, but most figure out how to adapt. For example, some will start moving if they are feeling lethargic. Teaching children's sensory strategies increases their repertoire of ways to regulate their bodies.

9. False. When children are losing control, you increase the likelihood of getting hit if you stand in front of them. Stay to the side and avoid getting in their personal space. Stay calm and firmly state what the children need to do.

10. True. After a crisis, it is good practice to reflect on your actions. Ask yourself whether your actions made the situation better or worse. The important thing is to learn from the situation so that you can grow as a therapist.

Chapter 13: Avoid Power Struggles

1. True. When you find yourself continually reprimanding a child, you need to find ways to interact more positively with that child. Make a conscious effort to continually identify what children are doing well. If they are being unsafe, you have to set limits, but also teach them what else to do. Some may need picture cues regarding how to stay safe.

2. Recess is the last activity of the day. The class goes in but a 4-year-old girl hides under a slide. When you move around the slide, she moves further away and laughs. Parents are watching. If you chase her, it becomes a game. Instead, stand still and do not move.

Calmly name an enticing element or activity that is inside. You could say, "Everyone is inside. Let's go join your friends," or, "Your backpack is inside. You need to get your backpack and then your mom will be here." Another option would be to say, "It's hot out here. Let's get a cool drink of water before you go home. Come on." If she does not move, repeat the same sentence two or three times every couple of minutes and wait patiently.

3. False. You must not expect children to immediately respond to all your directives. As long as they are being safe, you can choose to give the children more time to respond. Check to make sure the children understand what you are saying. Think of various reasons why the children might not be responding. Be empathetic if the children have to stop a favorite activity. You may want to use different words or try a different approach.

4. A 5 year old snatches the playground ball from a boy and runs away. Three boys chase him, grab the ball back, and kick it to each other. He goes to the door and sits down with his back to the playground. You saw what happened and can see that he is upset. You can say, "What were you trying to tell those boys when you took the ball?" When he replies, "I just wanted a turn," point to the boys and say, "Let's go over and talk with them. Use your words to tell them you want a turn too."

5. You see a preschooler walk to the center full of blocks to play with a new toy as the rest of his class sits at their tables. You could say, "I wonder if you are worried you will not get a turn to play with this during center time." When he nods, tell him you will make sure he gets a chance, and state when that will happen.

6. You are in the kindergarten classroom sitting at the table with Ashley. The teacher tells the class they need to color, cut, and glue four pictures on a science sheet showing a seed growing into a plant. Ashley looks at the paper and says, "I don't want to do this." Three approaches you could use are:

- Be empathetic by saying, "I wonder if you're worried that it looks like too much work."
- Offer help by saying, "Let me help you get started." You could then outline the shape of a seed and have her color inside.
- Break the task down to one picture and one step. Use a blank piece of paper to cover the last three pictures so she only sees one picture. State the one step, "First just color the seed." Then offer her two different-colored crayons for her to choose.

7. False. Children respond more positively when you use a playful rather than serious approach to avoid power struggles.

8. False. Give children more attention when they are demonstrating positive actions. Limit your attention to unwanted actions.

9. True. Diverting young children's attention is often effective in stopping unwanted actions. This helps them shift their thinking away from the unwanted actions.

10. Three possible questions that can help guide older children to think about better choices for their actions are:

- Are you making things better by…?
- Are you helping by doing that?
- What did you learn from doing…?

Chapter 14: Co-Create Educational Experiences That Are Challenging and Fun

1. Five ways to structure small groups are the following:

- Have children work parallel to each other doing the same or similar activity.
- Have half of the group help the others and then switch midway.
- Go around the circle and have each member take a turn while the others wait.
- Have half of the group do one activity and the other half do another. Switch midway so the group members end up doing two activities.
- Have the group work cooperatively on one activity.

2. True. It is common for young children to expect to finish a project in one session and leave with it. If the project takes longer, prepare the children before starting it.

3. True. Children will persist at an activity if the challenge factor is just right for their abilities. They will persist because they perceive success to be attainable.

4. Most children like challenges unless they have had multiple experiences of failure. Challenges can provide a sense of accomplishment or achievement.

5. True. Although there are some common themes, such as the enjoyment of toys, there are individual differences regarding the notion of fun.

6. False. If you want to make sure children hear the directions, get their attention before stating what to do.

7. True. If children are ignoring you when you give directions, it may be because they do not understand the words you are using. You will often lose children's attention if they do not comprehend what you are saying.

8. Five ways to call young children's attention to an activity, toy, or object are the following:

- Gently place a child's hand on the object
- Use toys or objects that emit sounds or music

- Add sound effects
- Incorporate surprise
- Use toys or activities that incorporate movement

9. True. Children who are nonverbal can indicate their activity choices by gestures, sounds, eye gaze, pointing to picture symbols, or communication devices.

10. False. Children are aware if you are being fair. They want to make sure you are giving each of them the same number of turns and materials as others in the group.

Chapter 15: Help Children Face Challenges

1. True. Children's beliefs regarding their abilities affect their confidence and motivation to try.

2. A kindergartner stares at a 10-piece puzzle of animal shapes. He looks at you and says, "I can't." To help him get started, you can say, "Just try this one," and point to where the piece goes. Another approach is to subtly rotate the puzzle pieces right side up so they will easily go in and then encourage him to try. You could also say, "Let's do it together. We can take turns."

3. It is better to let children try on their own before you give help; this allows them to ask for help if they need it. However, if their nonverbal language and inaction indicates they are afraid to start, then jump in and provide assistance.

4. It better to say, "Try…" instead of asking, "Can you…?" If you say, "Can you…?" they are more likely to respond, "No." They may think about past failures and not attempt the activity. By telling children to "Try…" you are conveying your belief in them and offering encouragement.

5. True. The longer children have to wait, the more likely they will do something that gets them in trouble. Children get bored when they have to wait. They will try to entertain themselves. Some may even draw on the table or fiddle with objects they are not supposed to touch. These types of actions often get them in trouble.

6. False. Pointing out what children are doing *right* will encourage them to continue. They may become discouraged if you keep pointing out what they are doing wrong.

7. True. Creating a just-right challenge is key to having all children experience success in therapy. Occupational therapists' expertise in creating just-right challenges enables all children to experience success.

8. When children want to quit an activity, you can encourage them to continue by saying:

- "It takes practice."
- "You did it once, you can do it again."
- "Just think about [name one step]."

9. To help children regain their focus on an activity you can:

- Tap or point to the activity as a cue to restart.
- Ask a question about the activity such as, "Which section are you going to do next?"
- Define an area or a number to complete and count down.

10. False. Older children do mind getting a lot of adult assistance in front of their peers. They only want adult assistance if you do not embarrass them or make them look too different from their peers.

CHAPTER 16: CREATE SMOOTH TRANSITIONS

1. It is good to prepare children for changes because it gives them time to mentally and emotionally adjust.

2. Approaches you can use to get children to rejoin a group are the following:

- Point to the group and say, "Look where all your friends are. Go join your friends." (You can add, "They are waiting for you," or, "They want you to come over.")
- Show a picture symbol of the group activity and point where to go.
- Name or show an enticing element in the group activity and point where to go.
- Have a peer the child likes guide him or her to the group.

3. False. Children tend to like predictable routines because then they know what to expect and feel safe with the structure.

4. False. It is much harder for children to stop an activity, especially a fun one, without knowing what is next.

5. False. Not all children like to start with a sitting activity before doing a movement one. Each group is different. You have to find the right mix to create a smooth transition. Some children need movement before sitting. Others become overstimulated with movement and do better starting with a sitting activity.

6. True. When children transition within groups or a class, the amount of sensory stimulation increases. With larger groups of people, there is typically more noise and commotion during transitions.

7. You can create bridges to create a sense of flow by (a) building upon the children's actions, (b) mak-

ing comments that connect a series of activities, or (c) connecting your conversation to the children's experiences.

8. A unifying theme creates a sense of flow in the session by using common elements to connect each activity.

9. True. Children will not always tell you when they are finished. Although many children will, you also have to watch for and respond to nonverbal signs of boredom or frustration.

10. True. It is easier for younger children to transition when they see or hold onto an object or picture representing the next activity. Some younger children, especially visual learners, do better with transitions when holding a representative object or picture. These provide a concrete cue of what is next and where to go.

CHAPTER 17: PROMOTE THERAPEUTIC ENDINGS

1. False. Children do mind stopping an activity abruptly. It is easier for them to stop if you prepare them before it is time to end.

2. If young children do not stop an activity when asked, you can show a picture symbol of cleaning up, move the storage container next to them, and/or make it a joint effort by helping them.

3. True. Giving a clear endpoint helps children mentally prepare to stop.

4. True. One reason children do not want to stop an activity is that they do not know when they can do it again.

5. True. Children are more willing to clean up if it is easy and part of the routine and if everyone else is helping.

6. To provide closure at the end of the session, you can ask children the following:

- What did you do well?
- What was your favorite part? What did you like best?
- What would you like to do next time?

7. False. Only saying, "Good job," is too vague. Instead, describe a specific incident or detail that is reflective of their progress.

8. True. Like closing a book, having closure on therapy helps the children, caregivers, and you reflect on what you have learned from each other.

9. Two possible feelings children who have bonded with you may have about stopping therapy are being proud of their accomplishments and being sad to say goodbye.

10. False. Children are more perceptive than many adults realize. They are aware of what they liked about therapy,

you, and your actions. If they feel comfortable, they can at least tell you what they liked. They also appreciate being asked for their suggestions on how to make therapy better, even if they do not have any ideas.

Chapter 18: Methods to Enhance Children's Participation in Research

1. Five reasons why it is beneficial to include children in research are the following:
   - It improves the meaningfulness of services.
   - It can make services more effective and efficient and therefore possibly more cost-effective.
   - It increases occupational therapy's knowledge base and informs theories.
   - It has the potential to influence social policies affecting their lives.
   - It may be a rewarding learning experience for them.

2. The approach Corsaro (2015) used to give preschoolers the message that he was an unusual adult was to sit and wait for them to react and approach him, which gave children control over the interactions.

3. True. Children's ability to participate in research is affected by the researcher's ability to communicate with them.

4. True. Researchers can use children's advisory boards to assist with all stages of research.

5. False. A child's age is not the best determinant for judging his or her competence to participate in research. Competencies vary and are based more on experiences and context, as well as the researcher's ability to talk with them.

6. False. Although children can give their consent by a signature, they also can convey their agreement by printing "OK" or circling a representative figure (e.g., a figure showing a thumbs-up, neutral face, or thumbs-down). Children with disabilities may also use communication devices.

7. False. Children have different preferences. Some like the privacy of an individual interview, whereas others like to be with their peers in a focus group.

8. True. Researchers need children's interpretations of the data when using visual or activity-based research methods.

9. False. If the researcher makes adaptations, children with disabilities can also participate in research and have a voice.

10. True. In child-led research, children are actively involved in all stages of the research process.

Index